CONTINUING PROFESSIONAL DEVELOPMENT *in* MEDICINE *and* HEALTH CARE

Better Education, Better Patient Outcomes

CONTINUING PROFESSIONAL DEVELOPMENT *in* MEDICINE *and* HEALTH CARE

Better Education, Better Patient Outcomes

Editors:

William F. Rayburn, MD, MBA

Associate Dean, Continuing Medical Education and Professional Development
Distinguished Professor and Emeritus Chair, Obstetrics and Gynecology
University of New Mexico School of Medicine
President Elect, Society for Academic Continuing Medical Education
Albuquerque, New Mexico

Mary G. Turco, EdD

Assistant Professor of Medicine
Geisel School of Medicine at Dartmouth
Immediate Past President, Society for Academic Continuing Medical Education
Consultant, Center for Learning and Professional Development
Dartmouth-Hitchcock Medical Center
Hanover and Lebanon, New Hampshire

David A. Davis, MD

Professor Emeritus
University of Toronto
Past President, Society for Academic Continuing Medical Education
Dundas, Ontario, Canada
Fort Myers Beach, Florida

OFFICIAL PUBLICATION OF

Society *for* ACADEMIC
Continuing Medical Education
LEADERSHIP · SCHOLARSHIP · COLLABORATION

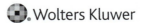 Wolters Kluwer

Philadelphia · Baltimore · New York · London
Buenos Aires · Hong Kong · Sydney · Tokyo

Executive Editor: Shannon Magee
Development Editor: Andrea Vosburgh
Editorial Coordinator: Emily Buccieri
Marketing Manager: Michael McMahon
Production Project Manager: David Saltzberg
Design Coordinator: Joan Wendt
Manufacturing Coordinator: Margie Orzech
Prepress Vendor: SPi Global

Library of Congress Cataloging-in-Publication Data
Names: Rayburn, William F., editor. | Davis, David A., M.D., editor. | Turco, Mary, editor.
Title: Continuing professional development in medicine and health care : better education, better patient outcomes / editors, William F. Rayburn, David A. Davis ; associate editor, Mary G. Turco.
Description: Philadelphia : Wolters Kluwer, [2018]
Identifiers: LCCN 2016053942 | ISBN 9781496356345
Subjects: | MESH: Education, Medical, Continuing | Clinical Competence
Classification: LCC R834 | NLM W 20 | DDC 610.71—dc23 LC record available at https://lccn.loc.gov/2016053942

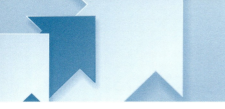

In Memory of

Karen V. Mann, PhD
We dedicate this book to the memory of Karen Mann, PhD, Professor Emeritus, Division of Medical Education, Faculty of Medicine, Dalhousie University, Halifax, Nova Scotia, Canada.

Karen's life and accomplishments were exemplary. She was a wonderful friend and mentor to members of the community of medical education researchers, teachers, and editors worldwide. A true scholar, she inspired peers and students alike. Her contributions over time to both the Society for Academic Continuing Medical Education (SACME), where she was the recipient of the SACME Award for Research in Continuing Medical Education, and to the *Journal of Continuing Education in the Health Professions* were greatly appreciated. Her authorship of the first chapter in this book with Jocelyn Lockyer, PhD, "Applying Educational Theory to Practice in Continuing Professional Development," is a testimony to her commitment to our field.

~ THE EDITORS

About the Editors

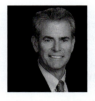 **William F. Rayburn, MD, MBA,** is a Distinguished Professor, Associate Dean of Continuing Medical Education and Professional Development, and emeritus chair of obstetrics and gynecology at the University of New Mexico School of Medicine in Albuquerque. He is the President-Elect of the Society for Academic Continuing Medical Education (SACME) and Vice Chairman of the Board, Accreditation Council of Continuing Medical Education (ACCME). Dr. Rayburn has voluntarily maintained his board certifications while being a long-standing examiner of the American Board of Obstetrics and Gynecology. A maternal–fetal medicine specialist, he is clinically active with patients having complicated pregnancies. Dr. Rayburn is the recipient of several teaching awards. His research in high-risk pregnancies, physician workforce issues, and faculty development has been continuously funded. His publications include several texts and professional books and more than 700 peer-reviewed journal articles, chapters, and abstracts presented at national medical meetings.

 Mary G. Turco, EdD, is Assistant Professor of Medicine at the Geisel School of Medicine in Hanover, New Hampshire and Learning Consultant at Dartmouth-Hitchcock Medical Center in Lebanon, New Hampshire, USA. She is Immediate Past President of the Society for Academic Continuing Medical Education (SACME) where she is Research Committee Vice Chair. Dr. Turco's scholarship and consultation services focus on health professions education and research (teaching and learning, evaluation and assessment, leadership, and professional development) across the continuum. She has contributed articles and chapters to various journals and books including *Continuing Medical Education: Looking Back, Planning Ahead* (Dartmouth College Press, Lebanon, New Hampshire, 2011). Dr. Turco earned her doctoral degree at the Harvard Graduate School of Education. She is a member of the Association of American Medical College's (AAMC) Competency Based Medical Education (CBME) Language Project and the Tri-Group Council (Association for Hospital Medical Education, Alliance for Continuing Education in the Health Professions, and SACME), which collaborates to support the *Journal of Continuing Education in the Health Professions* and World Congress on Continuing Professional Development in the Health Professions (which she co-chaired in 2016).

 David A. Davis, MD, is professor emeritus of family and community medicine and of health policy, management, and evaluation at the University of Toronto. Until May 2016 the AAMC's lead for continuing health care education and improvement, Dr. Davis was a family physician in Ontario, Canada, for nearly 40 years. Emphasizing a rigorous, outcome-based focus on CME, Dr. Davis has led or been an investigator on grants totaling several million dollars. This emphasis has seen the publication of over 150 peer-reviewed papers, dozens of abstracts, book chapters, and two major books on CME practices. His 1995 *JAMA* systematic review of the effect of CME interventions is widely cited as a seminal study in this field. Dr. Davis was the chair or president of national Canadian organizations, two North American organizations including the Society of Academic Continuing Medical Education and the Guidelines International Network. He is the lead editor of the book, Davis D, Barnes B, Fox R, eds. *The Continuing Professional Development of Physicians: From Research to Practice*. Chicago, IL: AMA Press, 2003.

Contributors

Lori L. Bakken, MS, PhD
Associate Professor, Civil Society and Community Studies, School of Human Ecology
Evaluation Specialist, University of Wisconsin Extension, Cooperative Extension
University of Wisconsin-Madison
Madison, Wisconsin

Barbara Barnes, MD, MS
Associate Vice Chancellor
Continuing Education and Industry Relationships
University of Pittsburgh
Vice President for CME and Director of the Health Professional Education Service Line
University of Pittsburgh Medical Center
Past President, Society for Academic Continuing Medical Education
Pittsburgh, Pennsylvania

Morris J. Blachman, PhD, FACEHP
Associate Dean, Continuous Professional Development and Strategic Affairs
Clinical Professor, Neuropsychiatry and Behavioral Science
University of South Carolina School of Medicine and Palmetto Health
Columbia, South Carolina

Paul Batalden, MD
Emeritus Professor
The Dartmouth Institute for Health Policy and Clinical Practice
Geisel Medical School at Dartmouth
Hanover, New Hampshire

Karyn D. Baum, MD, MSEd, MHA
Professor of Medicine
Executive Medical Director, M Health
University of Minnesota
Minneapolis, Minnesota

David A. Davis, MD
Professor Emeritus
University of Toronto
Past President, Society for Academic Continuing Medical Education
Dundas, Ontario, Canada
Fort Myers Beach, Florida

Nancy L. Davis, PhD
Assistant Dean, Faculty Affairs and Development
University of Kansas School of Medicine
Kansas City, Kansas
Past President, Society for Academic Continuing Medical Education
Wichita, Kansas

Mary A. Dolansky, PhD, RN
Associate Professor
Director, Quality and Safety Education in Nursing (QSEN) Institute
Frances Payne Bolton School of Nursing
Case Western Reserve University
Cleveland, Ohio

Todd Dorman, MD, FCCM
Senior Associate Dean for Education Coordination
Associate Dean for Continuing Medical Education
Professor and Vice Chair for Critical Care
Past President, Society for Academic Continuing Medical Education
Department of Anesthesiology and Critical Care Medicine
Joint Appointments in Medicine, Surgery and the School of Nursing
Johns Hopkins University School of Medicine
Baltimore, Maryland

Geoffrey M. Fleming, MD
Associate Professor of Pediatrics
Vanderbilt University School of Medicine
Vice President for Continuing Professional Development
Director, Pediatric Critical Care Fellowship Program
Vanderbilt University Medical Center
Nashville, Tennessee

Linda A. Headrick, MD, MS, FACP
Senior Associate Dean for Education
Helen Mae Spiese Professor in Medicine
University of Missouri School of Medicine
Columbia, Missouri

Eric S. Holmboe, MD, MACP, FRCP
Senior Vice President, Milestones Development and Evaluation
    of the Accreditation Council for Graduate Medical Education
Chicago, Illinois
Professor (adjunct) of Medicine
Yale School of Medicine
New Haven, Connecticut

Tanya Horsley, PhD
Associate Director, Research Unit
Royal College of Physicians and Surgeons of Canada and (adjunct) School of Epidemiology
Public Health and Preventive Medicine
University of Ottawa
Ottawa, Ontario, Canada

Ginny Jacobs-Halsey, M.Ed., MLS, CHCP
Director, Strategic Initiatives
Past President, Society for Academic Continuing Medical Education
Office of Medical Education
University of Minnesota
Minneapolis, Minnesota

Charles M. Kilo, MD, MPH
Vice President and Chief Medical Officer
Oregon Health & Science University (OHSU) Healthcare
Oregon Health & Science University
Portland, Oregon

Simon Kitto, PhD
Associate Professor
Department of Innovation in Medical Education and Director of Research at Office of
    Continuing Professional Development
University of Ottawa
Ottawa, Ontario, Canada

Mila Kostic, CHCP
Director of Continuing Medical Education
Perelman School of Medicine at the University of Pennsylvania
Co-Director, Continuing Interprofessional Education
Penn Medicine
Philadelphia, Pennsylvania

Karen Leslie, MD, MEd, FRCP(C)
Director, Centre for Faculty Development
Professor, Department of Paediatrics
Faculty of Medicine, University of Toronto
Toronto, Ontario, Canada

Jocelyn Lockyer, PhD
Senior Associate Dean, Education
Professor, Department of Community Health Sciences
Past President, Society for Academic Continuing Medical Education
Cumming School of Medicine
University of Calgary
Calgary, Alabama, Canada

Ellen Luebbers, MD
Assistant Professor
Center for Medical Education
School of Medicine
Case Western Reserve University
Cleveland, Ohio

Karen V. Mann, MSc, PhD, FCFPC (honorary), CAHS*
Professor Emeritus
Division of Medical Education, Faculty of Medicine
Dalhousie University
Halifax, Nova Scotia, Canada

Paul E. Mazmanian, PhD
Associate Dean
Assessment and Evaluation Studies
Professor
Department of Family Medicine and Population Health
School of Medicine, Virginia Commonwealth University
Richmond, Virginia

Allison T. McHugh, RN, BSN, MHCDS, MS, NE-BC
Associate Chief Nursing Officer, Heart and Vascular, Neuroscience,
    Medical Specialties, Critical Care and Acute Dialysis
Department of Nursing
Dartmouth-Hitchcock Medical Center
Lebanon, New Hampshire

Graham T. McMahon, MD, MMSc
President and Chief Executive Officer
Accreditation Council for Continuing Medical Education
Professor of Medical Education (adjunct)
Northwestern University
Chicago, Illinois

George Mejicano, MD, MS, FACP
Senior Associate Dean for Education
Professor of Medicine
School of Medicine
Oregon Health & Science University
Portland, Oregon

Bonnie M. Miller, MD
Professor of Clinical Surgery
Professor of Medical Education and Administration
Senior Associate Dean for Health Sciences Education
Vanderbilt University School of Medicine
Executive Vice President for Educational Affairs
Vanderbilt University Medical Center
Nashville, Tennessee

---

*Deceased

Donald E. Moore, Jr., PhD
Professor of Medical Education and Administration
Director of Evaluation, Office of Undergraduate Medical Education
Vanderbilt University School of Medicine
Director, Office for Continuous Professional Development
Vanderbilt University Medical Center
Nashville, Tennessee

Sarah Knox Morley, MLS, PhD
Principal Lecturer III
Clinical Services Librarian
Research, Education, and Distance Services
University of New Mexico Health Sciences Library and Informatics Center
Albuquerque, New Mexico

Curtis A. Olson, PhD
Assistant Professor of Medicine
Department of Medicine
Geisel School of Medicine at Dartmouth
Editor, Journal of Continuing Education in the Health Professions
Hanover, New Hampshire

David W. Price, MD, FAAFP, FACEHP
Senior Vice-President
American Board of Medical Specialties Research and Education Foundation
Chicago, Illinois
Executive Director
American Board of Medical Specialties Multi-Specialty Portfolio Approval Program
Chicago, Illinois
Professor, Family Medicine
University of Colorado School of Medicine
Denver, Colorado

William F. Rayburn, MD, MBA
Associate Dean, Continuing Medical Education and Professional Development
Distinguished Professor and Emeritus Chair, Obstetrics and Gynecology
University of New Mexico School of Medicine
President Elect, Society for Academic Continuing Medical Education
Albuquerque, New Mexico

Scott Reeves, PhD
Professor in Interprofessional Research
Centre for Health and Social Care Research
Kingston University and St. George's
University of London
St. George's Hospital
Cranmer Terrace, London, United Kingdom

Jonathan M. Ross, MD, FACP

Professor of Medicine
Geisel School of Medicine at Dartmouth
Dartmouth-Hitchcock Medical Center
Hanover and Lebanon, New Hampshire

Richard I. Rothstein, MD

Joseph M. Huber Professor of Medicine and Professor of Surgery
Senior Associate Dean for Clinical Affairs
Geisel School of Medicine at Dartmouth
Chair, Department of Medicine
Chief Academic Officer (interim)
Dartmouth-Hitchcock Medical Center
Lebanon, New Hampshire

Ajit K. Sachdeva, MD, FRCSC, FACS

Director, Division of Education
American College of Surgeons
Adjunct Professor of Surgery
Feinberg School of Medicine, Northwestern University
President, Society for Academic Continuing Medical Education
Chicago, Illinois

Ivan Silver, MD, MEd, FRCP(C)

Vice-President Education
Centre for Addiction and Mental Health
Professor, Department of Psychiatry
Faculty of Medicine, University of Toronto
Toronto, Ontario, Canada

Gary A. Smith, PhD

Assistant Dean of Faculty Development in Education, School of Medicine
Professor, Organization, Information, and Learning Sciences
University of New Mexico
Albuquerque, New Mexico

Audriana M. Stark, MBA

Professional Development Assistant, STEM Gateway
Doctoral student, Organization, Information, & Learning Sciences
University of New Mexico
Albuquerque, New Mexico

Dimitrios Stefanidis, MD, PhD, FACS, FASMBS

Vice Chair of Education
Chief, Minimally Invasive, Bariatric, and GI Surgery
Director of Simulation
Associate Professor of Surgery
Department of Surgery, Indiana University
Indianapolis, Indiana

Sharon Straus, MD, FRCPC, MSc
Director, Knowledge Translation Program
Li Ka Shing Knowledge Institute of St. Michael's
Professor, Department of Medicine
University of Toronto
Toronto, Ontario, Canada

Mary G. Turco, EdD
Assistant Professor of Medicine
Geisel School of Medicine at Dartmouth
Immediate Past President, Society for Academic Continuing Medical Education
Consultant, Center for Learning and Professional Development
Dartmouth-Hitchcock Medical Center
Hanover and Lebanon, New Hampshire

Dillon Welindt, BS
Research Assistant
Wales Behavioral Assessment
Lawrence, Kansas

David Wiljer, PhD
Senior Director, Transformational Education and Academic Advancement
Centre for Addiction and Mental Health
Associate Professor
Department of Psychiatry
Faculty of Medicine
Institute for Health Policy Management and Evaluation
University of Toronto
Toronto, Ontario, Canada

Brian M. Wong, MD, FRCPC
Associate Professor and Director, Continuing Education and Quality Improvement
Department of Medicine
Associate Director
Centre for Quality Improvement and Patient Safety
University of Toronto
Toronto, Ontario, Canada

Betsy White Williams, PhD, MPH
Clinical Associate Professor
Department of Psychiatry
School of Medicine, University of Kansas
Clinical Program Director
Professional Renewal Center
Lawrence, Kansas

Foreword

How Might Health Professional Development Contribute to Professional Competence, Joy, and Mastery in the Time Ahead?

This professional book *Continuing Professional Development in Medicine and Health Care: Better Education, Better Patient Outcomes* advances meaningful scholarship and innovation in continuing education to better prepare today's physicians and other health professionals for emerging complex health systems. It offers a foundation based on the power of tested theory and evidence to maximize a health provider's potential, by not only changing behavior and improving care, but in reducing serious illness for their patients and community. Its editors bring lifetimes of scholarship to the volume.

This book invites us to consider the fundamental proposition that health care professional development is never done—only ongoing. Though "never done" it is "due." Due when a professional meets a person seeking help, when a colleague depends on you, or when society assesses, validates the competence of a person claiming recognition as a "professional"…and in so many other situations.

The fundamental social claim of "professional" carries the promise of ongoing learning and improvement—of self and of the increasingly complex arrangements in health care professional work.

Historically, health professionals have had a commitment to science as a way of discovering the truth. We have been committed to destroying iconic thinking and acting to be able to embrace advances. We have lived in the paradox of pursuing better health for *individuals* and for *populations*—knowing that truth in a paradox becomes clearer as we work to strengthen both of its limbs. We have known that the best among us are "first class noticers" of the humanity in another and in self.

In that context, what might we recognize today that might be useful tomorrow?

- Health care work is composed of relationship and action
- Making a "service" is different than making a "product"
- Professional joy, mastery is inextricably connected to the systems and outcomes of the work done to benefit other individuals, communities, and populations in need.

Health Care Work: Relationship and Action

Two parties work together in some relationship, based on beneficiary need and the assumption that professional capability can help. In this relationship, an agreement on some discrete activities is made. This relationship/action is held together by knowledge, skill, habit, and the open pursuit of truth, which carries some willingness to be vulnerable to one another.[1]

Historically, improvement efforts may have distorted the situation. We have focused largely on the "actions." They are usually visible and bounded in time and context. Relationships have been assumed. What held relationship and action together was at best implicit. Improvement so conceptualized may have contributed to the impoverishment of those involved and to the diminishment of those truly seeking "professional" work. New, more complete models of the work and its improvement are needed.

Making "Service" and "Product"

Many years ago, Victor Fuchs invited people to notice that making a service and making a product are different. Services always involved two parties in the "making." Products are made by one party and "sold" to another.[2]

Health care professionals make both in their usual work. But in many ways, we have adopted the language of "product" when we talk about our work or its leadership. This "product dominant" logic has contributed to the ways we organize, pay for health care professional work. By focusing on "action" and "product," we have "machine-ified" our views of the job of a professional, leading to further diminishment and less joy.

Making a health care service involves discerning the individual or population need/ aim and coupling the generalizable scientific knowledge, which can help contribute to a shared aim of both the beneficiary and the professional. The diversity of these couplings is most clearly seen today in efforts to create "personalized" health care service, informed by the genomics of the match of the intended beneficiary and the intervention. The "particularity" that arises when combinations of the individual/population's aim, assets *and* the relevant, effective science able to serve that aim is likely no less heterogenous.[3,4] The coproduction of health care service is illustrated in Figure F.1.

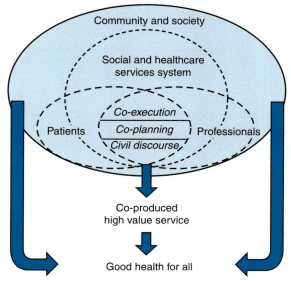

Figure F.1 A model of healthcare service coproduction. Reproduced from Batalden M, Batalden P, Margolis P, et al. Coproduction of healthcare service. *BMJ Qual Saf.* 2016;25:509–517; used with permission from BMJ Publishing Group Ltd.

TABLE F.1
Possible Future Professional Capabilities and Their Rationale

Possible Professional Capability	Relevance, Rationale
Difference between making a "service" and a "product"	Health care professionals make both. Service requires the coproductive work of professional and beneficiary
Aligning professional knowledge with individual, population aim	Health is not "outsourceable." Professional knowledge must be coupled with beneficiary aim
Eliciting "aim," "assets," "possible supports" of the intended beneficiary...and their "expertise"	Patients come with a variety of aims, assets, and supports available for the work of cocreating a health care service
"Nimbleness"	Beneficiaries, contexts, and the science of intervention design and efficacy are always in flux
Linkages involving knowledge, skill, habit, and vulnerability	The relationship and activity involved in any health care service are held together by the knowledge, skill, habit, and capacity to be vulnerable in the service of another's need
Reflection on patterns of interaction with self, diverse beneficiaries	Reflective practice can offer a professional the perspective necessary for legitimate pride, joy, and improvement
Ability to measure the "goodness" of the coproduced service—reflecting accurately what is important to the patient and what the expected application of "science" should produce	Outcome measures must reflect on both the attainment of the patient's goal(s) and the actual performance of the professional's science-in-practice
Ability to create a situation of trust and respect for the communication	Basic requirement for the coproductive work of health care service
Ability to learn from single cases as well as populations of experience	Just like the match of the genetics of the host and the design of a "personalized" intervention...the match of a particular patient's aim and a well-designed, scientifically grounded intervention will come in smaller groups. These single cases or small groups will express the heterogeneity of daily professional practice...and our patterns of knowledge building must be capable of work at that level

Leadership that understands and facilitates this work and the knowledge development it needs is likely to be key to creating work settings that nurture and contribute to a sense of joy and mastery in the health care professional of tomorrow.

Connecting Professional Development, System Performance, and Beneficiary Outcome

The ability to measure and improve the outcome of health care professional work has invited attention to the operating systems and the content of professional development that contribute to those outcomes. Sustainable, generative improvement of those outcomes in individuals and populations seems to invite attention to the connectedness of these elements (Figure F.2).[5]

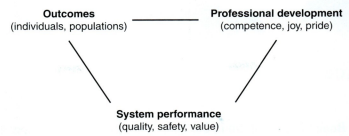

Figure F.2   Relationships necessary for sustainably generative improvement. (From Batalden P, Foster T, eds. *Sustainably Improving Health Care: Creatively Linking Care Outcomes, System Performance, and Professional Development.* London, UK: Radcliffe; [2012]; used with permission from CRC Press.)

Developing professionals capable of thriving in the complex systems that are currently emerging with these and other assumptions will invite attention to familiar and possibly some new capabilities (Table F.1).

This next chapter in professional formation and development offers a wonderful opportunity for fresh thinking and the identification of new forms of professional capability and sources of joy. The poet Rumi advised us to live our lives as "guesthouses"—welcoming all who come.[6] Savor this book and welcome the invitations to change that come to the "professional development guesthouse" of this time.

Paul Batalden, MD

Emeritus Professor

The Dartmouth Institute for Health Policy and Clinical Practice

Geisel School of Medicine at Dartmouth

July, 2016

REFERENCES

1. Leach DC. Personal reflection and correspondence in preparation of this foreword. July 14, 2016.
2. Fuchs V. *The Service Economy.* New York: National Bureau of Economic Research; 1968
3. Batalden M, Batalden P, Margolis P, et al. The coproduction of healthcare service. *BMJ Qual Saf.* 2016;25:509–517.
4. Davidoff F. Heterogeneity is not always noise: lessons from improvement. *JAMA.* 2009;302(23):2580–2586.
5. Batalden P, Foster T, eds. *Sustainably Improving Health Care: Creatively Linking Care Outcomes, System Performance, and Professional Development.* London, UK: Radcliffe; 2012.
6. Rumi J. *The Essential Rumi.* Coleman Barks, trans. Edison, NJ: Castle Books; 1997:109.

Preface

Why This Book? The Need, Goal, Content, Contributors, and Readers

So much about how medicine is practiced is learned beyond undergraduate and graduate training. Those fortunate to associate with young colleagues become quickly aware about innovations and newer means of inquiry and discovery that did not exist when senior physicians began practice. The power of prevention, the fruits of teamwork between physicians and other professionals, the growing diversity in the workplace, and the disruptions and empowerment of technology have brought important transformations in health awareness and health care delivery. Each of these issues derives from the forces for change and progress in health care systems around the world. Indeed, these forces will increase and intensify over the next several decades.

Why Write This Book?

Such dynamic forces compel us to consider a new role for continuing education and professional development. Much of what is currently designed and delivered as "continuing education" fails to influence or change medical practices or improve patient outcomes. Traditional classroom-based lectures are largely driven by the educator who lacked an objective assessment of the learners' needs.

Until the past decade, continuing medical education (CME) was viewed as an ineffective, unscrutinized, and often commercially driven stepchild to the heavily-studied undergraduate and graduate medical education. Its predominant "one and done," lecture-based model of knowledge transfer was evaluated as to whether it met the learners' "satisfaction index"—rather than whether it was effective in imprinting information that could be applied to practice, thus changing certain behaviors of participants.

Throughout this book, we use the term continuing professional development (CPD). In these times of rapid information generation and exchange, as well as team-based practice and patient empowerment to achieve quality outcomes, a repositioning of continuing education and professional development is needed to assure improved care at the bedside, in the clinic and hospital, and throughout the community. It calls for physicians to engage in a process of reflecting on their performance, identifying means to reduce practice gaps, engaging in formal and informal learning activities, and making changes in practice to eliminate those gaps in performance.

Goal of This Book

The goal of this professional book, *Continuing Professional Development in Medicine and Health Care: Better Education, Better Patient Outcomes*, is to address the need for better education to produce better clinical practice and improved health care outcomes. The text is intended to advance meaningful scholarship and innovation in continuing education that will develop our health professionals. The role of continuing education as a strategic resource that can transform delivery of care is explored at the beginning. This transformation must be multidirectional and, therefore, we provide modes as to how CPD can be reorganized and repositioned, to make more visible the many initiatives currently underway and to underscore issues and challenges in defining contributions for improving patient care. As a field of practice, we draw on theoretical frameworks and evolving evidence from numerous disciplines, for example, engineering, neuroscience, education, organization management, sociology, and psychology.

We strive to present evidence-informed theory and content. For far too long, much of CME lacked a grounding in accepted educational theory and research-generated evidence. This problem is not unique to health profession education, as teaching and learning theory evolve as new science emerges. The day has come to eradicate concerns about CME and establish the CPD tenets and examples reported in this book. This progressive text is a call for ending ineffective CME and starting an era of reform, an era that uses the power of proper theory and evidence to maximize the potential of CPD, not just to change behavior and improve care, but to reduce serious illness and hopefully save lives.

We realized that this professional book would be eclectic. There are many themes and voices, ranging from the practical to the theoretical, from current practice to future directions, from evidence-based to more philosophical. The intent of the book was not to follow any one approach but to select and use what we considered to be the best elements from a variety of health systems. Instead, it provided an opportunity to present subjects that applied to all fields of medicine and health care for readers interested in developing and/or continuing leadership roles in education.

Content of the Book

Physicians and other health professionals need education to gain guidance on how to judge the value of new diagnostic and therapeutic technologies. Delivering important topics in an evidence-informed way is the science of health care delivery, using informatics tools for assessing, evaluating, and managing data. An appreciation of the new learning environment is essential in understanding how knowledge can be gained, applied, and assessed in contemporary practice settings. Illustrated in each chapter are case scenarios and relevant questions that pertain to the chapter topic.

Techniques for maximizing educational benefits (learning, administrative, and otherwise) are described throughout the text. Topics and techniques range from the evolution of core competencies between and among teams of health care professionals to advances in simulation models (from high-tech complex mannequins to low-tech standardized patients and case scenarios). The chapters in total explain why todays' faculty must not only teach medical knowledge but also assess what and how they teach not only to improve competency and performance but also to ultimately align the teaching with patient outcomes.

Performance improvement through the use of data to impact practice is now a focus of CME and CPD. In the future, electronic health records and institutional and national quality and value metrics will inform targeted audiences' learning needs. There will be an emphasis on providing realistic, personal needs assessments to improve health outcomes. Data from improved coding, electronic health records, and other medical databases (e.g., disease registries, quality of care dashboards, patient experience surveys) will, over time, be readily available and better accepted by once skeptical clinicians.

Busy clinicians will want their education to be more flexible, efficient, effective, and accessible with less need to travel. Broad efforts are underway for lectures or seminars in auditoria or classrooms to be replaced by or complemented with self-paced, practice-based learning in the workplace setting. Accomplishing this requires hybrid (online and live) formats, primarily virtual (either asynchronous or real time) options paired with and face-to-face learning. Physicians will continue to adapt to innovative educational delivery systems such as multipoint videoconferencing, integrated web-based imaging tools, social networking, Internet information sites, and text messaging. Easier access to an expanding array of portable electronic devices is permitting information resources to be available for decision making at the point of care. Constant updating allows these virtual libraries to be more evidence based.

Improved communication by physicians and teams, and enhanced interprofessional, team-based care coincide with practice-based learning. This book describes how new competencies in clinician–patient communication and clinician cultural awareness are evolving. Patient education materials are becoming more available on the Internet and in social media. Patients, family, and friends of all ages and levels of education are gaining better understandings (and potentially misunderstandings) about preventive health and disease management from this information. Clarification of patients' medical literacy is becoming a feature of clinicians' professional development and personal communication skill sets.

A strong value of continuing education and professional development is advancing quality improvement and patient safety. Acquisition of skills by clinician educators for systems-based reform and performance improvement, along with their instructing about patient safety, are highlighted throughout the text. Practice-based learning is an effective means to demonstrate the systematic changes that many physicians have attempted or completed as they largely learned from experience after training. Delivery of care will require a continuous iterative process of reflective learning through many interventions that incorporate measureable and sustainable improvements.

We recognize the growing emphasis on quality care, patient experience, and cost reduction. The book describes means to develop faculty responsible for educating present and future health care providers about these topics. While medical knowledge remains essential to proper patient care, other core competencies (e.g., effective communication with patients and health care teams) are needed to escape from a "silo mentality." Patient-centered, team-based care can and should deliver value and safety along with efficacy. Strides in multidisciplinary and interprofessional collaboration are reforming a health care environment strapped by unnecessarily high costs and an uneven geographic distribution of physicians in most medical and surgical disciplines.

The text ends with discussions of methods for conducting research to measure the magnitude of effectiveness in professional education. Use of proper terminology and both qualitative and quantitative analyses for comparison are essential for the reader to appreciate and understand. The assessment of the complex issues including quality, value (quality divided by cost), and patient-provider satisfaction (in daily practice) require sophisticated research strategies and methods. As described in the book, rigor, scientific methodology, and appropriate tools are essential for assessing the effects from contemporary education approaches on physician performance and patient outcomes. We also address reasons and methods for developing strong leaders for the challenges of 21st century health systems and project the future of continuing professional development to help meet those challenges.

The Book's Authors

Several of the book's authors are members of the Society of Academic CME (SACME) and engaged with the Association of American Medical Colleges (AAMC). Throughout the book are references to advances in CPD, as fostered by these two organizations. SACME has supported studies of and developments in CPD/CME for nearly four decades. This book is regarded as an official SACME publication. The AAMC has sponsored two major, national initiatives with relevance to academic, effective CPD: the Aligning and Educating for Quality (ae4Q) and Teaching for Quality (te4Q) projects. Both initiatives are highlighted throughout this book. Much of the content and direction of CPD outlined in this text are a result of activities supported by the Josiah Macy Foundation over the last decade. By convening meetings and supporting the work of the Institute of Medicine, the Foundation has enabled a new, evidence-based and integrated vision of the field.

Many contributors to this book are recognized internationally in moving CPD in the health professions forward. Their assistance is invaluable to a large professional audience, including clinician faculty and health system leaders, CME deans and directors in academic CME offices, and quality and performance improvement experts at medical centers, academic institutions, hospitals and health systems throughout the United States, Canada, and internationally. The authors' balanced approaches in describing effective, professional education are intended to reflect upon and impact clinical practice behaviors to improve health care delivery. The future, as taught by these contributors, will be determined not only by physicians' and other health professionals' desires but by health needs of individual patients, communities, regions, or provinces globally. Other key stakeholders committed to creating healthy communities (i.e., payers, governments, regulatory agencies) will shape this change and place more importance on the continuing development of all physicians and health care professionals.

Who Should Read This Book?

The editors and authors of this professional book have created it with a primary view toward the needs of the CPD provider and their key stakeholders, for example, the dean or vice president of CME or CPD, the Chief Academic Officer, the Chief Learning

Officer, the Leaders of CPD and Quality Improvement in Professional Societies and so forth, and those physicians and health care professionals with whom the provider and key stakeholders work. This is a growing, worldwide community of educators, planners, and scholars stimulated in part by the Society for Academic Continuing Medical Education. Any number of health system leaders, such as Chief Medical and Chief Nursing Officers of Health Care Systems, will find the directions, effects, and potential role of CPD to be of interest, fulfilling certain needs in the ongoing changes in health care systems. Similarly, educators at all levels across the health professions will find messages in the book to be useful in their strategic planning and curricular needs. Finally, the book's contents will resonate with patients and patient advocacy groups whose primary interest is that CPD be developed and assessed on one critical measure—whether or not it ultimately provides better patient outcomes.

WILLIAM F. RAYBURN, MD, MBA
Albuquerque, New Mexico, USA

MARY G. TURCO, EDD
Hanover and Lebanon, New Hampshire, USA

DAVID A. DAVIS, MD
Dundas, Ontario, Canada and Fort Myers Beach, Florida, USA

Acknowledgments

Preparation of this professional book required the help and inspiration of many people and organizations in many ways.

Administrative colleagues, notably Jennifer Silva, offered much needed attention to communicating with our many authors. Sarah Morley, PhD, was invaluable in searching for very current references and abstracts on topics covered in each chapter to assist authors in including the most complete and applicable evidence-based information.

Department leaders at the University of New Mexico (WR) and at the Geisel School of Medicine at Dartmouth and Dartmouth-Hitchcock Medical Center (MT) provided time and support for our work, as we undertook our usual rigorous daily routines. The Association of American Medical Colleges permitted one of us (DD) the opportunity to engage with dozens of academic medical centers, their faculty and continuing medical education/continuing professional development (CME/CPD) divisions. This engagement enriched and provided a vision for much of this book.

The Wolters Kluwer Health publishers provided an excellent team led by Shannon Magee and Andrea Vosburgh, with marketing expertise and support from Michael McMahon. Emily Buccieri was an exceptional coordinator and a delight in her attention to detail. We are grateful for their timely responses to questions, regular communications, and overall encouragement for the project.

Paul Batalden was generous in agreeing to write the foreword and share his thoughts on changes in health care delivery and professional development.

Our 43 authors displayed considerable responsibility and energy in preparing their chapters. Collectively, their work represents innovative thinking, forward-looking concepts, practical tips, and sizable scholarship. We are grateful for their timely and enthusiastic responses. Those signs were highly encouraging, enabling us to meet strict deadlines and to be critical about necessary changes to make every chapter better. We were grateful for the dedication and professionalism displayed by these busy and very talented individuals.

A very special thanks goes to our spouses (Pam Rayburn, Jack Turco, and Maureen Davis). All were generous in their understanding about frequent interruptions and additional time away from our families.

Improving health care delivered to patients was the central theme of this professional book. It was an honor to edit and contribute. We dedicate this book to both the patients we have known and the patients worldwide from whom health care professionals and educators learn the most about improving education and outcomes.

Prologue

Monumental changes in health care, new imperatives and mandates, calls for greater accountability and transparency, impact of emerging technologies, and major advances in the science and practice of continuing professional development/continuing medical education (CPD/CME) underscore the need for a definitive text that addresses contemporary topics in CPD/CME and highlights the critical role of CPD/CME in providing health care of the highest quality, safety, and value. This book, "*Continuing Professional Development in Medicine and Health Care: Better Education, Better Patient Outcomes*," is a comprehensive text that focuses specifically on improving the learning environment, learning in the workplace, roles of the faculty, active involvement of learners, and evaluation of critical outcomes of CPD/CME.

The chapters are written by internationally renowned experts who are recognized as leaders and innovators in this field. This book should be of immense value to CPD/CME leaders, including CME deans at medical schools, vice presidents and directors of education of professional societies, and directors of CME offices, as well as to the teaching faculty and key stakeholders engaged in efforts to improve outcomes of patient care and demonstrate the value of new models of health care delivery. Individuals involved with a variety of regulatory organizations and agencies should also find this book interesting and helpful.

Over the past four decades, the Society for Academic CME (SACME) has remained on the forefront of steering national directions in CPD/CME and advancing the field of CPD/CME through cutting-edge scholarship. SACME continues to lead innovative efforts to harness a range of opportunities in CPD/CME that are aimed at positively impacting patient care and safety. This book is an official publication of SACME, and Members of the Board of Directors of SACME have strongly supported this book from the time of its inception through various stages of development and publication. SACME believes that this book will serve as the definitive resource in the rapidly evolving field of CPD/CME and will spawn future developments that will help physicians and health care teams provide the best care to patients now and well into the future.

On behalf of the SACME Board of Directors, I would like to express my profound gratitude to Drs. William Rayburn, Mary Turco, and David Davis for their outstanding work as co-editors of this important book. I would also like to thank the authors for their willingness to share expertise and volunteer precious time to write various chapters. SACME looks forward to collaborating with the entire CPD/CME community to take the field of CPD/CME to the next level!

AJIT K. SACHDEVA, MD, FRCSC, FACS
President, Society for Academic CME

Director, Division of Education
American College of Surgeons

Adjunct Professor of Surgery
Feinberg School of Medicine, Northwestern University

OFFICIAL PUBLICATION OF

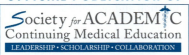

Society *for* ACADEMIC
Continuing Medical Education
LEADERSHIP · SCHOLARSHIP · COLLABORATION

Introduction: Integrating Continuing Professional Development with Health System Change[*]

David A. Davis, MD and William F. Rayburn, MD, MBA

A decade and a half ago, the Institute of Medicine (IOM), in its landmark report entitled "To Err is Human," cited widespread clinical failures leading to unacceptable mortality figures in the United States.[1] One year later, the IOM's companion piece "Crossing the Quality Chasm" issued its call for widespread health system reform.[2] This report and subsequent ones about reshaping the health care system identified several essential elements: (1) a focus on advances of evidence-based medicine, (2) an alignment of the multiple elements of the health care system, and (3) a means to overcome the financial, physician, and economic barriers to reform. Change has been slow or nonexistent, however, despite advances in information technology and decision support, and use of quality metrics and practice reorganization, performance incentives, and well-intended leadership.

Educational elements have been examined in an attempt to support this reform. Questions were raised about the effect of continuing medical education (CME) and continuing professional development (CPD) on health care quality and safety in general and on the maintenance of licensure and certification of independent practitioners in particular.[3,4] The presumption that board certification affects the quality of care is an ongoing interest intended to explain disparities in patient outcome.[5,6] Furthermore, discussions about accreditation requirements for graduate medical education programs have been revitalized and studied under the rubric of a New Accreditation System.[7] Finally, recent or future publications in *Academic Medicine* focus on the discrepancy between the minimum time commitments necessary to become licensed as a competent physician.[8]

Two Parallel Pathways of Change, One Direction

In response to this need for quality improvement and practice reorganization, two, parallel pathways have taken hold in medicine. Both share a commonly desired outcome, that is, the improvement of patient care and population health. Each has also shared a common fate—widespread dissemination without widespread implementation. Examples of characteristics of each pathway are identified in Table I.1.

---

[*]Reprinted from Davis D, Rayburn W. Integrating continuing professional development with health system reform: building pillars of support. *Acad Med*. 2016;91:26–29.

TABLE I.1
Examples of Characteristics of the Macro and Micro Pathways in Health System Reform

	Macro Pathway	Micro Pathway
Perspective	Entire health system	Individual provider or team in the system
Theoretical grounding	Organizational behavior	Individual and team-based learning, behavioral theory
Proponents	Health system leaders, health service researchers, others	Educationists, psychologists
Major competency	Systems-based practice	Practice-based learning
Key drivers	Finances, regulations, data/ evidence	Individual motivation, peer input, professional specialty societies, performance improvement

The first pathway, by far the larger and more visible, relates to a macro model, providing a system-wide lens enabling a view of the entire health system. One of the most widely disseminated visions of this worldview is the "continuously learning health system" consisting of several components. According to an IOM workshop summary, the learning health system embraces three key elements: (1) a vigorous and well-integrated electronic health record, (2) integrated learning and practice networks, and (3) widespread availability and use of data.[9] Central to these elements is a better understanding of "evidence" and a subsequent, rigorous evidence base (not necessarily on randomized controlled trials only), with which practice and other incentives are aligned. Leadership and culture in the institution are key ingredients in the success or failure of such systems.

In contrast to the macro perspective and predating it by at least a decade is a second pathway involving CME/CPD. Both CME and CPD deal with a much more micro perspective, that is, the individual clinician or team that are the major if not sole actors in the health system. Defined by a Macy Foundation Report on Continuing Education in the Health Professions, CME is the "last and longest phase of education undertaken by physicians, [consisting of] any activity undertaken to enhance competence, increase learning, and provide better care for patients."[10] CPD is seen as being broader than CME, encompassing all forms of learning and professional development, and relating to activities of all health professionals.

The CME/CPD pathway is barely noticeable in the discussion of health system reform. Like its macro cousin, this micro pathway influences patient and population health that include the following discrete elements: (1) interactivity, by which clinician learners truly engage with content; (2) multiple methods of learning strategies; (3) sequencing, by which learning and performance changes are reinforced; and (4) continued support for the learner.[11] Additional elements described as effecting positive outcomes include interprofessionalism; allowing for a greater team-based approach to learning; use of quality and other objective data (as opposed to subjective needs) to drive learning; and integration with the health care system.[12]

Dissemination without Implementation

It would appear that more thoughtful integration of the two pathways would effect change. So, why are these two pathways not better aligned? It is not as though players in, and students of, either pathway are unaware of each other. For example, the Accreditation Council for CME (ACCME) in its evaluation of systematic reviews focused on the types and methods of CME that affect physician performance or health care outcomes.[13] Furthermore, the Council issues accreditation with commendation to those CME providers who are able to demonstrate clinical linkages with improvement. Reciprocally, learning health system reports do reference broadly defined educational activities for physicians as "tools and systems that imbed evidence into practice, reshaping formal educational curricula for all health care practitioners, and shifting to continuing educational approaches that are integrated with care delivery."[9]

It is also not as though there are no examples of best practices in this area. Clear instances of educational activities, stimulated by the AAMC's Aligning and Educating for Quality (ae4Q) initiative, that exemplify the use of quality data in planning grand rounds, in more systems-based approaches to morbidity and mortality (M&M) conferences, and for interprofessional efforts to alter clinical performance and patient outcomes.[14,15] While growing in number, these activities remain sporadic and without widespread recognition, system support, and integration.

To the external observer, there are many answers to the question of dissemination without implementation. While changing culture, leadership, financial rewards, and other incentives are part of the answer to the question of reform, it appears obvious to think that the answer lies in a more complete, systematic marriage of the micro and macro pathways. On the one hand, profound and in depth professional development activities can attract the major players in the system, that is, the physicians and other clinicians. On the other hand, a robust commitment on the part of the health system to the training (and moreover retraining) of its major actors is an equal answer.

A small example illustrates the point. U.S. industry invests (the word is used in its most complete sense) over 80 billion dollars per year on training, an amount growing over a several-year period, and a recognition of the importance of continuing professional development to quality and consumer satisfaction.[16] In contrast, results from the AAMC's National Survey of Academic Health Centers (the Harrison Survey) indicate that only a small percentage of budgetary support from institutional (medical school, health system) sources and, in 2012, a slight decline in that support from previous years.[17] Furthermore, while nursing and other staff employed by health systems participate in system-driven education, physicians are generally not so directed, leaving the choice of continuing education in their hands.

A complete, systematic marriage between the macro and the micro pathways is not always the case. This lack of effective interaction is strikingly similar to the parallel play of toddlers, who play beside each other but do not attempt to modify the other's activity. This analogy is perhaps appropriate given the early state of health system reform in this and other countries.

Overcoming Parallel Play: Four Pillars of Support

What will it take for these parallel pathways to align more completely? We envision four pillars of support for better outcomes. As illustrated in Figure I.1, these four pillars involve (1) an acknowledgment that both pathways exist and are essential; (2) the faculty commitment to learn and educate about quality improvement and patient safety at undergraduate, graduate, and—in particular—practicing, postgraduate (career-long) levels; (3) reengineering tools of CME/CPD to serve as effective change agents; and (4) a development of standards to enforce and sustain this alignment of pathways.

First, both pathways need to *acknowledge* the importance of the other. Macropathways cannot change without a deep understanding of the individual and group human factors and the players who operate within it. Micropathways (in CME/CPD particularly) fail if they neglect the view and cooperation of the large, organizational systems in which they exist, with all their leadership and cultural distinctions. This union between pathways requires some sacrifice that can represent a hard but necessary first step. On the part of the health care system, it requires a deeper appreciation that "education" is more than boxes to be checked in a list of change strategies, particularly when those boxes indicate the need for merely a "lecture" or reminder in the newsletter. Instead, it requires a continuous, active experience based on several principles of educational effectiveness (relevance, interactivity, sequencing, and multiple methods). For the institution's CME/CPD office, it means abandoning the assumption that it is relatively independent from the health system. The day of the separate, externally funded cost-recovery "CME unit" is over, lost in an effort to birth a truly learning health system in which continuous professional development is imbedded and outcomes are studied in every action.

Secondly, and perhaps most importantly, this alignment calls for a profound reimagination of what it means to be a faculty member. For every faculty member, it means

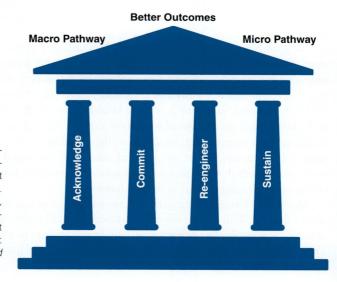

Figure I.1 Pillars of support for integrating continuing professional development with health system reform. (Reprinted from Davis D, Rayburn W. Integrating continuing professional development with health system reform: building pillars of support. *Acad Med.* 2016;91:26–29.)

to *commit* to quality improvement and patient safety thinking and processes in both the clinical and academic realm, a reconceptualizing of the role of the clinician and a goal of AAMC's 2013 Teaching for Quality report.[18] This is an important imperative for the CME/CPD enterprise in academic medicine. For the faculty member engaging in educational efforts—and possibly any faculty leader—it means the ability to guide professional learners, study and improve CME/CPD processes, utilize only those strategies with proven effectiveness, and envision the educational continuum as a whole.[19]

A third pillar is to *reengineer* tools of CME/CPD into more effective change agents. Less should be directed to didactic interaction and much more toward other tools: academic detail, reminders at the point of care, improvement strategies in morbidity and mortality conferences, team training in collaborative care, and communications training. Much more than traditional lectures and grand rounds, CME/CPD needs to encompass one-on-one training, performance improvement projects, patient safety initiatives, online simulation, learning from teaching, interactive courses, team-based learning, and many other approaches. The list is large, based on an equally large and growing literature base. It will also require a reimagination of the educational continuum that creates for faculty members a process in which the performance of the health system is the author of the curriculum.

Lastly, it will require development of external pressures and standards that recognize, acknowledge, support, and *sustain* this alignment. Advances in health system regulation point to ongoing and focused professional enhancement, commendation for health system linkage (ACCME), and maintenance of certification linked to performance.[20–22] These advancements require refinement and integration into the workflow of clinicians and the settings in which they practice and learn. Regulations about accreditation in this area also require redefinition and expansion in the unique and critical environment of the academic medical center. Perhaps a joint educational/clinical accreditation worldview is a necessary and logical next step.

With these pillars supporting the total integration of continuing professional development of its clinical members with health system reform, we envision a more outcomes-oriented and a mutually supportive academic medical center and learning health system. This effort should lead to better system functioning, improved metrics and value, and most importantly, more optimal patient care and population health.

Future Directions

Clinical failures leading to a widespread desire for health system reform has resulted in changes that are either slow or nonexistent. In response, academic medicine has moved in two directions: (1) system-wide reform using electronic health records, practice networks, and use of widespread data (macro pathway) and (2) professional development of individual clinicians through continuous performance improvement (micro pathway). Both share the desire to improve patient care and population health, yet each suffers from limitations in widespread implementation. We envision a better union between these two parallel pathways through four pillars of support: (1) an acknowledgement that both pathways are essential to each other and to the final outcome they intend to achieve; (2) a strong faculty commitment to educate about quality improvement and patient safety at all education levels; (3) a reengineering of tools for professional development to serve as effective change agents; and (4) the development of standards to sustain this alignment of pathways. With these pillars of support integrating continuing professional development with health system reform, we envision a better functioning system, with improved metrics and value to enhance patient care and population health.

REFERENCES

1. Institute of Medicine. *To Err Is Human*. Washington, DC: National Academies Press; 2000.
2. Institute of Medicine. *Crossing the Quality Chasm*. Washington, DC: National Academies Press; 2001.
3. Tzeng DS, Chung WC, Lin CH, et al. Effort-reward imbalance and quality of life of healthcare workers in military hospitals: a cross-sectional study. *BMC Health Services Research*. 2012;12:309–314.
4. Eric SH, Yun W, Thomas PM, et al. Association between maintenance of certification examination scores and quality of care for medicare beneficiaries. *Intern Med*. 2008;168(13):1396–1403.
5. Curtis JP, Luebbert JJ, Wang Y, et al. Association of physician certification and outcomes among patients receiving an implantable cardioverter-defibrillator. *JAMA*. 2009;301(16):1661–1670.
6. Fleischut P, Eskreis-Winkler J, Gaber-Baylis L, et al. Provider board certification status and practice patterns in total knee arthroplasty. *Acad Med*. 2016;91:79–86.
7. Thomas JN, Ingrid P, Timothy B, et al. The next GME accreditation system: rationale and benefits. *N Engl J Med*. 2012;366:1051–1105.
8. Rosenbluth G, Tabas J, Baron R. What's in it for me? Maintenance of certification as an incentive for faculty supervision of resident quality improvement project. *Acad Med*. 2016;91:56–59.
9. Institute of Medicine (US) Roundtable on Evidence-Based Medicine; Olsen LA, Aisner D, McGinnis JM, eds. *The Learning Healthcare System: Workshop Summary*. Washington, DC: National Academies Press; 2007.
10. Josiah Macy Foundation. *Continuing Education in the Health Professions*. Hager M, Russell S, Fletcher SW, eds. New York: Josiah Macy Jr. Foundation; 2008.
11. Marinopoulos SS, Dorman T, Ratanawongsa N, et al. Effectiveness of continuing medical education. *Evid Rep Technol Assess* (Full Rep). 2007;149:1–69.
12. Davis DA, Baron RB, Grichnik K, et al. Commentary: CME and its role in the academic medical center: increasing integration adding value. *Acad Med*. 2010;85:12–15.
13. *Improving Genetics Education in Graduate and Continuing Health Professional Education: Workshop Summary*. Washington, DC: The National Academies Press; 2015.
14. Davis NL, Davis DA, Johnson NM. Aligning academic continuing medical education with quality improvement: a model for the 21st century. *Acad Med*. 2013;88(10):1437–1441.
15. Pingleton SK, Carlton E, Wilkinson S, et al. Reduction of venous thromboembolism (VTE) in hospitalized patients: aligning continuing education with interprofessional team-based quality improvement in an academic medical center. *Acad Med*. 2013;88(10):1454–1459.
16. 2014 Industry Training Report. Training Magazine. Nov/Dec 2014. http://pubs.royle.com/publication/?i=233369&p=18. Accessed September 3, 2016.
17. Association of American Medical Colleges and the Society for Academic CME Harrison survey 2013 of academic CME https://members.aamc.org/eweb/upload/Academic%20CME,%20The%202012%20AAMC-SACME%20Harrison%20Survey.pdf. Accessed September 3, 2016.
18. Headrick LA, Baron RB, Pingleton SK, et al. *Teaching for Quality: Integrating Quality Improvement and Patient Safety across the Continuum of Medical Education*. Washington, DC: Association of American Medical Colleges. Available at www.aamc.org/te4q. Accessed August 31, 2016.
19. Bennett LN, Davis DA, Easterling, EW Jr, et al. Continuing medical education: a new vision of the professional development of physicians. *Acad Med*. 2000;75(12):1167–1172.
20. Martin AM, Elizabeth Wick, Julie AF, et al. Complying with the new alphabet soup of credentialing. *Arch Surg*. 2011;146(6):642–644.
21. McMahon GT. Advancing continuing medical education. *JAMA*. 2015;314(6):561–562.
22. Hawkins RE, Lipner RS, Ham H, et al. American Board of Medical Specialties Maintenance of Certification: Theory and Evidence Regarding the Current Framework. *J Cont Ed Health Prof*. 2013;33:S7–S19.

Contents

PART **I**

Improving the Learning Environment   1

PART **II**

Learning in the Workplace   67

Abbreviations

Like most professions, those in health care have a wide assortment of abbreviations. Shown below are standard abbreviations of common terms or organizations found throughout this professional book and more generally in the study of Continuing Professional Development.

Common Terminology

AE4Q	aligning and educating for quality
AHC	academic health center
AHS	academic health system
AMC	academic medical center
CAO	chief academic officer
CBME	competency-based medical education
CDSS	computerized decision support system
CE	continuing education
CEO	chief executive officer
CHAPS	customer assessment of healthcare providers and systems
CIPD	continuing interprofessional development
CIPE	continuing interprofessional education
CLER	clinical learning environment review
CLO	chief learning officer
CME	continuing medical education
CMO	chief medical officer
CNE	continuing nursing education
CNO	chief nursing officer
CPD	continuing professional development
CPE	continuing pharmacy education
CQO	chief quality officer
CSA	clinical skills assessment
EBHC	evidence-based health care
EBM	evidence-based medicine
EHR	electronic health record
EMR	electronic medical record
EPA	entrustable professional activity
GME	graduate medical education (residency/fellowship training)
FPPE	focused professional practice evaluation
HCP	health care professionals
HPE	health professions education

IPE	interprofessional education
IPLC	interprofessional learning continuum
IT	information technology
KT	knowledge translation
LOS	length of stay (in hospital)
M&M	morbidity and mortality
MMIC	morbidity, mortality, and improvement conference
MOC	maintenance of certification
OPEQ	outpatient experience questionnaire
OPPE	ongoing professional practice evaluation
PDSA	plan, do, study, act (cycle)
POC	point of care
PS	patient safety
QI	quality improvement
RCT	randomized controlled trial
RSS	regularly scheduled series (of M&M conferences, rounds, etc.)
SDL	self-directed learning
SMART	specific, measurable, achievable, relevant, time bound (objectives)
SPAR	situation, background, assessment, recommendation
SQUIRE	standards for quality improvement reporting excellence
SRL	self-regulated learning
SWOT	strengths, weaknesses, opportunities, threats
Te4Q	teaching for quality
UME	undergraduate medical education

Agencies, Associations, Councils, Institutes, Organizations, and Societies

AACH	American Academy on Communication in Healthcare
AACN	American Association of Colleges of Nursing
AAMC	Association of American Medical Colleges
AANC	American Nurses Credentialing Center
ABMS	American Board of Medical Specialties
ACCME	Accreditation Council for Continuing Medical Education
ACGME	Accreditation Council for Graduate Medical Education
ACPE	American College of Physician Executives
AFMC	Association of Faculties of Medicine in Canada
AHA	American Hospital Association
AHME	Association for Hospital Medical Education
AHRQ	Agency for Healthcare Research and Quality
ACEhp	Alliance for Continuing Education in the Health Professions
AMEE	Association for Medical Education in Europe
AOA	American Osteopathic Association
AONE	American Association of Nurse Executives
CACME	Committee on Accreditation of Continuing Medical Education (Canada)
CFPC	College of Family Physicians of Canada

EACCME	European Accreditation Council for Continuing Medical Education
GAME	Global Alliance for Medical Education
GMC	General Medical Council of the United Kingdom
IHC	Institute of Healthcare Communication
IHI	Institute for Healthcare Improvement
IOM	Institutes of Medicine
JCAHO	Joint Commission on Accreditation of Healthcare Organizations
JCEHP	Journal of Continuing Education in the Health Professions
JCI	Joint Commission International
NHS	National Health Service (of the United Kingdom)
RCPSC	Royal College of Physicians and Surgeons of Canada
SACME	Society for Academic Continuing Medical Education
WFME	World Federation of Medical Education
WHO	World Health Organization

PART I

IMPROVING THE LEARNING ENVIRONMENT

APPLYING EDUCATIONAL THEORY *to* PRACTICE *in* CONTINUING PROFESSIONAL DEVELOPMENT

Karen V. Mann and Jocelyn Lockyer

Case

You have assumed responsibility for educational planning in obstetrical care for a population of 1.3 million people. The family physicians, obstetricians, and nurse midwives work alongside nursing staff to deliver babies in three health facilities, as well as provide perinatal care in their offices and clinics. Comparative statistics for your region have identified several areas where patient care could be improved, but the changes will require new knowledge and skills, behavioral changes in the ways that the providers work together, and likely system changes.

Questions

Your goals in planning educational programs for the health care team include improving the individual competence of all of the health care professionals involved in obstetrical care, ensuring that all of the professionals engage in ongoing learning, and making a contribution to new and effective systems of care. As you reflect on these lofty goals, you ask yourself the following questions: What theories exist to help you understand how learning and change occur both for individuals as well as within social groups and communities of practice? How can you draw on what is known about changing behavior to improve patient outcomes? What are the new directions in adult and medical education that might inform your next steps?

INTRODUCTION

Theory can be an essential resource in our educational work and contribute to improvements in practice that our interventions aim to achieve. In short, it can help us to do our work better. In medical education, theories are drawn from several fields and disciplinary perspectives, including cognitive psychology, sociology, and anthropology, among others. Theory can guide our focus in developing our interventions, inform how we may understand our outcomes, and help us to design educational interventions that are more reliably likely to have the intended effect.[1]

A theory may be thought of as a system of ideas that is intended to explain something, for example, an event or a phenomenon. Theory can inform our practice at several levels.[2,3] *Grand or overarching theories* cannot directly guide our intervention; however, they can provide a framework and a language for thinking and talking about it. For example, *social learning theories* help us to think broadly about how learning occurs with and from others and the environment.[4] Secondly, *midrange theories* can guide our thinking more specifically about concepts and frameworks within which to place our interventions. An example of a midrange theory in continuing professional development (CPD) is the *Theory of Physician Learning and Change*,[5] which informs our thinking about the influences on physicians' decisions to change and how they integrate change into their practice. Theories can shorten the time it takes us to develop an intervention, and help to maximize the learning that results.

A third level is *program theory*, which includes our beliefs and assumptions about why a planned intervention or strategy will work in a particular setting, or with a specific group. Frequently, this theory is expressed through a flowchart or logic model, or an evaluation plan. It is intended to be feasible and practical. An elegant example of a program theory is found in a report by Stamer and colleagues[6] of the development, implementation, and dissemination of a handoff curriculum. Through program theory, we can make explicit our implicit theories and develop a shared understanding of what we are trying to achieve in an intervention. We also can explain our work in ways that allow others to see its wider application. This is especially relevant in the settings of health care and education, as the contexts and systems in which physicians learn and work are complex and vary widely. Theory promotes the transfer of learning from one project and one context to the next.[2]

We begin the chapter by describing theories about how physicians and other health professionals learn and change; we next explore models for change that help us understand how educational interventions can influence learning. The theories and models we have chosen to present apply broadly beyond medicine, and we believe they have relevance to learners in all health professions. In presenting them, we have focused deliberately on their relevance to physicians as learners, to underline their importance in physician ongoing learning, and professional development. We then return to the case we have presented above and discuss how these theories can be used to create effective programs and support physicians' independent and self-directed learning. We conclude with future directions.

PHYSICIAN LEARNING

We present six theoretical approaches that describe how physicians learn and change. All have found their way into the CPD literature and have informed educational programming. These include an overall model of learning and change in practice, as well as theories that illuminate how learning occurs from experience, through reflection, through informed self-assessment and feedback, and through social learning and within communities of practice. The theories and their main focus are summarized in Table 1.1.

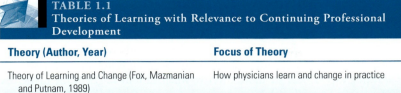

TABLE 1.1
Theories of Learning with Relevance to Continuing Professional Development

Theory (Author, Year)	Focus of Theory
Theory of Learning and Change (Fox, Mazmanian and Putnam, 1989)	How physicians learn and change in practice
Experiential learning (Kolb, 2014)	How learning occurs through a cycle of experience
The Reflective Practitioner (Schön, 1983, 1987)	How learning occurs through reflection in and on practice
Informed self-assessment (Sargeant et al., 2010)	How individuals gather and respond to external feedback to judge how they are performing
Social Learning Theory (Bandura, 1986)	How learning occurs through interaction with others and the environment
Communities of Practice (Lave and Wenger, 1991)	How learning occurs through gradually increasing participation in the activities of the community

The Theory of Learning and Change

The *Theory of Learning and Change*, developed by Fox et al.[5] was an outcome of "the change study." The study goal was to understand how physicians learn and change in practice. Through interviews with 340 physicians who provided data about 775 recent changes, the role of personal, professional, and social forces in stimulating change was identified. Professional forces, including a desire for competence, or changes in the clinical environment, were the most likely to lead to change. Personal factors, such as personal growth, and social forces, such as relationships with colleagues, were also important. Changes ranged in scope from very minor accommodations, often in response to regulatory changes, through larger more substantial and sometimes transformative changes. Three stages of change were identified: preparing to change, making the change, and sustaining the change. This model allows administrators and program planners with a goal of facilitating changes in practice to consider what forces in physicians' lives will facilitate or act as barriers to change. Similarly, when changes are complex, it highlights that developing a staged approach to facilitating the innovation can enable physicians to prepare for and ultimately adopt and sustain the innovation.

Learning from Experience

Learning from experience is fundamental both to acquiring the knowledge, skills, and dispositions required for practice and in maintaining competence throughout the practice lifetime.[7] Kolb's *Theory of Experiential Learning*[8] can provide a helpful framework for planning educational activities, both formal and informal. Kolb's model is an iterative model, which consists of four stages, as follows: (1) concrete experience, where the individual has an opportunity, either directly or indirectly, to experience a learning event (in the case of physician education, the event might be caring for a patient or discussing a patient's health problem(s), as examples); (2) observation and reflection, where the individual can reflect on the experience he or she has had or observed; (3) abstract generalization, during which the experience can be supplemented through self-directed exploration, or through formal teaching, and general principles can be abstracted; and (4) application and testing of new concepts, and evaluating them, so that they can be incorporated into future practice. Learners may enter the cycle at different stages; for example, while some may prefer to grasp new experiences head-on, others may prefer to begin their experiential learning with reading and preparation using formal knowledge. Generally, learning experiences are more effective when all four stages of the model are involved.[8] The model fits well with how physicians learn and can help in framing interventions and educational programs that allow opportunities for experiencing all aspects of the learning cycle.

Learning through Reflection

Reflection is increasingly recognized as a critical component of learning. One of the best-known approaches to reflection in CPD is the model of reflective practice developed by Schön,[9,10] which draws on observations and study of professionals in several fields of education and professional practice. Schön's model of reflection was based on his view that the problems encountered in "the messy lowlands of practice" were not readily solved by applying formal knowledge. Solving these problems requires a fund of practical knowledge accrued from formal knowledge, and from past experience that Schön called "knowing in action." The model involves an iterative cycle that begins when the physician's accumulated knowledge, skill, and experience (knowing-in-action) are challenged by the realization that the problem in front of him or her is not exactly like those encountered before, which generates a "surprise." The surprise requires that he/she "take stock in the moment," a process Schön called "reflection-in-action." Reflection-in-action usually involves some weighing of options, which usually lead to a decision guiding how to act at that time. This stage Schön called "active experimentation." We have all experienced such reflection-in-action ourselves, in both our professional and personal lives. Schön described a more considered and critical revisiting and analysis of the event after it occurred, which he labeled "reflection-on-action." This revisiting of the experience and extracting what has been learned then add to the physician's knowing-in-action and may be applied in future situations. Through this iterative cycle, ongoing learning occurs in and from practice.

Informed Self-assessment Theory and Feedback

Self-assessment is recognized as critical to ongoing maintenance and growth of competence; it is a key element of self-regulation, and as such is of great relevance to physician learning and practice. It has received considerable attention in medical education, as studies have shown that physician self-assessment is variable.[11]

Self-assessment has been described as a process of interpreting data about one's own performance and comparing it to practices or data that are explicit or implicit standards. Self-assessment thus lies in two major domains—the integration of high-quality external and internal data to assess current performance and promote future learning, and the capacity for ongoing self-monitoring during everyday clinical practice.[12] In this description, self-assessment moves from unguided self-reflection into a domain in which one's assessment is guided by data. As developed further by Sargeant et al.[13] the theory of "informed self-assessment" describes a process in which people receive information (or data) about themselves from others and from processes around them (e.g., audit and feedback, patient feedback) as well as through their own internal beliefs and feelings. These data are interpreted through reflection, calibration, filtering, and assimilation. The end result is to ignore, reject, accept, or seek more data. Within this environment, there are conditions that influence data sources used, interpreted, and responded to including the learning and practice climate, personal attributes, relationships in the workplace, and the credibility of the information and processes providing the data. Similarly, tensions between and within people and in the learning or practice environment also impact on how people use, interpret, and respond to data.

External feedback appears to be a fundamental element in enhancing the accuracy of self-assessment. Feedback comes from many sources including colleagues and patients as well as data from audits and multisource feedback systems. Recent work on providing feedback using an evidence-based model that incorporates building a relationship, seeking reactions to data, focusing on content, and coaching for change (the R2C2 model) shows promise in settings in which there are opportunities for physicians to discuss their feedback with a trusted peer or supervisor.[14]

While needs assessment has been considered integral to program development, it is often done at a group level. Individual participants do not always acknowledge or know how they perform. The theory of "informed self-assessment" and the R2C2 model for providing feedback[14] remind us that it is important to engage the individuals in providing their own data, to compare it to a standard and enable them to explore the gap between their performance and desired performance, so that they can identify and commit to changes that will mitigate the gap, and lead to performance improvement.

Social Learning Theory

Social learning theory explains how we learn from and with others and in interaction with our environment. Bandura's *social cognitive theory*[15] sets forth important principles that can inform how we plan for and support effective learning. A fundamental principle is that we are always in a dynamic reciprocal interaction with our environment: individuals' actions affect the environment, which in turn affects the individual and the behavior. Individuals interact with their environment based on their values, beliefs, and their existing knowledge and experience. Secondly, learning occurs very powerfully through observation of people's actions and of the consequences of their action. Through observation, people acquire knowledge and learn skills, attitudes, and values. In other words, learning occurs powerfully from role models. A third key concept embedded in social learning theory is that of self-efficacy—the individuals' perception of their ability to successfully execute a particular task.[15] Self-efficacy perceptions are a strong predictor of what tasks individuals take on, the goals they set for themselves, and how long they will persevere with a task.[16] Self-efficacy is developed most powerfully by experience, followed by observation of others. Fourth, individuals have basic capabilities that enable them to set goals and to monitor their progress toward them. They also have innate capabilities to reflect on and evaluate their progress. Bandura[15] emphasized the importance of goal setting, demonstration, practice, and feedback to support learners in developing and using these basic capabilities. Each of these principles has implications for supporting physician learning and for learning that will occur both in formal and informal settings. For example, recognizing the importance of observation of others to facilitate change highlights the importance of demonstrations with feedback, role modeling, and mentorships.

Learning in Communities of Practice

Communities of practice (CoPs) theory has emerged from anthropological studies demonstrating how practical learning is situated within practice and occurs through social interactions and in settings as close to the actual practice as possible.[17,18] This theory has particular relevance for physician learning as it was originally described in an effort to better understand learning through apprenticeship, which remains a pervasive method of learning in medical education. Wenger defined a CoP as a "group of people who share a concern, set of problems, or a passion about a topic, and who deepen their knowledge and expertise in this area by interacting on an ongoing basis"[17] (p. 4). This involves adopting shared, tacit understandings; developing competence in the skilled pursuits of the practice; and assuming a common outlook on the nature of the work and its context.[17] Newcomers to the group become legitimate practitioners and develop their identities within CoPs by participating in practice.[17] In the traditional perspective of CoPs, they were informal naturalistic groups that formed to share tacit and explicit knowledge as well as to create and disseminate knowledge.[19,20] However, CoPs can also be groups that are intentionally brought together or deliberately started by an organization as a knowledge management tool.[21,22] They may be face-to-face or virtual.[23,24] Work within practice-based small group learning groups, a form of CoPs, demonstrates the power of the CoP to effect change in a social setting.[25]

APPROACHES TO BEHAVIOR CHANGE

In the previous section of the chapter, we have discussed selected theories of learning, which we believe are relevant for understanding how physicians learn. The theoretical perspectives we have presented describe processes through which learning occurs that can inform our planning and implementation of educational interventions. In this section, we highlight theories, concepts, and models that explain factors that influence learning and decisions to change practice. Readers will see elements of the theories we have presented previously in the approaches discussed in this section.

We present four approaches to enabling behavior change that have been found useful and have high relevance for CPD. These are the *PRECEDE* model: the *theory of planned behavior*, the *transtheoretical model* also called *"stages of change,"* and *domains of behavior change*, recently labeled the *COM-B* model. The main focus of each of these models is shown in Table 1.2.

The PRECEDE Model

This evidence-based model of behavior change originated in the health promotion literature[26] as a guide to systematic planning implementation and evaluation of educational

TABLE 1.2
Models of Behavior Change with Relevance to CPD

Model of Change (Author, Year)	Focus of Model
The PRECEDE model (Green and Kreuter, 1981)	The factors that predispose, enable, and reinforce the effectiveness of education in bringing about behavioral change
The theory of planned behavior (Ajzen, 1991)	The influences of individual's perception of norms, and attitudes of others, and perceived agency, on the intention to change behavior
The transtheoretical model of change (stages of change) (Prochaska and Diclemente, 1984)	The stages of change that individuals must negotiate to make sustained behavioral change
The COM-B model (Michie et al., 2011)	The factors that influence behavioral change and the importance of capability, opportunity, and motivation

interventions intended to bring about change. PRECEDE stands for Predisposing, Reinforcing, and Enabling factors in educational diagnosis and evaluation. Factors affecting change in behavior fall into three groups: Predisposing factors are those that predispose an individual to undertake an action and include knowledge, attitudes, values, and perceptions. Enabling factors enable the individual to undertake the change and include the individual's skills and access and availability of resources. Reinforcing factors help to maintain a new behavior and include feedback on the action, positive effects for the individual, or some other reward or reinforcement. The *PRECEDE* model is very useful in both identifying relevant factors and how they might be optimized for an educational intervention to have its desired effect. Educational planners can consider which factors may or may not be amenable to change and which might be facilitators or barriers for the intervention. An additional benefit afforded is that the same analysis can be applied to other stakeholders beyond the physician, including patients and communities. The model has been used widely in health promotion and patient education and also in medical education studies particularly in CPD.[27,28]

The Theory of Planned Behavior

Developed by Ajzen in 1991,[29] the *theory of planned behavior (TPB)* highlights major influences on an individual's decision to change a behavior. Because the goal of CPD interventions is to bring about behavior change, this theory is very appropriate to consider. It has been one of the most commonly used behavioral theories used in the context of health professional education.[1] Three main influences are identified: attitudes, perceived norms, and perceived agency. Attitudes are influenced by our feelings about the behavior and our beliefs about the outcomes of the behavior. Perceived norms include what we believe others in the group believe and our personal motivation to comply, and perceived agency reflects the amount of control we believe we have to effect the change and the relevant skills we have. Together, these factors influence the intention to perform the behavior. Although the actual performance of the behavior may be influenced by environmental and interpersonal factors, one's intention to change is thought to be the most proximal and strongest influence. This model has been used by Grimshaw and colleagues[30] in a randomized trial of CPD intervention designed to change physician behavior. Although the *TPB* does not explain completely the changes that have or have not occurred, it offers planners an important way to understand the factors that might be involved and to identify points of influence.

The Transtheoretical Model and Stages of Change

The *transtheoretical model*[31,32] views change as a dynamic process, rather than an event. Originally described in relation to addictions, the model has also proven useful in understanding and motivating individuals to change other behaviors. It forms the basis for motivational interviewing, which many physicians use in helping their patients to make important lifestyle changes. The model identifies five stages in behavior change: these are precontemplation, contemplation, preparation, action, and maintenance. The model allows planners to identify at which stage their learner audience may be and can inform selection of strategies to enable movement from stage to the next. This model also focuses on the critical stage of maintaining change. For example, physician learners may need appropriate evidence to allow them to contemplate how they might change their practice in a particular area; similarly, considerable preparation may be required before a change is made.

Domains of Behavior Change: The COM-B Model

Health psychologists employ a range of approaches to assist people to make and maintain change. Twelve domains of behavior change have been identified to enable effective use of evidence-based approaches to more reliably effect change.[33] These domains include knowledge; skills; social or professional role or identity, beliefs about capabilities; beliefs about consequences; motivation and goals; memory, attention and decision processes; environmental context and resources; social influences, emotion, action plans, and the nature of the behaviors. Understanding these domains enables us to also understand influences that may lie outside our control and those where change can be accomplished. Most recently, these authors have reduced these 12 factors to a 3-factor model, which they have called COM-B.[34] In this model, Behavior (B) emerges from the interaction of three necessary conditions: Capability, Opportunity, and Motivation (COM). Capability refers to the individual's psychological or physical ability to enact the behavior; opportunity describes the factors in the physical and social environment that hinder or enable the individual's ability to perform the new behavior, and motivation includes the mechanisms, both conscious and unconscious, that encourage or inhibit behavior. Each of these conditions can clearly apply to the goal of helping practitioners to make change in their practice. Competence, or the ability to execute the behavior, is fundamental, as is motivation, which may involve both intrinsic and extrinsic factors. However, even in the presence of these two conditions, practice cannot change without opportunities to perform the new behavior and to sustain it. These strategies may be particularly important to assist physicians in transferring their formal learning to their practice.

The four models above, the *PRECEDE model*,[26] the *theory of planned behavior*,[29] the *transtheoretical model*,[31,32] and the *COM-B* model,[33,34] offer similar and important benefits: they each provide conceptual frameworks for thinking systematically about how to accomplish desired behavior/practice change. They are each both informed by theory and evidence based, making the likelihood of their resulting in the desired change greater than would be the case without. They allow for the inclusion and consideration of the complex environments into which change is to be introduced and also for the inclusion of a wide range of factors that may be relevant at both the individual and the group level.

USING THEORIES TO CREATE EFFECTIVE PROGRAMS AND SUPPORT PHYSICIANS' INDEPENDENT AND SELF-DIRECTED LEARNING

With so many theories and frameworks available to us, some readers will be wondering how best to select and use them. We suggest that theory be used judiciously; educational programming requires careful consideration of the theories and available empirical research to develop educational activities in a logical and strategic way. It may be helpful to consider such questions as: What is the problem we are addressing? What are the goals of the program? What do our learners need to know and be able to do as a result of participating? What kind of learning will best meet the learners' needs? Answers to these questions will point us to those theories that can best inform our planning. Sometimes more than one theory might be relevant; combining aspects of frameworks is also possible.[35,36] Using theory appropriately helps ensure that our programs are suited to their goals; that is, they have "validity" and we can have confidence in their likelihood of effectiveness.

We now return to the obstetrical case scenario that began the chapter. Using that as a focus, we explore how the theories and models we have discussed above might inform and be applied to enhance learning and change. We'll first discuss overall approaches to learning: program design and teaching and learning strategies. The case presents opportunities for professionals to improve their individual practices; it also suggests the use of group learning strategies that occur as one-time or longitudinal opportunities; lastly, it recognizes that there are potential ways in which groups as well as systems that might be enhanced.

While motivation to learn and change, learning from experience, and reflection are individually driven activities, professionals are driven by professional, social, and personal forces.[5] Recognizing that professionals learn through their social interactions and strive to fit into the "norms" of the groups in which they work can be helpful in designing educational programs and structures for ongoing learning.

Social learning theories suggest that opportunities to learn together with colleagues can increase motivation to learn, provide valuable opportunities to learn from observing others, and build shared understanding and experience. Research findings have shown that courses including certain design elements are more likely to be effective. These elements include multiple exposures to content; a longitudinal design; use of didactic, interactive, and active learning strategies; and engagement of learners.[37–40] Further, including opportunities for self-assessment and reflection on learning can hone and support self-regulatory capacity. Including testing to enhance longer-term retention of learning is also effective[41] as is done with structured resuscitation courses.[42] Adding an opportunity for commitment to change statements on an evaluation or as a separate course component can be helpful. This strategy enables participants to identify commitments (changes) they intend to make following the intervention and are later followed up to see which changes they actually make.[43,44] These strategies have been shown to increase motivation and enhance transfer to practice and also to contribute to the impact that courses can have in supporting learning.[26,37,43] It is important to consider which strategies are best suited to the context and for the learners to achieve the course outcomes.

Beyond individual courses, it is also possible to create longitudinal networks or communities of practice. As noted earlier, these can be naturalistic groupings of professionals or can be created, as demonstrated by Balint groups,[45] practice-based small groups,[25,46] and research groups.[21,24,47] CoPs will provide informal (and sometimes formal) CPD, enable the professional to gain tacit and practical knowledge, and determine the "norms" and evidence base for practice. All group members may contribute to these activities. CoPs also allow for more senior members of the group to act as mentors and role models for younger or more junior members. Communities of practice may also be interprofessional, depending on the goals of the community.[19]

Using CoPs effectively requires attention to the establishment of a recognized and trained leader, development of relationships between members, evolution of communication pathways, collaboration in developing shared goals and objectives, and evaluation of the community to improve it.[23,24,48] They also require a comprehensive support infrastructure that enables collaborative work across organizational and professional barriers; they must link individual and group CPD to the implementation of evidence-based standards and practice to facilitate quality improvement initiatives and to reframe performance measurement metrics.[21,24,47]

In Table 1.3, we have drawn on the obstetrics case at the beginning of the chapter, to suggest which theories might be helpful in informing educational planning and evaluation.

Two other general principles are important to consider—these are context and learning as a process.

Context is critical. An essential element of planning, intervening, and evaluation of change is understanding the context. Context includes a wide range of influences: it influences knowledge retention and recalls practice in authentic contexts, simulated or real, and encourages transfer to the context of the physician's practice setting.[49] The context of the learning environment also includes emotional and social elements, relationships with colleagues, safety to learn, and sense of belonging to the community and competence. The complexity of the practice environment both underlines and complicates the notion of context. Assessing the context both for learning and for practice is important in planning. Physicians also need skills in analyzing their environment and how they will implement and manage the process of change there.

Learning is a process. Learning and change are the result of many factors and appear to happen in stages or cycles. For example, the *theory of learning and change* identifies stages of preparing for, making, and maintaining change. Reflective practice occurs in a cycle from identifying surprise to reflecting on action, which lays the ground for an ongoing series of learning cycles. Moore et al.[50] have also identified four stages of change. They have grouped several approaches to learning and change into the four stages of recognizing and evaluating an opportunity for learning; engaging in learning; trying out what was learned; and incorporating what was learned. They note that at each stage physicians will use different learning resources to access information and will stop when they feel they have answered their questions to move to the next stage or to discontinue learning completely. As CPD educators, this idea of stages and cycles can inform our

TABLE 1.3
Educational Planning to Improve Obstetrical Care: Potential Theories to Consider

Goals of the Program	Theoretical Framework or Model	Use	Theory-Based Design
Analysis of the problem	PRECEDE model	Identify factors that may influence the ability to meet goals and which are within the scope of educational change	Provide opportunities to complete a self-assessment related to their practice, beliefs, and values
Improve individual competence	Social learning theory	Design of program	Provide opportunities to learn with others Include opportunities to observe peers and teachers Opportunities to practice and to receive and provide feedback Opportunities to set goals and plan for meeting them
	Learning from experience	Design of program	Active, experiential learning Opportunities to reflect on experience Provision of knowledge and resources to supplement experience Longitudinal programs, allowing participants to try out changes and reflect on their effectiveness
Recognize the need for ongoing learning	Informed self-assessment and feedback	Design of program	Opportunities to draw on and reflect on own experience Opportunities to consider data on their performance (group or individual) Identifying sources of feedback Setting goals for learning
Contribute to new systems of care	Communities of practice	Design of programs	Longitudinal programs Support creation of ongoing groups Encourage interprofessional, multidisciplinary groups

work through reminding us that any intervention will have greater likelihood of success if it attends to all stages in the process. Making these stages explicit for learners can also enhance their skills in approaching their self-directed learning activities.

FUTURE DIRECTIONS

There are several new directions in the context of medicine that will have an impact on CPD and the application of theory and research. Being strategic and efficient in program design will be critical. While major conferences and didactic courses are unlikely to disappear, astute planners will recognize that they need to temper their expectations of such activities and to consider more their role in bringing people together, facilitating the creation of networks, and introducing novel concepts. Several phenomena are likely to impact on CPD in the future: technological change, workplace learning, interprofessional care, and competency-based education.

Technological advances are being integrated into CPD, and their presence is likely to grow. For example, the Internet can provide pre- and postcourse material, test learners, provide resource material, and enable discussion groups. It also transcends geographic and time zone barriers enabling people greater access to experts and peers. These advances enable program developers to be more effective in recognizing and acting upon stages of learning, structuring communities of practice, and creating reflective exercises.

Learning in the workplace and learning in conjunction with other professionals is increasingly recognized as an optimal approach to managing chronic disease and delivering safe and appropriate care in surgical suites, and for the preterm infant and the frail elderly. In these settings, providing educational opportunities within the workplace at lunch, or at a designated time within the workday, can enable natural groupings of people to learn socially, to develop evidence-based procedures and policies, and to support newcomers in learning about approaches to care that have been adopted. It also facilitates staged approaches to learning, particularly, if resources (e.g., simulation equipment, diagnostic equipment, health record systems) are being acquired or upgraded that require new learning and practice. Lastly, it facilitates the development of relationships that can further strengthen the community of practice and support for individuals within it.

As competency-based medical education (CBME) is increasingly adopted for undergraduate and postgraduate education and attention is paid to the broader competency frameworks (e.g., those developed by the Accreditation Council for Graduate Medical Education or the Royal College of Physicians and Surgeons of Canada, CanMEDS roles), CBME will play a role in CPD. In this sphere, the individual's competencies will be determined involving an interplay between the competencies of the specialty, the health needs of the community in which the physician works, and the physician's scope of practice.[51] Physicians will have to demonstrate they meet the expected standards through learning and assessment activities that are specifically designed around the competencies and the entrustable professional activities that enable the practitioner to independently perform the task or activity.

Last, patient safety will require more attention to both delivery of education and assessment of individuals providing care. This will require attention to the theory and research undergirding learning, particularly in high acuity situations and for handovers. These strategies may draw on experiential learning, assessment, and feedback. For example, for new surgical procedures, surgeons may engage in educational programming that includes a staged approach to learning with simulation using task trainers, mannequins, and later biological material along with precise feedback for improvement before they perform the procedure in the operating room. Similarly, for those struggling to communicate effectively with patients demanding opiates, training with standardized patients may be a requirement for continued practice. Where skills in patient handovers are lacking, role playing within a team may be a helpful way of ensuring continuity of care.

REFERENCES

1. Cilliers F, Schuwirth L, van der Vleuten C. Health behaviour theories: a conceptual lens to explore behaviour change. In: Cleland J, Durning S, eds. *Researching Medical Education*. Chichester, UK: John Wiley & Sons, Ltd.; 2015:143–153.
2. Davidoff F, Dixon-Woods M, Leviton L, et al. Demystifying theory and its use in improvement. *BMJ Qual Saf*. 2015;24:228–238.
3. Green J, Thorogood N. *Qualitative Methods for Health Research*, 3rd ed. Los Angeles, CA: SAGE; 2014.
4. Bandura A. *Social Foundations of Thought and Action: A Social Cognitive Theory*. Englewood Cliffs, NJ: Prentice-Hall; 1986.
5. Fox RD, Mazmanian PE, Putnam RW. *Changing and Learning in the Lives of Physicians*. New York: Praeger; 1989.
6. Stamer AJ, O'Toole JK, Rosenbluth G, et al. Development, implementation and dissemination of the I-PASS handoff curriculum: a multisite educational intervention to improve patient handoffs. *Acad Med*. 2014;89:876–884.
7. Billett S. Readiness and learning in health care education. *Clin Teach*. 2015;12:367–372.
8. Kolb DA. *Experiential Learning: Experience as the Source of Learning and Development*, 2nd ed. Upper Saddle River, NJ: Pearson Education Inc; 2014.
9. Schön DA. *The Reflective Practitioner: How Professionals Think in Action*. New York: Basic Books; 1983.
10. Schön DA. *Educating the Reflective Practitioner: Toward a New Design for Teaching and Learning in the Professions*. San Francisco, CA: Jossey Bass; 1987.
11. Davis DA, Mazmanian PE, Fordis M, et al. Accuracy of physician self-assessment compared with observed measures of competence: a systematic review. *JAMA*. 2006;296(9):1094–1102.
12. Epstein RM, Siegel DJ, Silberman J. Self-monitoring in clinical practice: a challenge for medical educators. *J Contin Educ Health Prof*. 2008;28(1):5–13.
13. Sargeant J, Armson H, Chesluk B, et al. The processes and dimensions of informed self-assessment: a conceptual model. *Acad Med*. 2010;85(7):1212–1220.
14. Sargeant J, Lockyer J, Mann K, et al. Facilitated reflective performance feedback: developing an evidence-and theory-based model that builds relationship, explores reactions and content, and coaches for performance change (R2C2). *Acad Med*. 2015;90(12):1698–1706.
15. Bandura A. *Social Foundations of Thought and Action*. Englewood Cliffs, NJ: Prentice-Hall; 1986.
16. Cervone D. Thinking about self-efficacy. *Behav Modif*. 2000;24:30–56.
17. Lave J, Wenger E. *Situated Learning: Legitimate Peripheral Participation*. Cambridge, UK: Cambridge University Press; 1991.
18. Bertone MP, Meessen B, Clarysse G, et al. Assessing communities of practice in health policy: a conceptual framework as a first step towards empirical research. *Health Res Policy Syst*. 2013;11:39.
19. Wenger E, McDermott R, Snyder WM. *Cultivating Communities of Practice A Guide to Managing Knowledge*. Boston, MA: Harvard Business School Press; 2002.
20. Meagher-Stewart D, Solberg SM, Warner G, et al. Understanding the role of communities of practice in evidence-informed decision making in public health. *Qual Health Res*. 2012;22(6):723–739.
21. Fung-Kee-Fung M, Boushey RP, Morash R. Exploring a "community of practice" methodology as a regional platform for large-scale collaboration in cancer surgery-the Ottawa approach. *Curr Oncol*. 2014;21(1):13–18.
22. McKellar KA, Pitzul KB, Yi JY, et al. Evaluating communities of practice and knowledge networks: a systematic scoping review of evaluation frameworks. *Ecohealth*. 2014;11:383–399.
23. Dijkmans-Hadley B, Bonney A, Barnett SR. Development of an Australian practice-based research network as a community of practice. *Aust J Prim Health*. 2015;21(4):373–378.
24. Swift L. Online communities of practice and their role in educational development: a systematic appraisal. *Community Pract*. 2014;87(4):28–31.
25. Armson H, Elmslie T, Roder S, et al. Is the cognitive complexity of commitment-to-change statements associated with change in clinical practice? An application of Bloom's taxonomy. *J Contin Educ Health Prof*. 2015;35(3):166–175.
26. Green LW, Kreuter MW. *Health Promotion Planning: An Educational and Environmental Approach*. Toronto, ON: Mayfield Publishing Group; 1991.
27. Mann KV. Increasing physician involvement in cholesterol-lowering practices: the role of knowledge, attitudes and perceptions. *Adv Health Sci Educ Theory Pract*. 1997;2:237–253.
28. Mann K, Sargeant J, Hill T. Knowledge translation in interprofessional education: what difference does IPE make to practice? *Learn Health Social Care*. 2009;8:154–164.
29. Ajzen I. The theory of planned behavior. *Organ Behav Hum Decis Process*. 1991;50(2):179–211.

30. Grimshaw JM, Eccles MP, Steen N, et al. Applying psychological theories to evidence-based clinical practice: identifying factors predictive of lumbar spine x-ray for low back pain in UK primary care practice. *Implement Sci.* 2011;6:55.

31. Prochaska JO, DiClemente CC. *The Trans-theoretical Approach: Crossing the Traditional Boundaries of Therapy.* Homewood, IL: Dow Jones/Irwin; 1984.

32. Lipschitz JM, Yusufov M, Paiva A, et al. Transtheoretical principles and processes for adopting physical activity: a longitudinal 24-month comparison of maintainers, relapsers, and nonchangers. *J Sport Exerc Psychol.* 2015;37(6):592–606.

33. Michie S, Johnston M, Abraham C, et al. "Psychological Theory" Group. Making psychological theory useful for implementing evidence based practice: a consensus approach. *Qual Saf Health Care.* 2005;14(1):26–33.

34. Michie S, van Stralen MM, West R. The behaviour change wheel: a new method for characterising and designing behaviour change interventions. *Implement Sci.* 2011;23(6):42. doi:10.1186/1748-5908-6-42.

35. Bordage G. Conceptual frameworks to illuminate and magnify. *Med Educ.* 2009;43(4):312–319.

36. Wenger-Trayner E, Fenton-O'Creevy M, Hutchinson S, et al. *Learning in Landscapes of Practice: Boundaries, Identity, and Knowledgeability in Practice-based Learning.* Abingdon, UK: Routledge; 2015.

37. Forsetlund L, Bjørndal A, Rashidian A, et al. Continuing education meetings and workshops: effects on professional practice and health care outcomes. *Cochrane Database Syst Rev.* 2009;(2):CD003030.

38. Marinopoulos SS, Dorman T, Ratanawongsa N, et al. *Effectiveness of Continuing Medical Education, Report for Agency for Healthcare Research and Quality.* Publication No 07-E006. Rockville, MD. 2007. http://archive.ahrq.gov/downloads/pub/evidence/pdf/cme/cme.pdf. Accessed July 18, 2016.

39. Steinert Y, Mann K, Centeno A, et al. A systematic review of faculty development initiatives designed to improve teaching effectiveness in medical education: BEME Guide No. 8. *Med Teach.* 2006;28(6):497–526.

40. Steinert Y, Mann K, Anderson B, et al. A systematic review of faculty development initiatives designed to enhance teaching effectiveness: a 10-year update. *Med Teach.* 2016;38(8):769–786.

41. Larsen DP, Butler AC, Roediger HL III. Test-enhanced learning in medical education. *Med Educ.* 2008;42(10):959–966.

42. Mosley C, Dewhurst C, Molloy S, et al. What is the impact of structured resuscitation training on healthcare practitioners, their clients and the wider service? A BEME systematic review: BEME Guide 20. *Med Teach.* 2012;34(6)e349–e385.

43. Evans JA, Mazmanian PE, Dow AW, et al. Commitment to change and assessment of confidence: tools to inform the design and evaluation of interprofessional education. *J Contin Educ Health Prof.* 2014;34(3):155–163.

44. Mazmanian PE, Waugh JL, Mazmanian PM. Commitment to change: ideational roots, empirical evidence, and ethical implications. *J Contin Educ Health Prof.* 1997;17:133–140.

45. Koppe H, van de Mortel TF, Ahern CM. How effective and acceptable is Web 2.0 Balint group participation for general practitioners and general practitioner registrars in regional Australia? a pilot study. *Aust J Rural Health.* 2016;24(1):16–22.

46. Armson H, Kinzie S, Hawes D, et al. Translating learning into practice: lessons from the practice-based small group learning program. *Can Fam Physician.* 2007;53(9):1477–1485.

47. Fung-Kee-Fung M, Goubanova E, Sequeira K, et al. Development of communities of practice to facilitate quality improvement initiatives in surgical oncology. *Qual Manag Health Care.* 2008;17(2):174–185.

48. Jakubec SL, Parboosingh J, Colvin B. Introducing a multimedia course to enhance health professionals' skills to facilitate communities of practice. *J Health Organ Manag.* 2014;28(4):477–494.

49. Regehr G, Norman GR. Issues in cognitive psychology: implications for professional education. *Acad Med.* 1996;71:988–1001.

50. Moore DE Jr, Cervero RM, Fox R. A conceptual model of CME to address disparities in depression care. *J Contin Educ Health Prof.* 2007;27(suppl 1):S40–S54.

51. Lockyer J, Bursey F, Richardson D, et al. Competency-based medical education and continuing professional development: a conceptualization for change. *Med Teach.* 2016. [In Press].

Chapter 2

REGULARLY SCHEDULED SERIES: IMBEDDED EDUCATION *for* CHANGE

Jonathan M. Ross and Lori L. Bakken

Case

For years, the Department of Medicine in your institution has had two outstanding weekly events, Grand Rounds and Morbidity and Mortality Conference. The former features external speakers who are knowledge experts, and the latter involve resident presenters, a faculty facilitator, and audience participation. You have noticed that despite the high quality of external speakers, attendance at Grand Rounds has been declining, while the M&M conference is valued by participants as the high point of the week. You and your education colleagues decide to understand why the M&M conference appears to be more effective and if some of its successes could be applied more broadly.

Questions

What unique characteristics of regularly scheduled series make them particularly useful in promoting clinician behavior change and improved patient outcomes? How would you go about understanding the elements of M&M that are so effective? Can they be applied more broadly to other regularly scheduled series, such as grand rounds, tumor boards, and journal clubs?

INTRODUCTION

Continuing professional development (CPD) has been undergoing remarkable change, buffeted by clinicians' needs and preferences, regulatory requirements, and patient expectations. "Clinicians" is used broadly and includes nurses, allied health professionals, students, and training physicians as well as academic and practicing physicians. Some have argued for more clarity in the definitions of CPD as compared to continuing medical education (CME), with the former defined as systematic ongoing self-directed learning, while the latter is defined as organized learning activities focused on the development of skills, attitudes, and knowledge to maintain clinical proficiency.[1,2] Because there is much overlap, CPD will be used here to denote those activities and interventions designed to promote, enhance, and maintain clinical excellence. Historically, CME has been seen as separate from quality improvement (QI) and patient safety (PS) training, but in CPD, synergies in these fields of expertise are important although the need for cooperation and integration remains an outstanding challenge.[1,3]

The Society for Academic Continuing Medical Education has recently issued a series of guidelines focusing on important educational interventions including (1) performance measurement and feedback, (2) practice facilitation, (3) educational meetings, and (4) interprofessional education.[4–7] They define an educational meeting "as an intervention used for quality improvement and other professional purposes. The essence of the intervention is that a group of professionals assembles to communicate about important information relevant to patient care as part of a series of meetings and/or as part of a multifaceted intervention. Generally, an educational meeting will include a brief didactic component (recommended to be brief), such as an expert facilitator's perspective on a clinical case, new or revised guideline, and/or latest evidence. An educational meeting should include an interactive component (recommended to predominate the session), which allows participants to evaluate new information and to consider how it relates to (ideally, to the extent possible) higher-order educational outcomes, such as clinician competence, clinician performance, and patient outcomes."[6] They then go on to highlight some specific components of an educational intervention such as starting with a case discussion, sharing best practices, consideration of barriers to implementing change, and encouraging the development of outcomes measurements. The effort to sculpt the format, process, and evaluation of educational interventions is a valuable one as we continue to move from purely content-focused education to instructional methods aimed at improving patient outcomes.

In many academic health centers, there are a panoply of CPD offerings, including single or episodic multiday conferences (updates in a specialty, review boards, e-learning, Internet-enduring materials, courses, section meetings, and the like), which are heavily content or skill acquisition focused. Their efficacy and efficiency in promoting CPD can vary widely. Another format is the regularly scheduled series (RSS), which has the putative advantage of being longitudinal, emphasizes evidence-based medicine, shares wisdom, and provides role modeling and socialization. It also can be multidisciplinary, interprofessional, and multigenerational and often has repeating attendees week to week (grand rounds, morbidity and mortality conference, autopsy review, tumor board, journal club, and the like). The use of real-time interaction (e.g., live polling, team-based care, interdisciplinary collaboration, critical discussion) can also enhance learning. Additionally, simulation technology has improved skills acquisition and maintenance, such as for CPR and central line competency. Newer modalities involving social networks, virtual communities, and Web-based education are becoming more prevalent as the Millennial generation brings their comfort to bear within the digital age.

There also is a persistent tension between institutional and organizational definitions of CPD and the newer focus on learner-centric methodologies, spurred on by the ubiquitous availability of information on the Internet.[8] The need to more clearly define CPD in the context of high-value learning (i.e., learning that is likely to change clinician behavior and impact patient outcomes) has become ever more important. Indeed, a thorough examination of the very purpose of CPD remains an important one in the era of measurement, lest such education be defined almost exclusively on the measurement and comparison of educational outcomes.[9] Simply stated, CPD should support the development and sustenance of clinicians who are patient centered, highly skilled, adaptive, resilient, and reflective.

This chapter focuses on the RSS, and particularly morbidity and mortality conferences, as a particularly high-value learning opportunity for a host of learners. The RSS, in addition to being content focused, has other potentially more enduring impacts on professional development that will be explored. Given the commitment of nearly all stakeholders to promoting patient safety, improving health outcomes, and reducing costs (the triple aim in health care delivery today), the RSS may offer a particularly effective teaching and learning environment in which to help achieve these goals. Indeed, it has been recognized that changing physician behavior (performance) and patient outcomes is more likely to be achieved when it is interactive, employs learner-centric pedagogical approaches, and reinforces desirable cognitive pathways and behaviors.[10] Other RSS, such as grand rounds, journal club, or autopsy review, also offer a multilayered educational experience beyond content experts' presentations, such as socialization in the professional culture, communication, inspiration, and stimulation, and contribute to a subsystem of education in health care, each with unique characteristics. Medical education in this context can be understood to require a necessarily highly variable set of pedagogies that aspire to a common goal.

QUALITY IS THE GOAL OF CONTINUING PROFESSIONAL DEVELOPMENT

Quality is central to patient safety, improved health outcomes, and lower costs. Defining quality is quite challenging, as it resides in the eye of the beholder. Different people (e.g., patients) may define quality in different ways, and various stakeholders, be they physicians, nurses, administrators, financial officers, corporate leaders, politicians, or others, may each offer their version of quality. Each individual or group defines quality in his or her own interests. Yet, it matters that it be made explicit, because no matter what the perspective, virtually everyone in health care wants safety, better outcomes, and lower costs—the key ingredients of quality. Being clear about what constitutes quality both in the complex world of health care and in designing education best suited to attain it requires a thoughtful analysis of quality.

Concepts of Quality

One way to conceptualize quality is to describe it as having two dimensions—professional activities and patient experience. Professional activities include technical excellence, encompassing everything that resides within a system of care delivery: clinicians, their competencies, and the hardware on which they depend, such as testing, pharmaceuticals, and procedures. The second is the experience of patients, who seek enhancement of a sense of well-being and relief from suffering.[11] Another conceptualization includes access to care as well as satisfaction in the patient experience, with continuity, comprehensiveness, prevention, and compliance supplementing the importance of accurate diagnosis and effective treatment on the technical dimension.[12,13] Notably, these constructs exclude concerns with cost and efficiency. Others discuss a classic quality triad, with structure (bricks and mortar of care delivery), process (the way care is delivered), and outcomes as being the pillars of quality. Still others posit a triple aim of better care for individuals, better health for populations, and lower per capita costs of health care[14,15] but focus almost exclusively on health care systems more broadly, rather than individual clinician behavior. Systems redesigns (including the Affordable Care Act [ACA], Accountable Care Organizations, and Medical Homes)[16] are attempting to create engineered as well as incentivized momentum to achieve these aims.

Kitto et al.[3] have discussed the intersections and discontinuities between four academic domains that attempt to address the triple aim, namely (1) continuing education, (2) knowledge translation, (3) patient safety, and (4) quality improvement.[3] They analyzed each of these domains to define their mission, theoretical underpinnings, platform, and desirable outcomes and endpoints. Each domain shares an interest in collaboration and patient care and has a shared stakeholder and interdisciplinary focus and a shared change agenda with a focus on positivist research. However, there is lack of integration of these domains complicated by competition for scarce resources—this creates a real opportunity for collaboration across domains going forward and a need for greater emphasis on systems thinking and its associated strategies for ongoing and adaptive learning.

Creating a workforce that is capable of delivering high-quality care has been aided by concerted efforts of many accrediting and quality-oriented organizations. For example, a guiding set of principles has been created by the Accreditation Council on Graduate Medical Education, which identifies six core competencies.[17] New systems of accreditation have been devised to ensure that learners achieve "milestones" that are measurable and well defined. Maintenance of certification (MOC) and state licensure requirements mandate achieving other metrics that seek to ensure that physicians are effective, safe, and current. Hospitals and care organizations are assessed by state, federal, and quality organizations that seek to protect patients, promote quality, and reduce costs. The Accreditation Council on Continuing Medical Education seeks to maintain high standards by requiring needs assessments and evaluations of accredited conferences and workshops. The Institute of Medicine has identified five competencies that promote proficiency in the health professions.[18] The medical field's strong focus on performance standards suggests one that values excellence and adherence to high-quality performance indicators, but often this level of standardization inhibits the type of learning that is necessary for personal and organizational growth and professional development.[19]

Yet, quality gaps persist, with startling statistics demonstrating harm throughout the care systems, tremendous waste and inappropriate testing, a business model in medicine that rewards doing more rather than getting more (value), and the creation of distorted incentives toward profits rather than patients. The quality improvement (QI) movement begun in the 1950s by Edward Deming in the Japanese automotive industry has penetrated deeply into the fabric of medicine, although it is far from certain whether QI in its present version is equipped to address the crisis in health care today. Deming is credited with the familiar Plan–Do–Study–Act cycle for QI.[20] QI is embedded in the ACA, which has supported pilots and created incentives for improving health care delivery and promoting quality improvement. All agree that clinician engagement is essential to success in improvement efforts, although quality improvement is sometimes felt as something mandated from without, rather than as confluent with, actual practice. Yet tremendous efforts are being made to "get everyone on board" with QI, including accrediting and MOC bodies. Clinicians vary in what they know, do, and experience and in how they learn. Any definitions of quality must take into account personal attributes (of patients and of clinicians), systems of health care delivery, financial incentives or disincentives, external mandates, resource constraints, and numerous other contextual and mechanistic variables that contribute to quality health care. In other words, definitions of quality must take into account a broader system of care that goes beyond clinicians' knowledge and behavior alone.

Defining Quality

In our current system of health care, there is an increasing emphasis on Value. In this context one expresses Value as:

$$\text{Value} = \text{Quality} / \text{Cost}$$

Some[12] place focus on structure, process, and outcomes (or values, vision, and mission) as necessary for delivering quality. This focus tends to emphasize linear thinking and processes that assume static change.[21] However, complex systems, such as those of health care, are continuously changing and readily adapting to the needs of its various stakeholders. Therefore, linear thinking patterns and associated methods and models are oversimplified and inadequate for understanding complex systems, such as health care delivery, and its associated outcomes.

From the clinician's perspective, these concepts and variables are highly interactive. Value is defined from patient, system, and payer perspectives. Costs are market driven, supply and preference driven, regulated, incentivized, and highly dependent on clinician behavior. Clinician quality includes a myriad of complexities and falls into three main categories: clinician competence, delivery system support, and patient experience. Clinician competence includes the ability to take a history; perform physical diagnosis; generate and refine differential diagnoses; make accurate assessments and recommendations; demonstrate appropriate and patient-centered diagnostic and treatment decisions; engage in clear communication with patients, family, and staff; and be committed to continuous improvement through self-reflection or formal QI projects. Patient experience includes a sense of well-being, relief of suffering, adequate education, and preferences both elicited and honored. For the purposes of this paper, a focus on the clinician is emphasized, given the central role such individuals have within the health care matrix, but it is acknowledged that other individuals, systems, and socioeconomic, demographic, health equity, and other factors play critical roles in achieving quality. In addition, clinician influence on promoting and achieving quality is a generally neglected part of the conversation concerning quality. Quality improvement generally focuses on what Leykum et al.[22] emphasize as low-uncertainty situations, that is, those that allow for routine, standardized processes. Examples of those might be in screening and prevention protocols. In high-uncertainty situations, such as in acute hospitalized or chronic disease management scenarios, process improvement, the typical mechanism for current QI efforts, is less likely to be effective, requiring instead more emphasis on clinician relationships and how they make sense of what is happening, solve problems, improvise, and learn from and with one another. Clinicians also must modulate their behavior due to shared decision making required by understanding patient preferences and values. Indeed, there is growing support for formal education in delivering and assessing shared decision making as critical to improving quality.[23]

If one accepts the foregoing definition of clinician quality, including in both low- and high-uncertainty situations, then a number of important questions arise. First, if population-based metrics of quality are necessary but insufficient bases for measuring value, what other measures may be used to understand and improve clinician behavior? Second, since clinician behavior has such a large impact on health care utilization, how then can one educate and then track the effects of interventions to promote excellence in such behavior? Indeed, how can improvement occur in real time, rather than as feedback temporally removed from actual care? Further, how does one acquire such skills, continue to develop them over time, and monitor them in meaningful ways? The answer to these questions requires attention to the entire medical education subsystem, which includes medical school education as well as graduate and CME. A complete discussion of undergraduate, graduate, and CME is beyond the scope of this chapter, but attention to a number of conceptual models for educational programming and evaluation of their associated impacts is important. Quality techniques like Six Sigma do not lend themselves well to solving problems that are nonlinear and complex, unlike the linear environments that such techniques were designed for in the first place. "None of these techniques can independently succeed in improving the quality of healthcare delivery because… healthcare is a complex, non-linear system, fundamentally different from the linear processes from which the underlying quality concepts were derived."[24] (p. 3) Thus, in order for value to be maximized, quality must include both traditional QI and formal and informal education as part of a system to deliver the care that patients need and want.

EDUCATION AS QUALITY IMPROVEMENT

The central supposition of this paper is that CPD requires continuing education of the clinician as a partner to traditional QI and patient safety efforts. Broadly speaking, clinical excellence may be viewed as possible when four main domains are particularly well developed: communication and interpersonal skills; knowledge and technical skills; professionalism and humanistic skills; and reasoning and judgment.[25] Education in this area can be seen as promoting another group of processes: knowledge/skills, socialization, and individuation.[9]

Education can also be viewed as focused on promoting such excellence in these areas, including an emphasis on such specific skills as seen in Table 2.1. This is not meant as an exhaustive list, but an attempt to explicitly delineate the essential components that form the core attributes of a clinician who is then capable of delivering quality care. Because much of what clinicians working in high-uncertainty situations do requires these skills, it is essential that education supports real development and

TABLE 2.1
Specific Attributes of the Clinician in Medicine

Clinical presentation—how to listen and elicit and integrate information from patient stories
Clinical findings—skills of physical and psychological diagnosis
Empathy and compassionate care
Etiology—considering causality
Epidemiology—understanding probabilities
Pathophysiology—a necessary skill for clinical therapeutics
Differential diagnosis—creating and refining possibilities
Clinical reasoning—organizing and revising complex information
Risk assessment—combining population and individual risk
Prognosis—learning natural history with and without treatment
Diagnostic tests—understanding test characteristics and limitations
Documentation—coherent management of information and communication
Therapy/Procedures—competence in choosing therapy, and performing procedures
Prevention and screening—understanding benefits and risks of diverse interventions
Motivational interviewing and shared decision making
Continuity—promoting the value of relationship and commitment to knowing patients over time
Experience and meaning—understanding of self and of the patient's experience of illness
Self-improvement—learning and practicing mindfulness
Practice improvement—encompassing both practice improvement and systems thinking
Communication—with learners, colleagues, patients, and families
Teaching—facilitating learning by others, narrative medicine

maintenance of expertise over time. Evidence that most accredited CPD activities are not designed to promote clinical behavior change is concerning.[26] Further, emphasis has been heavily weighted by accrediting organizations toward attaining competencies as a goal, as opposed to emphasizing skills needed to go beyond, and which are necessary to move from those who are experienced to those who attain expertise.[27] In essence, in reconsidering the value equation $V = Q/C$, the extent to which clinician behavior contributes to Q and to C has been underestimated. Some have posited that " … up to one-third of the over $2 trillion that we now spend annually on healthcare is squandered on unnecessary hospitalizations; unneeded and often redundant tests; unproven treatments; overpriced, cutting-edge drugs; devices no better than the less expensive products they replaced; and end-of-life care that brings neither comfort care nor cure."[28] (p. 32) A study by Thompson Reuters in 2009 estimated that 40% of the $700 billion dollars spent annually in unwarranted care is attributable to erroneous clinical decision making.[29] It is possible that improving training and CPD would have a greater impact on improving quality and controlling costs than the current top-down and often intrusive mandates that are now widespread.[15]

CPD AND LEARNING IN A HEALTH CARE SYSTEM

The different perspectives just described (i.e., value, quality improvement, and education) represent different mental models for how quality health care should be delivered and evaluated. These mental models reflect three elements that are fundamental to and characteristic of all systems, namely (1) distinctive components, (2) interrelationships among components, and (3) multiple perspectives, known as simple rules of systems.[21,30] From a physician's perspective, a system might include patients, pharmacy, nursing, social services, and other components necessary to perform and function in his/her role. From a CEO's perspective, a system might include financial specialists and resources, health care staff, organizational structures (e.g., departments, clinics, hospitals), and other administrative components. Medical, graduate, CME, CNE (nursing), CPE (pharmacy), and CPD might all be thought of as part of a formal educational system. These are just three examples of perspectives that can shape a system and demonstrate that each system will look different based on these perspectives. Moreover, the interrelationships among components will also vary. These different "mental models" exhibit separate and autonomous forms of thinking that must be brought together if a complex system, such as health care, is to function effectively, efficiently, and sustainably. In doing so, the role of education, specifically CPD, can be clearly defined and play a significant role in advancing the systems vision for high-quality health care.

However, this is not an easy task. As already pointed out, health care is characterized by rapid change, shifting priorities, and high levels of uncertainty—it is a highly complex system. In complex systems, such as those of health care delivery and acquisition, change is not static, but highly dynamic, and therefore, the system must be adaptive. Dynamic change is characterized by multiple factors that influence events, reciprocal causes and effects, and fluid or open boundaries.[21] To be adaptive to this form of change, organizations, such as academic medical centers, must become learning organizations. Ways of thinking must be shifted from those that support linear and autonomous models and static change to those that support nonlinear and adaptive models and dynamic change. In adaptive systems, performance indicators (e.g., competencies, quality benchmarks, educational outcomes, value equations) become monitors of change, rather than targets for change. Viewed this way, they become information that informs learning and can be used to leverage collective actions in favor of quality health care. With respect to CPD/CME education, systems thinking requires that physicians and other stakeholders (e.g., administrators, financial specialists, public health officials) abandon autonomous ways of thinking and doing their work and shift toward more collaborative and shared ways of knowing that help to shape high-quality health care. Simultaneously, they must be adaptive to declining quality so that the system can react in favor of improving care. The RSS described in the section that follows provides one example of a CPD activity that reinforces organizational learning from multiple perspectives, adaptive action, and systems thinking.

AN EXAMPLE OF AN RSS THAT PROMOTES QUALITY IMPROVEMENT IN EDUCATION—MMIC

Morbidity and mortality conferences are a major exemplar of an education forum that seeks to integrate many of the aspects of quality and value referenced above. The goals highlight the four areas noted by Kitto et al.,[3] notably (1) continuing education, (2) knowledge translation, (3) patient safety, and (4) quality improvement. In some institutions such as the Dartmouth-Hitchcock Medical Center, the weekly Morbidity, Mortality and Improvement Conference (MMIC) serves as both a quality assurance and a CME conference, highlighting systems issues, promoting evidence-based practice, and identifying quality improvement opportunities. This type of RSS has increasingly been seen as a vehicle for quality improvement,[31] patient safety,[32,33] and systems-based practice competency.[34–36]

The MMIC is an educational intervention focused on improving patient care and which can be deconstructed to learn about how it promotes these goals, a process that has been particularly illuminating at the Dartmouth-Hitchcock Medical Center. It is an environment in which multidisciplinary, multigenerational, interprofessional learning occurs and in which many participants experience as occurring in a psychologically and professionally safe environment.[37] Participants include residents, attending physicians, faculty, medical students, community physicians, retired physicians, nurses, physician assistants, and trainees from various programs. In reaction to patient cases presented by residents, the facilitator engages the audience to generate differential diagnoses, discuss the selection of and interpretation of ancillary tests, and model patient-centered decision making. Identification of evidence supporting critical needs in improving communication (e.g., between providers and providers and patients, particularly during critical illness and end-of-life care) suggests a rich opportunity for care improvement.

Using Logic Analysis to Understand an Educational Intervention

To gain a clearer understanding for how the MMIC contributes to high-quality patient care, its theory of change was analyzed. This inquiry was approached by asking the question, "What works for whom and under what conditions?"[38] To do this, a direct logic analysis[39] was performed to examine an MMIC's practices and espoused theory for improving patient care. Logic analysis provides a means for evaluating an educational intervention's underlying theory of action, allowing for a critical examination of the hypothesized linkages between an intervention (i.e., the MMIC) and intended outcomes (e.g., improved patient care). This analysis provides a means for gaining insight into the validity of the theory of action and can help in planning evaluations that are well aligned with an educational program's characteristics and context. It is important that logic *analysis* not be confused with logic *modeling*, which is a visual technique for conceptualizing a program's theory of change and is the first of three steps in a logic analysis. Therefore, a logic analysis begins by working with a program's stakeholders to create a logic model that visually illustrates and describes how a program is *currently organized to produce its desired outcomes*.

In step two, the opinions of experts are consulted and a targeted literature review is performed to create a conceptual framework that will "clarify stakeholders' representations [of the program's theory] using scientific knowledge."[39] (p. 71) For the purpose of the MMIC logic analysis, the evaluation team (including the MMIC's director) sought the insights of local experts (e.g., the department's advisory committee for education) and conducted a targeted literature review of research on MMICs, organizational learning, diagnostic reasoning and critical thinking, interprofessional education, human factors science, and systems thinking to address gaps in the program's current theory as identified in step one of the logic analysis. In the third and final step of the logic analysis, the evaluation team compared the MMIC's current theory of change (i.e., logic model) to the one suggested by the literature review and information gleaned from the consulted experts (i.e., conceptual framework). This step revealed ways that the MMIC, its assessment approaches, and/or its theory could be enhanced to achieve the desired impact of improving patient care.

Three major findings emerged from this logic analysis: (1) the MMIC involved multiple units of analysis (i.e., resident, participants, facilitator, and clinical case); (2) the program's current implementation, assessment, and evaluation process were focused almost entirely on program delivery and its immediate outputs; and (3) mechanisms (effector arms) and pathways that could facilitate the translation of knowledge from conference activities into changes in clinical practice or patient care were limited. The new model that emerged from this logic analysis suggested additional pathways for improved patient outcomes and revealed a level of contextual complexity greater than originally theorized. The four hypothesized quality improvement pathways that emerged were as follows: (1) an MMIC participant changes his or her own practice; (2) a participant initiates a change involving a clinical team; (3) the department's Vice Chair of Quality draws on what he or she learns from the conference to inform quality initiatives at the department level; or (4) a participant communicates what is learned at the conference to decision makers at DHMC's Value Institute, which organizes quality initiatives at the organizational level. These pathways provided anchoring points where one could begin to understand the underlying mechanisms and context for how the MMIC was contributing to high-value and high-quality patient outcomes.[38]

What the Logic Analysis Revealed

As these pathways were analyzed, a variety of important outcomes of the MMIC were discovered as reported by the participants themselves (Table 2.2).[37]

1. *Elaboration of illness scripts*: Studies of expert clinical performance demonstrate that clinicians build up illness scripts based on their personal experience with patients. For at least some participants, it appears that the MMIC may serve a similar function, allowing participants to enhance and refine their mental schemas by drawing on the experiences of others as well.
2. *Situational understanding*: Participants acquire new knowledge about the context in which they provide care for patients. They described developing greater awareness of the resources available to them for providing patient care.

TABLE 2.2
Participant-Reported Outcomes of Morbidity, Mortality, and Improvement Conference

Elaboration of illness scripts
Situational understanding
Gains in medical knowledge
Deeper understanding of problems and opportunities
Critical reflection on one's own practice
Mental models of effective communication
Better understanding of social and interpersonal dimensions of care
Greater empathy for and sensitivity to patient and family experiences of care
Greater acceptance of the uncertainties of medical practice

3. *Gains in medical knowledge*: These knowledge gains during the MMIC, or reactivation of previously learned and forgotten knowledge, can translate into a change in clinical practice at the individual level. New knowledge might comprise a deeper understanding of a disease process, but it can also occur when the conference provides a participant with a better understanding of the organizational context and an opportunity to become more familiar with the people who inhabit it.

4. *Deeper understanding of problems and opportunities*: The longitudinal nature of the MMIC provides a deeper, more integrated understanding of the frequency, nature, causes, and consequences of problems, challenges, and opportunities to improve patient care. Insight into how systems issues cause or exacerbate problems and how systems might be used to address problems and for a better understanding of the challenges around communicating with patients and families were all noted.

5. *Critical reflection on one's own practice*: All learners at the MMIC can compare one's clinical reasoning and knowledge with that of the team that cared for the patient and that of the attending faculty, providing opportunities to recognize biases and habits of thought that might reflect poorly or well in patient care.

6. *Mental models of effective collaboration*: The MMIC provides an example of joint inquiry and collegial critique of practice in the context of respectful communication between health care providers. It helps to establish the value of multiple perspectives not only as useful for a given case but also as a general principle.

7. *Better understanding of social and interpersonal dimensions of care*: The MMIC leads to better understanding of these dimensions (especially as they relate to having goals of care discussions with patients and families) and to the importance of a shared understanding among members of the care team concerning what those goals of care are.

8. *Greater empathy for and sensitivity to patient and family experiences of care*: The MMIC heightens empathetic feelings, especially in regard to patients during end of life.

9. *Greater acceptance of the uncertainties of medical practice*: The MMIC validates the uncertainty that is experienced by participants, even senior faculty. The conference provides role models who have dealt with and who are more comfortable with medical uncertainty.

Thus, using a case-based, problem-based, and team learning approach in meticulously understanding and discussing the care of an individual, we have found that learning in an experiential way and collaborating with others provide a rich, repetitive, and reinforcing process that increases the likelihood of getting optimal patient outcomes. Importantly, the RSS promotes systems thinking that leverages the unique contributions of a multigenerational, multidisciplinary and problem-centered approach that brings together multiple perspectives focused around the care of individual patients.

Conceptually, one can formulate the relationship of this educational intervention with traditional QI and PS efforts as seen in Figure 2.1. In this formulation, it is suggested that patient outcomes are affected by multiple processes, including from the quality improvement and patient safety fields, as well as by quality-focused educational interventions such as the RSS described. Participants (learners) inevitably engage in integrated processing, a concept referring to those cognitive, emotional, and reflective qualities that underlie learning and behavior change.

This model attempts to define CPD in the setting of MMIC as an effort to allow individual clinicians to learn from many domains of expertise, to identify gaps in knowledge,

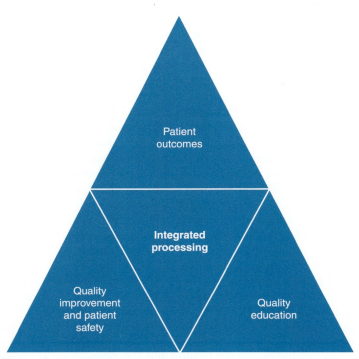

FIGURE 2.1. A model for merging quality improvement/patient safety, quality education, and integrated processing to attain optimal patient outcomes as promoted by the RSS.

and to engage in repetitive and reinforcing behaviors that have effects on patient care. In order to do this, they must, in participating, engage in active learning and integrated processing from diverse sources—for example, knowledge, attitudes, problem solving, communication, self-reflection, and continual revising of their mental models of right or constructive behavior. The figure could be made more complex, of course, but its intent is to emphasize the important synergies that quality improvement, patient safety, and quality education offer both the learner and the educator committed to professional development.

Finally, there are two additional factors that play a role in the effectiveness of the RSS, namely the role of the director or facilitator and that of the learner attending the RSS. The former must be a champion who feels responsible for the quality of the series much the same way as having a clinician who accepts responsibility for the care of a patient is crucial for optimal health outcomes. A committed champion or leader is also one element that is necessary for supporting the collaborative dynamics of groups involved in systems change.[40] Many of the same characteristics of the director are shared with those that are associated with excellence in clinical care. Some of these are seen in Table 2.3. The facilitator must have a broad appreciation for the relevance of the content, adult learning behavior, and a long-term commitment to improvement in both patient care and self-development. No less important is the learner her/himself. Someone who attends the RSS must be committed to being an active learner. Examples of critical attributes for being a successful learner include engagement, curiosity, and being open-minded and

TABLE 2.3
Attributes of the RSS Director/Facilitator

Awareness of participants' learning needs
Mentoring colleagues, residents, and students
Creating a culture of safety in group learning
Skilled at facilitating and coaching
Flexible, willing to vary format, pedagogies, and technologies
Reflective regarding self, interpersonal relationships, and clinical issues
Able to move between individual and systems factors
Skilled at evaluation and feedback
Identification of quality improvement opportunities
Collaboration with others
Love of medicine
Humility in the face of uncertainty

RSS, regularly scheduled series.

self-directed. Learners who understand the need to pursue understanding diligently are more likely to enjoy the fruits of such a conference. For example, if an important concept, therapy, or ethical issue is raised during the conference, a learner who pursues a deeper understanding following the conference is more likely to engage in changed behavior in the future. The ability to reconfigure mental constructs and the ability to tolerate the inevitable uncertainty in medical practice are additional attributes of importance. These are listed in Table 2.4 and have been explored earlier in this chapter.

FUTURE DIRECTIONS

CPD requires a multidimensional approach to learning and practice that employs a multiplicity of disciplines and pedagogies. An integrated application of diverse areas of expertise and experiential learning includes a commitment to lifelong learning, knowledge acquisition, systems thinking, adaptation action, patient safety, and quality improvement. The RSS described has a remarkable ability to combine all of these diverse goals in a patient-centered and learner-centric way. A simple construct is presented that also addresses an unfortunate gap that has developed between two committed groups of experts dedicated to improving patient outcomes. Quality improvement (QI) and patient safety (PS) efforts have grown in expertise, methodology, and measurable process

TABLE 2.4
Attributes of the Successful Learner

Self-directed
Engaged
Curious
Pursues learning diligently
Tolerates uncertainty
Able to reconfigure mental constructs
Open-minded

outcomes since their introduction. An impressive literature, dedicated and innovative training and implementation strategies, and prestigious centers of excellence have arisen to promote better value, increase quality, and lower costs. Quality education (QE), particularly CPD, has not had a similarly recognizable base with which to advance the same agenda, yet all are necessary to achieve better patient outcomes in the complex environment that is health care. To better understand how and to what extent educational programs contribute to these outcomes, it is important that their underlying mechanisms and context for change be understood as part of a larger health care system.[38] An example of one such conference (a complex educational intervention in a complex environment) at the Dartmouth-Hitchcock Medical Center is presented, which addresses the role of the clinician as a vital component in the effort to improve value. The value equation should explicitly reflect the need to strengthen and integrate the processes of QI/PS and QE. Neither is sufficient. Both are necessary.

From the foregoing, it should be clear that a variety of educational techniques, pedagogies, and assessments are currently applied to CPD. This effort is international, with innovations seen from all parts of the world. Most of the anticipated change and improvement will come in the following areas: (1) the generation, availability, and organization of information; (2) demonstration and practice of skills; (3) local and distance consultation; (4) communication at every branch point of clinical decision making; and (5) shared decision making. The ubiquitous availability of information (e.g., UpToDate, DynaMed, PubMed), demonstration of skills (YouTube), and consultations (ask Mayo, eConsults) have fundamentally altered the delivery of information, although evidence of efficacy and outcomes is lacking. The effort to improve the quality, efficiency, and effectiveness of these interventions continues to evolve as newer technologies and formats are developed. Online journal clubs are uniting faculty and residents in a medical center[41] and hundreds of medical practitioners from around the world[42] in order to enhance knowledge translation of the medical literature without the limitations of geography. In addition, social media are beginning to be employed in order to include expertise from geographically discontinuous participants with various levels of expertise. One group has employed a Twitter-augmented journal club in anesthesiology.[43] They cite the benefits of Twitter as (1) easy adoption; (2) access to experts, peers, and patients across the globe; (3) 24/7 connectivity; (4) creation of education-based communities using hashtags; and (5) crowdsourcing information using retweets. Another group created a Twitter journal club for nephrology that primarily provides postpublication peer review of high-impact nephrology articles, but additionally helps Twitter users build a network of engaged people with interests in academic nephrology. By following participants in the nephrology journal club, users are able to stock their personal learning network.[44] An experiment using a multimodal e-learning platform to facilitate a journal club and the development of critical appraisal skills, a virtual journal club, was reported by Oliphant et al.[45]

Web-based interactive conferences also have united rural or multisite clinicians without the necessity for a single meeting site, expanding the geography and resource offering in real time.[46,47] These innovations seek to expand a learner-centric approach while utilizing social media or live teleconferencing. Furthermore, no single educational activity or intervention, in and of itself, is responsible for high-quality patient care, but, as part of an educational subsystem, they may be extremely effective. Their impact on patient outcomes has yet to be demonstrated even as clinician acceptance appears to be growing. New technologies and innovative approaches to medical education and professional development create great opportunities to capture information and learning in real time in ways that facilitate adaptation to rapidly changing environments and conditions in health care systems. It will be important for education researchers and evaluators to assess the contributions of these new efforts using a systems perspective in order to fully understand how education can be linked to better quality and lower costs that define high-value health care. Although the fundamentals remain the same (knowledge informing the humane care of individuals), the paths to improved patient outcomes will continue to be varied, complex, and creative and will depend not only on innovation and evaluation but on thoughtful and caring clinicians.

REFERENCES

1. Sockalingam S, Tehrani H, Lin E, et al. Integrating quality improvement and continuing professional development: a model from the mental health care system. *Acad Med.* 2016;91(4):540–547.
2. Austin Z, Marini A, Glover N, et al. Continuous professional development: a qualitative study of pharmacists' attitudes, behaviors and preferences in Ontario, Canada. *Am J Pharm Educ.* 2005;69:25–33.
3. Kitto S, Bell M, Peller J, et al. Positioning continuing education: boundaries and intersections between the domains continuing education, knowledge translation, patient safety and quality improvement. *Adv Health Sci Educ Theory Pract.* 2013;18(1):141–156.
4. Van Hoof TJ, Grant RE, Miller NE, et al. Society for Academic Continuing Medical Education Intervention Guideline Series: Guideline 1, Performance Measurement and Feedback. *J Contin Educ Health Prof.* 2015;35(suppl 2):S51–S54.
5. Van Hoof TJ, Grant RE, Campbell C, et al. Society for Academic Continuing Medical Education Intervention Guideline Series: Guideline 2, Practice Facilitation. *J Contin Educ Health Prof.* 2015;35(suppl 2):S55–S59.
6. Van Hoof TJ, Grant RE, Sajdlowska J, et al. Society for Academic Continuing Medical Education Intervention Guideline Series: Guideline 3, Educational Meetings. *J Contin Educ Health Prof.* 2015;35(suppl 2):S60–S64.
7. Van Hoof TJ, Grant RE, Sajdlowska J, et al. Society for Academic Continuing Medical Education Intervention Guideline Series: Guideline 4, Interprofessional Education. *J Contin Educ Health Prof.* 2015;35(suppl 2):S65–S69.
8. McMahon GT. What do I need to learn today?—the evolution of CME. *N Engl J Med.* 2016;374(15): 1403–1404.
9. Biesta G. Good education in an age of measurement: on the need to reconnect with the question of purpose in education. *Educ Assess Eval Account.* 2009;21:33–46.
10. Cervero RM, Gaines JK. The impact of CME on physician performance and patient health outcomes: an updated synthesis of systematic reviews. *J Contin Educ Health Prof.* 2015;35:131–138.
11. Ransom SB, Griffith JR, Campbell DA, et al. Conceptualizing and improving quality: overview. In: Nash NB, Goldfarb NI, eds. *The Quality Solution.* Sudbury, MA: Jones and Bartlett; 2006:49–72.
12. Donabedian A. Quality and cost: choices and responsibilities. *Inquiry.* 1988;25(1):90–99.
13. Gerber PD, Smith DS, Ross JM. Generalist physicians and the new health care system. *Am J Med.* 1994;97(6):554–558.
14. Berwick DM, Nolan TW, Whittington J. The triple aim: care, health, and cost. *Health Aff.* 2008; 27(3):759–769.
15. Berwick DM. Measuring surgical outcomes for improvement: was Codman wrong? *JAMA.* 2015; 313(5):469–470.
16. US Department of Health and Human Services. Patient Protection and the Affordable Health Act. December 2009. http://www.hhs.gov/sites/default/files/patient-protection.pdf. Accessed June 23, 2016.
17. Accreditation Council for Graduate Medical Education. Next Accreditation System (NAS) Competency Definitions and Recommended Practice Performance Tools. 2015. http://www.acgme.org/acgmeweb/Portals/0/PFAssets/ProgramResources/430_CompetencyDefinitions_RO_ED_10182007.pdf. Accessed June 2, 2016.
18. Institute of Medicine (US) Committee on the Health Professions Education Summit, Greiner AC, Knebel E, eds. *Health Professions Education: A Bridge to Quality.* Washington, DC: National Academies Press; 2003. http://iom.nationalacademies.org/Reports/2003/Health-Professions-Education-A-Bridge-to-Quality.aspx. Accessed December 5, 2015.
19. Dweck C. *Mindset: The New Psychology of Success.* New York: Random House; 2006.

20. Deming Cycle, PDCA. 2000. https://www.isixsigma.com/dictionary/deming-cycle-pdca/. Accessed December 7, 2015.
21. Eoyang GH, Holladay RJ. *Adaptive Action: Leveraging Uncertainty in Your Organization.* Stanford, CA: Stanford University Press; 2013.
22. Leykum LK, Lanham HJ, Pugh JA, et al. Manifestations and implications of uncertainty for improving healthcare systems: an analysis of observational and interventional studies grounded in complexity science. *Implement Sci.* 2014;19(9):165.
23. Elwyn G, Barr PJ, Grande SW, et al. Developing CollaboRATE: a fast and frugal patient-reported measure of shared decision making in clinical encounters. *Patient Educ Couns.* 2013;93(1):102–107.
24. Chapman W, Hutchinson C, Bialek D. *Medical Quality Systems: The Elusive Goal of Quality in Complex Systems.* 2011. http://www.mwestonchapman.com/medical-quality-systems-the-elusive-goal-of-quality-in-complex-medical-systems/. Accessed January 15, 2016.
25. Christmas C, Kravet SJ, Durso SC, et al. Clinical excellence in academia: perspectives from masterful academic clinicians. *Mayo Clin Proc.* 2008;83(9):989–994.
26. Legare F, Freitas A, Thompson-Leduc P, et al. The majority of accredited continuing professional development activities do not target clinical behavior change. *Acad Med.* 2015;90(2):197–202.
27. Ericsson KA. Deliberate practice and the acquisition and maintenance of expert performance in medicine and related domains. *Acad Med.* 2004;79(10):S70–S81.
28. Mahar M. The state of the nation's health. *Dartm Med.* 2007;31(3):26–35.
29. Kelley B, Fabius R. A Path to Eliminating $3.6 Trillion in Wasteful Healthcare Spending. https://outlook.office365.com/owa/?realm=wisc.edu&exsvurl=1. Accessed December 20, 2015.
30. Cabrara D, Cabrara L. *Systems Thinking Made Simple: New Hope for Solving Wicked Problems.* Ithaca, NY: Odyssean Press; 2015.
31. Gerstein WH, Ledford J, Cooper J, et al. Interdisciplinary quality improvement conference: using a revised morbidity and mortality format to focus on systems-based patient safety issues in a VA hospital: design and outcomes. *Am J Med Qual.* 2016;31(2):162–168.
32. Frey B, Doell C, Klauwer D, et al. The morbidity and mortality conference in pediatric intensive care as a means for improving patient safety. *Pediatr Crit Care Med.* 2016;17(1):67–72.
33. Sellier E, David-Tchouda S, Bal G, et al. Morbidity and mortality conferences: their place in quality assessments. *Int J Health Care Qual Assur.* 2012;25(3):189–196.
34. Gonzalo JD, Yang JJ, Huang GC. Systems-based content in medical morbidity and mortality conferences: a decade of change. *J Grad Med Educ.* 2012;4(4):438–444.
35. Gonzalo JD, Bump GM, Huang GC, et al. Implementation and evaluation of a multidisciplinary systems-focused internal medicine morbidity and mortality conference. *J Grad Med Educ.* 2014;6(1):139–146.
36. Rabizadeh S, Gower WA, Payton K, et al. Restructuring the Morbidity and Mortality Conference in a Department of Pediatrics to serve as a vehicle for system changes. *Clin Pediatr (Phila).* 2012;51(11):1079–1086.
37. Bakken LL, Olson CA, Ross JM, et al. *The Department of Medicine Morbidity, Mortality and Improvement Conference: Phase I Report.* Lebanon, NH: Dartmouth-Hitchcock Medical Center; 2015:70.
38. Pawson R, Tilley N. *Realistic Evaluation.* Thousand Oaks, CA: Sage Publications, Inc.; 1997.
39. Brousselle A, Champagne F. Program theory evaluation: logic analysis. *Eval Program Plann.* 2011;34:69–78.
40. Emerson K, Nabatchi T, Balogh S. An integrative framework for collaborative governance. *J Public Admin Res Theory.* 2012;22(1):1–29.
41. Yang PR, Meals RA. How to establish an interactive eConference and eJournal club. *J Hand Surg [Am].* 2014;39(1):129–133.
42. Chan TB. Ten steps for setting up an online journal club. *J Contin Educ Health Prof.* 2015;35(2):148–154.
43. Udani A, Moyse D, Peery C, et al. Twitter-augmented journal club: educational engagement and experience so far. *A Case Rep.* 2016;16(6):253–256.
44. Topf J, Hiremath S. Social media, medicine and the modern journal club. *Int Rev Psychiatry.* 2015;27(2):147–154.
45. Oliphant R, Blackhall V, Moug S, et al. Early experience of a virtual journal club. *Clin Teach.* 2015;12(6):389–393.
46. Pletcher SN, Rodi SW. Web-based morbidity and mortality conferencing: a model for rural medical education. *J Contin Educ Health Prof.* 2011;31(2):128–133.
47. Falcone JL, Watson AR. Surgical Morbidity and Mortality Conference using teleconferencing allows for increased faculty participation and moderation from satellite campuses and saves costs. *J Surg Educ.* 2012;69(1):58–62.

Chapter 3

Advances *in* Simulation-Based Continuing Professional Development *and* Training

Dimitrios Stefanidis and Ajit K. Sachdeva

Case

Concerns regarding decrease in attendance at grand rounds and morbidity and mortality conferences have prompted you to pursue other options to address the learning needs of surgeons in practice. One of these approaches makes great sense to you: the more we provide the learner–participant with hands-on, practical experience, the more he or she can acquire new knowledge and skills and then apply them in practice. You have also been speaking with your surgical colleagues who complain that their residents are getting less clinical and operating room experiences than they did in training; their concerns relate to major operations, outpatient procedures, and less exposure to pre- and postoperative care.

Questions

Could simulation technologies help both of these problems? What does simulation mean? Can the technologies only be applied effectively in surgery and other procedural specialties?

INTRODUCTION

Simulation has been used in medical training for centuries, but its widespread use in medical education did not occur until the past few decades.[1,2] Simulation-based education in health care refers to any intervention that replicates clinical situations, processes, actions, or behaviors and may include devices, computer programs, technologies, standardized patients, case scenarios, and other methods of depicting clinical conditions (Table 3.1). For medical educators, simulation affords increased control over the training environment and ability to manipulate it; for learners, it provides greater opportunities for experiential learning in a nonthreatening environment and the ability to learn from their errors, which is paramount for learning.[3]

Indeed, a systematic review by Davis and colleagues[4] that assessed the effect of formal continuing medical education (CME)/continuous professional development (CPD)

| TABLE 3.1 |
| Simulation modalities used in healthcare |

- Clinical examination models
- Part task trainers
- Realistic procedural simulators
- Virtual reality simulators
- Hybrid simulators
- Live animal models
- Cadaveric models
- Cut suit
- Screen-based simulation
- Human patient mannequins
- Standardized patients
- Virtual patients
- Virtual environments

interventions on physician performance and health care outcomes identified that interactive CME/CPD sessions that actively involve participants and provide the opportunity to practice skills can affect change in professional practice and, on occasion, health care outcomes. The benefits of experiential learning and the fact that simulation helps decrease the risks associated with on-the-job training have propelled the use of simulation in today's health care environment that has no tolerance for patient harm. In this chapter, we will review the current application of simulation in CME/CPD and provide suggestions for how it may best be incorporated into CME/CPD programs to maximize their impact.

APPLICATION OF SIMULATION IN HEALTH CARE

Simulation Centers

Technologic advances and development of new simulators along with recognition of the benefits of experiential learning provided by simulation have sparked the establishment of skills laboratories and simulation centers that aim to bring these effective training approaches to a diverse group of health care learners. Such centers allow for training and assessment of health care providers in a safe environment that focuses on the individual learner or teams and provides significant control of the training and testing conditions. As outlined in the next sections of this chapter, such centers can offer structured, effective, evidence-based skills curricula to their learners, include use of a variety of valid and reliable assessment tools and performance metrics, and provide effective performance feedback through structured debriefing that can have a lasting effect on learning. Nevertheless, the undisciplined proliferation of simulation centers around the country led to the implementation of training strategies that lacked consistent quality and evidence of effectiveness.

In an effort to improve standardization of simulation practices, steer the simulation community to design and adopt innovative education and training programs, and advance the field of simulation-based surgical education and training, the American College of Surgeons (ACS) Division of Education launched a program to accredit simulation centers in 2005.[5] A consortium of accredited education institutes (ACS-AEI) has been created and now includes 94 such institutes. Key leaders and experts from the

ACS-AEI Consortium meet regularly, share advances and best practices, exchange ideas, and develop collaborative simulation research projects. Realizing the importance of this approach in leveraging the standards in simulation use across the health care professions, the Society for Simulation in Healthcare has followed suit and implemented its own accreditation process.[6] Challenges associated with the establishment of major simulation centers include the need for sufficient resources (i.e., space, simulation equipment, personnel, supplies), institutional commitments relating to these resources, and the limited capacity of the centers to educate and train learners dictated as a result of finite resources.

In Situ Simulation

Given that the effectiveness of the health care delivery system and quality of patient care are determined not solely by the competency of a single provider or team (mainly targeted by simulation centers), but rather by a constellation of factors, such as interactions of the provider with patients, other providers, the tools and technologies used while providing care, higher-level organizational work processes, policies, and cultural factors, other uses of simulation such as in situ have also been popularized.[7,8] With in situ simulation, besides individuals and teams, additional factors within the health care delivery systems can be analyzed and improved by bringing learners to real clinical environments where simulations may be conducted.[9] According to a systematic review from 2012 studies on in situ simulation addressed team competencies of staff members (28%), unit- or system-level latent errors (28%), a combination of individual and teamwork competencies (17%), a combination of teamwork competencies and unit or system issues (14%), or a combination thereof (14%).[9]

While most of the available literature on the effectiveness of in situ simulation has focused on learner reactions and attitudes, a few studies have also demonstrated its effectiveness in regard to organizational performance.[10–12] The ability to study health care systems, savings in staff time (e.g., no travel time to a physically separate training environment), and reductions in the overhead and physical footprint of a simulation center are all advantages of in situ simulation. Nevertheless, this approach requires different resources, planning, and data capture methods than do programs conducted in traditional simulation settings. For in situ simulations to become a robust learning strategy in the continuing education toolbox, additional work is needed to address faculty development, learner assessment and feedback, incorporation of structured needs assessments, and collection of data on return on investment.[9,12]

Distributed Models

Critics of current simulation practices have argued that simulation remains a "toy of the rich" that makes training impossible for large parts of our world that need it the most but cannot afford access to expensive simulators, state-of-the-art facilities, complex simulations, and even clinical experts.[13] Distance simulation-based medical education and training have therefore been proposed as solutions to the unequal distribution of training across the globe and are feasible today as a result of rapid advances in technology. The dissemination of knowledge and expertise via online platforms (telesimulation, telepresence) and e-learning can close the gaps in not only physical but also intellectual terms and can help to address needs relating to knowledge and skills across a broad range of learners independent of their location in relation to a simulation center.[13] While initial reports support the feasibility and effectiveness of distributed simulation, additional high-quality

TABLE 3.2
Advantages and Disadvantages of various Simulation Delivery Options

	Advantages	Disadvantages
Simulation center	Enables training in a safe, unrushed environment	Costly
	Provides excellent control of the training and testing conditions	Requires significant resources (personnel, space)
	Maximizes training efficiency	Limits access to training when number of learners outgrow resources
In-situ simulation	Enables system probing	Disruptive to clinical workflow
	Training takes place in working environment	Difficult to standardize training and testing environment
	No inconvenience to the learner traveling to a center	Requires permission/ cannot occur anytime
	Reduced overhead of physical space	
Distributed simulation	Low cost	Technology dependent
	Affords simulation training to remote learners and those who have no ability to access a center	Potential for communication break downs between host and remote site
	Makes lacking clinical expertise available	Reliance on availability of remote expertise

studies are needed for this promising approach to become a major component of simulation center operations in the future.[14,15] Distributed simulation training is also aligned with the needs of CME as it is likely to bring an effective education strategy closer to the learner, minimizing the burden of time and money required to attend distant courses. Advantages and disadvantages of each simulation delivery method are listed in Table 3.2.

SIMULATION-BASED CONTINUOUS PROFESSIONAL DEVELOPMENT AND TRAINING

Simulation-based training has been applied and studied across the continuum of professional development in medicine in regard to a variety of skills, including clinical, technical, and nontechnical skills, as well as teamwork. A 2011 survey of the American Association of Medical Colleges on the use of simulation in medical education revealed that all responding medical schools and teaching hospitals used simulation at some point during the 4 years of undergraduate medical education, over 85% used it with residents, over 60% with clinical fellows, and over 84% with other health care professionals. Of the programs using simulation, 86% used simulation for educational purposes, 71% for assessment, and 40% for quality improvement. A broad range of competencies was addressed by these programs, including medical knowledge, patient care, interpersonal and communication skills, professionalism, practice-based learning and improvement, systems-based practice, psychomotor skills, leadership, team training, and critical thinking and decision-making.[16] Two main categories of simulation are currently being used for the training of health care providers: scenario-based and procedural.

Scenario-Based Simulations

Scenario-based simulations enable training and assessment of clinical knowledge, judgment, and nontechnical skills. Scenarios typically are based on real or fictitious patient cases and are driven by learning objectives. The learning objectives define the flow of the scenario. As an example, if the learning objective is to teach appropriate diagnosis and management of a patient with a pulmonary embolism, then a relevant scenario may include an early postsurgical patient who experiences acute onset shortness of breath, desaturation, and tachycardia. The learner is asked to evaluate and treat the patient for the underlying problem and to demonstrate through a series of actions that he or she is able to address the problem expeditiously by taking the appropriate diagnostic steps, establishing the diagnosis, and providing timely and appropriate treatment. Most (but not all) learner actions can be anticipated, and case algorithms developed to define the simulated patient's "clinical" state as a consequence of those actions. Even when learner actions do not go as planned, instructors have the ability to change scenarios "on the fly" to accommodate any unexpected occurrences and still achieve the learning objectives. This creates a very powerful learning environment as it provides insight not only into the knowledge base of the learner but also into his or her decision-making ability, and skills in developing appropriate differential diagnoses and appropriately and efficiently managing the situation.

Most importantly, scenario-based training not only allows teachers to objectively assess learner performance but affords them the opportunity to debrief with the learners after the session and review all their actions in detail. The debriefing session that follows each scenario provides learners with feedback on their performance, and this is where most of the learning occurs.[17] Instructors can explore in-depth learner knowledge and understanding of clinical conditions, teach to address the identified deficiencies, and share take-home points. Thus, teaching can be individualized to target those topics most in need of being addressed rather than adopting a blanket approach to a topic, which characterizes traditional lectures. Further, through the use of video (scenario-based sessions are typically video recorded), learners can review their performance with their instructors and learn from their actual actions rather than from a discussion about their actions, maximizing the effectiveness of teaching.[18] It is not uncommon for learners to be unaware of or even deny specific actions during a scenario until they see themselves on the video. Such experiences leave lasting memories that cement learning.

The value of scenario-based training goes beyond clinical knowledge and decision-making. It provides an ideal environment to also effectively teach and assess nontechnical skills such as leadership, communication, collaboration, situational awareness, and teamwork.[19,20] Such scenarios include learning objectives that focus on the requisite nontechnical skills and are structured specifically to address them in a clinical context. Learners remain interested and focused on "solving" the clinical problem. In the authors' experiences, trainees are less interested in scenarios that only address nontechnical skills and more eager to learn when clinical and technical elements are also addressed. An additional benefit of scenario-based training is that they can be focused on teams rather than an individual. Given that effective teamwork in health care is critical to improving quality and safety, such scenarios facilitate training and assessment of clinical teams and development of shared mental models among health care professionals and promote improvements in patient care and clinical processes.[21,22]

Procedural Skill Acquisition

Simulation also provides an optimal environment for procedural skill acquisition. Multiple simulators have been developed and are being used for training, from low-cost task trainers to expensive virtual reality training platforms. While validity evidence for use of available simulators is accumulating rapidly, there is widespread recognition that acquiring a simulator does not by itself yield the desired training outcome; rather, a robust curriculum needs to be built around the simulator.[23] Proficiency-based curricula that focus on training outcomes rather than solely on education delivery have emerged as the preferred training paradigm for procedural skill acquisition.

Proficiency-based training is grounded in learning theory and incorporates goal-oriented training, deliberate practice, frequent objective assessments of performance, and formative feedback relating to performance.[23] Such curricula tailor training to individual needs, support acquisition of skills uniformly across learners, and have been shown to result in robust skill acquisition and retention that translates to the real environment, such as the operating room.[24,25] They represent a more effective training paradigm compared with the traditional time-based training that is pervasive in medical education today.[23,26]

This type of training is frequently referenced in the simulation literature as mastery learning. According to McGaghie and colleagues,[27] mastery learning is characterized by baseline testing, the definition of clear learning objectives sequenced in units of increasing difficulty, deliberate practice of the desired skills, the setting of minimum pass standards with frequent formative testing to assess when those standards have been achieved in order to advance to the next level of difficulty, and the continuation of training until the mastery standard has been reached. One of the most important elements of these curricula is deliberate practice, a concept that was popularized by the work of Ericsson KA and refers to a highly structured repetitive practice of cognitive or psychomotor skills that learners engage in, with the specific goal of improving their performance and developing expertise through specific feedback and rigorous skills assessment.[28,29] Duvivier et al. from Maastricht University in the Netherlands described the general skills learners need to exhibit during various stages in order to be successful in developing their clinical skills. These include planning (organize work in a structured way), concentration/dedication (higher attention span), repetition/revision (strong tendency to practice), and study style/self-reflection (tendency to self-regulate learning).[30]

Along with procedural skills, many principles of mastery learning can also be applied to scenario-based training. A systematic review of the best available evidence identified 10 features and uses of high-fidelity simulations that lead to effective learning. These included feedback provided during learning experiences, learner engagement in repetitive practice, use of clearly defined outcomes or benchmarks, integration of simulation into an overall curriculum, task practice with increasing levels of difficulty, use of multiple learning strategies, implementation of simulation experiences in a controlled environment, reliable representation of clinical practice and incorporating clinical variation, and promotion of individualized learning.[29]

Simulation and the curricula that have been developed around them offer educational opportunities that can lead to significant positive changes in the domain of CME/CPD through mastery learning, deliberate practice, and valid and reliable performance assessment coupled with specific feedback. The benefits of such interventions can extend across the continuum of medical education, from early stages of skill development to expertise.

ROLE OF SIMULATION-BASED TRAINING TO ENHANCE PATIENT CARE AND IMPROVE PATIENT SAFETY

Several papers, systematic reviews, and meta-analyses have demonstrated the effectiveness of simulation in enhancing patient care and improving patient safety.[31,32] At the level of the individual, a series of observational studies by Barsuk et al.[33,34] at Northwestern University in Chicago, United States, assessed the impact of simulator-based mastery learning of central line placement by internal medicine residents on patient outcomes and demonstrated 85% reduction in central line–associated bloodstream infections (CLABSI) resulting from this training. Further, the decreased complications led to significant medical care cost savings, which resulted in a 7:1 ratio of return on investment.[35] In a follow-up report, the authors also demonstrated the generalizability of their findings by showing a 74% reduction in the incidence of CLABSI at other institutions that adopted their intervention.[36] These findings have also been replicated by Khouli and colleagues[37] who used a randomized design to demonstrate a 70% reduction in the incidence of ICU CLABSI for residents trained on simulators compared with a video only trained group.

Rogers and colleagues[38] implemented a structured simulation-based curriculum for ophthalmology residents that incorporated deliberate practice of capsulorhexis and formative feedback. These authors demonstrated a statistically significant reduction in sentinel events (defined as posterior capsule tears or vitreous loss) in the operating room from 7.2% before to 3.8% after the introduction of the simulation-based curriculum. In a randomized study of general surgery residents, the group that trained to proficiency on a laparoscopic extraperitoneal (TEP) hernia repair simulator performed TEP repairs in the operating room faster, achieved higher operative performance scores, and had fewer intraoperative complications (peritoneal tear, procedure conversion) and postoperative complications (urinary retention, seroma) as compared with controls.[39] Also noteworthy is that the need for overnight stay of patients after surgery was less likely in the simulator trained group.

A systematic review of simulation-based training in laparoscopic surgery skills confirmed that simulation was an effective method to teach laparoscopic surgery skills and resulted in increased translation of these skills to the OR, as well as improved patient safety.[40] Another systematic review and meta-analysis found that simulation-based education in gastrointestinal endoscopy was associated with improved performance in a test setting and in clinical practice and in improved patient outcomes, when compared with no intervention.[41] Similar findings have been reported by many other systematic reviews and studies for a variety of skills and from a variety of institutions and continents.[42–46]

For teams and systems of care, Andreatta and colleagues[47] conducted a study using simulation-based pediatric mock codes and identified improved survival rates (from 33% before to 56% after the intervention) for pediatric cardiopulmonary arrest (CPA) patients (pulseless survival rate improved from 15% to 56%). Draycott and colleagues[48,49] from the University of Bristol in the United Kingdom demonstrated that introduction of obstetric emergencies training courses incorporating simulation was associated with a significant reduction in low 5-minute Apgar scores, a decrease in neonatal hypoxic–ischemic encephalopathy, and improved management and neonatal outcomes of births complicated by shoulder dystocia. Riley et al. compared perinatal outcomes using a randomized design in three separate hospitals among a TeamSTEPPS trained group, a TeamSTEPPS with adjunct simulation training group, and a control group and demonstrated a 37.4% decrease in adverse event rates in the simulation group. In another study, the implementation of simulation-based TeamSTEPPS in the trauma resuscitation bay led to improved team performance (including leadership, monitoring, mutual support, and communication) and in-hospital patient mortality was reduced from 13.1% pretraining to 8.5% posttraining.[50,51]

Two systematic reviews have confirmed the benefits of simulation team training in regard to patient safety. Hesselink et al.[52] assessed the value of simulation in emergency departments (ED) and found that use of simulation-based training programs and well-designed incident reporting systems led to a statistically significant improvement of safety knowledge and attitudes by ED staff and an increase of incident reports within EDs. In addition, Fung et al.[53] reviewed simulation-based crew resource management (CRM) for interprofessional and interdisciplinary teams and identified significant improvements in CRM skills compared with didactic case-based CRM.

USE OF SIMULATION TO ADDRESS SPECIFIC CHALLENGES AND OPPORTUNITIES

The introduction of new technologies and techniques in medicine has the potential to dramatically improve patient outcomes; however, it also poses risks to patients while physicians and surgeons are learning the safe use of new technologies and performance of new procedures.[54] To address new skill acquisition, CME/CPD courses are typically offered at annual national meetings or at academic institutions. Such courses may include didactics and observation of live cases and often include a hands-on experience with the new technology or procedure.

Simulation is playing an increasingly important role in these courses as the use of simulators, animal models, or cadavers enables experiential learning, thus maximizing training effectiveness. Recognizing the value of simulation for skill acquisition, professional organizations, such as the American College of Surgeons through its Division of Education, have incorporated simulations and simulators into several CME/CPD courses.[55] Further, the Australian government has developed the National Health Education and Training in Simulation (NHET-Sim) program that utilizes simulation to train health care professionals and their educators across the country aimed at improving clinical training capacity.[56,57] Challenges with CME/CPD courses for new skill acquisition relate to their short duration and often limited objectives, and they typically do not enable development of proficiency. The limited hands-on exposure participants are provided is not sufficient to promote robust skill acquisition, which typically leads participants to either abandon the technology or pursue additional courses before adopting it. In addition, objective assessment of participant performance, which can easily be achieved using simulators, is rarely used making it impossible to affirm competency or proficiency of participants in the new technique or procedure.

Evidence for the need for objective assessment and robust reorganization of such courses was recently provided by Pugh and colleagues[58] who, using a laparoscopic ventral hernia simulator during a CME/CPD course with 30 surgeon participants, identified a surprisingly low level of competence in the quality and completeness of hernia repairs (average score, 3.9 on a scale of 16 points) by surgeons who had previously performed these procedures clinically. Thus, there appears to be a need for the implementation of CME/CPD courses that objectively assess and provide longitudinal experiences to learners to assure achievement of the predetermined level of proficiency. The ACS Division of Education has developed a five-level model for objective assessments of surgeons in the use of new technologies and performance of new procedures.[59] Guidelines for the safe and effective introduction of new technology and techniques in practice have been published, and efforts to accomplish this are already being pursued by professional organizations such as the ACS, the Society of American Gastrointestinal and Endoscopic Surgeons, and others. Simulation remains central to such efforts.[58,60–62]

Equally important to initial skill acquisition using simulators is maintenance of these skills. This is especially important for skills that are infrequently performed and practiced in the clinical environment. Indeed, several studies have demonstrated that skills decay over time in the absence of practice.[63,64] While the grade of skill decay is dependent on a number of factors, such as the length of retention interval, degree of overlearning, certain task characteristics (i.e., physical vs. cognitive tasks), methods of testing and conditions of retrieval, instructional strategies, training methods, and individual variations, a systematic review by Arthur indicated that factors that influence retention the most are the quality of initial training and the amount of overtraining (i.e., amount of training after proficiency has been initially achieved) (Arthur 1998 Hum Perf). Fortunately, simulators not only enable robust initial training using effective training paradigms (i.e., proficiency-based training and overlearning) but also make maintenance of skills through retraining possible. Such retraining has been shown to minimize skill degradation and can help to ensure skill retention over time.[65]

This use of simulation can be very helpful to address needs during changes in practice patterns and reentry of physicians into practice. Simulation can be employed when physicians change the focus of their practices or reenter clinical practice after a period of absence. It can provide objective assessment of the physician's skill and to enable training in skills found to be deficient.[66]

Simulation can also be used for leadership training and other nontechnical skills as previously mentioned within a team context. The simulated environment has been used for both diagnosing leadership problems in a team and correcting them through scenario-based training. Studies employing simulation have shown improvements in resident leadership during trauma care and cardiopulmonary resuscitations and in senior medical students' leadership during codes.[67–69] In a randomized controlled trial from the university of Göttingen in Germany using a simulated environment, team leader crisis resource management training in addition to advanced life support training led to improved adherence to resuscitation guidelines, shorter no-flow times, and improved planning, task assignment, and order verbalization compared with teams that only received advanced life support training.[70] Thus, initial evidence suggests that leadership training can be effectively accomplished using simulation and should be used within the domain of CME/CPD.

Another application of simulation has been to address disclosure of errors. Given that medical errors are the third leading cause of mortality in the United States, error disclosure is an important skill that health care professionals need to master. A scoping review of curricula targeting error disclosure by physician trainees identified 21 studies, several of which incorporated simulation, that demonstrated improvements in learners' knowledge, skills, and attitudes.[71,72] Simulation scenarios on medical error disclosure typically use standardized patients as patients and family members and have been used both to diagnose error disclosure problems and to effectively teach error disclosure skills. The importance of error disclosure in medicine warrants additional better quality study of the use of simulation to inform CME/CPD practices.[73–78]

NEW FRONTIERS IN THE USE OF SIMULATION

Simulation is well suited for high-stakes assessments that can be used in processes of credentialing and privileging. It enables objective assessments of performance in controlled environments. Simulation provides a platform that can be consistently reproduced within a variety of health care settings and offers opportunities for valid and reliable summative assessments of a spectrum of skills. Incorporation of simulation into Licensure, Initial Certification, and Maintenance of Certification (MOC) processes could therefore be very useful.[79] A good example where simulation has been used for a number of years in high-stakes assessments is the Clinical Skills Assessment (CSA) exam initially implemented in the Educational Commission for Foreign Medical Graduates certification process and later adopted by the United States Medical Licensing Examination. A study that examined the effectiveness of CSA over a 6-year period found that standardized patients with proper training and a benchmarked scoring rubric could provide accurate and defensible ratings of physicians' interpersonal skills and suggested that these findings could generalize to other CSAs.[80] In Israel, high-stakes simulation-based assessments have been demonstrated to be effective in the evaluation of the personal and interpersonal qualities of medical school candidates.[81] Further, low-fidelity simulation has been used for years as an adjunct to Advanced Cardiac Life Support (ACLS) certification. As a result of studies that demonstrated poor knowledge and skill retention after traditional ACLS training, high-fidelity mannequins and full environment simulations were introduced into ACLS training and have proven effective in improving knowledge and skills retention.[82–85]

In surgery, certification in Advanced Trauma Life Support and Fundamentals of Laparoscopic Surgery that include simulation-based assessments are now required for Initial Certification by the American Board of Surgery.[86] The American Board of Anesthesiology (ABA) was the first Certifying Board to require participation in a simulation-based experience as part of their Maintenance of Certification program, Maintenance of Certification in Anesthesiology (MOCA).[87,88] Results from the first 2 years of experience with this program, including 583 physician participants, demonstrated that participants transferred knowledge and skills from the simulated experiences into real-world practice, consistently found the experience educationally valuable and clinically relevant, and reported that it led to changes in their practices.[89] Nevertheless, while early results of the use of simulation have shown promise for certification and formal credentialing in medicine, its use has been limited. The ABA MOCA program simply requires participation in the simulation-based course but does not include any assessment of participant skill. Further, the ABA has recently made the simulation-based experiences an optional MOC Part 4 activity.[90]

In general, current credentialing and privileging of physicians to practice in a particular field or to perform specific procedures is based primarily on documentation of prior formal (specialty) training in the field and/or documentation of prior experience in those procedures and documentation of participation in specific continuing education and training programs. The main surrogates of competency used frequently are duration of training, number of procedures performed, and number of CME/CPD credits. Unfortunately, this information, while easy to collect and document, is not objective in assessing competence.[91] Further, while today licensure and certification require minimal and infrequent formal reevaluations of most providers, in the future, demonstration of provider commitment to lifelong learning and sustained competence through participation in simulations may occur.[92]

In the opinion of the authors of this chapter, multimodality assessment of physician performance that takes into account physician's patient outcomes should be the hallmark of credentialing and privileging. Physicians' cognitive, technical, and non-technical skills should all be assessed using a variety of validated methods, including simulation. Simulation can provide objective, reliable, and reproducible assessments of physician performance and can be used for retraining and remediation of skills that are found deficient during such assessments. Such a process would document competence and help to identify any existing needs and deficiencies that may need to be addressed. Further, it can serve to determine whether the educational intervention positively impacts patient outcomes and whether it needs modification.

CHALLENGES AND LIMITATIONS REGARDING USE OF SIMULATION IN CME/CPD

Despite the anticipated benefits, there are several challenges that need to be overcome to incorporate simulation into teaching, learning, and assessment programs. These include simulation cost, fidelity, and physician acceptance. The application of simulation in medical training is associated with a substantial cost estimated to be approaching $1 million for the establishment of a simulation center and additional fixed costs of at least $350k annually.[93] Such costs consist of space acquisition, personnel to administer the simulations, simulation equipment acquisition, and supplies. The costs can be highly variable across institutions.

A significant variability in the cost of simulators is related to their fidelity. Fidelity is the resemblance of a simulation/simulator to the intended real-world context it is replicating.[94] While fidelity is typically referred to in the literature as a unidimensional construct ranging from low to high, Curtis and colleagues[95] have defined simulation fidelity as a multidimensional construct consisting of physical, functional, and psychological components. They argue that while there is some overlap among these three components, by understanding their differences and learning to manipulate them, educators can achieve different training outcomes.[95]

By extending beyond simulator appearance and feel, which attract practitioners and policy makers alike due to the parallels that can easily be drawn to real-world application, educators can better select the appropriate simulator that matches the training objective and skills to be addressed and offers a cost-effective training solution. Therefore, the authors advocate for the judicious use of simulation that should be grounded in contemporary education and training principles, considers the intended audience, and takes into account the available budget and simulation fidelity.[95] The cost-conscious application of simulation in CME/CPD programs is imperative given current budget constraints and insufficient data on return on investment of simulation. This has often led to reluctance of administrators to embrace the use of simulation with enthusiasm. Additional work in this area is needed to advance the use of simulation in CME/CPD.

Besides cost, motivation of learners has been highlighted as a prerequisite for simulation effectiveness. Learner motivation drives deliberate practice and optimizes skill acquisition and retention.[96] While the majority of trainees are internally motivated to improve their skills and can also be influenced by external motivators, it may be harder to motivate practicing physicians because of the multiple external pressures they face in the changing health care environment. Time constraints and costs of participation in experiential training and retraining programs remain major deterrents.[59] Further, high-stakes assessment of skills using simulation can cause additional stress and be disconcerting to practicing physicians and surgeons.

Another challenge affecting practicing physicians relates to their roles as teachers. Given all the expectations that exist for faculty today, will they have the willingness and time to engage in simulation activities to help learners improve their competency?[97] To motivate faculty, innovative approaches that account for the time they spent teaching with simulation may be necessary such as the concept of educational relative value units.[98]

For simulation to achieve its full potential, the challenges and limitations outlined above will need to be addressed. Additional evidence of effectiveness of simulation in improving outcomes in the domain of CME/CPD needs to be defined and the value proposition clearly articulated.

FUTURE DIRECTIONS IN ADVANCING SIMULATION-BASED EDUCATION AND TRAINING

The potential for simulation-based education and training in CME/CPD to enhance patient outcomes and promote patient safety is tremendous. A variety of simulations and simulators could be used effectively in innovative education and training models to address the spectrum of clinical skills, technical skills, nontechnical skills, and teamwork. Latent conditions and vulnerabilities within systems of care could also be identified and addressed through the use of simulation to promote patient safety. Specific challenges and opportunities that focus on acquisition of new skills, acquisition and maintenance of expertise, retraining and reentry, error reduction and disclosure of errors, and training in leadership could all be addressed through innovative simulation-based CME/CPD programs. The use of simulation in credentialing, privileging, and MOC needs to be explored further. For the full potential of simulation-based CME/CPD to be realized, major efforts need to be made to demonstrate the added value of the use of simulation. This should lead to widespread use of simulation in CME/CPD.

The mission of professional organizations dedicated to continuing professional development is to promote the highest quality of patient care and health of the public and demonstrate the value of CME/CPD through scholarship and research in the field. Given the major benefits of simulation-based education and training outlined in the previous sections of this chapter, professional organizations should embrace simulation to increase the effectiveness of CME/CPD programs as a strategic priority. These efforts should include multimodal competency development and assessment using simulation.[97]

The use of simulation will inform the design of specific interventions to address needs of individual health care providers and teams. Patient outcomes should be used to define needs for such training. Simulation can be employed as the sole training tool or as part of a comprehensive training strategy that will effectively address the providers' learning needs through proficiency-based, mastery learning. Ongoing monitoring of patient outcomes, training in new skills, training to address skills rarely used, and training to address skills found to be deficient could maximize the effectiveness and impact of simulation-based CME/CPD programs.

Professional organizations need to play key leadership roles in applying research findings from undergraduate medical education and graduate medical education to the domain of CME/CPD. The specific needs in CME/CPD across various specialties and disciplines should be addressed, and special emphasis placed on interprofessional education and practice. For example, the Society for Academic Continuing Medical Education (SACME) should lead major national efforts to design effective training and assessment methods in simulation-based CME/CPD, using contemporary education and training methodologies. It could also catalyze further innovation in CME/CPD and play a pivotal role in pursuing large-scale research to demonstrate the added value and return on investment of the use of simulation in CME/CPD. Culture change could also be fostered through simulation-based CME/CPD, which should help to promote excellence in patient care and increase patient safety. Further, SACME and other professional organizations should help to disseminate best practices and special experiences. Such efforts would advance the use of simulation in CME/CPD and, through these efforts, positively impact patient care on a large scale. The combined expertise in SACME and other professional organizations could be a major asset in achieving optimal outcomes.[99] Partnerships between professional organizations and other stakeholders should be of great help in this regard.

REFERENCES

1. Khan K, Pattison T, Sherwood M. Simulation in medical education. *Med Teach*. 2011;33:1–3.
2. Owen H. Early use of simulation in medical education. *Simul Healthc*. 2012;7:102–116.
3. Fischer MA, Mazor KM, Baril J, et al. Learning from mistakes. Factors that influence how students and residents learn from medical errors. *J Gen Intern Med*. 2006;21(5):419–423.
4. Davis D, O'Brien MA, Freemantle N, et al. Impact of formal continuing medical education: do conferences, workshops, rounds, and other traditional continuing education activities change physician behavior or health care outcomes? *JAMA*. 1999;282(9):867–874.
5. Sachdeva AK, Pellegrini CA, Johnson KA. Support for simulation-based surgical education through American College of Surgeons-Accredited Education Institutes. *World J Surg*. 2008;32(2):196–207.
6. Society for Simulation in Healthcare Web site. http://www.ssih.org/Accreditation. Accessed August 20, 2016.
7. Pronovost PJ, Goeschel CA, Marsteller JA, et al. Framework for patient safety research and improvement. *Circulation*. 2009;119(2):330–337.
8. Donabedian A. *An Introduction to Quality Assurance in Healthcare*. New York: Oxford University Press; 2003.
9. Rosen MA, Hunt EA, Pronovost PJ, et al. In situ simulation in continuing education for the health care professions: a systematic review. *J Contin Educ Health Prof*. 2012;32(4):243–254.
10. Steinemann S, Berg B, Skinner A, et al. In situ, multidisciplinary, simulation-based teamwork training improves early trauma care. *J Surg Educ*. 2011;68(6):472–477.
11. Hunt EA, Heine M, Hohenhaus SM, et al. Simulated pediatric trauma team management: assessment of an educational intervention. *Pediatr Emerg Care*. 2007;23(11):796–804.
12. Villemure C, Tanoubi I, Georgescu LM, et al. An integrative review of in situ simulation training: implications for critical care nurses. *Can J Crit Care Nurs*. 2016;27(1):22–31.
13. von Lubitz DKJE. Distributed simulation-based clinical training: going beyond the obvious. In: Kyle R, Murray WB, eds. *Clinical Simulation. Operations, Engineering, and Management*, Vol. 64. Cambridge, MA: Academic Press; 2010:591–622.
14. Ohta K, Kurosawa H, Shiima Y, et al. The effectiveness of remote facilitation in simulation-based pediatric resuscitation training for medical students. *Pediatr Emerg Care*. 2016. doi: 10.1097/PEC.0000000000000752.
15. Maertens H, Madani A, Landry T, et al. Systematic review of e-learning for surgical training. *Br J Surg*. 2016;103(11):1428–1437.
16. Association of American Medical Colleges Web site. *Medical Simulation in Medical Education: Results of an AAMC Survey*. September 2011. https://www.aamc.org/download/259760/data. Accessed August 20, 2016.
17. Levett-Jones T, Lapkin S. A systematic review of the effectiveness of simulation debriefing in health professional education. *Nurse Educ Today*. 2014;34(6):e58–e63.

18. Hamilton NA, Kieninger AN, Woodhouse J, et al. Video review using a reliable evaluation metric improves team function in high-fidelity simulated trauma resuscitation. *J Surg Educ.* 2012;69(3):428–433.
19. Dedy NJ, Bonrath EM, Ahmed N, et al. Structured training to improve nontechnical performance of junior surgical residents in the operating room: a randomized controlled trial. *Ann Surg.* 2016;263(1):43–49.
20. Hull L, Sevdalis N. Advances in teaching and assessing nontechnical skills. *Surg Clin North Am.* 2015;95(4):869–884.
21. Cumin D, Boyd MJ, Webster CS, et al. A systematic review of simulation for multidisciplinary team training in operating rooms. *Simul Healthc.* 2013;8(3):171–179.
22. Merién AE, van de Ven J, Mol BW, et al. Multidisciplinary team training in a simulation setting for acute obstetric emergencies: a systematic review. *Obstet Gynecol.* 2010;115(5):1021–1031.
23. Stefanidis D. Optimal acquisition and assessment of proficiency on simulators in surgery. *Surg Clin North Am.* 2010;90(3):475–489.
24. Seymour NE, Gallagher AG, Roman SA, et al. Virtual reality training improves operating room performance: results of a randomized, double-blinded study. *Ann Surg.* 2002;236(4):458–463; discussion 463–464.
25. Gallagher AG, Ritter EM, Champion H, et al. Virtual reality simulation for the operating room: proficiency-based training as a paradigm shift in surgical skills training. *Ann Surg.* 2005;241(2):364–372.
26. Madan AK, Harper JL, Taddeucci RJ, et al. Goal-directed laparoscopic training leads to better laparoscopic skill acquisition. *Surgery.* 2008;144(2):345–350.
27. McGaghie WC, Siddall VJ, Mazmanian PE, et al.; American College of Chest Physicians Health and Science Policy Committee. Lessons for continuing medical education from simulation research in undergraduate and graduate medical education: effectiveness of continuing medical education: American College of Chest Physicians Evidence-Based Educational Guidelines. *Chest.* 2009;135(3 suppl):62S–68S.
28. Ericsson KA. Deliberate practice and the acquisition and maintenance of expert performance in medicine and related domains. *Acad Med.* 2004;79(10 suppl):S70–S81.
29. Issenberg SB, McGaghie WC, Petrusa ER, et al. Features and uses of high-fidelity medical simulations that lead to effective learning: a BEME systematic review. *Med Teach.* 2005;27:10–28.
30. Duvivier RJ, van Dalen J, Muijtjens AM, et al. The role of deliberate practice in the acquisition of clinical skills. *BMC Med Educ.* 2011;11:101.
31. Cox T, Seymour N, Stefanidis D. Moving the needle: simulation's impact on patient outcomes. *Surg Clin North Am.* 2015;95(4):827–838.
32. McGaghie WC, Draycott TJ, Dunn WF, et al. Evaluating the impact of simulation on translational patient outcomes. *Simul Healthc.* 2011;6(suppl):S42–S47.
33. Barsuk JH, Cohen ER, Feinglass J, et al. Use of simulation-based education to reduce catheter-related bloodstream infections. *Arch Intern Med.* 2009;169(15):1420–1423.
34. Barsuk JH, McGaghie WC, Cohen ER, et al. Simulation-based mastery learning reduces complications during central venous catheter insertion in a medical intensive care unit. *Crit Care Med.* 2009;37(10):2697–2701.
35. Cohen ER, Feinglass J, Barsuk JH, et al. Cost savings from reduced catheter-related bloodstream infection after simulation-based education for residents in a medical intensive care unit. *Simul Healthc.* 2010;5(2):98–102.
36. Barsuk JH, Cohen ER, Potts S, et al. Dissemination of a simulation-based mastery learning intervention reduces central line-associated bloodstream infections. *BMJ Qual Saf.* 2014;23(9):749–756.
37. Khouli H, Jahnes K, Shapiro J, et al. Performance of medical residents in sterile techniques during central vein catheterization: randomized trial of efficacy of simulation-based training. *Chest.* 2011;139(1):80–87.
38. Rogers GM, Oetting TA, Lee AG, et al. Impact of a structured surgical curriculum on ophthalmic resident cataract surgery complication rates. *J Cataract Refract Surg.* 2009;35(11):1956–1960.
39. Zendejas B, Cook DA, Bingener J, et al. Simulation-based mastery learning improves patient outcomes in laparoscopic inguinal hernia repair: a randomized controlled trial. *Ann Surg.* 2011;254(3):502–509; discussion 509–511.
40. Vanderbilt AA, Grover AC, Pastis NJ, et al. Randomized controlled trials: a systematic review of laparoscopic surgery and simulation-based training. *Glob J Health Sci.* 2014;7(2):310–327.
41. Singh S, Sedlack RE, Cook DA. Effects of simulation-based training in gastrointestinal endoscopy: a systematic review and meta-analysis. *Clin Gastroenterol Hepatol.* 2014;12(10):1611–1623.e4.
42. Dilaveri CA, Szostek JH, Wang AT, et al. Simulation training for breast and pelvic physical examination: a systematic review and meta-analysis. *BJOG.* 2013;120(10):1171–1182.
43. Shin S, Park JH, Kim JH. Effectiveness of patient simulation in nursing education: meta-analysis. *Nurse Educ Today.* 2015;35(1):176–182.
44. Mileder LP, Urlesberger B, Szyld EG, et al. Simulation-based neonatal and infant resuscitation teaching: a systematic review of randomized controlled trials. *Klin Padiatr.* 2014;226(5):259–267.

45. Cheng A, Lang TR, Starr SR, et al. Technology-enhanced simulation and pediatric education: a meta-analysis. TES for pediatric education is associated with large ESs in comparison with no intervention. *Pediatrics.* 2014;133(5):e1313–e1323.
46. Mundell WC, Kennedy CC, Szostek JH, et al. Simulation technology for resuscitation training: a systematic review and meta-analysis. *Resuscitation.* 2013;84(9):1174–1183.
47. Andreatta P, Saxton E, Thompson M, et al. Simulation-based mock codes significantly correlate with improved pediatric patient cardiopulmonary arrest survival rates. *Pediatr Crit Care Med.* 2011;12(1):33–38.
48. Draycott T, Sibanda T, Owen L, et al. Does training in obstetric emergencies improve neonatal outcome? *BJOG.* 2006;113(2):177–182.
49. Draycott TJ, Crofts JF, Ash JP, et al. Improving neonatal outcome through practical shoulder dystocia training. *Obstetr Gyn.* 2008;112(1):14–20.
50. Riley W, Davis S, Miller K, et al. Didactic and simulation nontechnical skills team training to improve perinatal patient outcomes in a community hospital. *Jt Comm J Qual Patient Saf.* 2011;37(8):357–364.
51. Capella J, Smith S, Philp A, et al. Teamwork training improves the clinical care of trauma patients. *J Surg Educ.* 2010;67(6):439–443.
52. Hesselink G, Berben S, Beune T, et al. Improving the governance of patient safety in emergency care: a systematic review of interventions. *BMJ Open.* 2016;6(1):e009837.
53. Fung L, Boet S, Bould MD, et al. Impact of crisis resource management simulation-based training for interprofessional and interdisciplinary teams: a systematic review. *J Interprof Care.* 2015;29(5):433–444.
54. Peltola M, Malmivaara A, Paavola M. Introducing a knee endoprosthesis model increases risk of early revision surgery. *Clin Orthop Relat Res.* 2012;470(6):1711–1717.
55. American College of Surgeons. *Clinical Congress. 2016.* https://www.facs.org/clincon2016. Accessed August 18, 2016.
56. National Health Education and Training in Simulation (NHET-Sim) Web site. http://www.nhet-sim.edu.au/#. Accessed August 24, 2016.
57. Nestel D, Bearman M, Brooks P, et al. A national training program for simulation educators and technicians: evaluation strategy and outcomes. *BMC Med Educ.* 2016;16:25.
58. Pugh CM, Arafat FO, Kwan C, et al. Development and evaluation of a simulation-based continuing medical education course: beyond lectures and credit hours. *Am J Surg.* 2015;210(4):603–609.
59. Sachdeva AK. Acquiring skills in new procedures and technology: the challenge and the opportunity. *Arch Surg.* 2005;140(4):387–389.
60. Sachdeva AK, Russell TR. Safe introduction of new procedures and emerging technologies in surgery: education, credentialing, and privileging. *Surg Clin N Am.* 2007;87(4):853–866.
61. Stefanidis D, Fanelli RD, Price R, et al.; SAGES Guidelines Committee. SAGES guidelines for the introduction of new technology and techniques. *Surg Endosc.* 2014;28(8):2257–2271.
62. Society of American Gastrointestinal and Endoscopic Surgeons Web site. *SAGES ADOPT Program.* http://www.sages.org/sages-adopt-program/. Accessed August 20, 2016.
63. Arthur W Jr, Bennett W Jr, Stanush PL, et al. Factors that influence skill decay and retention: a quantitative review and analysis. *Hum Perform.* 1998;11(1):57–101.
64. Stefanidis D, Korndorffer JR Jr, Sierra R, et al. Skill retention following proficiency-based laparoscopic simulator training. *Surgery.* 2005;138(2):165–170.
65. Stefanidis D, Korndorffer JR Jr, Markley S, et al. Proficiency maintenance: impact of ongoing simulator training on laparoscopic skill retention. *J Am Coll Surg.* 2006;202(4):599–603.
66. DeMaria S Jr, Samuelson ST, Schwartz AD, et al. Simulation-based assessment and retraining for the anesthesiologist seeking reentry to clinical practice: a case series. *Anesthesiology.* 2013;119(1):206–217.
67. Gregg SC, Heffernan DS, Connolly MD, et al. Teaching leadership in trauma resuscitation: immediate feedback from a real-time, competency-based evaluation tool shows long-term improvement in resident performance. *J Trauma Acute Care Surg.* 2016;81(4):729–734.
68. Burden AR, Pukenas EW, Deal ER, et al. Using simulation education with deliberate practice to teach leadership and resource management skills to senior resident code leaders. *J Grad Med Educ.* 2014;6(3):463–469.
69. Reed T, Pirotte M, McHugh M, et al. Simulation-based mastery learning improves medical student performance and retention of core clinical skills. *Simul Healthc.* 2016;11(3):173–180.
70. Fernandez Castelao E, Boos M, Ringer C, et al. Effect of CRM team leader training on team performance and leadership behavior in simulated cardiac arrest scenarios: a prospective, randomized, controlled study. *BMC Med Educ.* 2015;15:116.
71. Makary MA, Daniel M. Medical error-the third leading cause of death in the US. *BMJ.* 2016;353:i2139.
72. Stroud L, Wong BM, Hollenberg E, et al. Teaching medical error disclosure to physicians-in-training: a scoping review. *Acad Med.* 2013;88(6):884–892.
73. Leone D, Lamiani G, Vegni E, et al. Error disclosure and family members' reactions: does the type of error really matter? *Patient Educ Couns.* 2015;98(4):446–452.

74. Stroud L, McIlroy J, Levinson W. Skills of internal medicine residents in disclosing medical errors: a study using standardized patients. *Acad Med.* 2009;84(12):1803–1808.

75. Brown SD, Callahan MJ, Browning DM, et al. Radiology trainees' comfort with difficult conversations and attitudes about error disclosure: effect of a communication skills workshop. *J Am Coll Radiol.* 2014;11(8):781–787.

76. Sukalich S, Elliott JO, Ruffner G. Teaching medical error disclosure to residents using patient-centered simulation training. *Acad Med.* 2014;89(1):136–143.

77. Raper SE, Resnick AS, Morris JB. Simulated disclosure of a medical error by residents: development of a course in specific communication skills. *J Surg Educ.* 2014;71(6):e116–e126.

78. Tobler K, Grant E, Marczinski C. Evaluation of the impact of a simulation-enhanced breaking bad news workshop in pediatrics. *Simul Healthc.* 2014;9(4):213–219.

79. Ross BK, Metzner J. Simulation for maintenance of certification. *Surg Clin North Am.* 2015;95(4):893–905.

80. van Zanten M, Boulet JR, McKinley D. Using standardized patients to assess the interpersonal skills of physicians: six years' experience with a high-stakes certification examination. *Health Commun.* 2007;22(3):195–205.

81. Ziv A, Rubin O, Moshinsky A, et al. MOR: a simulation-based assessment centre for evaluating the personal and interpersonal qualities of medical school candidates. *Med Educ.* 2008;42(10):991–998.

82. Wollard M, Whitfeild R, Smith A, et al. Skill acquisition and retention in automated external defibrillator (AED) use and CPR by lay responders: a prospective study. *Resuscitation.* 2004;60:17–28.

83. O'Steen DS, Kee CC, Minick MP. The retention of advanced cardiac life support knowledge among registered nurses. *J Nurs Staff Dev.* 1996;12:66–72.

84. Wayne DB, Butter J, Siddall VJ, et al. Simulation-based training of internal medicine residents in advanced cardiac life support protocols: a randomized trial. *Teach Learn Med.* 2005;17(3):210–216.

85. Wayne DB, Siddall VJ, Butter J, et al. A longitudinal study of internal medicine residents' retention of advanced cardiac life support skills. *Acad Med.* 2006;81(10 suppl):S9–S12.

86. Buyske J. The role of simulation in certification. *Surg Clin North Am.* 2010;90:619–621.

87. American Board of Anesthesiology. *Maintenance of Certification in Anesthesiology (MOCA).* http://www.theaba.org/Home/anesthesiology_maintenance. Accessed August 10, 2016.

88. Gallagher CJ, Tan JM. The current status of simulation in the maintenance of certification in anesthesia. *Int Anesthesiol Clin.* 2010;48:83–99.

89. McIvor W, Burden A, Weinger MB, et al. Simulation for maintenance of certification in anesthesiology: the first two years. *J Contin Educ Health Prof.* 2012;32(4):236–242.

90. American Board of Anesthesiology. *ABA MOCA 2.0 Pilot to Launch Jan. 1, 2016.* http://www.theaba.org/ABOUT/News-Announcements/ABA-MOCA-2-0-Pilot-to-Launch-Jan-1,-2016. Accessed August 19, 2016.

91. Ahmed K, Wang TT, Ashrafian H, et al. The effectiveness of continuing medical education for specialist recertification. *Can Urol Assoc J.* 2013;7(7–8):266–272.

92. Levine AI, Schwartz AD, Bryson EO, et al. Role of simulation in US physician licensure and certification. *Mt Sinai J Med.* 2012;79:140–153.

93. McIntosh C, Macario A, Flanagan B, et al. Simulation: what does it really cost? *Simul Healthc.* 2006;1(2):109.

94. Hays RT, Singer MJ. Simulation fidelity in training system design. In: Hays RT, Singer MJ, eds. *Bridging the Gap between Reality and Training.* New York: Springer-Verlag; 1989.

95. Curtis MT, DiazGranados D, Feldman M. Judicious use of simulation technology in continuing medical education. *J Contin Educ Health Prof.* 2012;32(4):255–260.

96. Ste-Marie DM, Vertes KA, Law B, et al. Learner-controlled self-observation is advantageous for motor skill acquisition. *Front Psychol.* 2013;17(3):556.

97. Moore DE Jr. CME Congress 2012: improving today's CME and looking toward the future of CEHP. *J Contin Educ Health Prof.* 2013;33(1):4–10.

98. Stites S, Vansaghi L, Pingleton S, et al. Aligning compensation with education: design and implementation of the Educational Value Unit (EVU) system in an academic internal medicine department. *Acad Med.* 2005;80(12):1100–1106.

99. Society for Academic Continuing Medical Education Web site. http://www.sacme.org/About. Accessed August 20, 2016.

Chapter 4

DESIGNING *and* DELIVERING EFFECTIVE CONTINUING EDUCATION ACTIVITIES

Ginny Jacobs-Halsey and David A. Davis

Case

You are the recently named chair of your specialty society's largest annual program a significant honor. In the time spent thinking about the program (as a participant, as a member of the planning committee, and as an observer), you have noticed a "same old, same old" phenomenon and you are anxious to make changes. While you are interested in attracting more participants, you are primarily intent on making the program more meaningful to participants and creating more impact on their patients and health systems.

Questions

How do you proceed? What are effective ways to improve these activities? How can they be improved at a time when there are so many other offerings, some of them online?

INTRODUCTION

According to the American speaker and conference organizer, Roger von Oech, "It's easy to come up with new ideas; the hard part is letting go of what worked for you two years ago, but will soon be out of date."[1] A formal, planned activity*—the hallmark of CME/CPD in most physicians', nurses', and other health professionals' minds—presents the stereotypical picture of a series of lectures and an array of professional participants more or less engaged in the learning experience. These activities incorporate a wide variety of formats, to include, conferences, courses (live and online), regularly scheduled series (e.g., grand rounds or morbidity and mortality sessions), workshops, symposia, refresher courses, and enduring mate-

---

*NOTE: The word "activity" in this chapter is used to describe a wide variety of CPD formats, including conferences, courses (live or online), regularly scheduled series, workshops, symposia, refresher courses, enduring materials (printed or online), and other educational programs.

rials (printed or online). It is also true that while didactic lectures may not work to effect practice change or health care outcomes, they do offer a relatively efficient way of developing and delivering educational content.[2] There is certainly an abundance of accredited activities: in the United States alone; the ACCME 2015 annual report indicates that nearly 2,000 providers developed 71,000 courses, attracting 2 million physician–participants and a slightly smaller number of other health professionals.[3]

While assuming the role as chair of specialty society's annual conference may be invigorating, there are barriers to change. The chair's role is time-consuming, problematic for busy clinicians. Further, introducing change and innovation requires time and energy to overcome the objections of those planners and participants who have grown accustomed to certain patterns and practices. It requires even more time and energy to sustain those changes. In contrast, it is relatively easy to repeat what has been done in the past—an approach that could be described as "resting on your laurels," a phrase whose origin is drawn from ancient Greece, where laurel wreaths were symbols of victory and status. Translated to the contemporary world of health care educational planning, this expression would imply someone is satisfied with their past success and considers further effort for improvement unnecessary. As the chair of the planning group, that would be the equivalent of repeating last year's conference with the same format, program, instructional methods, and even the same marketing/promotion messages.

REASONS TO CHANGE: EVIDENCE, ACCREDITATION, AND MANDATE

A static approach would mean ignoring several key ingredients in the evolution of continuing professional development (CPD): (1) the evidence, (2) the evolving health care landscape, (3) a heightened emphasis on team performance, (4) new insights regarding the science of learning, (5) modifications in the accreditation system, and (6) a need for the integration of CME/CPD into health care reform. Published studies call for more effective, innovative methods and design in formal, planned activities.[4] It is clear that teaching methods need to be pushed beyond the traditional didactic and to find ways to engage clinician–learners. Contemporary learners demand new approaches that leverage available tools, teams, and technology. Further, data are required in order to track and assess the impact of the variety of educational activities. At least in the context of North America, reporting activities to accreditation systems requires a focus on changes in competence, performance, or patient outcomes. While such an accreditation process is not universal, its principles are widely understood and can apply more broadly to CME/CPD planning on a global basis. Perhaps most importantly, a compelling argument exists in the Macy Report for the closer alignment and integration of CME/CPD with health care, the health system, and a patient's needs.[5] CPD outside of that framework appears isolated and less effective.

Despite these forces for change, planning groups often still rely on traditional teaching and evaluation methods. Learners are still viewed as passive (and sometimes anonymous) attendees, interested in earning the credits required of them to maintain their license as a practicing health care provider. Further, physicians (and others) are self-directed and participate in selected educational opportunities that appeal to them, possibly not involving innovative methods that are the most effective in changing physician behavior.[6] Even if the last specialty society conference (or annual medical school refresher day, or medical society course) was considered "a success" by earlier standards, undertaking a continuous review and improvement cycle is of benefit. Given that the field of health care is in a state of continual change, aligning educational initiatives with a health care improvement model is a useful and compatible way to approach CME/CPD realignment.

The field of CPD itself has undergone significant changes over the past several years. It continues to evolve in response to the demands for educational initiatives strategically aligned with the shifts in the health care system. Appendix A provides a brief historical perspective on each element of educational activity planning while outlining current trends and future directions.

THE DEMING APPROACH: PLAN, DO, STUDY, ACT

Only by raising expectations to meaningfully engage learners in their assessment and learning will much attention be paid to the process of change. One such approach, using the processes outlined by W. Edwards Deming, offers a way to overcome these barriers and to develop effective, patient care–focused CPD activities. This chapter attempts to harness the enthusiasm for introducing necessary changes in the educational planning process by providing a road map that applies the Plan–Do–Study–Act (PDSA) cycle, a useful, structured framework derived from the field of quality improvement (QI).[7]

The PDSA cycle is a systematic series of steps that enables the continual improvement of a product or process. Also known as the Deming Wheel, it was originally used to help instill a continuous QI culture in manufacturing settings in Japan. Figure 4.1 displays the components of the PDSA cycle as they relate to the educational planning process. Each phase of the PDSA cycle offers questions designed to address each of the underlying elements. Examples of key questions for each phase are also shown in more detail in Table 4.1.

The "Plan" phase is intended to design an effective educational activity. In the *Do* phase, the CPD planner delivers the educational content in a manner that engages learners and that intends a positive impact on their knowledge, skills, and behaviors, thus meeting established educational goals. The *Study* phase involves measuring the effectiveness of the educational activity, relying on earlier planning to have established appropriate goals and objectives by which to assess impact. Finally, the *Act* phase promotes a reflective state in which CPD planners and other stakeholders review and analyze outcomes and incorporate lessons into an ongoing, iterative improvement process. This phase is best accomplished by applying QI principles to the overall educational program planning and/or curriculum development process.

"PLAN" PHASE

The initial or *Plan* phase in designing effective educational activities addresses two key aspects of change. The first focuses on leading the change process, useful when considering the case of the annual conference planner. The second focuses on the educational planning process itself.

CME/CPD Planning Process

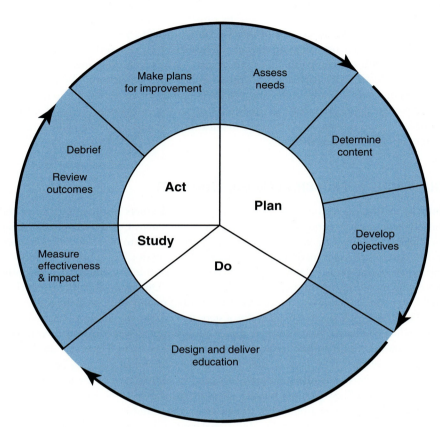

FIGURE 4.1.   CME/CPD educational planning process (PDSA).

Leading Change: Brief Lessons from the Literature

While the topic of managing and leading change is addressed in Chapters 22 and 23, a few critical steps address the challenge of converting standard educational activities into those considered more effective, engaging, and integrated with the needs and settings of health care delivery. These steps include the need to identify a champion, assemble a team, and frame the problem with a sense of urgency.

While many take on a singular role as a champion for change, the task of change can be made easier by viewing it as a team activity. This is an iterative process requiring ongoing commitment, stakeholder involvement, and support. Here, the process benefits from an effective coach to articulate a clear vision, strategically align staff and resources, and judge progress toward the ultimate goal of the CPD activity. Effective planners usually recruit and engage a devoted, diverse team of colleagues and stakeholders to share

	Key Question(s)	**Element(s)**
	TABLE 4.1	
	Plan–Do–Study–Act Cycle Applied to the Educational Planning Process	
Plan	Who is responsible for identifying gaps in care or outcomes that fall short of our goals?	Assess Needs
	Who is responsible for translating those issues into educational needs?	Ensure Alignment (determine appropriate topics and objectives)
	What are we doing to ensure the patient's voice is incorporated into our planning process?	
	What educational objectives are we trying to accomplish?	
	How can we align educational efforts to ensure learners are held accountable for applying the learning to improve their practice?	
Do	What are the underlying educational topics?	Develop Content
	What competencies are core to the issues that have been identified?	Determine Competencies
		Select Format
	What is the best instructional approach to deliver this content?	Identify Strategies for Learner Engagement
	How do we engage learners?	Focus on Special Needs of Target Audience
	What can be done to frame educational content in a way that promotes reflection and performance improvement?	Assess and Address
	Who do we target for our educational activities?	Learner Motivation
	What is the draw for our learners?	Develop Faculty Skills
	What expectations do we have of our faculty?	Select Delivery Methods
	What are we doing to ensure preceptors are well equipped to identify and address learner's needs?	• Level of Interactivity • Use of Technology
	How do we ensure faculty are skilled coaches and able to provide constructive feedback?	• Sequencing • Materials (Type and Timing)
	How do we equip our faculty to effectively introduce innovative approaches to instructional design and delivery?	• Physical Space
Study	Did we accomplish our program goals?	Measure Effectiveness and Impact
	Did we achieve our educational objectives?	
	How do we know if we achieved the desired change(s)?	
	Was the effort part of a larger initiative?	
Act	What can we do to measure and help sustain the desired change(s)?	Review Outcomes
		Debrief
	How can we incorporate what we have learned for future improvements?	Make Plans for Improvement
	What can we do to ensure our faculty are well equipped to meet the evolving needs of today's learners?	

their vision for change and leverage their unique skill sets and perspectives. Patients may be useful (and intelligent) contributors to the process.

Kotter outlined eight steps for change, the first of which is to create a sense of urgency and the subsequent communication of a vision for change.[8] The latter requires the articulation of the issue in real (and often personal) terms, clarifying its importance and framing it in a manner that makes the "call to action" clear, and thus more likely to spur action.

In turn, this requires framing the issues in ways that help colleagues and team members understand the larger picture and where this issue (in this case, reshaping an activity to be more effective) fits within it. In the case presented at the beginning of this chapter, one might frame a new model for the annual meeting in terms of addressing known and widely broadcast gaps in care and the urgent role of the specialty in addressing them.

Envisioning the end result or outcome of an educational activity—and determining the metrics by which its achievement can be measured—may be the most important step in the process. It certainly is the first. This is done with the intention of clearly defining and driving toward outcomes (i.e., ultimate changes in behavior).

A useful way to think about the outcome of an educational activity in CPD is to align educational effort with the patient-centered Quadruple Aim.[9] As shown by the rubric and table in Figure 4.2, the Quadruple Aim is an extension of the so-called Triple Aim, a framework developed by the U.S. Institute for Healthcare Improvement (IHI). The Triple Aim calls for health care systems to improve population health, enhance the patient experience, and reduce the cost of care. The subsequently added fourth aim addresses the need to be mindful of the health care provider's well-being as a critical part of the delivery system. This four-pronged approach is designed to help keep patient-centered care as the focus of each encounter. While designed for use in the United States, the model and its message have global relevance and are reflected in similar international health care reports.

Accomplishing the first three goals calls attention to the need to partner with institutional QI initiatives in order to maximize workflow and performance in practice.[10] Additionally, CPD activities provide support for continuous improvement and learning as clinicians address gaps in their professional practice. In most developed nations, this process is required of physicians (and other health care professionals) for renewal of license, maintenance of specialty board certification, credentialing, membership in professional societies, and other professional privileges.[11] Given the nature of education as a means to develop, reflect, and learn, the fourth goal or aim is a distinct call to CPD providers. Health care is a demanding field with high stakes. It is especially critical for health care professionals to take the time needed to update their knowledge and experience, renewing their energy through meaningful continuous professional development.

Contemporary Educational Planning Methods

Several contemporary elements are important to education planning. These include triangulating educational need with clinical performance gaps, broadening the participant base, and establishing clear goals and specific learning objectives,

Triangulating Educational Needs with Clinical Performance Gaps

Relative to the process of course planning itself, much is written on the subject of needs assessment. Most CME/CPD providers are familiar with needs assessments, or "gaps in professional practice," terms that essentially reflect the question, *What is the difference between the actual (what is) and ideal (what should be) performance of health care professionals and/or patient outcomes?* A critical element in initial planning is a needs

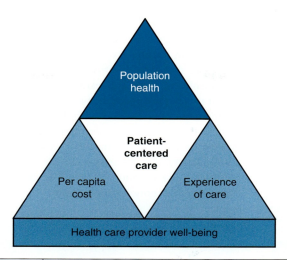

Improvements in:	Measured by: (partial list of examples)
Population health	• Decreasing trend in modifiable risk factors for chronic conditions (tobacco use, obesity, physical inactivity, unhealthy eating, and alcohol consumption). • Increasing uptake of strategies to prevent illness/disease (health screening, vaccinations, infection prevention). • Decreasing number of heart attacks and strokes.
Experience of care	• Fewer people hospitalized for conditions that could be treated elsewhere. • Increased use of telemedicine for appropriate clinical patient consultation. • Fewer return visits to the emergency department for a mental health or substance abuse condition. • Improvements in patient satisfaction scores related to communication and shared decision-making.
Per capita cost	• Efficient level of laboratory test and prescription orders. • Decreased number of emergency room visits and/or hospitalizations for individuals with diabetes, COPD, or heart disease.
Health care provider well-being	• Reduction in health care provider depression and burn-out. • Improvements in satisfaction and overall quality of healthy work life (individuals experiencing joy and meaning in their work). • Increase in the number of impactful professional development activities and/or meaningful opportunities for individual and team reflection. • Improvements in team effectiveness and/or coordination of care.

FIGURE 4.2. Ultimate goal to align education efforts with the Quadruple Aim.

assessment to enable course directors to align their efforts with specific measurable outcomes. Planners can use several strategies to increase the motivation or readiness of health care professionals to engage in learning by assisting them in reflecting on their current performance and patient outcomes.[12] Effective needs assessment strategies include multimethod feedback from educators and learners.[13] At best, they amalgamate subjective needs (what a health professional *thinks* he or she needs) with objective data (*actual* information based on patient or population health data) and (often) with a third perspective such as patient input or health system information. Some term this activity "triangulating needs," described by Kuper and Lingard to reflect multiple sources of information.[14] There are a wide variety of needs assessment data available to help identify targeted educational needs requiring attention. Table 4.2 describes examples of data resources to assess needs across three categories: people, reports (to include studies and guidelines), and new developments.

TABLE 4.2
Needs Assessment Data Sources

Data Sources	Examples
People	• Activity directors/planning committee members
	• Departmental faculty and/or staff
	• Experts (thought leaders) in the field
	• Hospital/clinic administrators
	• Leaders of relevant medical societies
	• Past participant evaluations
	• Patients (satisfaction surveys, advocacy groups)
	• Potential participants and their health care team members (formal/informal requests or surveys)
	• Researchers
Reports/Studies/Guidelines International, national, regional, and/or local levels	• Accreditation reports (Association of Canadian Medical Colleges and Accreditation Council for Continuing Medical Education audits and site visit reports)
	• Clinical Learning Environment Review (CLER) visit feedback
	• Debriefing notes from previous related educational activities
	• Electronic health record data/incident reports
	• Epidemiological/public health data
	• Government sources/consensus reports (outlining health care practice gaps and educational needs)
	• Institutional performance metrics, quality improvement reports
	• International health care quality organizations
	• World Health Organization (WHO) http://www.who.int/en/
	• African Regional Organization (AFRO)
	• Pan American Health Organization (PAHO)
	• United Nations Foundation
	• Mortality/morbidity data (e.g., AHRQ Patient Safety Network—M&M Review) www.webmm.ahrq.gov
	• National clinical guidelines
	• National/international health care quality and patient safety organizations
	• Agency for Healthcare Research and Quality (AHRQ) www.ahrq.gov
	• Center for Disease Control and Prevention www.cdc.gov
	• Department of Health and Human Services www.dhhs.gov

TABLE 4.2 **Needs Assessment Data Sources (*Continued*)**	
Data Sources	**Examples**

	• Health Finder—A service of the national health information center http://www.healthfinder.gov/
	• Healthy People 2020 www.healthypeople.gov/2020/Leading-Health-Indicators
	• Institute for Healthcare Improvement www.ihi.org/ihi
	• Institute of Medicine: Healthcare and Quality www.iom.edu
	• Institute for Clinical Systems Improvement www.icsi.org
	• Joint Commission Patient Safety goals www.jcaho.org (has information on hospital accreditation findings from recent surveys—you can search for your institution by zip code or name)
	• Leapfrog Group www.leapfroggroup.org
	• MedLine Plus http://medlineplus.gov/
	• National Center for Interprofessional Practice and Education https://nexusipe.org/informing/resource-center
	• U.S. Preventive Services Task Force www.uspreventiveservicestaskforce.org/
	• Peer-reviewed articles and systematic reviews
	  • EBSCO host links to MEDLINE, CINAHL, and Cochrane Library
	  • http://search.epnet.com
	  • http://www.cochranelibrary.com/
	• PubMed links to MEDLINE
	  • http://www.ncbi.nlm.nih.gov/entrez/query.fcgi

New Developments	• Advances in use of technology • Board examinations and/or recertification requirement insights • Evidence-based improvements in health care team performance • Health care practice trends • Legislative and regulatory updates • Organizational changes affecting patient care • Updated guidelines and/or specialty society practices

Broadening the Participant Base: What Teams Would Benefit from CPD?

Frequently, CPD planners consider a single-dimensional audience (e.g., physicians only) when planning an activity. In reality, however, much of health care is provided by teams of health professionals, a phenomenon that can be addressed by including various representatives of the health care team on a planning committee and on the agenda as presenters and/or facilitators. The composition of the planning team has a significant impact on the quality and outcome of continuing nursing education programs.[15] Such interprofessional planning may lead to activities structured to improve team functioning, in addition to new knowledge and skills adopted by individual participants.

Establishing Clear Goals and Specific Learning Objectives

The new CPD planner moves from the larger-picture "goal" of the program or activity to specific learning objectives. In some ways, learning objectives are the take-home messages, articulating the connection between the identified need and the desired result.

They address the question "What should the learner be able to accomplish in his or her practice setting after the activity?" and need to attend to all aspects of clinical competence. This range of competencies includes areas such as communication skills, professionalism (e.g., dealing with ethical dilemmas), and interprofessional collaboration skills, among others.

In the 1950s, Benjamin Bloom and colleagues published a framework for categorizing educational goals.[16] Known as Bloom's taxonomy, this framework has become a staple in educational planning, applied by generations of educators when developing effective learning objectives. The framework consisted of six major categories: knowledge, comprehension, application, analysis, synthesis, and evaluation. The categories following "knowledge" were presented as "skills and abilities," with the understanding that knowledge was the necessary precondition for putting these skills and abilities into practice.

During the 1990s, a former student of Bloom's, Lorin Anderson, led a group assigned the task of updating the taxonomy. They established a modified version of this tool (published in 2001), which draws attention away from the somewhat static notion of "educational objectives" (found in Bloom's original work) and points to a more dynamic conception of classification.[17] Table 4.3 utilizes the revised Bloom's taxonomy in writing effective learning objectives. A description is given for each cognitive-processing dimension, followed by suggested instructional strategies for use and examples of appropriate action verbs to use.

"DO" PHASE

The "Do" phase of educational planning asks the course planner to design and deliver the content in a manner that engages learners. The effort should have a positive impact on the learner's knowledge, skills, and behavior and serve to achieve established educational goals. This phase incorporates three often overlapping elements: multiple methods, interactivity, and sequencing. Evidence from the systematic reviews of randomized controlled trials points to an increased likelihood of improved clinical performance or health care outcome changes when one or more of these educational elements are used.[18]

Multiple Methods

The evidence is clear that the use of multiple methods to communicate concepts and facts increases the uptake and application of knowledge.[19] In the instance of an annual refresher program, examples might include online materials distributed before or after the course, case discussions using video or audio methods, and small group methods (outlined below). What is unclear is *why* the use of multiple approaches is effective. Success in using multiple methods relates to the variety of learning styles of health professionals, increased engagement of the learner, and reinforcement of learning.

TABLE 4.3
Writing Effective Learning Objectives Using Principles from Bloom's Taxonomy

Cognitive-Processing Dimensions (Listed from Low-level to High-level Thinking)	Description	Suggested Instructional Strategies for Use at this Level	Examples of Appropriate Action Verbs to Use as Learning Objectives (Words to Help Complete the Following Sentence)
			Upon completion of this educational activity, participants will be able to:
Remembering	Recalling information	Lecture, video or audio clips	Define List Recall Repeat Retrieve
Understanding	Explaining ideas or concepts	More interactive lectures with opportunity for Q&A, discussion, review, tests, small group presentations	Describe Discuss Explain Identify Recognize
Applying	Using information in another familiar situation	Practice, demonstrations, exercises, projects, simulations, role play	Demonstrate Experiment Interpret Perform Use
Analyzing	Breaking information into parts to explore understandings and relationships	Team problem-solving, case studies, critical incidents, discussions, test questions	Classify Compare Contrast Differentiate Distinguish
Evaluating	Justifying a decision or course of action	Case studies, projects, appraisals, constructs, critiques	Assess Choose Decide Justify Rate
Creating	Generating new ideas, products, or ways of viewing things	Creative exercises or projects, simulations, case studies	Constructing Designing Inventing Planning Producing

NOTE: A well-written learning objective gives maximum structure to the instruction and helps define a concise, explicit, measurable learner outcome. Vague or ambiguous words *should be avoided*, such as appreciate, know, learn, and understand.

Adapted by Jacobs & Davis from Pohl M. *Learning to Think, Thinking to Learn*. Cheltenham, UK: Hawker Brownlow; 2000.

In turn, Pohl's work was adapted from Bloom BS, Engelhart MD, Furst EJ, et al. *Taxonomy of Educational Objectives: The Classification of Educational Goals. Handbook 1: Cognitive Domain*. New York: David McKay; 1956.

Interactivity

Arising from the literature of adult education, *interactivity* is seen as a way to increase engagement of the learner. Interactivity may exist between (1) the presenter or faculty member and the audience (e.g., using audience response systems, other polling devices, or questions and answers), (2) the audience members (in buzz or small groups, in dyads, while engaged in case discussion), or (3) resource materials and the audience (the critique of a video of, say, a communications issue). Steinert and Snell outlines more complete descriptions of interactive techniques.[20]

Sequencing

Complex topics deserve an approach that enables learners to integrate information into their practices by *sequencing* educational elements over a period of time. For example, the same content may be better assimilated by learners as a result of two 3-hour workshops than by one 6-hour session. Learners absorb knowledge initially, reflect on (or apply) it over the intervening period, and consolidate it in follow-up sessions. If course logistics do not permit such sequencing, alternative methods exist for planners to provide access to materials for review in advance of the activity as a primer and to follow up with case and other materials at the activity itself. Such methods, including skill acquisition, can offer a longitudinal experience that fosters ongoing discussions and follow-up with peers. Similar to shampoo instructions to "lather, rinse, and repeat," it is best to anticipate the need to adopt beneficial educational reinforcement strategies as part of the learning cycle.

Reflection and Self-assessment

While evidence from randomized controlled trials in this area may be nonexistent currently, there is strong theoretical support for allowing clinicians to *reflect on and self-assess* their learning. This permits them to determine which facts or new knowledge they will apply in practice, to examine their own practice needs and care gaps and to make plans to integrate new knowledge into practice. One way to facilitate this is the commitment to change model,[21] in which the learner indicates his/her intended adoption of a clinical practice objective at the end of an educational activity. Other ways of enabling reflection and self-assessment include dedicating a section of a program to "reflection," encouraging small groups to discuss the implications of new findings or creating communities of practitioners to participate in online or live discussions after an activity.

Developing Faculty

Each of the key elements in the "Do" phase—multiple methods, interactivity, and sequencing—is important for faculty (teachers, presenters, workshop leaders) to understand and incorporate. In doing so, they will be better equipped to keep pace with the demands of a new learning environment and adapt their teaching methods to align with the expectations of today's learners. Comprehensive development programs to foster the growth of teachers, presenters, and other faculty are described in Chapters 14 and 15.

"STUDY" PHASE

Answering the question "Was this course successful?" is relatively easy. The immediate metrics available to CME planners include such items as course attendance, evaluations of speakers and presentations or workshops, and even—for those with an interest in the business side of CPD—income and expense reports. However, in the context of this book and (more importantly) in the current context of health care, this construct is insufficient. More important considerations anchor our work in improvements in health care systems and in patient outcomes, including attention to issues of quality and safety.

It is easier to study the success (or failure) of a program in this context by using a framework such as Moore's model.[22] It highlights the need to integrate strategies for assessing outcomes. This model has been modified for the purposes of this chapter. Figure 4.3 portrays the definition and scope of each outcome level, in addition to the corresponding tools and examples useful in assessing the impact of that educational activity. For example, learner exams could serve to measure changes in competence. Clinical activities could be measured as a means to assess changes in performance. Individual measures assess patient health, while public health measures assess changes at the

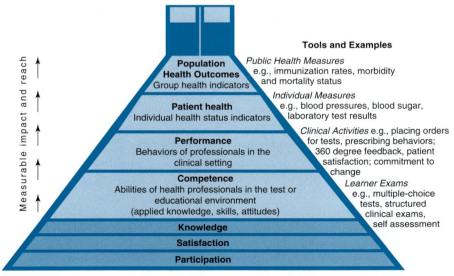

FIGURE 4.3. Studying the outcome: definition and scope, tools, and examples useful in assessing the impact of educational activities. (Original pyramid by Moore DE, Green JS, Gallis HA. Achieving the desired results and improved outcomes: integrating planning and assessment throughout learning activities. *J Contin Educ Health Prof.* 2009;29:1–15, adapted by Jacobs and Davis [July, 2016].)

population health level. Details about lower levels of change representing participation and satisfaction (the classical happiness index) have been bypassed in this discussion in order to focus on higher-level outcomes.

The question of assessing competence as a result of a single CPD intervention—in comparison with higher levels of assessment—is relatively easy to establish. "Competence" reflects the knowledge, skills, and attitudes of health professionals as assessed in the *test* environment. Declarative knowledge may be the simplest to assess, for example, using multiple choice examinations postcourse. There is evidence, as noted in the AHRQ studies,[18] that most formal courses have increased use of these written examinations. The more important question, especially in the context of health care systems, is "does health professional performance change in the workplace?"

Here the evidence is slightly less impressive. Many randomized controlled trials and their systematic reviews indicate that formal CPD activities, especially if designed in the integrated and interactive manner described in this chapter, can enhance the performance of participating health professionals. There are many ways to assess performance (e.g., utilization data, chart review, and other methods), but these may prove problematic in the context of a periodic educational activity. Given these difficulties, many CPD providers use the commitment to change model, referred to above as a means to promote reflection and to document intended changes. There is reasonable concordance between what is indicated as a planned change and an actual one. The process of care can be enhanced through guided reflection and feedback and use of elements to facilitate the change itself.[23] The question of improving clinical or patient outcomes is more difficult still, given the complexities of health care delivery. These outcome measures are outside the realm of the CPD provider and speak to the need—as does much of this book—to develop a working relationship with the health care system (see Chapters 24 to 26).

While this framework offers a continuum of outcomes from professional satisfaction to community or population-based changes, there appears to be a need for a larger framework by which to assess the overall impact of an educational activity. Several ways exist in which to frame such an examination. Of these, the Logic Model is perhaps the best known and most widely used.[24] It involves assumptions integral to developing an educational activity, the context in which it is offered, the resources deployed in its development, and outcomes (short, medium, and long term).

"ACT" PHASE

It is easy to think of evaluation or the "study" stage as a "one and done" activity. While such an approach is convenient, it is not sufficient for the process leading to a learning health system (i.e., one that feeds forward, aligns, and integrates with the health system). In the PDSA cycle, the verb "act" implies action at several levels: (1) internally, within the cycle of planning a CPD activity; (2) externally, in the context of the health care system; and (3) globally.

Improvement of internal planning is familiar territory for most CPD planners and leaders. Here, postcourse evaluations and other data are employed in a thoughtful manner leading to improvements in subsequent conferences and meetings. This step assumes greater weight when coupled with the new, broader vision of CPD and its role relative to the organization and with the ability to track outcomes as improvements in health care. This step is "external" in the sense that the CPD provider and/or the organization (specialty society, medical school, hospital) begins to realize the potential for its impact on health care and thus integration with the system. Finally, the "act" step in the Deming cycle calls us to begin to communicate findings of an improved CPD presence more globally in publications and at international/national/regional gatherings of health care education professionals, groups of CPD professionals, and specialty societies.

FUTURE DIRECTIONS

While predicting the future is clearly not evidence based, certain trends are visible and can be used to project a vision of the future of health care–integrated CPD activities. These trends relate to the learner, the content, the educational methodology, and the context and integration of CPD.

The Learner

Learners will continue to expect CPD activities to provide meaningful, relevant insights and practical skill development, which they can readily apply to their work; changes will arise in the consideration of the nature of the learner. Among the trends documented by the Harrison survey of the AAMC and SACME is one that suggests that increasing numbers of nurses and other health professionals attend "CME" activities.[25] Although these professionals may be attending as individuals, it is clear that many participate as members of interprofessional teams, carrying the possibility of enhanced communication between team members and thus better outcomes. Special new learners may also become participants in future CPD planning and development processes—among them, patients, public members, and health system leaders. These additional learners will require some creativity when seeking to maintain their engagement among an even more diverse group of participants with varying levels of experience on a given topic. Perhaps a flipped classroom approach (e.g., using precourse readings and/or video clips) will help provide the necessary orientation for productive group discussions. Further, as noted by Wenger, communities of practitioners exist, in which knowledge and skills are communicated and shared.[26] The thoughtful CPD planner of the future will heed the rise and power of such communities, enabling their growth both during and after a CPD educational activity. A further shift is occurring in process as well: learners will be the holders of, in increasing numbers, educational portfolios. These act as learning logs, collecting educational activity participation (e.g., blended learning activities, courses, and other interventions) along with performance records and other achievements. They may be used to demonstrate alignment with an organization's strategic priorities, among other functions (see Chapter 26).

The Content

The content of CPD activities in the United States, and to some extent globally, has already demonstrated a decreased reliance on commercial support: a heavily therapeutic focus has shifted to one more holistically dedicated to disease management. Further, the content of CPD will be expanded to incorporate a more robust complement of competencies such as contextual elements (systems-based practice) and team effectiveness (interprofessional collaboration and interpersonal communications). QI and patient safety–specific learning opportunities will be increasingly used to ensure relevant application of key principles to "real" work. It is anticipated there will be an even greater emphasis on measurement of impact and results of an educational activity. This will spur further refinement of performance metrics in accordance with the health care system's collective interests, further driving the content of CPD. It will also drive health system interest in efficient data collection and meaningful data review and follow-up.

The Educational Methodology

Other chapters in this book (see Chapters 3 and 9) deal with advances in educational technology and simulation. There is no doubt that the future of activity planning will see an expanded use of technology to make the learning process more integrated with social media and other technical tools. These changes have the potential of making learning more responsive to immediate needs—offering point-of-care learning, bringing the clinical and educational venues closer together, and supporting learning reinforcement strategies. These enhanced technical components, coupled with improved data management strategies and heightened interest in tracking longitudinal progress (on both an individual and system level), will increase the level of learner accountability and (hopefully) their level of engagement in the reflection and development process. It will become more difficult for a learner to be a passive, isolated attendee, since there will be increased focus on their accountability to their patients as a contributing member of a health care team.

Context and Integration: The New CPD

Finally, several major themes emerge in response to the chapter's opening case and to the questions of the future of formal, planned CPD. First, it is clear that the purely didactic course or conference have the potential to develop more complete planning processes, use a broader array of educational methods and technologies, and—in the process—achieve greater impact. Second, the QI process used as a framework in this chapter holds potential, not only for the health care system but also for the improvement of CPD activities. Finally, the future holds promise for a professional world in which the CPD process increasingly aligns with the needs of the health care system thus integrating patient care and education.

REFERENCES

1. Von Oech R. Quotation from book by Attong M and Metz T. *Change or Die: The Business Process Improvement Manual.* 2012:196. https://books.google.com/books?isbn=1466512512
2. Forsetlund L, Bjorndal A, Rashidian A, et al. Continuing education meetings and workshops: effects on professional practice and health care outcomes. *Cochrane Database Syst Rev.* 2009;(2):CD003030.
3. Accreditation Council for Continuing Medical Education (ACCME) Annual Report. 2015. www.accme.org/annualreport. Accessed July 1, 2016.
4. Marinopoulos SS, Baumann MH. Methods and definition of terms: effectiveness of continuing medical education: American College of Chest Physicians Evidence-Based Educational Guidelines. *Chest.* 2009;135:17S–28S. doi:10.1378/chest.08-2514.
5. Hager M, Russell S, Fletcher SW, eds. *Continuing Education in the Health Professions: Improving Healthcare Through Lifelong Learning, Proceedings of a Conference Sponsored by the Josiah Macy Jr Foundation; 2007 Nov 28–Dec 1; Bermuda.* New York: Josiah Macy Jr Foundation; 2008. Accessed at www.josiahmacy-foundation.org
6. Bower EA, Girard DE, Wessel K, et al. Barriers to innovation in continuing medical education. *J Contin Educ Health Prof.* 2008 Summer;28(3):148–156. doi:10.1002/chp.176.
7. Langley G, Moen R, Nolan K, et al. *The Improvement Guide,* 2nd ed. San Francisco, CA: Jossey-Bass; 2009:24.
8. Kotter JP. *Leading Change.* Boston, MA: Harvard Business School Press; 1996. ISBN 978-0-87584-747-4.
9. Bodenheimer T, Sinsky C. From triple to quadruple aim: care of the patient requires care of the provider. *Ann Fam Med.* 2014;12:573–576. doi:10.1370/afm.1713.
10. Davis NL, Davis DA, Johnson NM, et al. Aligning academic continuing medical education with QI: a model for the 21st century. *Acad Med.* 2013;88(10):1437–1441. doi:10.1097/ACM.0b013e3182a34ae7.
11. Combes JR, Arespacochaga E. *AHA Report. Continuing Medical Education as a Strategic Resource.* Chicago, IL: American Hospital Association's Physician Leadership Forum; 2014.
12. Campbell CM, Tunde Gondocz S. Identifying the needs of the individual learner. In: Davis D, Barnes B, Fox R, eds. *The Continuing Professional Development of Physicians: From Research to Practice.* Chicago, IL: AMA Press; 2003:81–96.
13. Keister D, Grames H. Multi-method needs assessment optimises learning. *Clin Teach.* 2012;9(5):295–298.
14. Kuper A, Lingard L, Levinson W. Critically appraising qualitative research. *BMJ.* 2008;337:a1035. doi:http://dx.doi.org/10.1136/bmj.a1035.
15. Lubejko BG. The planning team—who belongs? *J Contin Educ Nurs.* 2014;45(6):244–245. doi:10.3928/00220124-20140527-11.
16. Bloom BS, Engelhart MD, Furst EJ, et al. *Taxonomy of Educational Objectives: The Classification of Educational Goals. Handbook 1: Cognitive domain.* New York: David McKay; 1956.
17. Pohl M. *Learning to Think, Thinking to Learn: Models & Strategies to Develop a Classroom Culture of Thinking.* Cheltenham, Australia: Hawker Brownlow; 2000.
18. Marinopoulos SS, Dorman T, Ratanawongsa N, et al. *Effectiveness of Continuing Medical Education. Evidence Report/Technology Assessment No. 149.* Rockville, MD: Agency for Healthcare Research and Quality; 2007.
19. Davis DA, Galbraith R. Continuing medical education effect on practice performance: effectiveness of continuing medical education: American College of Chest Physicians Evidence-based Educational Guidelines. *Chest.* 2009;35(suppl 3):42S–48S.
20. Steinert Y, Snell L. Interactive lecturing: strategies for increasing participation in large group presentations. *Med Teach.* 1999;21(1):37–42.
21. White MI, Grzybowski S, Broudo M. Commitment to change instrument enhances program planning, implementation, and evaluation. *J Contin Educ Health Prof.* 2004;24:153–162.
22. Moore DE, Green JS, Gallis HA. Achieving the desired results and improved outcomes: integrating planning and assessment throughout learning activities. *J Contin Educ Health Prof.* 2009;29:1–15.
23. Sandars J. The use of reflection in medical education: AMEE Guide No. 44. *Med Teach.* 2009;31(8):685–695.
24. Serowoky ML, George N, Yarandi H. Using the Program Logic Model to evaluate ¡Cuídate!: a sexual health program for latino adolescents in a school-based health center. *Worldviews Evid Based Nurs.* 2015;12(5):297–305.
25. AAMC-SACME Harrison Survey Report. 2015. http://sacme.org/resources/Documents/SurveyResults/2015_survey_report.pdf
26. Wenger-Trayner E, Wenger-Trayner B. *Video link—What is Learning? A Model for Challenging Times. Social Learning: Planning, Implementing, Evaluating.* January 2015. http://wenger-trayner.com/introduction-to-communities-of-practice. Accessed July 7, 2016.

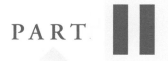

LEARNING IN THE WORKPLACE

Chapter 5

Drivers *of* Change *and* Advancing *the* Clinical Learning Environment

Barbara Barnes

Case

Administrators of a primary care practice that educates students from many different professional disciplines have advised providers that they might not be able to continue to teach in the office setting based on the need to increase clinical productivity and allocate additional staff time to administrative responsibilities. There has also been feedback from trainees and students that physicians and nurse practitioners do not consistently follow accepted guidelines for care and are sometimes disrespectful to patients and other staff members. The major college of health professions in the city considers this site to be critical to its mission, and it is very concerned that other practices may decline to teach students. You, as the continuing professional development (CPD) director of the health system, have been asked to attend a meeting, along with other key stakeholders, to discuss the ongoing viability of education in the outpatient setting.

Questions

How does the practice environment influence learning among practitioners, trainees, and students? How do clinical learning environments, learning organizations, and learning health care systems relate to one another? What has been learned from the Accreditation Council for Graduate Medical Education's Next Accreditation System requirements for clinical education? How are trends in the health care system impacting the clinical learning environment? What is the role of CPD in improving the clinical learning environment?

INTRODUCTION

The clinical environment, whether it is inpatient or outpatient, is inherently the place where patient care occurs. However, it has been less obvious that this is also the milieu in which individuals at all levels of the continuum of health care education and practice learn and implement competencies to improve care for individuals and populations. The Next Accreditation System introduced by the Accreditation Council for Graduate Medical Education (ACGME) in 2012[1] represents the most comprehensive attempt to date to examine and assess the impact of the clinical environment on learners,[2] stimulating hospitals and clinics to examine the quality, resources, and culture of the settings in which young physicians train. However, there has been much less discussion about these issues outside of graduate medical education (GME) and the degree to which the practice setting impacts continuing professional development (CPD).

All clinical sites, regardless of the presence of students and trainees, are, in reality, learning environments in which care is continuously modified by the structure, staffing complement, and culture of the individual hospital or office, as well as the nature of the micro and macro systems of care delivery in which the facilities are embedded. To achieve desired outcomes, learning should occur in highly performing sites that efficiently provide effective care.[3] Functioning in a suboptimal clinical setting minimizes opportunities to acquire knowledge and improve practice, and it may actually have a negative effect on students', trainees', and clinicians' behaviors and attitudes. For example, a young physician joining colleagues who base decisions on individual preference rather than the best available evidence may, over time, develop her own practice patterns that are not in conformance with accepted guidelines. Similarly, if a nurse manager in a hospital unit demeans his staff and other employees, resident trainees may believe that this behavior is acceptable and eventually adopt similar attitudes toward other clinicians.

As educators, we have traditionally looked at learning in the clinical setting through the discrete lenses of the individual health care professions and parts of the continuum. The concept of the clinical learning environment (CLE) reconfigures our focus to the setting of care in which we view all individuals and teams who work and learn there. From this perspective, we are better able to recognize the contribution of the organizational structure, resources, culture, and professional complement to the work and education that is occurring at the practice level. The concept of the CLE fosters the alignment of education with quality, patient safety, and redesigned models of care, preparing current and future clinicians for practice in our ever-changing health care environment. In addition, we can better understand the contributions that learners make to one another. This includes not only the exposure of students to individuals from other professions but also the learning undertaken by the preceptor in the process of teaching.

Within CPD, the concept of the CLE is critical, given that practicing health care providers spend most of their time in patient care rather than in formal learning venues. In addition, educational needs are best derived from actual competence and performance gaps, determining one's capabilities as an individual provider, participant in a team, and member of a health care organization. Traditionally, learning in practice, being temporally and spatially separate from formal activities, has occurred in reaction to issues encountered in practice ("incidental" learning[4]) or through personal reflection,[5] which is not necessarily deliberate nor congruent with what is actually desirable to improve competency and patient outcomes. In addition, this informal process is usually not shared among the various individuals who work together or with the system of care in which practitioners function.

The concept of the CLE helps us to understand how we can integrate, formalize, and enhance the learning that occurs in practice.[6] To accomplish this, we can draw on many of the principles employed in accredited CPD, such as the systematic identifica-tion of performance gaps within and among the health care team and organizations in which they work, the development of interventions to address them, and the creation of opportunities for clinicians to reflect on outcomes. Through collaboration with clinical sites and other educators to implement these initiatives, CPD professionals can signifi-cantly contribute not only to the improvement in care provided by clinicians but also to the training of students and residents. To accomplish this, it is important to understand the broader context in which the CLE operates.

THE LEARNING HEALTH CARE SYSTEM

Development of an optimal CLE is determined by the institution in which it operates, which, in turn, is driven by national policy for health care delivery. The US health care system is experiencing rapid and significant change as we struggle to simultaneously optimize cost, quality, and access in the face of ever-changing laws, regulations, finan-cial constraints, and competition. We will be successful as a society and as health care organizations only if we continuously and systematically assess the impact of our policies and strategies, understanding how they affect patient care. To accomplish this, we must create a "learning" environment that facilitates translation of policy into practice and uses the outcomes to inform future policy related to quality and safety, access to services, models of care, reimbursement strategies, and workforce needs.

Nelson et al. describe the interrelationships among the setting of front-line care delivery (a "microsystem") and the larger "mesosystems" (health care organizations) and "macrosystems" (national health care systems) in which they operate.[7] This model helps us to understand the role of the CLE within these broader contexts and underscores the importance of communication and feedback among all three of the levels (Fig. 5.1), with each one informing the others in a continuous feedback loop that fosters desired change and creates cohesion between policy and practice. Drawing on the principles of perfor-mance improvement, gaps in quality, cost, and access are identified (planning), interven-tions undertaken (doing), results assessed (studying), and improvements implemented (acting). Input to and from the clinical learning environment is a particularly critical part of this process, as we attempt to change practice and prepare future professionals to function in redesigned systems of care.

The concept of a learning health care system advanced by the Institute of Medicine (IOM)[8] codifies the strategies required to address our current inadequacies for incorporat-ing available knowledge to improve care and using information generated from care to improve the system. The IOM stresses the need to consistently inform and modify the broader health care system in order to address the complexities associated with containing costs and enhancing quality. They encourage us to teach health professionals how to access, manage, and apply evidence; facilitate participation in lifelong learning; and deliver care in an interdisciplinary manner. In turn, incentives, policy, culture, and leadership at the macro health system level foster integration of information from the scientific literature, evidence, and care delivery, as well as feedback from patients, clinicians, and communities.

Drawing on the principles put forth by the IOM, Chambers and colleagues[9] describe how the learning health care system can interface with implementation science

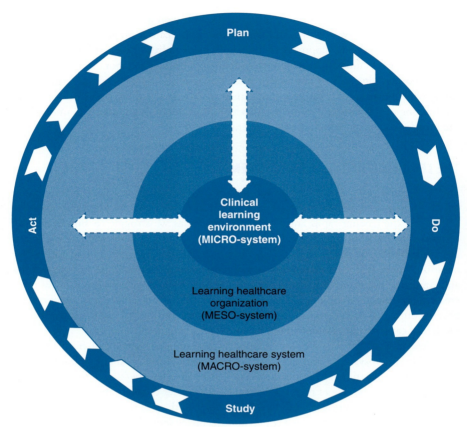

FIGURE 5.1. A model for learning and improving in health care. (Adapted from Nelson et al. © Joint Commission Resources: *Jt Comm J Qual Pt Safety*. Oakbrook Terrace, IL: Joint Commission on Accreditation of Healthcare Organizations, 2008:34(7);367–378, reprinted with permission.)

and precision medicine to generate data from practice, applying the best available evidence and appropriate tools to determine what strategies actually improved the health of individuals and populations. The use of diverse clinical settings helps to demonstrate the generalizability and practicality of applying research findings, as well as institutional and practice characteristics that correlate with better outcomes. Such a model informs the dynamic relationship among research, implementation science, and practice to provide ongoing feedback and adaptation to the rapidly changing health care environment. The CLE is the "laboratory" in which this process occurs, advancing translation into practice and educating our next generation of providers.

THE HEALTH CARE SYSTEM AS A DRIVER OF THE LEARNING ORGANIZATION

The United States and many other countries around the world are struggling to address the Institute for Healthcare Improvement's (IHI's) "Triple Aim" of simultaneously improving population health, enhancing the patient experience, and reducing costs, which is dependent on learning systems to drive and sustain change over time.[10] It has become evident that achievement of the IHI's goals will require disruptive thinking about the way we deliver and pay for health care, leading to a focus on the value rather than the volume of services delivered.[11] In some new models, reimbursement is provided as "bundled" payments encompassing the continuum of a patient's care across sites and providers, placing health care organizations and providers at mutual risk for achieving desirable outcomes at the lowest cost. To support this, organizations are creating much more cohesive relationships with providers through structures such as service lines that bring together various health professionals and administrators to develop clinical pathways, guidelines, and financial models to improve quality and decrease cost. These activities are another form of a learning environment, including constituents drawn from many practice settings and professions. There has been much less involvement of students and trainees in these initiatives, which is a missed opportunity to educate them on new delivery mechanisms and for the delivery systems to gain fresh perspectives from young professionals on how we can improve care.

For us to translate the initiatives of the learning health care system into practice, the structure and function of our hospitals and clinics must be flexible, adaptive, productive, and responsive.[12] These are all characteristics of what Senge calls the learning organization "where people continually expand their capacity to create the results they truly desire, where new and expansive patterns of thinking are nurtured, where collective aspiration is set free, and where people are continually learning to see the whole together."[13] The five components he sets forth are highly relevant to health care organizations and the CLE:

- *Personal Mastery:* Members of health care teams and organizations must be competent in their own domain in order to contribute to the quality of the institution in which they work. Models of interprofessional practice expect that everyone in the team function at the maximum scope of their scope of practice.
- *Mental Models:* People form assumptions about their roles and work environment. In the educational realm, this is relevant to the concept of the "hidden curriculum," which is reflective of the personal and collective values of the care team. Organizations must imbue core values, such as diversity and inclusion, professionalism, and safe culture to align values and promote institutional loyalty.
- *Shared Vision:* It is the responsibility of organizations to promulgate a vision and set a strategic direction. In regard to education, this relates to advancing the academic mission and training students and residents to gain agreed-upon competencies required of the future work force.
- *Team Learning:* Individuals who work together must learn together. This is the heart of the clinical learning environment and interprofessional education and practice.
- *Systems Thinking:* The capstone of the learning organization addresses systems-based learning and practice in which all individuals understand the structures and processes in which they work, have the competencies to improve care, and function within the broader environment of practice to promote quality and safety. New ACGME requirements are drawn from this perspective.

In our evolving health care environment, it is critical for organizations to continuously learn and adapt to new and unexpected events. To accomplish this, there must be a supportive milieu, concrete learning processes and practices, and leaders who advocate for and reinforce improvement.[14] Institutional culture should cultivate diverse perspectives and allow employees to feel safe to raise difficult issues and admit mistakes. Time has to be provided for reflection on personal, departmental, and organizational experiences, with the establishment of mechanisms to share information at all levels. Managers and executives must be open to new ideas and underscore the importance of systematically identifying and addressing opportunities for improvement.

Virtually all health care institutions have employed tools such as process improvement processes and information technology to improve clinical care. However, a learning health care organization also requires a culture that fosters and rewards excellence, development of effective clinician–educator relationships, and provision of adequate educational resources and facilities.[15,16] All of these elements must be coordinated along the continuum of education and across professional disciplines to produce and support a workforce that is able to improve and adapt to ever-changing societal demands for better quality, lower cost, and enhanced access to care.

THE CLINICAL LEARNING ENVIRONMENT WITHIN THE LEARNING ORGANIZATION

Traditionally, the practice–learning environment has formed and functioned in an organic manner, without sufficient explicit thought being given to the structure, processes, culture, or resources required to support clinicians, students, and trainees. Learning among the clinical team is commonly informal, with various degrees of cohesion with other clinical units and the broader organization. Education of students and trainees still has elements of the "apprenticeship" model, often with the preceptor having little knowledge of or regard for curricular objectives and desired competencies to be gained during the rotation. To be effective, learning on the part of clinicians and emerging professionals must be explicit and conscious, through the mutual determination of goals, structure, processes, and expected outcomes. Institutional leadership has to acknowledge the value of education through the dedication of both facilities and release time from clinical responsibilities. Senior clinicians and administrators of the CLE have responsibility for facilitating communication between the institution and the clinical staff, prioritizing quality and educational initiatives and developing a work environment that fosters excellence in care and learning. They must also determine the complement of students who can reasonably be trained within their setting and create effective working relationships with partnering educational institutions to understand curricular objectives and expected learning outcomes.

New models of care have driven the employment of an increasingly diverse health care professionals in both inpatient and outpatient settings. However, the degree to which these individuals work together in a complementary and synergistic manner can vary considerably. Moving from multidisciplinary to interprofessional practice requires definition of relative roles, establishment of effective communication processes, and group decisions about key clinical issues. The establishment of core competencies for collaborative practice provides a framework for educating both practitioners and students about how to maximally function as a clinical team.[17]

THE ROLE OF AN ACCREDITATION SYSTEM IN ADVANCING THE CLINICAL LEARNING ENVIRONMENT

Although the concept of the CLE seems intuitive, until recently it has not been systematically deployed or assessed. The ACGME's CLER program, which is a part of its Next Accreditation System, represents a significant expansion in the scope of accreditation review, extending beyond individual training programs to the clinical settings where residents and fellows learn and work.[18] The ACGME has defined the CLE as: "any and all such clinical settings where residents and fellows learn to care for patients." The clinical learning environment is much more than a set of places and resources. It also includes the people who work there, their values, and the sense of team and community. The CLER program is a landmark attempt to assess and improve the learning environment, placing considerable responsibility on the sponsoring health care organization to demonstrate a culture of quality and safety and to support excellence in education through interactions among the preceptor, learner, and patient. At the heart of the CLER program is the belief in the congruence and interdependency of the educational mission, care mission, and overall institutional success.

The CLER framework reinforces the importance of placing educational programs within a highly performing and reliable delivery system and that quality of education is positively correlated with the quality of care provided. GME programs are expected to develop explicit curricula, particularly in the core competencies associated with systems-based practice, and offer dedicated experiential learning opportunities. Requirements of the CLER program are organized in six key areas addressing quality and safety, supervision, care transitions, duty hours and fatigue, and professionalism (Table 5.1). Surveys are conducted on 10 days' notice and consist of interviews with executive leadership of the health care facility, quality improvement leadership, residents and fellows, and program directors, as well as "walking rounds" on inpatient and outpatient units to gain feedback from various clinical staff members.

In 2015, the ACGME concluded CLER visits to clinical facilities associated with 297 accredited institutions, with the intent of providing formative feedback and identifying common issues that need to be improved within individual institutions as well as across the accreditation system. Surveys revealed variability in the approach to and capacity for training on quality and safety and the degree to which residents are actually

TABLE 5.1
Key Elements of the ACGME CLER Requirements

- Quality and safety
- Supervision
- Care transitions
- Duty hours and fatigue
- Professionalism

engaged in these activities. It was observed that this was not only a missed opportunity for the trainees but also for the sponsoring institutions, which could greatly benefit from the input and perspectives provided by the trainees. In addition, the principles and practices of quality and safety were not well incorporated into day-to-day clinical care or into faculty development activities.

The ACGME also found structural and operational challenges associated with the degree to which GME is strategically aligned and integrated into the clinical delivery system, often functioning as a unique and discrete entity within the hospital or health system, lacking key relationships important to achieving the educational mission. This observation indicates that institutions marginalize GME from the rest of the enterprise, which minimizes opportunities for hospital leadership to inform the GME program and for trainees to learn about and contribute to adaptations for the emerging health care system in which they will practice. Even within the domain of education, GME was found to be poorly aligned with other parts of the medical education continuum and other health professional training. In addition, there was fragmentation and lack of centralized planning for important instructional resources (Table 5.2).[19]

The ACGME is in the process of conducting a second round of CLER visits, which focus on many of the issues identified in the first surveys. While the feedback from the initial reviews was intended to be largely formative in nature, it is likely that ongoing deficiencies within institutions will affect accreditation standing as the ACGME's requirements evolve and mature. Future areas of emphasis may address issues such as resident resilience and burnout, interprofessional learning and practice, and the degree to which GME programs are addressing the Institute for Healthcare Improvement's Triple Aim. The ACGME has also convened a collaborative with other major US organizations representing professional and educational constituencies, the Pathway to Clinical Excellence, to reflect on the CLER process and outcomes, with the intent to continuously refine the criteria and assessment methodology and to share best practices.[20]

The ACGME's experience with the CLER program is instructive for the continuum of medical education as well as other health professions. Although it has focused heavily on quality and safety and less so with some of the other systems-based competencies, findings demonstrate the marginalization of education and failure to recognize the importance of the systems and cultures in which people learn. The CLER program is a positive force in motivating hospitals and health care organizations to become learning organizations and to align with what will hopefully be our learning health care system.

TABLE 5.2
Relevant Findings of the ACGME's Initial CLER Visits

- Variability in training and engagement of residents in quality and safety
- Principles of quality and safety not well integrated into clinical care or faculty development
- Lack of strategic alignment between GME and the clinical delivery system
- Poor alignment of GME with the continuum of health professional education
- Fragmentation and poor central planning for institutional educational resources

OTHER APPROACHES TO ASSESSMENT OF THE CLINICAL LEARNING ENVIRONMENT

Other than the CLER program, most efforts to assess the quality of the learning environment have drawn on feedback from students about their particular clinical rotations. Some of these studies have identified the negative impact of low staff morale and lack of teamwork on the educational experience.[21] Schönrock-Adema and colleagues reviewed a number of instruments designed to assess the quality of medical education settings based on student evaluations, attempting to identify a theoretical framework on which these types of tools can be based.[22] Reviews of very diverse sites of professional education and relevant models led to the identification of the following key elements as being critical for an effective CLE: clear educational goal development as it relates to curricular objectives, content, and feedback; favorable relationships among all individuals within the learning setting; and a supportive organizational setting that includes physical comfort and allocation of clinician time for teaching.

The Victoria State Government in Australia, through its initiative to improve the quality of clinical placements, has developed the Best Practice Clinical Learning Environment (BPCLE) framework, a web-based tool that helps organizations assess their current CLE to identify opportunities for improvement, develop strategies to address these issues, and choose indicators to monitor progress over time.[23,24] Based on health services data and input from seven professional disciplines, it offers a diagnostic instrument as well as a variety of resources to assist institutions implement improvements (using plan–do–study–act methodology) and assess outcomes. Similar to the CLER program, major domains include organizational culture, quality of clinical practice, nature of the learning environment, relationships between the clinical entity and educational partners, communication processes, and adequacy of resources and facilities. Self-reported assessments are analyzed and benchmarked against other institutions, with recommendations and resources to help individual sites address areas needing improvement. The tool has been deployed in 125 organizations in Victoria with high levels of satisfaction. There is limited published information about common challenges across different institutions or the degree to which this tool has actually improved the effectiveness of the CLE. The availability of additional instruments of this nature would be very useful in helping educators and their institutions throughout the world assess and improve their health care systems and educational programs.

OPERATIONALIZING THE CLINICAL LEARNING ENVIRONMENT

As noted earlier, the CLE can be effective only if it is embedded within a highly functioning learning organization that is committed to excellence in clinical care and education. Early results of the ACGME's CLER process are informative in regard to the strengths and challenges seen in GME, particular as related to advancement of clinical quality and patient safety. It is not known how these findings relate to other professions, levels of training, or to practicing health care professionals, but it is likely that these issues permeate the rest of the learning environment. So what can organizations do to create an effective CLE? Requisite tactics build on the core principles espoused by Senge and others, including a shared vision of the learning mission, common values of professionalism and achievement of excellence, learning in teams, and systems thinking.

The majority of health care organizations do not have central structures and leaders to manage education across the continuum and disciplines, creating a lack of cohesion between the "mesosystem" of the academic medical center and the "microsystem" of the clinical learning environment. Instead, different departments are charged with CPD, GME, and clinical rotations for health professional students. There is insufficient coordination of placements in practices, without explicit consideration of how well the complement of students aligns with that of the practice's staff and patient population. As a result, opportunities for acquisition of core interprofessional competencies are significantly limited. Integration between clinical delivery systems and educational institutions is increasingly challenged as the health care enterprise is becoming more complex and, in many cases, creating structures with varying degrees of separation from the university.[25]

There is an emerging supply–demand inequality between the number of students and trainees who need clinical placements and the educational capacity of hospitals and outpatient sites. As health care resources become scarcer, there will be more pressure for clinical productivity, leaving less time for teaching. Unlike GME in the United States where federal money is provided to support the institutional resources required to teach, clinical sites have traditionally received little or no reimbursement for practice-based teaching. As clinical revenues decline as a result of payment reform, health care systems will have to justify the cost of education through metrics such as fulfillment of workforce needs and improved preparedness of graduates to function in the clinical domain. Alternately, health systems will likely explore mechanisms to share tuition revenue with universities or to receive other forms of remuneration for teaching. The shortage of clinical training sites is a looming reality given the increasing number of health professional training programs. In one study of 685 allopathic, osteopathic, nurse practitioner, and physician assistant programs, 80% of respondents experienced difficulty in obtaining clinical placements.[26] This issue is likely to worsen, as the number of health professional students increases and the duration of training resulting from specialization lengthens. Health care organizations must develop explicit strategies to define the congruence of education with workforce needs, determine the numbers and complement of students and trainees it can accept, develop processes for allocating these individuals to the most appropriate sites, and provide appropriate resources to support teaching, including professional development to improve efficiency and effectiveness in the CLE. In the ideal situation, interprofessional students and practitioners will learn together to tackle the challenges associated with balancing cost, quality, and access, addressing all professional competency areas.

To address these issues, health care systems must establish more centrally organized structures to direct and assess the CLE within the entire organization, aligning the educational mission of the CLE with that of the strategic imperatives of the institution. An innovative approach being implemented at UPMC (the University of Pittsburgh Medical Center) is a health professional education service line designed to strategically coordinate the clinical education of individuals throughout the continuum of interprofessional education and practice. This paradigm is modeled after clinical services lines that are increasingly being used to support the continuum of care, creating a more coordinated patient experience and addressing new payment models. As applied to education, the overarching structure of a service line does not subsume operational authority of the many administrative units involved with teaching and learning but rather provides strategic direction and alignment for student placement with the capabilities of particular offices and hospital units, assuring adequate enterprise-wide infrastructure and resources, and promoting innovation such as creative teaching methods.

THE ROLE OF CONTINUING PROFESSIONAL DEVELOPMENT IN THE CLINICAL LEARNING ENVIRONMENT

CPD is in a unique position to be a driver for change in the CLE, given that the field is responsible for improving the competency of clinicians who also serve as faculty for students and residents. As we reflect on the case at the beginning of the chapter, we can understand the pressures confronting education in the clinical setting, highlighting the need for practitioners to learn how to efficiently teach during their routine practice and to assure that they are modeling professional behaviors and delivering high-quality care. However, in many academic medical centers, the CPD unit is not positioned to collaborate across disciplines and the continuum based on its resources and reporting structure.

Although the CLER program requirements provide an excellent example of how institutions can integrate education with quality improvement and patient safety, these efforts are limited to one profession and to a system that is unique in terms of its funding, giving its financial and strategic importance to the sponsoring institution. In order for CPD units to assume similar influential positions with health care organizations, they must be led by individuals who possess the gravitas to reach beyond the traditional domain of continuing education (e.g., courses and series) to effect change in the setting in which most learning occurs: the CLE. In addition, these individuals need the educational credibility to be able to work effectively with their academic partners. To achieve this, CPD leaders will have to strategically collaborate with other senior educators to put forth the value proposition for education in order to garner the requisite support, infrastructure, and resources. Key initiatives will include faculty development related to interprofessional competencies; efficient teaching in the clinical setting; training on QI skills, delivery systems, and models of care; and collaboration with drivers of change such as senior leadership.

Accreditation can create a barrier or opportunity to effect these changes. Traditionally, each profession and sector of the continuum has had to comply with its own sets of standards and requirements. Formation of the single GME accreditation through collaboration between the ACGME and the American Osteopathic Association is a significant step forward in this regard. Similarly, the Joint Accreditation Program sponsored by the Accreditation Council for Continuing Medical Education (ACCME), the Accreditation Council for Pharmacy Education, and the American Nurses Credentialing Center positions CPD professionals to meet the needs of interdisciplinary teams, not only for their clinical roles but also as teachers in the practice setting. The ACCME has created incentives for CME units to become more engaged with the larger environment in which it operates, through its requirements for accreditation with commendation. Further iterations of these criteria are likely to provide even greater impetus for these departments to integrate across the continuum and with other professions.

In order to play a significant role in improving the CLE, the field of CPD must develop leaders who have broad knowledge of health professional education and who can effectively engage with diverse constituents at national and international levels, advancing scholarly activities that critically assess learning in the clinical setting as well as the science of implementing effective learning activities that are concurrent with day to day clinical practice. These individuals must possess a fundamental understanding of the forces that are shaping the macro systems of care delivery, as well as the increasing challenges that are being placed on front-line providers who must balance clinical service, their own professional development, and the education of students and residents.

FUTURE DIRECTIONS

The quality and effectiveness of the clinical learning environment will be increasingly important in the upcoming decades. In the face of health professional shortages and rising student loan debt, there is great pressure to prepare young professionals to be as competent as possible when they enter the workforce. To accomplish this, accreditation systems such as the Licensing Committee on Medical Education (LCME) and the ACGME have established criteria for competencies that should be achieved at different levels of training, as defined and measured by entrustable professional activities (what students should be able to do with minimal supervision at various stages of their education) and milestones that address all core competency areas. These initiatives are reframing clinical education from a time-based to a proficiency-based perspective, establishing clear expectations for the knowledge and skills should be gained from the CLE. Consequently, much more responsibility is being placed on clinical faculty to understand curricular objectives and to design experiences to address them, exposing students to appropriate patients and populations, addressing competency areas that go beyond medical knowledge and clinical care, and overseeing performance on core skills. This trend requires much closer interaction between educational institutions and the CLE, providing ongoing faculty development and feedback on the degree to which teaching has produced the desired changes in competency and performance. These relationships are likely to become more challenging as many universities are either divesting their delivery systems or creating parallel structures for their academic and clinical enterprises.

Concurrent with the increased demands placed on clinical educators, changes in the health care delivery system are transforming clinical practice. Economic pressures and initiatives to make services more convenient for patients are creating shifts from inpatient to outpatient sites, altering the availability of certain teaching locations. These changes also affect practicing professionals, as many individuals are tending to concentrate their time into either ambulatory or hospital-based settings, altering their ability to interact with colleagues and diverse aspects of the delivery system. Such shifts affect the nature and availability of teaching sites as well as the opportunities for practitioners to learn from colleagues. Although the ACGME's CLER program currently focuses on hospitals, the scope of these accreditation standards will have to steadily adapt over time, extending beyond the inpatient setting to locations representing the entire continuum of care. Similar forces will impact CPD, requiring that lifelong learning be incorporated into the day-to-day clinical duties of the care team, regardless of whether they are in a hospital, office, or long-term care facility. The principles of a learning organization and learning health care system create a framework to operationalize this, creating coherence with quality improvement, value-based care delivery, patient engagement, and other strategic imperatives at the local and national levels.

In order to achieve the optimal clinical learning environment, educators must develop a compelling argument to justify the resources and institutional commitment that will be required. While accreditation requirements are a useful driver to effect change, it is ultimately up to local organizations and clinicians to determine how these efforts will be supported. It is critically important that we, as the field of CPD, amass a body of evidence to demonstrate the benefit of learning within the care setting in regard to quality, cost, access, and patient satisfaction. Educational leaders must interface with thought leaders, policy makers, and other key stakeholders to understand how the CLE can be optimized to achieve these ends. The significant issues facing health care delivery will be addressed only if we can learn from what we do and incorporate that knowledge into improvements among the clinical learning environment, learning organizations, and the learning health care system.

REFERENCES

1. Nasca TJ, Philibert I, Brigham T, et al. The next GME accreditation system—rationale and benefits. *N Engl J Med.* 2012;366(11):1051–1056.
2. Thibault GE. The importance of an environment conducive to education. *J Grad Med Educ.* 2016;8(2s1):134–135.
3. Famiglio LM, Thompson MA, Kupas DF. Considering the clinical context of medical education. *Acad Med.* 2013;88(9):1202–1205.
4. Schneider FW, Kintz BL. An analysis of the incidental-intentional learning dichotomy. *J Exp Psychol.* 1967;73(1):85–90.
5. Schön D. *The Reflective Practitioner: How Professionals Think in Action.* New York: Basic Books. 1983.
6. Barnes BE. Creating the practice-learning environment: using information technology to support a new model of continuing education. *Acad Med.* 1998;73(3):278–281.
7. Nelson EC, Godfrey MM, Batalden PB, et al. Clinical microsystems. Part 1. The building blocks of health systems. *Jt Comm J Qual Improv.* 2008;34(7):367–378.
8. Smith M, Saunders R, Stuckhardt L, et al. *Best Care at Lower Cost: The Path to Continuously Learning Health Care in America.* Washington, DC: Institute of Medicine; 2013.
9. Chambers DA, Feero WG, Khoury ML. Convergence of implementation science, precision learning, and the learning health care system. *JAMA.* 2016;315(18):1941–1942.
10. Whittington JW, Nolan K, Lewis N, et al. Pursuing the triple aim: the first 7 years. *Milbank Q.* 2015;93(2):263–300.
11. Miller HD. From volume to value: better ways to pay for healthcare. *Health Aff (Millwood).* 2009;28(5):1418–1428.
12. Wickramasinghe N. Critical factors for the creation of learning healthcare organizations in human resources in health informatics and healthcare systems. In: Kabene SM, ed. *Medical Information Science Reference.* Hershey, PA: IGI Global; 2011.
13. Senge PM. *The Fifth Discipline. The Art and Practice of the Learning Organization.* New York: Doubleday/Currency; 1990.
14. Garvin DA, Edmondson AC, Gino F. Is yours a learning organization? *Harvard Bus Rev.* 2008;86(3):109–116.
15. Tess A, Vidyarth A, Yang J, et al. Bridging the gap: a framework and strategies for integrating the quality and safety mission of teaching hospitals and graduate medical education. *Acad Med.* 2015;90(9):1251–1257.
16. Melrose S, Park C, Perry B. *Factors Influencing the CLE.* 2015. https://keats.kci.ac.uk.pluginfile.php/1137317/mod_resourcece/content/1/page_05.htm
17. Interprofessional Education Collaborative Expert Panel. *Core Competencies for Interprofessional Collaborative Practice: Report of an Expert Panel.* Washington, DC: Interprofessional Collaborative; 2011.

18. The Accreditation Council for Graduate Medical Education (ACGME). *CLER Pathways to Excellence: Expectations for an Optimal Clinical Learning Environment to Achieve Safe and High Quality Patient Care.* https://www.acgme.org/Portals/0/PDFs/CLER/CLER_Brochure.pdf. Accessed June 20, 2016.
19. Bagian JP, Weiss KB. The overarching themes from the CLER national report of findings. *J Grad Med Educ.* 2016;8(2s1):21–24.
20. Wagner R, Koh NJ, Palow C, et al. The overview of the CLER program: CLER National Report of Findings 2016. *J Grad Med Educ.* 2016;8(2s1):35–54.
21. Nursing and Midwifery Board of Ireland. *Quality Clinical Learning Environment.* 2015. http://www.nmbi.ie/nmbi/media/NMBI/Publications/quality-clinical-learning-environment-professional-guidance.pdf?ext=.pdf. Accessed July 31, 2016.
22. Schönrock-Adema J, Bouwkap-Timmer T, va Hell EA, et al. Key elements in assessing the educational environment: where is the theory? *Adv Health Sci Educ Theory Pract.* 2012;17(5):727–742.
23. The BPCLE Framework. https://bpcletool.net.au/bpcle-framework/. Accessed June 6, 2016.
24. Darcy Associates. *Development of an Evaluation Framework for Well-Placed. Well-prepared: Victoria's Strategic Plan for Clinical Placements 2012–2015.* 2013. https://www2.health.vic.gov.au/getfile/?sc_itemid=%7bFC43E6A0-4C4C-44AB-A562-02D30651437F%7d&title=Final%20report%20-%20Development%20of%20an%20evaluation%20framework%20-%20Victoria%27s%20strategic%20plan%20for%20clinical%20placements%202012-15. Accessed July 31, 2016.
25. Enders T, Conroy J. *Advancing the Academic Health System for the Future: A Report from the AAMC Advisory Panel on Health Care.* Washington, DC: Association of American Medical Colleges; 2014.
26. American Association of Colleges of Nursing, American Association of Colleges of Osteopathic Medicine, Physician Assistant Education Association, Association of American Medical Colleges. *Recruiting and Maintaining US Clinical Training Sites: Joint Report of the 2013 Multi-Disciplinary Clerkship/Clinical Training Site Survey.* 2014. https://members.aamc.org/eweb/upload/13-225%20WC%20Report%202%20update.pdf

LEARNING *in the* PRACTICE SETTING: A SYNTHESIS *of* RESEARCH *and* THEORY *and* SUGGESTIONS *for* STRENGTHENING CPD

Donald E. Moore Jr, Geoffrey M. Fleming, and Bonnie M. Miller

Case

Dr. Lerner is board certified in Internal Medicine and has a busy general practice in the community. One of her patients, Mrs. Smith, has arrived today in clinic with a chief complaint of "high blood pressure." Dr. Lerner's nurse hands her the chart and says "Isn't she a bit young for hypertension?" and a quick look at the chart reveals she is a 35-year-old, otherwise healthy female who was in the office for a routine check 8 months ago. Review of the vital signs reveals her pulse is 65 beats per minute with a blood pressure (BP) of 145/90 mm Hg. The patient reports that at a recent visit to the dentist her BP was noted to be elevated and it was recommended that she see Dr. Lerner. During the visit an exam, medication review, and general review of systems do not reveal any obvious etiology for the hypertension. Although the blood pressure is elevated, Dr. Lerner recommends a return visit in 3 to 5 days for recheck prior to starting antihypertensive medications. Although this could be essential hypertension, the variety she sees daily in her older patients, Dr. Lerner reflects that it is unusual in young healthy patients and is concerned that further evaluation for the etiology is warranted. Dr. Lerner intends to reeducate herself prior to the return visit regarding hypertension and its usual and unusual causes.

Questions

What are the three general types of learning that a clinician could pursue? How does thinking about learning in practice change our conception of how learning occurs? What strategies does a clinician use to learn in the practice setting? What should be considered to support a clinician learning in practice?

INTRODUCTION

Despite the many years of training to reach certification in Internal Medicine, practitioners like Dr. Lerner will encounter opportunities for learning on a daily basis. For most practitioners, this ongoing lifelong learning generally occurs in three different ways.[1] The most recognized way is participating in formal learning activities, which could include regularly scheduled series (grand rounds, patient care conferences, tumor boards, etc.) or daylong conferences on managing a specific disease. In addition, one could also participate in informal learning, which might include reading published journal articles or synthesized data sources such as Up-To-Date or communicating with an expert colleague to answer a question about a specific patient. A third type of learning activity is incidental, which is generally defined as a by-product of some other activity, such as managing a patient in a clinical encounter or interacting with colleagues while working. Dr. Lerner and other practitioners may not always be aware that they are learning in these incidental situations.

Both the setting and context affect and influence learning in the practice setting. The settings in which informal and incidental learning take place include busy inpatient wards, emergency departments, operating rooms, ambulatory clinics, and anywhere that a clinical encounter occurs between a clinician and a patient. Each of these settings have a particular context that influences how learning occurs.[2] The context of a practice setting includes people, processes, technology, artifacts, and sociocultural influences. Practice theory has emerged in the field of organizational studies that examines the dynamic interactions that occur in practice settings.[3]

In this chapter, we will examine theories of learning and how the recognition that learning occurs in nonclassroom settings has modified generally accepted notions of learning. We will also specifically examine new knowledge that elucidates learning in those settings and tie theory to how we believe learning occurs in the practice setting. Finally we will conclude the chapter with implications for practice and suggestions for the future.

LEARNING THEORIES

In this section, we will briefly explore four learning theories to help us understand how learning likely occurs in the practice setting. *Behaviorist learning* theory sees learning as the formation of associations between stimuli and responses. The learner is essentially passive, reactively responding to stimuli from his or her environment, and focuses on the reactive behavior that results. According to this theory, a response to a stimulus is more likely to occur in the future because of the consequences of previous responding. Reinforcing consequences make the response more likely to occur. Behaviorist theories were influential in the first part of the 20th century but have largely fallen out of favor and been replaced by cognitive theories. Consequently, we will not say much more about behaviorist theories.[4–7] We will focus on two cognitive theories and constructivism. Cognitive theories stress the acquisition of knowledge and skills, the formation of mental structures, and the processing of information. A central theme is of the first cognitive theory, *information processing theory*, in the mental processing of information that includes its acquisition, organization, coding, rehearsal, storage in memory, and retrieval or nonretrieval from memory. The second cognitive theory, *social cognitive theory*, which stresses the idea that learning occurs in a social environment whereby observing others people can acquire knowledge and understanding about the usefulness, appropriateness, and consequences of behavior.[4-8] Finally, constructivism describes learning as a process of an individual constructing meaning from experience. In this theory, people create meaning as opposed to acquiring it and there is not an objective reality that learners strive to know. *Social constructivist theory* describes learning that occurs when an individual has attained a level of knowledge and skill that provides him or her with the conceptual power to deal with complex and unstructured problems.[4-7,9] For a summary of distinguishing characteristics for these learning theories, see Table 6.1. There is some overlap between and among theories of learning. Even with overlap, however, the usefulness of a learning theory to explain learning reflects the level of the learner and the nature of the content.

Cognitive Learning Theory—Information Processing

The information processing theory of learning is based on the idea that humans actively process the information they receive. Learners select and attend to features of the environment, transform and rehearse information, relate new information to previously acquired knowledge, and organize knowledge to make it meaningful.[4,10] Proponents of information processing theories focus more on the mental processes that occur between stimuli and responses.

While there are many different perspectives represented among scholars and researchers in the information processing perspective, most will agree with the general portrayal of how learning happens depicted in Figure 6.1. An individual learner will sense and pay attention to auditory and visual stimuli in his or her surroundings, select words and images and organize them into categories, and then encode categories into patterns that are stored in long-term memory. Individuals pay attention to certain words and images because they have had experience with them or similar words and images. If the incoming categorized words and images match parts of an already existing pattern, a learner will retrieve the pattern from memory and merge incoming words and images to modify the pattern. If novel input does not match parts of an existing pattern, a new pattern will form. Some words and images are deemphasized and ultimately ignored, while others become more important as associations grow. There is considerable interaction between working memory and long-term memory to construct associations among representations of new knowledge and prior knowledge. Surviving associations are encoded as patterns in long-term memory. Vital to this process and essential to the information processing theory are three components: sensory memory, working memory, and long-term memory.

Sensory memory utilizes information gathered via the senses and their receptor cell activity that is transformed and processed to form memories. These memories, usually subconscious, last for seconds and are transient unless transferred to working memory.[4] Our senses are constantly bombarded with large amounts of information, and sensory memory acts as a filter by focusing on what is important and relevant, and discarding what is unnecessary. When sensory information catches our attention, it progresses into working memory, but only if it is interpreted as relevant or familiar.

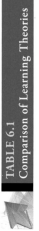

TABLE 6.1
Comparison of Learning Theories

Distinguishing Features	Behaviorist Theories	Cognitivist Theories		
		Information Processing	Social Cognition	Social Constructivist
How is learning defined?	Learning is a process of reacting to external stimuli.	Learning is a process of acquiring and storing information.	Learning is a process of acquiring information by observing others in social interactions, experiences, and/or media.	Learning is a process of an individual constructing meaning from experience.
How does learning occur?	Learning is accomplished when a proper response is demonstrated following the presentation of a specific environmental stimulus.	Learning occurs when information is stored and organized in long-term memory so it can be retrieved when necessary.	Learning occurs by doing and by observing, reading, and listening. The setting in which learning takes place is important, and the term situated cognition is used to characterize how learning emerges from the interaction of an individual and his/her surroundings.	Learning occurs when an individual creates meaning from experience and that meaning is stored in memory. People create meaning as opposed to acquiring it. They build personal interpretations of the world based on their experiences and interactions.
What factors influence learning?	The most critical factor is the association between stimulus and response and strengthening it through repetition, selective reinforcement, and consequences.	These theories focus on how mental activities of the brain process information in response to perceiving stimuli in an individual's environment.	The learner is central to social cognitive theory in that he or she can learn to set goals and self-regulate cognition to achieve them. The quality of the interaction between an individual and his/her surroundings (people, process, technology, and social–cultural influences) is extremely important.	Both learner and environmental factors are critical to the constructivist; it is the interaction between the two that creates knowledge. Situations (along with cognition) also create knowledge through activity.
What is the role of memory?	Memory is not typically addressed by behaviorists who do not study internal processes.	Information is stored in two memories: short term and long term. Learning results when information is coded in short-term memory and stored in long-term memory.	Social cognitive researchers have not investigated in depth the role of human memory. Social cognitive theory predicts that memory includes information stored as images or symbols.	Memory is always under construction as a cumulative history of interactions.
What types of learning are best explained by the theory?	Lecture	Discussion, active learning	Demonstration, hands-on experiences	Inquiry-based learning

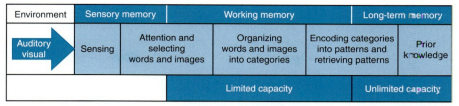

FIGURE 6.1. Learning from information processing perspective (adapted from Mayer[11] with permission from Wiley) Components of brain function are portrayed in the top row, and what those components do is displayed in the middle row. The capacities of working memory and long-term memory are shown in the third row.

Working memory consists of three components.[12] The executive controls system is responsible for selection of information and method of processing, assigning meaning, and determining relevance. Two counterparts of this system are the auditory loop, where auditory information is processed, and the visual–spatial check-pad, where visual information is processed. Sensory memories transferred into working memory will last for 15 to 20 seconds, with a capacity for 5 to 9 pieces or chunks of information. Information is maintained in working memory through maintenance such as repetition or elaborative rehearsal (organizing information as in chunking or chronological order). This processing is affected by a number of factors that become relevant in the practice setting. First, individuals have varying levels of cognitive load determined by individual characteristics and intellectual capacities, which affects maximal mental effort in a given moment. Second, information that has been repeated many times becomes automatic and thus does not require much cognitive resources (e.g., driving home from work). Third, individuals may use selective processing to focus attention on highly relevant and necessary information to the task at hand.

Long-term memory includes various types of information: declarative (what to do), procedural (how to do something), and dispositional (values and attitudes). As opposed to the previous sensory and working memory constructs, long-term memory has unlimited space but selective retrieval. Recall of information from long-term memory is affected by its organizational structure. Information stored simultaneously in different areas of the brain is interconnected as a network, and the number of connections to a single piece of information affects the ease of retrieval. Proper encoding (elaboration processes in transferring to long-term memory) and retrieval processes (scanning memory for the information and transferring into working memory so that it could be used) determine the usability of long-term memory. The degree of similarity between the way information was encoded and the way it is being accessed will shape the quality of retrieval processes.[13] That is, information processed and encoded in the practice setting will be more easily retrieved in a similar setting and may be "triggered" by familiar patterns in a case presentation.

Perceptual learning is increasingly regarded as important because it operates at the interface of the individual and his or her surroundings, and is a source of "triggers" for later recall. It is the process by which the ability of the sensory systems to recognize stimuli is improved through experience. Experienced clinicians, for example, largely use pattern recognition and other thought processes that are faster and more accurate than those of novices. Learning involves domain-specific changes in the way the brain extracts relevant information from the environment. Two functions of perception are important in perceptual learning. Discovery is finding (sensing) information relevant to categorizations. Fluency is efficiency in extracting and encoding relevant information.[14,15]

Social Cognition Theory and Situated Learning

Studies of learning in medicine have been cognitively oriented and draw predominantly on information-processing theories where the focus has been on what is going on in the brain of an individual learner. Knowledge is perceived to be a "substance" that is acquired, processed, and stored for later use. A number of theories characterized as social cognition theories arose in the 1980s as an alternative understanding of learning, focusing more on how individuals learn by observing models and model behavior as well as the setting within which observation takes place. In this perspective, referred to as situated cognition, thinking, participating, and learning are thought to be "situated" or located in the specifics of events of a clinical transaction.[8] This is considered to be the context of learning and includes locations, individuals, activities (processes), technology, artifacts, and sociocultural influences that are in continuous dynamic interaction.[16]

In the situated cognition perspective, knowing* and learning are perceived as relationships between an individual and the situations (processes, individuals, artifacts, technology, sociocultural influences) that he or she is in (Fig. 6.2). In this situation, "knowing" is the ability to interact with other people and things in a situation; learning is improving that ability—getting better at participating in a situated activity.[18] As described in the earlier section on information processing, a learner's cognition is represented as sensing, attending to, and selecting words and images; organizing words and images into categories; encoding the categories into patterns; and storing those patterns in long-term memory until they are retrieved for learning and/or performance. Out of this cognitive process emerge capacities and intentionalities,† which enable an individual to experience a situation by performing activities while interacting with factors in his or her environment. Capacities can be described in terms of the declarative, procedural, and dispositional knowledge stored in working memory and activated by suggestions and affordances‡ projected by the environment. The suggestions and affordances are projected from the dynamic interaction of the people, processes, technology, artifacts, and sociocultural influences in the environment.

What constitutes a learning experience in the situated cognition perspective? When an individual encounters an event by performing activities and interacting with the situation, he or she selectively perceives elements of the physical and sociocultural environment in which the event is occurring.[14,19] This selective perception is due to prior experience with key elements in similar events. These elements are the product of the

---

*The use of the term "knowing" signifies an activity and process which unfolds over time and led to its consideration as an activity situated in time and space and as taking place in work practices by both individuals and the larger interconnected system. We first encountered the term in Billett's 2009 article "Conceptualizing learning experiences…"

†Intentionality is being consciously aware that there is potential for action in a current situation.

‡Affordances are opportunities for potential action in a situation.

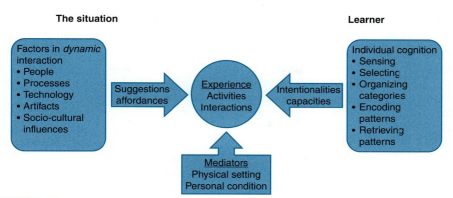

FIGURE 6.2.   Situated cognition (adapted from Billett[17] with permission) represents a learner, a situation, an experience, and mediating factors.

dynamic contextual interaction of people, processes, technology, artifacts, and the socio-cultural influences. Prior learning will shape the perception of the current event and dictate new learning. The elements that the individual perceives *projects* an opportunity for learning in the form of affordances and suggestions. He or she approaches these opportunities with intentionalities and capacities. Learning involves a negotiation between the opportunities projected by the situation and his or her perception of that projection. Institutional factors as well as physical and emotional conditions of the learner will mediate his or her ability to engage with the situation and its opportunities for learning.

Social Constructivism Perspective

Social constructivism is a more recent perspective on learning that combines elements of the information processing, social cognition, and situated cognition theories.[9] Individuals develop cognitive schemata or patterns as they make meaning of their surroundings. Schemata become increasingly complex as people learn through thinking and participating in their world. Learners construct and expand these schemata as they engage in new experiences and test what they perceive in these new experiences against what they know, adjusting or expanding their knowledge or integrating new knowledge into existing structures. A schema consisting of declarative, procedural, and dispositional knowledge encapsulated around a particular diagnosis is called an illness script.[20]

It has become increasingly recognized that the dynamic interactions that occur among an individual and the context of his or her surroundings inform what learning occurs. Learning is more and more considered to be a social process. All learning occurs in a relation to people, processes, technology, artifacts, and the sociocultural influences and is closely associated with that context.[8] The idea of learning in a social context expands the notion of learning from an individual, internal process to a collective process that occurs through participation in the authentic, real-life practices of a community.[9] The salient characteristics of learning in a social context include the agency of an individual learner (capacities and intentionalities) and the dynamic interaction of the factors in the situation (suggestions and affordances; Fig. 6.2). Learning in the social constructivism perspective includes declarative, procedural, and dispositional knowledge as well as professional identity formation.

Lave and Wenger have developed the concept of communities of practice as a way of describing learning as a social, collaborative, and interactive process.[8,21,22] As learning takes place in a community of practice, members share resources and experiences and develop relationships that form a social entity. The community of practice develops around mutual goals and interests over time, such as caring for a group of patients with a specific diagnosis. A community of practice develops methods, ideas, knowledge, and practices to solve problems in the community. In many ways, a community of practice becomes a self-organized and self-sustained entity that shares practices and models of approaching challenges among members.

Regardless if a community of practice exists, distributed cognition occurs across people, processes, technologies, and artifacts in any situation. Distributed cognition extends beyond the cognition of the individual to encompass interactions between people and resources and materials in the environment.[23] As opposed to traditional views of cognition where the unit of analysis is the thinking of an individual, the unit of analysis in distributed cognition is the entire system. In bedside rounds, for example, the units of analysis would be each individual team member, the patient, the environment, the technology, the artifacts, and the sociocultural influences, and the interactions among them. The distributed cognition perspective enables us to recognize the importance of the interactions among all the components of the situation.[8] Although an individual may be embedded in an environment of learning, he or she is no longer central.

Now that we have developed a notion of learning that combines individual mental processing equally with a collective situational experience, let us examine the situation through the lens of practice theory to see if it will help us understand learning in the practice setting in a more meaningful way.

Practice Theory

At the same time that social constructivist perspective was gaining increasing acceptance, "practice theory" was becoming increasingly important in the field of organizational studies. Social constructivist perspective focuses on cognition in learning and practice theories focus on action, yet there is a shared dialectic between social structure and human agency working back and forth in a dynamic relationship in both sets of theories. Practice theorists have attempted to resolve the apparent contradictions between structuralist approaches that explain social phenomena in terms of the relationships among things, and individual-oriented approaches that attempt to explain social phenomena in terms of the motivations and actions of individual agents. They have described three ways that learning at work involves individual agents and their work environment. First, opportunities for learning are created from the tension between individual engagement and organizational affordances.[24] Second, learning occurs through the dual reciprocal relationship between individuals and the work environment[25] Third, learning results from contingently formed patterns of understandings and interactions when actors enact the practical and situated work activities with others, often using material resources in their environment.[26]

"Practice" is a commonly used term to refer to a site of healthcare delivery, but in practice theory it references both the situation and context of a profession. Practice consists of people, activities (processes), technology, artifacts, and sociocultural influences that are in continuous dynamic interaction. A practice of medicine consists of the following:

- People: health care professionals and office staff
- Activities/processes: what they do to provide health care services to people who seek those services
- Artifacts and technology: the things they use to plan, coordinate, deliver, record and monitor the provision of those services
- The sociocultural factors that influence patterns of work and interpersonal relations

Medicine as a "practice" is characterized by four main elements.[27] First is the structure of a range of agreed-upon and hierarchically ordered ends, projects, and tasks focused on a goal. The activities of the practice of medicine are focused on accomplishing the goal of providing the best possible health care services to patients. Second, the activities are characterized by a practical understanding of knowing what to do, how to do it, when to do it, and why to do it. Third are the explicit "rules" that direct people to perform certain actions through formulations, principles, precepts, and instructions. Fourth are the implicit "rules" governing actions through a collective system of dispositions and understandings. Within each practice, there is agency, the human capacity to act, that emerges from the complex interaction of these four elements.

Practices of medicine are local professional complex adaptive systems: dynamic bounded webs of diverse agents interacting nonlinearly.[28-30] They are dynamic due to the continual presence of multiple interactions and their accompanying surprises, challenges, and responses, both within the practice and between the practice and its environment. Practices are bounded by their defining purpose of delivering the best possible health care services, but within that boundary is a web of multiple interconnections between people, processes, technology, artifacts and sociocultural influences. Practices are considered to be professional because their agents apply socially defined professional values and professionally defined expertise to the health problems presented by patients. Individuals within the system have the capability to adapt through information exchange, learning, and adjusting behaviors. No single agent can understand and/or do everything that is happening in the practice, yet each plays a vital role of interconnectivity in a complex web of interactions.

Practices are viewed as the locus of knowing, working, learning, and innovating, enacted by those participating in practice, mobilizing resources, using instruments, and employing a contingent and goal-directed rationality. Knowing is not only an activity that is situated in a practice; it is also actively distributed among humans, artifacts, and technology. Artifacts and technology anchor practices in their physical nature and serve as extensions of human memory. Knowing is not an object captured by means of mental schemes; it is a practical and collective activity, acquired not only through thought but also through the perceptual and "aesthetic" learning. In the practice of medicine, "aesthetic" learning is awareness of the immediate situation, seated in immediate practical action; including awareness of the patient and his or her circumstances as uniquely individual, and of the combined wholeness of the situation.[31,32]

Practices are not stable, homogeneous or ahistorical. Practices exist and evolve in social and historical context. A practice is emergent in the sense that the ways it exists change from one moment to the next and it is not always fully specifiable in advance. A practice emerges from the interaction of the social and historical context, people, processes, technology, and artifacts in unanticipated and unpredictable ways. As the practice evolves so does the practitioner's professional identity, which is constructed and reconstructed in an ongoing process. The emergent character of practices means that there is a close link between learning and becoming a proficient practitioner. Learning is directly implicated in practice, and learning can be represented as an outcome of participating in practice. Learning is discovered and generated together with others from a complex web of contextual, interactional, and expectational factors.

LEARNING IN PRACTICE

Earlier we mentioned that Billett has created an expanded definition of knowledge in the term *knowing*.[17] Reference to his definition will help us understand learning in the practice setting. Knowledge in this expanded definition is "knowing," "doing," and "disposition," or, declarative, procedural, and dispositional knowledge, with some combination of these required for successful work experiences. Declarative knowledge is the collection of facts, concepts, and propositions that can be expressed as a statement. Procedural knowledge is the variety of skills that people use to achieve goals through thinking and acting. Dispositional knowledge comprises attitudes, values interests, and intentions that direct and guide an individual's conscious thinking and acting, and therefore learning. Billett suggests that this expanded definition of knowledge is more comprehensive than Bloom's taxonomies and continues the modification of them as research in the learning sciences produces better understandings of how people learn.[§]

We will use this expanded definition of knowledge to describe how a clinician learns in the practice setting. Our description of learning in practice will follow the social constructive perspective of learning. Learning occurs when a clinician engages in a clinical transaction with a patient and uses what she knows and can do, and her disposition to participate in that situation, and by doing so expands what the clinician knows, can do, and is disposed to know through that participation and defines the clinician's learning potential in that situation. The clinician's potential can be described as the difference between what he or she knows at a given moment and what he or she needs to know to perform effectively in his or her practice domain, which is sometimes called a "professional practice gap."

[§]We think Billett's expanded definition is an important addition to the learning sciences' pursuit of understanding how people learn. In particular, his identification of "dispositional knowledge" appears to us to "activate" the term "attitudes" that many theorists have ignored in their thinking about workplace learning because it is a "static" term. "Having a disposition to" is much more dynamic and fits nicely in the tripartite "knowing," "doing," and "disposed to knowing and doing."

The clinical encounter is an activity that is embedded in a situation of the practice of medicine. As the clinician engages with that situation, he or she notices projected clues and cues (affordances and suggestions) that enable the clinician to understand what he or she needs to know and needs to do and what disposition he or she should exhibit towards the situation. Returning to the case that we described at the beginning of this chapter, Dr. Lerner has a great deal of experience with hypertension in her practice. But she and her nurse have recognized that Mrs. Smith does not fit the typical profile of hypertension, triggering recognition of a practice gap.

Dr. Lerner's learning experience describes what might go on in a primary care clinic, but we feel that a similar experience would occur in any clinician's practice when he or she engages in a clinical encounter.

"Knowing-in-practice" is always a combination of declarative, procedural, and dispositional knowledge: knowing, doing, and having an appropriate disposition to knowing and doing. Dr. Lerner is one of the "agents" in the practice and engages to perform an activity, such as the clinical encounter with Mrs. Smith. A relationship forms with Mrs. Smith who is also one of the agents in the practice in which the encounter takes place. Dr. Lerner is expected to have "knowing" (the integration of what to do, how to do it, and disposition) to perform her role in accomplishing the goal of the practice (provide the very best possible health care services to Mrs. Smith with a novel presentation of hypertension).

Dr. Lerner and Mrs. Smith are not the only agents in the practice. The nurse, the receptionist, and Dr. Lerner's clinician partners are also agents. There are technology and artifacts in the practice that are serving as extensions of the Dr. Lerner's "knowing," such as the electronic health record (EHR) and the variety of instruments that the nurse or clinicians may use to elicit and record data from the patient. Artifacts include the paperwork provided by the receptionist and completed by the patient as well as the furniture in the examination room.

Dr. Lerner is faced with an undifferentiated diagnostic problem (practice gap) and will begin problem solving by generating one or more diagnostic hypotheses. She will then begin searching for additional clinical information to confirm or rule out one or more of the hypotheses during the clinical encounter.[33] Dr. Lerner will use her well-established learning scripts for hypertension and begin to compare Mrs. Smith's data with these reference standards.[34] As she works through the list, she will likely begin to categorize data from working memory and compare it to items in long-term memory (see Fig. 6.1). There are two dominant theories that explain the process of categorization: the prototype theory and the exemplar theory. In the prototype theory, it is proposed that Dr. Lerner's experience with individual objects is "averaged" into a prototype of the category. A new object that appears in working memory is classified by identifying the category in memory that contains most features in common with the new object.[4] For example, Dr. Lerner may draw upon a memory of renal artery stenosis and see that Mrs. Smith fits many of the features, while simultaneously thinking about hyperthyroidism as a cause and realizing that Mrs. Smith did not describe important defining symptoms. In exemplar theory, it is proposed that Dr. Lerner is able to identify category members effortlessly and without apparent feature analysis because in the course of her experience, she has acquired a large number of examples, or exemplars, of each natural category and is able to carry out the categorization by making an unconscious similarity match with a particular prior example of the category.[34] For exemplar theory to fit here, Dr. Lerner would need to have a practice with numerous young adults with hypertension such that her experience would allow her to match more holistically to the case at hand.

These two theoretical perspectives imply different mental processes. Croskerry has called feature by feature matching against a prototype System 2 and the holistic match to a prior example as System 1.[35] Recent evidence suggests that most use a mixture of the two strategies.[36,37] Custers has referred to the mixture of two strategies as a cognitive continuum.[38] Dr. Lerner is an experienced clinician and will more than likely be reasoning at several points along the prototype–exemplar clinical reasoning continuum.

In addition to the learning that situates her in the clinical encounter, there are at least three possible learning experiences for Dr. Lerner as the result of the activities that she performs and the relationships that develop in this clinical encounter. In one example of a possible learning experience, her "knowing" is reproduced in the clinical encounter. In other words, what she knew, what she could do, and her disposition matched what the patient needed. She is reasoning automatically at the exemplar space on the cognitive continuum, and her learning is *reinforcing* her knowing. This would be the case if Dr. Lerner routinely managed the full spectrum of hypertension and had developed specific expertise in this arena. Alternatively, if Dr. Lerner incorrectly categorized Mrs. Smith as having essential hypertension and treated her as a routine older patient, she would have incorrectly reinforced her "knowing." Failure to recognize practice gaps is the initial maladaptive feature of a learner the practice setting who does not have an opportunity to receive feedback.

In a second example of learning, Dr. Lerner's "knowing" is *modified* in the clinical encounter. That is, what she knew, what she could do, and her disposition did not exactly meet what the patient needed. Dr. Lerner recognized her practice gap and reasoned in the middle portions of the cognitive continuum trying to perceive features in this situation that would match her existing knowing. She is retrieving and adjusting her existing "knowing" to match a slightly different pattern of signs and symptoms. This learning expands her options for patients in a specific disease domain if she is able to call upon infrequently used memories through categorization and feature matching to expand her conscious "knowing" in the case of Mrs. Smith.

In a third example of learning, Dr. Lerner recognizes her practice gap and knows that she will need to create new "knowing" because what she knew, what she could do, and her disposition do not match what the patient needs. With a novel patient presentation, she reasons in the prototype space of the continuum and uses resources to search for new "knowing" during the clinical encounter or decides to undertake a more substantial search at another time. Dr. Lerner, who will use the interval between Mrs. Smith's visits to expand her knowing to include features of her case. Dr. Lerner will access resources such as review articles or textbooks with a specific question that represents her practice gap and will attempt to create new illness scripts for hypertension that fit Mrs. Smith's case. She will then return to the subsequent patient visit and reenter the cycle of categorization likely using Croskerry's systems.

Dr. Lerner engages in each clinical encounter with existing knowing. Existing knowledge is her combination of declarative, procedural, and dispositional knowledge that provides her with capacities and intentionalities to engage with the patient in the clinical environment.** What she perceives is a patient embedded in the clinical encounter situation, which is projecting suggestions and affordances that create an opportunity for activity and learning. If her existing knowledge does not perceive a recognizable exemplar, she will have to recognize the gap and then review the suggestions and affordances feature by feature until there is a match between her knowing and what she is perceiving. In some situations, Dr. Lerner will be able to sense a match, and in other situations, she will have to learn new knowing.[17,34]

In a complex adaptive system like a practice of medicine, clinicians such as Dr. Lerner must navigate situations where they are at the edge of their existing "knowing." In the situations just described, Dr. Lerner had to decide whether she could work with her existing "knowing" or whether she had to learn new "knowing." Clinicians who can rely on their existing "knowing" or modify it in the clinical encounter are using "routine" expertise. Clinicians who recognize that current "knowing" is not working and search for new "knowing" are demonstrating "adaptive expertise."[39] Recent work suggests that a clinician who demonstrates the use of adaptive expertise follows a staged process to pursue new "knowing."[40] When a clinician encounters a novel presentation or receives a summary of unexpected results as part of performance review, she may experience what Schon has called "surprise."[41] Mindful practitioners attend, in a nonjudgmental way, to their own physical and mental processes during everyday professional tasks and have a receptive disposition to acknowledge practice gap. They engage in metacognition, self-monitoring, and reflecting in and on action that allows the practitioners to recognize errors, refine their technical skills, make evidence-based decisions, and clarify their values so that they can act with compassion, technical competence, presence, and insight.[42] Mindful practice is essential for a clinician to sense a performance gap through either self-assessment or acceptance of external performance feedback.[43] The recognition of a gap creates the essential component of cognitive dissonance, a feeling of mental discomfort that is the motivation to pursue new knowing.[44]

When Dr. Lerner has identified her cognitive dissonance from a practice gap, she next engages in the four steps of critical thinking to bring forth a resolution.[45,46] In the first two steps, she identifies and analyze the assumptions that supported the knowing, doing, and valuing that would not work in the specific patient encounter. After completing the first and second step, she pursues alternative perspectives. The fourth step would involve investigating an approach to pursue new "knowing."

Dr. Lerner's approach to pursuing new "knowing" about Mrs. Smith's hypertension would begin by determining what she needed to learn. Although it is well known that most physicians have difficulty self-assessing, Dr. Lerner is sufficiently mindful that she is receptive to her nurse's comment that Mrs. Smith is in an unusual demographic for hypertension.[47] Hence, even if a clinician were practicing mindfully, he or she would find it difficult to engage in critical thinking effectively without help.

**One of the significant benefits of using the term "dispositional" knowing with reference to the clinical encounter is that it allows us to demonstrate that there is a knowledge base for issues like equity and that it has a recognizable and legitimate place in a clinician's knowing.

Sargeant has suggested that informed self-assessment is an important alternative to consider.[48] Two types of assistance could be provided to help clinicians with informed self-assessment. First, performance data organized by clinical domains would highlight where gaps in a clinician's knowing, doing, and disposition existed. Second, a compendium of evidence in clinical domains relevant to a clinician's practice would enable convenient access to resources for learning. However, for Dr. Lerner performance data and a compendium of evidence from practice would likely be insufficient to recognize the specific learning need in the case of Mrs. Smith, making the internal sense of cognitive dissonance so important. Opportunity to engage with a coach would help clinicians create and stick to a plan, interpret performance data and determine learning needs, identify evidence-based resources and select opportunities for learning, try out what was learned, and incorporate what was learned into routine practice.[49,50]

FUTURE DIRECTIONS

This synthesis of theories and research from a variety of fields suggests that we are beginning to understand how clinicians learn in practice. The image that emerges is one of active clinicians "knowing" what to do, how to do it, and what disposition to display. Additionally, learning (improving their "knowing") likely has three objectives: reproducing or reinforcing "knowing," modifying existing "knowing," or creating new "knowing."

We propose that this emerging understanding be used to inform how opportunities for learning are made available to clinicians in each of the types of learning: incidental learning (learning in the practice setting); informal learning (self-directed learning); and formal learning (classroom education).

For clinician "*incidental*" learning, we propose that efforts be made to support his or her use of "routine expertise" where a clinician's "knowing" is reproduced (reinforced) or modified. There are two concerns about the quality of learning in this venue. Often incidental learning is focused on efficiency rather than a deeper understanding of one's practice or practitioner development. Second, because incidental learning may occur without feedback or reflection, the resulting changes may be maladaptive and described as "practice drift," an inappropriate shortcut or erroneous approach to practice rather than an approach based on evidence.[51] To strengthen routine expertise in incidental learning, performance feedback is essential for the clinician and can be derived from dashboards and reports in EHRs. Recognition of practice performance/gap precedes critical thinking and learning. Advanced decision support technology in practice would provide both feedback and incidental learning, such as a prompt for Dr. Lerner that Mrs. Smith's hypertension is atypical given an age and blood pressure variable in the EHR. Bringing practice feedback to the consciousness of the clinician frequently leads to a transition to informal learning.

A clinician engages in *informal learning* when his or her "knowing in practice" does not meet the needs of a patient. The effort is typically referred to as self-directed learning and encompasses the majority of a clinician's posttraining learning efforts. There are at least three barriers that prevent these efforts from being as successful as they could be.

First, as mentioned in the paragraph on incidental learning, clinicians are poor self-assessors and require feedback to recognize learning opportunities.[47] The dashboards used to support incidental learning can also be used to create dashboards to support informal learning. Even when a gap is identified, however, a second barrier that emerges is that many physicians do not know a credible source for practical evidence to address the identified performance gap.[47] Synthesized expert reviews of primary knowledge on a subject have increasingly become available in recent years. These include sources of expert data such as the Cochrane Library and Up-To-Date that make access to reliable evidence more feasible. In most practice settings, clinicians need to access the Cochrane Library and Up-To-Date on their own. Including these and similar resources within an EHR as decision support would improve access and convenience. Another approach would be to embed a coach in the practice setting. A practice coach could work with each clinician using an electronic portfolio that includes a performance dashboard and tracking of decision support use to facilitate a clinician's personal learning plan.[49,50] The third barrier is time. Many physicians find it difficult to self-direct an assessment and learning project in their busy practices.[52] The use of dashboards and personal learning plans facilitated by a coach may create an opportunity for effective learning to occur with the clinician's workflow.

There continue to be challenges in typical *formal learning activities* for clinicians, which is often accomplished by attending conferences or lectures in which topics are for the most already determined. While information about the most recent research evidence may be presented in conferences and other similar formal venues, there is little evidence that clinicians use what is presented in these settings in practice.[53,54] Two potential reasons have suggested. First, the research that is being presented does not meet the needs of practicing clinicians. Second, clinicians have not developed, nor have they been helped to develop, the critical clinical decision-making skills to discern how the research being reported could be relevant to their patients.[55,56] It may be time for high-level policy conferences between researchers and clinicians to determine what needs to be researched and how it can be formulated for relatively easy implementation in practice.[57]

At the same time, continuing education in the health professions as a field should begin to develop approaches to planning learning activities that will help clinicians develop the critical clinical decision-making skills they need. A recent synthesis of systematic reviews of CME effectiveness provides some guidelines for this effort. Cervero and Gaines found that learning activities in CME lead to greater improvement in physician performance and patient outcomes if they are more interactive, use multiple methods, involve multiple exposures over a greater period of time, and are focused on outcomes that physicians consider important.[58] An approach that has shown success is the strategy followed by Project ECHO, which was launched in 2003 at the University of New Mexico and utilizes technology to bring community and academic practitioners together for a case-based educational forum focused on specific patient problems and outcomes[59] A recent systematic review provides evidence of important impact on provider performance and patient outcomes.[60] This model focuses on real-world practice gaps for clinicians and decentralizes the source of knowledge from a single individual expert to a peer cohort of practitioners. As larger medical networks develop, such virtual learning communities will become more frequent.

In this chapter, we have examined notions of learning and how recognizing that learning occurs in settings that are not classrooms have modified these notions. We also looked at what has been learned about practice in those settings and how that has helped us understand what learning is in those settings. We then described briefly how we think learning occurs in the practice setting. And we finished by making proposals about how learning could be strengthened in each of the three venues where learning takes place.

In preparing this chapter, we have been influenced by two articles. One was by Boud and Hager, which suggested that a reconceptualization of continuing professional development was in order and that the new concept of CPD should be focused on practice.[61] Another article by Webster-Wright suggested that professional development should be reframed through understanding authentic professional learning.[62] We have attempted to come to an understanding of what authentic professional learning is through the lenses of social cognitivist and practice theory and have come to the conclusion that Billett's reconceptualization of "knowing-in-practice" is authentic professional learning.[17]

We are also concerned that many in the CME/CPD world have assumed that the reconceptualization and reframing have taken place because the term "continuing professional development" is being used more frequently now than the term "continuing medical education." Unfortunately, we have observed that the term "continuing professional development" is being used interchangeably with "continuing medical education" without much thought about the important difference between the two terms. Campbell and his colleagues have created a useful definition for CPD. It calls for physicians to engage in a process of monitoring and reflecting on professional performance, identifying opportunities to improve professional practice gaps, engaging in both formal and informal learning activities, and making changes in practice to reduce or eliminate gaps in performance.[63] While some CPD programs are moving in that direction because of their involvement in Maintenance of Certification activities, most are focused only on the formal activities in Campbell's definition without the other crucial components. Campbell's definition is knowing and learning in practice as we have described. The CME profession needs to work on reconceptualizing and reframing CME so it truly becomes CPD as Campbell and his colleagues have described.

We made three suggestions to strengthen learning. We think that when these suggestions are implemented and developed, a true health care learning system will emerge.[64] Demonstration projects and research needs to begin in each of the three areas using our suggestions or others to initiate the development of a health care system that will provide the very best possible health care services to our patients.

REFERENCES

1. Marsick VJ, Watkins KE. Informal and incidental learning. *New Dir Adult Contin Educ.* 2001;89:25–34.
2. Durning SJ, Artino AR, Pangaro LN, et al. Perspective: redefining context in the clinical encounter: implications for research and training in medical education. *Acad Med.* 2010;85(5):894–901.
3. Schatzki TR, Centina KK, von Savigny E. *The Practice Turn in Contemporary Society.* New York: Routledge; 2001.
4. Schunk DH. *Learning Theories: An Educational Perspective*, 6th ed. Boston, MA: Pearson; 2011.
5. Ertmer PA, Newby TJ. Behaviorism, cognitivism, constructivism: comparing critical features from an instructional design perspective. *Perform Improv Q.* 2013;26(2):43–71.
6. Mann KV. Theoretical perspectives in medical education: past experience and future possibilities. *Med Educ.* 2011;45(1):60–68.

7. Kaufman DM, Mann KV. Teaching and learning in medical education: how theory can inform practice. In: Swanwick T, ed. *Understanding Medical Education: Evidence, Theory, and Practice*. Malden, MA: Wiley Blackwell; 2014.
8. Torre D, Durning SJ. Social cognitive theory: thinking and learning in social settings. In: Cleland J, Durning SJ, eds. *Researching Medical Education*. Chichester, West Sussex, UK: Wiley Blackwell; 2015.
9. Mann K, MacLeod A. Constructivism: learning theories and approaches to research. In: Cleland J, Durning SJ, eds. *Researching Medical Education*. Chichester, West Sussex, UK: Wiley Blackwell; 2015.
10. Mayer RE. Learners as information processors: legacies and limitations of educational psychology's second metaphor. *J Educ Psychol*. 1996;31(3–4):151–161.
11. Mayer RE. Applying the science of learning to medical education. *Med Educ*. 2010;44:543–549.
12. Baddeley A. Is working memory still working? *Am Psychol*. 2001;56(11):851–864.
13. Bransford JD. *Human Cognition: Learning, Understanding, and Remembering*. Belmont, CA: Wadsworth Publishing Company; 1979.
14. Kellman PJ, Massey CM. Perception, cognition, and expertise. *Psychol Learn Motiv*. 2013;58:118–165.
15. Krasne S, Hillman JD, Kellman PJ, et al. Applying perceptual and adaptive learning techniques for teaching introductory histopathology. *J Pathol Inform*. 2013;4:34.
16. Durning SJ, Artino AR. Situativity theory: a perspective on how participants and the environment can interact: AMEE Guide no. 52. *Med Teach*. 2011;33(3):188–199.
17. Billett S. Conceptualizing learning experiences: contributions and mediations of the social, personal, and brute. *Mind Cult Act*. 2009;16(1):32–47.
18. Greeno JG, Moore JL, Smith DR. Transfer of situated learning. In: Detterman DK, Sternberg RJ, eds. *Transfer on Trial: Intelligence, Cognition, and Instruction*. Norwood, NJ: Ablex Publishing Company; 1993.
19. Goldstone RL. Perceptual learning. *Annu Rev Psychol*. 1998;49:585–612.
20. Schmidt HG, Rikers RMJP. How expertise develops in medicine: knowledge encapsulation and illness script formation. *Med Educ*. 2007;41:1133–1139.
21. Lave J, Wenger E. *Situated Learning: Legitimate Peripheral Participation*. Cambridge, UK: Cambridge University Press; 1990.
22. Wenger E. *Communities of Practice: Learning, Meaning, and Identity*. Cambridge, UK: Cambridge University Press; 1998.
23. Hutchins E. Distributed cognition. In: Smelser NJ, Baltes P, eds. *The International Encyclopedia of the Social & Behavioral Sciences*. Oxford, UK: Elsevier; 2001:2068–2072.
24. Billett S. *Learning in the Workplace; Strategies for Effective Practice*. Sydney, Australia: Allen & Unwin; 2001.
25. Bryson J, Pajo K, Ward R, et al. Learning at work: organisational affordances and individual engagement. *J Workplace Learn*. 2006;18(5):279–297.
26. Johnsson MC, Boud D, Solomon N. Learning in-between, across, and beyond workplace boundaries. *Int J Hum Resour Dev Manage*. 2010;12(1/2):61–76.
27. Schatzki TR. *The Site of the Social: A Philosophical Exploration of the Constitution of Social Life and Change*. State College, PA: Pennsylvania State University Press; 2002.
28. Crabtree BF, Miller WL, Stange KC. Understanding practice from the ground up. *J Fam Pract*. 2001;50(10):881–887.
29. Miller WL, Crabtree BF, McDaniel R, et al. Understanding change in primary care practice using complexity theory. *J Fam Pract*. 1998;46(5):369–376.
30. Miller WL, McDaniel RR Jr, Crabtree BF, et al. Practice jazz: understanding variation in family practices using complexity science. *J Fam Pract*. 2001;50(10):872–878.
31. Gherardi S. Knowing and learning in practice-based studies: an introduction. *Learn Organ*. 2009;16(5):352–359.
32. Heath H. Reflections and patterns of knowing in nursing. *J Adv Nurs*. 1998;27:1054–1059.
33. Elstein AS, Shulman LS, Sprafka SA. *Medical Problem-Solving: An Analysis of Clinical Reasoning*. Cambridge MA: Harvard University Press; 1978.
34. Norman G, Young M, Brooks L. Non-analytical models of clinical reasoning: the role of experience. *Med Educ*. 2007;41(12):1140–1145.
35. Croskerry P. A universal model of diagnostic reasoning. *Acad Med*. 2009;84(8):1022–1028.
36. Minda JP, Smith JD. Prototypes in category learning: the effects of category size, category structure, and stimulus complexity. *J Exp Psychol Learn Mem Cogn*. 2001;27(3):775–799.
37. Minda JP, Smith JD. Comparing prototype-based and exemplar-based accounts of category learning and attentional allocation. *J Exp Psychol Learn Mem Cogn*. 2002;28(2):275–292.
38. Custers EJFM. Medical education and cognitive continuum theory: an alternative perspective on medical problem-solving and clinical reasoning. *Acad Med*. 2013;88(8):1074–1080.
39. Hatano G, Inagaki K. Two courses of expertise. In: Stevenson H, Azuma H, Hakuta K, eds. *Child Development and Education in Japan*. New York: W.H. Freeman and Company; 1986:262–272.

40. Cutrer WB, Miller BM, Pusic M, et al. Fostering the development of the master adaptive learner: a conceptual model to guide skill acquisition in medical education. *Acad Med.* 2016. doi: 10.1097/ACM.0000000000001323.
41. Schon DA. *The Reflective Practitioner: How Professionals Think in Action.* New York: Basic Books; 1983:21–73.
42. Epstein RM. Mindful practice. *JAMA.* 1999;282(9):833–839.
43. Moore DE Jr. Needs assessment in the new health care environment: combining discrepancy analysis and outcomes to create more effective CME. *J Contin Educ Health Prof.* 1998;18(3):133–141.
44. Festinger L. *A Theory of Cognitive Dissonance.* Stanford, CA: Stanford University Press; 1957.
45. Mulnix JW. Thinking critically about critical thinking. *Educ Philos Theory.* 2012;44(5):464–479.
46. Scriven M, Paul R. *Defining Critical Thinking.* 2008. http://www.criticalthinking.org/aboutCT/definingCT.cfm
47. Davis DA, Mazmanian PE, Fordis M, et al. Accuracy of physician self-assessment compared with observed measures of competence: a systematic review. *JAMA.* 2006;296(9):1094–1102.
48. Sargeant J. Toward a common understanding of self-assessment. *J Contin Educ Health Prof.* 2008;28(1):1–4.
49. Gifford KA, Fall LH. Doctor coach: a deliberate practice approach to teaching and learning clinical skills. *Acad Med.* 2014;89(2):272–276.
50. Iyasere CA, Baggett M, Romano J, et al. Beyond continuing medical education: clinical coaching as a tool for ongoing professional development. *Acad Med.* 2016;91:1647–1650.
51. Regehr G, Mylopoulos M. Maintaining competence in the field: learning about practice, through practice, in practice. *J Contin Educ Health Prof.* 2008;28(suppl 1):S19–S23.
52. Artino AR, Brydges R, Gruppen LD. Self-regulated learning in healthcare professional education: theoretical perspectives and research methods. In: Cleland J, Durning SJ, eds. *Researching Medical Education.* Chichester, West Sussex, UK: Wiley Blackwell; 2015:155–166.
53. Davis D, Bordage G, Moores LK, et al. The science of continuing medical education: terms, tools, and gaps: effectiveness of continuing medical education: American College of Chest Physicians Evidence-Based Educational Guidelines. *Chest.* 2009;135(3 suppl):8S–16S.
54. Marinopoulos SS, Dorman T, Ratanawongsa N, et al. *Effectiveness of Continuing Medical Education.* Rockville MD: Agency for Healthcare Research and Quality; 2007. AHRQ Publication No. 07-E006.
55. Thomas A, Menon A, Boruff J, et al. Applications of social constructivist learning theories in knowledge translation for healthcare professionals: A scoping review. *Implement Sci.* 2014;9(1):54.
56. Mylopoulos M, Brydges R, Woods NN, et al. Preparation for future learning: a missing competency in health professions education? *Med Educ.* 2016;50(1):115–123.
57. Graham ID, Logan L, Harrison MB, et al. Lost in knowledge translation: time for a map? *J Contin Educ Health Prof.* 2006;26(1):13–24.
58. Cervero RM, Gaines JK. The impact of CME on physician performance and patient health outcomes: an updated synthesis of systematic reviews. *J Contin Educ Health Prof.* 2015;35(2):131–138.
59. Arora S, Thornton K, Komaromy M, et al. Demonopolizing medical knowledge. *Acad Med.* 2014;89(1):30–32.
60. Zhou C, Crawford A, Serhal E, et al. The impact of project ECHO on participant and patient outcomes: a systematic review. *Acad Med.* 2016;91(10):1439–1461.
61. Boud D, Hager P. Re-thinking continuing professional development through changing metaphors and location in professional practices. *Stud Contin Educ.* 2012;34(1):17–30.
62. Webster-Wright A. Reframing professional development through understanding authentic professional learning. *Rev Educ Res.* 2009;79(2):702–739.
63. Campbell C, Silver I, Sherbino J, et al. Competency-based continuing professional development. *Med Teach.* 2010;32(8):657–662.
64. Friedman CP, Wong AK, Blumenthal D. Achieving a nationwide learning health system. *Sci Transl Med.* 2010;2(57):57cm29.

Chapter 7

IMPROVING COMMUNICATION SKILLS *of* HEALTH CARE PROVIDERS

Mila Kostic

Case

The most recent patient safety report in your institution—and in fact almost all patient safety reports nationally—indicates that communication failures top the list of primary causes of poor quality and safety incidents. Some of the instances of such failure are tragic, resulting in adverse events and unnecessary loss of life. You realize that these issues are common in the hospital, but the link between safety and ineffective communication is also becoming evident in the outpatient setting.

Questions

How can you find out more about effective communication between physicians and patients and between physicians and other health care providers and staff members in your organization? What kinds of CPD programs have the potential to effect change in these important skills? Does the training show evidence of impact on the functioning of teams and clinical units? Are patients' needs better served and is there evidence that effective communication training may improve patients' experience and health outcomes?

INTRODUCTION

Patient-centered care is a term we hear and use every day as a goal of today's health care delivery irrespective of the specific context of that care. The term was coined in 1988 as a call to shift focus of health care providers (HCPs) and health care systems from disease management back to the patient and the families.[1] The concept of involving patients in designing, implementing, and evaluating health care was then introduced in the land-mark 2001 Institute of Medicine (IOM) Report *Crossing the Quality Chasm*. The IOM defined patient-centered care as "care that is respectful of and responsive to individual patient preferences, needs and values" and that ensures "that patient values guide all clinical decisions."[2,3] The IOM's 2003 report *Health Professions Education: A Bridge to Quality* identified health care communication as an essential feature of the patient-centered approach to care. Consequently, training in core communication skills became critically important as the report emphasized the need for educators and licensing bodies to strengthen HCPs' training requirements in the delivery of patient-centered care.[4]

Why Communication Skills Matter in Health Care

The quality of the interactions that patients experience in their clinical encounters highly influences the perception of the overall quality of health care they receive. Many studies have established that the connection and the perceived relationship that patients have with their HCPs can have a considerable effect, both positive and negative, on their engagement in health care, making positive changes in lifestyle behaviors, recall of information, adherence to treatment plans, and overall satisfaction, outlook, and attitudes toward their well-being.[5,6]

At the same time, there is evidence about patients not sharing their problems with their health care providers, such as not being able to afford the prescribed medication or avoiding treatments because of fear of side effects. In addition, there is often a disconnect between what patients report and what providers believe to be true. For example, one study reported that 83% of patients surveyed indicated that they would never tell their provider if they did not plan on buying a prescribed medication,[7] while between 75% and 89% of physicians surveyed in other studies believed that the majority of their patients were adherent.[8,9] In fact, *adherence* to prescribed treatment plan is an issue for an estimated 25% of Americans as reported by the Commonwealth Fund in 2002. Reasons cited for nonadherence have been shown to be related to concerns about the cost, finding instructions too difficult to follow, disagreements with what the clinicians recommended, and feelings that the treatment was in conflict with their personal beliefs.[10] As is seen in Table 7.1, it has been established that risk of nonadherence rises with patients whose providers are poor communicators and the opposite is true—good communication results in a 2.16-fold greater patient adherence.[6] Most importantly, evidence suggests that adherence is improved significantly with physician communication training when compared to those patients whose physicians received no training.[6]

During history-taking encounters, patients are routinely interrupted after a few seconds, their concerns or understanding of their own disease often dismissed and rarely enquired about. This lack of trust, or opportunity to address concerns with their

TABLE 7.1
Impact of Provider–Patient Communication

Effective provider–patient communication is linked to **improved patient satisfaction, health status, recall of information, and adherence**[6].
- **Poor communication** results in 19% higher risk of nonadherence.
- **Good communication** results in 2.16-fold greater patient adherence.
- **Communication training** results in 1.62-fold greater odds of patient adherence.

HCPs, contributes to missed diagnosis and other safety concerns—too often, very serious ones. Patients' experience is one of the composite measures that all hospitals and health care systems are concerned about. The core elements of what patients care about are in the communication domain and are related to meeting their expectations. Specifically, being allowed to tell their story, to communicate effectively with all members of the health care team across key areas of the encounter, to have shared control over the treatment plan, to have their time honored, and to be treated with respect is an important issue to patients.[11] One recent study involving more than 1,000 patients reported that 88% of patients interviewed believed that working with their health care professionals AS A PARTNER would help them manage and improve their overall health.[12]

It is now broadly accepted that effective communication is critical for quality and safety in health care. Communication failures are among the most frequently identified root causes of sentinel events in hospital settings as reported by the Joint Commission on Accreditation of Healthcare Organizations between 1995 and 2015, representing up to 70% of serious adverse health outcomes in hospitals, and rates are trending upward.[13] The failures of effective and accurate information sharing involve both patients and providers at the critical points in patient's hospital stay: the intake, any transfer of care, and discharge. Such problems are not unique to the US health care system and have prompted the Joint Commission International to include "Improving effective communication among clinical staff" in the International Patient Safety Goals.[14] These gaps in practice represent well-documented opportunities for quality and performance improvement as part of continuing professional development (CPD).

With the rising cost of health care, the cost of medical errors has also been studied. The *Journal of Healthcare Management* reported a 2010 study that developed a model for calculating the economic burden of poor communication in US hospitals. Agarwal and colleagues conceptualized a model that quantified efficiency of resource utilization as a function of physician and nurse time, effectiveness of care operations as being related to the length of stay (LOS) and incidence of medical errors, quality of working life as measured by stress and satisfaction with job, and service quality as determined by patient experience and provider job satisfaction.[15] They calculated the waste in time spent and increase in LOS as an outcome of communication errors and estimated that in 2009, this cost US hospitals ~$12.4 billion annually in waste alone, of which over 50% was attributable to an increase in LOS.

The quality of communication with other health care team members has a significant influence on the quality of the working relationships, reduction in nurse turnover, improvements in job satisfaction, and decrease in burnout.[16] "Interpersonal and communication skills" that result in effective information exchange and teaming with patients, their families, and other health professionals have been one of the core competencies of the Accreditation Council for Graduate Medical Education (ACGME) and American Board of Medical Specialties (ABMS) since 1999 in the United States. The Royal College of Physicians and Surgeons of Canada (RCPSC) released updated "CanMEDS 2005 Physician Competency Framework" that defines "communicator" as one of the key physician competencies. Similarly defined communication competency is part of the General Medical Council (GMC) system in the United Kingdom.[17–19]

Effective training methods and successful techniques for teaching and improving communication skills have been studied and linked to improvements in patient experience and health outcomes, safety of health care delivery overall, and HCP satisfaction and self-efficacy. Unfortunately, most physicians receive limited, if any, training in communication skills. The American Hospital Association 2012 report entitled *Lifelong Learning: Physician Competency Development* identified communication skills as one of the key competency gaps for physicians.[20] While continuing medical education (CME) and CPD are well suited to provide this type of training, very few skill development and training communication courses of any kind are provided as part of CME programs in the United States and in other parts of the world.[21]

THEORETICAL AND CONCEPTUAL FRAMEWORKS FOR COMMUNICATION IN MEDICAL EDUCATION

The current focus on patient-centered, collaborative, and team-based approach to care emphasizes the social context of communication in health care and positions it as a skill and competence to be mastered as part of a provider's professional identity. Bandura's social learning theory (SLT)[22] served as a theoretical background for developing training for communication with cancer patients in the late 1990s and early 2000s. The studies conducted with nurses at the time concluded that there was insufficient evidence about the effectiveness of the communication training on social and emotional needs of cancer patients because the focus had been on patients' physical needs. A demand for better designed studies that would incorporate assessment of transfer of learned communication skills into practice was articulated by Heaven, Clegg, and Maguire who also concluded that direct observation and supervision were associated with better transference of communication skill to practice.[23]

A major benefit of the *collaborative care model*, particularly in the context of chronic diseases such as diabetes, hypertension, or cancer, is the focus on promoting a patient's engagement in self-management. In contrast to *traditional* and often more paternalistic approaches to care, interactions between the patient and the provider are based on shared agenda, and the behavioral change comes from not just knowledge, but self-efficacy as well. In addition, decisions are made by the provider and the patient in partnership, and the aim is not just compliance with the provider's goals for the patient but also includes realizing self-efficacy and empowerment of patients and the provider.[9]

There are several *frameworks* for organizing provider communication skills training. Some methods have organized skills and strategies based on the components of the medical encounter—such as setting a shared agenda, building rapport, telling the diagnosis meaningfully, behavioral change counseling, and negotiating and implementing a treatment plan. Most existing frameworks can be classified based on whether they are oriented toward the *information exchange* as is the case with some frameworks focused on building communication skills of clinical teams and in hospital setting or *relationship development* as is the central goal of many modern physician–provider communication techniques. Both approaches have been shown to be effective for meeting patients' needs and values and both are important.

In his perspective on conceptual framework for communication in medical education, Martin applies Habermas' concepts of *communicative ethics* and the *theory of communicative action* to better understand the true nature of how to arrive at mutual understanding and agreement that establish the communicative goal as a product of a *democratic dialog*. A key characteristic of this type of dialog is that it is not influenced by power of intimidation as was the case in earlier, more traditional patient–physician encounters that focused solely on the biomedical world that dominated in medicine.[24,25] Martin contrasts "respectful communication" that includes arts of listening, translation, and interpretation to simply "gaining trust" or "information gathering" as skills that are not truly relationship building. A tension exists between the patient's need to understand complex medical issues and his or her right to make informed choice—the physician is then called upon to act truly in the best interest of the patient by first fully understanding the patient's needs and then acting to best meet them by never losing sight of professional biomedical expertise. In this context, the communication is seen as *medical epistemic competency*—as a way of developing an understanding of the interests and needs of others that enables physicians to bridge the "world of the patient" and the "world of medicine" in a delicate dance. Medical education in communication requires thoughtful training that marries communication skill building with contextual clinical situations and allows for the balancing act that meaningfully influences clinical decision-making. This includes acting in the best interest of the patient even when the patient is not capable of articulating his or her needs and it may, at times, be at odds with simply defined patient satisfaction or adherence.

The teaching methodology is critically important as faculty should model this approach of democratic dialog rather than trying to teach the learners to simply follow along by achieving the set goals and completing assignments based on the power of authority alone—such a method would instruct learners to only value communication with patients as a manipulative practice.[25]

PEDAGOGICAL BASES FOR COMMUNICATION SKILL TRAINING

We now have considerable evidence about what works in designing effective training in clinical communication skills. Courses that are structured, are longer in duration, and include identifying, demonstrating, practicing, and evaluating specific skills and strategies have been shown to be more effective than shorter and more didactic presentation type of educational interventions.[26] Other general principles of effective teaching and learning apply here as well. Ensuring relevance of the material to the learners in selection of cases and scenarios, using multiple and varied instructional methods, devoting more time to experiential and interactive elements in the learning environment, and ensuring proper sequencing in the predisposing, reinforcing, and enabling of elements as well as designing formative assessments that drive learning are all important.[27–29]

Simulation

Use of simulation approaches in designing clinical communication training has proven to be very effective in not only demonstrating skills in clinical encounters but also providing opportunity for direct practice and assessment of skill and competence. Academic medical institutions may benefit from access to *standardized patient programs*—these employ professional actors or specially trained patients who can provide authentic patient–provider encounter experience and are trained to respond skillfully to any provider clues as well as to provide credible feedback about the encounter episode.[30] In the absence of standardized patients (SPs), *role-play*, when structured correctly, has proven very effective, as well.[31] While there have been few studies that provide a direct comparison between SPs and role-play, some data suggest comparable results with one study finding peer role-play superior in achieving higher self-efficacy and better objective performance of content and process skills in communication.[32] One of the benefits of these training methods is the ability to allow learners to practice specific skills or scenarios in a safe environment, away from peer or administrative judgment and fear of harming patients. Both of these techniques work best when practiced in small groups—ideally 6 to 8 participants, or less, and it is recommended not to exceed 12 members in a group. Sequencing of training and materials should be evidence based and cases relatable to providers' practice needs.

Faculty training is critical as simulations require skilled facilitators who can design and guide the practice and facilitate feedback and debrief within the group. In training institutions, hospitals, and professional societies, this is an opportunity to partner with experts from other fields such as behavioral and social scientists.[26] Several organizations can provide high level of faculty training and support, for example, the American Academy on Communication in Healthcare (AACH), the Institute for Healthcare Communication (IHC), and the University of Calgary. Most experts agree that it is beneficial if faculty facilitators in small group simulation-type training are also clinical subject experts. In interprofessional, team-based training, it is recommended that perspectives of different relevant professions are represented.

Debriefing is a critical element of any simulation strategy and can be very impactful in teaching and learning if used as a developmental and not an administrative tool. It is equally powerful when used for individual and team performance, and it provides a structure for reflection, discussion, and goal setting in experiential learning. Debriefing is a form of structured feedback—it is considered an element of *active learning*—some active self-learning or self-discovery is required on the part of the learner, or a team, for it to be considered truly debriefing. These interventions are not time intensive or expensive, but they do require skillful facilitation and careful alignment of participants with the focus of intervention and the level of measurement. It is estimated that, if used properly, organizations can use debriefing as a means of improving individual and team performance by 20% to 25%.[33]

Shared Decision-making and Shared Presence in Physician–Patient Communication

Shared decision-making is one of the principal goals of effective communication in a patient-centered approach to the delivery of health care and is a process by which a decision is made about a clinical course of action in a collaborative manner that includes, at a minimum, a patient and a provider and may include patient's family, friends, and other members of the clinical team. The process includes sharing of information where the provider explains best options, risk, and benefits and the patient is able to ask questions and share values and needs so that the decision is made in the best interest of the patient. Patients have endorsed this concept worldwide. Shared decision-making assumes that patients are educated about the essential role they play in decision-making and that they are provided with useful decision support resources. It is also important that clinicians relinquish their power as the only authority in their interactions with patients, train to become effective coaches and partners in this process, and start asking patients "What matters to you?" and not only "What is the matter?".[3]

Shared Presence

Ventres and Frankel conceptualized how communication between a provider and a patient leads to *shared presence* as a fundamental characteristic of effective clinical communication.[34] The concept is defined as "shared state of being" in which both providers and patients share a deep sense of trust, respect, and knowing that facilitates healing.

This complex conceptual framework includes *interpersonal skills* by which physicians first "develop awareness and inquisitiveness for exploring patients' concerns by reflecting upon self and other, accepting diversity of perspectives, considering differences in expectations, and adjusting approach as needed." Integrating *relational context* into their clinical encounters is the next step in the process and includes understanding of influential factors and development of new consciousness that is focused on building relationships (with family, caregivers, and others), employing organizational structure to affect health literacy and benefits from IT/EHR, and understanding how cultural issues such as social determinants, illness understanding, and religious beliefs all contribute to patient resilience and strengths and integrate contextual issues into clinical inquiry and plan development. *Actions in clinical encounters* are about developing "habits of practice" by which a provider builds connections with patients, routinely elicits patients' perspectives, demonstrates empathy, educates patients, and motivates positive behavioral change. This is then the practice that leads to addressing clinical issues by identifying symptoms and concerns. Ventres and Frankel state that *shared presence* will, through optimizing process and therapeutic outcomes, lead to *healing outcomes*. This model positions physician–patient relationship at the core of what medicine should be about as a moral function of healing outcomes.

About Power

In a recent qualitative study about perceived issues of power in physician–patient relationships, Bourdien's social theory served as a framework for understanding of physicians' perception of power in their interactions with patients.[35] The authors propose education at all levels of training and in particular in the CME context to consider including opportunities in ongoing professional development for (1) cultivating awareness and building capacity to be reflective of physician power and how it plays out in various interactions with patients and other members of the clinical team and (2) developing communication strategies to "handle" the power with "insightful deliberation" in different clinical encounters by exerting, sharing, moderating, and relinquishing that authoritative power based on a specific context.

COMMUNICATION STRATEGIES FOR FACILITATING PROVIDER–PATIENT RELATIONSHIP

One of the criticisms of the "communication in health care literature" is that inadequate information is often reported about specific communication skills taught in a training or education program.

One approach to training often taken is to structure specific strategies across the key communicative and clinical points of a patient–provider encounter. Table 7.2 provides an example of those critical points in the encounter and strategies to use in the

TABLE 7.2
Common Communication Strategies for Facilitating Provider–Patient Relationship in a Typical Encounter

Negotiating a Shared Agenda
- Negotiating the agenda to include both the patient's and the provider's items
- Conveying interest in patient's priorities and inviting patient to take part in discussion
- Ensuring that patient's questions are being addressed ("What would you like to discuss today?")
- Research estimates that agenda setting adds just 1.9 min on average to the length of visit

Building Rapport with Patients
- Asking open-ended questions
- Eliciting patient's explanatory model of his/her illness
- Showing interest in the patient as a person
- Making empathic and reflecting statements (**NURS, PEARLS, RESPECT**) (see Table 7.3)

Telling the Diagnosis Meaningfully–(Ask–Tell–Ask)
- Asking the patient what he/she already knows or wants to know about his/her illness
- Telling the patient what he/she needs to know
- Asking or ascertaining whether the patient understands the information or has additional questions

Behavioral Change Counseling
- Assessing Readiness to Change
- Motivation: How important is it to make this change? (Using a 1–10 scale)
- Self-efficacy: How confident is the patient that he/she is able to make the change? (Using a 1–10 scale)

Negotiating and Implementing a Treatment Plan for Self-Management
- Coming up with a list of actions for self-management
- Setting Self-Management Plan (**SLAM**)
- Confirming patient's understanding of the plan
  - Ask the patient to repeat the important points and instructions to ensure correct understanding
  - Correct any misunderstandings before they become errors

Based on Boxer H, Snyder S. Five communication strategies to promote self-management of chronic illness. *Fam Pract Manag.* 2009;16(5):12–16.

Adapted with permission from the Office of Continuing Medical and Interprofessional Education at Penn Medicine, University of Pennsylvania from *Talking Diabetes with Your Patients: Practical Strategies for Overcoming Barriers and Improving Care with Effective Communication Strategies* online continuing education activity.

context of a chronic disease, such as a follow-up visit of a patient with hypertension or diabetes. This example is taken from the University of Pennsylvania CPD communication skills building workshop *Talking Diabetes with Your Patients: Practical Strategies for Overcoming Barriers and Improving Care with Effective Communication Strategies.*[39] The structure of the entire encounter can be organized around the following steps[9]:

1. *Negotiating a Shared Agenda*—Research estimates that agenda setting in a collaborative way adds just 1.9 minutes on average to the length of visit.[40]
2. *Building Rapport with Patients*—This is the time to build trust by inviting the patient's opinions and getting to know the patient as a person and to show care and understanding by using empathic and reflecting statements. Several methods and mnemonics for communication strategies that foster creation of more empathic relationships in clinical encounters were developed to help providers practice these skills. Providers usually pick one that resonates with them such as PEARLS,[37] NURS,[36] or RESPECT[38] and, once they master it, tend to always use the same approach in their practice. More information about how to best use these strategies is available in Table 7.3.
3. *Telling the Diagnosis Meaningfully*—"Ask–Tell–Ask" format provides a structure for the provider to tailor information to the patient's needs by providing chunks of clinical information that the patient needs to know and checking in to gauge understanding and answer any additional questions that a patient may have.
4. *Behavioral Change Counseling*—*Motivational interviewing* is a goal-directed method of counseling that is used for eliciting behavior change by helping patients to explore and resolve ambivalence. Helping patients assess their readiness to make changes in behaviors that will improve their management of their own disease by assessing their motivation, self-efficacy, or confidence that they can actually make the change can be accomplished with two simple questions: *On a scale from 1 to 10, how important is it to you to make this change?* followed by *On a scale from 1 to 10, how confident are you that you will be able to make this change?* If a patient is sufficiently motivated, it is still important to help him or her be realistic about it. If patient's confidence is below 6 or 7, the goals may need to be adjusted and the providers can usually help the patients problem-solve based on their experience. Investing time to do these steps properly can make a significant difference in patients' adherence to treatment and overall experience.
5. *Negotiating and Implementing a Treatment Plan for Self-Management*—This final and closing step in the encounter is focused on summarizing and negotiating the plan of action. It is important to incorporate a patient's concerns when coming up with a list of actions for self-management (to include adherence to taking medications as prescribed) and to confirm his or her understanding of the plan. The SLAM mnemonic is useful at this stage.

   Specific—the more specific the plan, the more likely it is that the patient will follow it

   Limited—both in the number of goals (1 or 2) and the timeline (no more than a few weeks)

   Achievable—must be realistic

   Measurable—the goal should be measurable so the patient and the provider can determine whether the plan was effective at the next visit

TABLE 7.3
Helpful Mnemonics and Communication Strategies for Building Empathic Relationships

Mnemonic	Example
NURS[36]	
Naming the emotion	*"You seem frustrated."*
Understanding	*"I would be frustrated too if I had to choose between paying for electricity or my medications."*
Respect	*"Thank you for telling me your dilemma."*
Support	*"I will do as much as I can to help you work on a solution to this."*
PEARLS[37]	
Partnering statements	*"I'd like to work together to figure out why you are not feeling like your usual self."*
Empathy	*"I can only imagine how hard it must be keeping these feeling bottled up inside."*
Appreciation/apology	*"I am sorry that you have been feeling down in the dumps."*
Respect	*"I know it must be hard to talk about this. I appreciate your openness."*
Legitimization	*"Your problem is common and I have helped others in similar situations."*
Support	*"Taking medicine to deal with this does not mean you have given up."*
RESPECT[38]	
Respect the patient →	By attentive listening, affirming comments, and nonverbal behaviors
Explanatory model →	Understand the patients' perspective, what thoughts and/or beliefs do they have about their disease, and self-management issues
Social context →	Understand the framework the patients are working within and what type of support systems they have in place
Power →	Share the power; do not dominate the conversation
Empathy →	Pause to imagine how the patient might be feeling and state your perception of the feeling, legitimizing the feeling
Concerns and fears →	Often very patient-specific and must be addressed to promote adherence
Trust/Therapeutic alliance →	Build by finding common ground

Adapted with permission from the Office of Continuing Medical and Interprofessional Education at Penn Medicine, University of Pennsylvania from *Talking Diabetes with Your Patients: Practical Strategies for Overcoming Barriers and Improving Care with Effective Communication Strategies* online continuing education activity.

TRAINING MODELS AND FRAMEWORKS

A number of communication models and frameworks have been described in recent published studies on effective communication training approaches in health care. Most models are based on live 2- to 5-day-long skill-building courses that combine information about communication as a competence, its relevance, and evidence about what works and why, with experiential learning—work with simulated patients directly or role-play—that allows for practicing demonstrated skills and strategies in a safe environment, ideally with a skilled facilitator. Feedback or debriefing is another important intervention that promotes deeper learning as part of the whole experience.

Several models have been well studied and validated in different environments. Table 7.4 provides examples and a quick reference guide to main features of eight well-known and frequently used communication training and evaluative models and frameworks across the health care professions. These include *SEGUE*,[41] *Calgary–Cambridge Guide*,[42,43] *the Four Habits model*,[44,45] *REDE model*,[46] *SAGE & THYME*,[47] *SPIKES*,[48] *SBAR*,[49] and *Team STEPPS*.[50] All of these models are linked to positive performance outcomes, use a similar approach to training design, and provide strong evaluative strategies—SPs and direct observation using checklists are commonly used to assess whether specific tasks were accomplished during the clinical encounter in a variety of health care professionals and trainees as well as in different clinical settings.

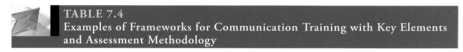

TABLE 7.4
Examples of Frameworks for Communication Training with Key Elements and Assessment Methodology

Framework	Key Elements	Assessment Methodology +/−
SEGUE[41]	Checklist-based method for teaching, assessing, and studying communication skills organized in five sections: **S**et the stage **E**licit information **G**ive information **U**nderstand the patient's perspective **E**nd the encounter	+ Checklist
Calgary–Cambridge Guide[42,43]	Structured patient–provider encounter approach for relationship building and assessment using a basic stepwise approach 1. Initiating the session 2. Gathering information 3. Physical information 4. Explanation and planning 5. Closing the session	+ Observational Guides
The Four Habits model[44,45]	Originally designed for outpatient setting, organized around 4 behaviors or habits: **HABIT 1:** Invest in the beginning of the encounter to create rapport and set the agenda. **HABIT 2:** Elicit the patient's perspective. **HABIT 3:** Demonstrate empathy to provide opportunity for patients to express emotional concerns. **HABIT 4:** Invest in the end to provide information and closure.	+ Four Habits Coding Schema (4HCS)
REDE model[46]	A framework for teaching and evaluating relationship-centered health care communication skills organized in three primary phases of **R**elationship: **E**stablishment **D**evelopment **E**ngagement	+ Checklist
SAGE & THYME[47]	Structured approach to improving knowledge and communication skills such as effective listening, clarifying concerns of patients, and responding to patient's concerns with empathy used in health and social care patient-focused support. **S**etting, **A**sk, **G**ather, **E**mpathy, **T**alk, **H**elp, **Y**ou, **M**e, End	+ Multiple Questionnaires

(Continued)

TABLE 7.4
Examples of Frameworks for Communication Training with Key Elements and Assessment Methodology (*Continued*)

Framework	Key Elements	Assessment Methodology +/–
SPIKES[48]	Six-step protocol for disclosing unfavorable information to patients with cancer **STEP 1: S**etting up the interview **STEP 2:** Assessing the patient's **P**erception **STEP 3:** Obtaining the patient's **I**nvitation **STEP 4:** Giving **K**nowledge and information to the patient **STEP 5:** Addressing the patient's **E**motions with **E**mpathic responses **STEP 6: S**trategy and **S**ummary	+ Questionnaires
SBAR[49]	Situational briefing communication technique: **S**ituation (a concise statement of the problem) **B**ackground (pertinent/brief information related to the situation) **A**ssessment (analysis and considerations of options—what you found/think) **R**ecommendation (action requested/recommended—what you want)	+ Observer Checklist
Team STEPPS[50]	**Team S**trategies and **T**ools to **E**nhance **P**erformance and **P**atient **s**afety is a comprehensive training system incorporates SBAR, check-back, closed communication loop, simulation and feedback.	+ Multiple

Two recent randomized control studies from Denmark have been reported where the *Calgary–Cambridge Guide* methodology was implemented across both inpatient and outpatient departments of a large hospital. In the first study, significant improvements were achieved in clinicians' self-efficacy in specific communication tasks. In addition, parents' (pediatric study) satisfaction increased overall and was sustained for 3 years.[51]

The second study focused on the improvements of communication with patients, as well as with colleagues, and found that the gains were more evident in the interprofessional than in the intraprofessional communication and that they persisted for 6 months after the training.[52] Based on this demonstrated clinical confirmation of implementing evidence-based programs for improving patient–provider and collegial communication, it was decided that the entire 3,000-large clinical staff would receive mandatory training based on this model.

The Four Habits model was developed at Kaiser Permanente, the largest health care organization in the United States by Frankel, Stein, et al. The same authors developed and validated the Four Habits Coding Scheme (4HCS), a compendium communication behavior assessment instrument for systematically evaluating the quality of physician–patient-centered communication across the structured elements of the "four habits."[44,45]

Subsequently, in 2011, the Four Habits model was successfully implemented in an inhospital setting in Norway and studied in a randomized controlled trial.[53] These researchers then conducted a follow-up observational study to examine the long-term effect and relationship of reported self-efficacy and actual performance.[54] The results of this study confirmed previous findings by Davis and colleagues about physicians' limited ability to self-assess their skills and needs for education and improvement, which is a particularly troubling issue since most CPD is self-directed.[55] Physician performance and self-efficacy were assessed in this Norwegian study with different instruments, including 4HCS, before and after the standard Four Habits 2-day course and at follow-up. Patient evaluation data were also obtained using the Customer Assessment of Healthcare Providers and Systems (CAHPS) and the Outpatient Experience Questionnaire (OPEQ) and captured both in-hospital and outpatient setting. It was found that not only did the long-term (up to 3.5 years) communication skills and self-efficacy of physicians improve with the communication skills training, but the actual performance as observed by experts (based on structured review of the videotaped performance) also improved. It is also noteworthy that these measured improvements were sustained for up to 1 year posttraining for the study duration. Because there was no observed association between the performance and self-efficacy prior to training, this study suggests a positive correlation between the increased confidence as a result of the training and the actual improvements in performance.[54]

The Boissy et al. study published in 2016 was an observational study designed to assess impact of a CME-accredited physician training intervention on patient satisfaction and physician experience across a large multispecialty academic medical center with almost 3,500 physicians using REDE, a relationship-centered communication training framework.[46] Data were collected using both inpatient (Hospital Consumer Assessment of Healthcare Providers and Systems [HCAHPS]) and outpatient (Clinician and Group Consumer Assessment of Healthcare Providers and Systems [CGCAHPS]) scores as well as Jefferson Scale of Empathy (JSE), Maslach Burnout Inventory (MBI), self-efficacy, and postcourse satisfaction. Their findings showed significant improvements in overall outpatient communication scores, the "respect domain" on the inpatient measures, as well as empathy and burnout. The results were sustained at 3 months.

Another significance of this study is that it included system-wide training, and it associated positive outcomes of a relatively short intervention (compared to previous studies with similar findings) with positive economic impact in the current environment of value-based incentives in health care.

A study assessing effectiveness of a foundational-level 3-hour workshop that teaches nurses and other hospital staff a structured approach to discussing patients' concerns was conducted in Manchester, United Kingdom. The SAGE & THYME model is a mnemonic for a sequential approach to listening and responding to patients' concerns. It is based on SLT and was designed to teach basics of providing emotional support.[47] The Connolly et al. study reported positive outcomes in self-efficacy as perceived sense of mastery over communication skills, motivation, and perceived usefulness. Qualitative data indicated that those who had an opportunity to use the skill in practice found it helpful in making communication more patient-focused and that, in turn, left patients more satisfied and empowered.

Communication skills training is very important in oncology and in particular for the way that providers "deliver bad news." Based on the SPIKES framework six-step protocol, there are four goals in disclosing bad news: gathering information from the patient, providing culturally and health literacy competent information in accord with patients' needs, supporting the patient using skills that will help reduce emotional impact of the bad news, and developing a collaborative treatment approach.[48] Because patients regard their oncologists as one of the key sources of their psychological support, it is critical that these physicians and other clinicians are comfortable and skilled in combining empathy with exploratory and validating statements. Several videos of the patent–provider encounters based on this six-step protocol are available from the MD Anderson Cancer Center Web site, some for CME credit.[56]

OVERCOMING BARRIERS TO EFFECTIVE TEAMWORK IN HEALTH CARE

Core Competencies of Collaborative Practice

The ability to work with professionals from other disciplines and specialties has been identified as a key skill set necessary for delivering collaborative, patient-centered high-quality and safe care. A review of the literature about collaborative practice and teamwork has identified a number of key competencies needed to enable professionals in health care to work effectively as part of an interprofessional team. A specific set of competencies required as part of professional practice was described by the Interprofessional Education Consortium (IPEC).[57] Possibly, the most significant competency domain is in the communication area.

A Health Canada–funded project published in 2009 sought to identify what professionals on the front line considered to be the most important competencies for collaborative practice. This qualitative study identified important elements for practice as well as interprofessional training. Negotiations between different perspectives and different professional role–based cultures as well as reaching consensus within the team, promoting understanding of different perspectives, treating others with respect and dignity, adjusting terminology and the communicative approach to different practice environments, and willingness to learn and change as needed were some of the foundational themes identified as necessary for successful collaboration by different HCPs interviewed in this study.[58]

Information Breakdowns in Handoff Communications

When the care of a patient is transferred from one care provider to the next one, we refer to this process as a "patient handoff" or a "transition of care"—and implied is the transfer of information, responsibility, and authority. This complex process is critical in health care and is also open to communication failures that can produce issues with quality and safety at any point of transfer. A patient's stay in the hospital can be looked at as a series of continuous handoffs at all levels, individual (between nurses as the shifts change) departments (from emergency department to admission and the ward or surgery to intensive care unit), and between hospitals (e.g., during transfers from a community setting to the specialty center).

Communication challenges have been identified as one of the three main barriers to effective handoffs, together with lack of standardization of the handoff as a system issue, and the absence or shortage of specific handoff training for health care professionals.

Abraham et al. studied the causes of the information breakdown in group handoff communication in an academic hospital setting using several qualitative methods such as direct observation, shadowing of providers during work, and audio recordings of handoffs and provider interviews.[59] They found that lack of face-to-face communication, double sign-outs, illegible notes and other issues that could all be classified as some form of deficiency in standardization of handoff communication events and unsuccessful completion of pre-turnover coordination activities were key areas of concern.

Abraham et al. suggested three interventions as strategies for improvement and for overcoming these barriers:

1. Incorporating standardized communication methods, templates, and tools for handoffs—body system format familiar to residents focused on patient statues including cardiovascular, neurologic, and pulmonary.
2. Development of education sessions to train providers interprofessionally in teams about effective handoffs using simulation and other active experiential communicative teaching and learning strategies. The training needs to be provided at the system level to minimize omissions.
3. System-based intervention focused on incorporating IT-supported tools, such as online forms, checklists, and other computerized technology, to provide structure to share relevant information across EMRs.

To address the issue of differences in communication styles of different professions and perception of teamwork where physicians tended to view the health care environment as much more collaborative than nurses, Kaiser Permanente developed a communication tool that was adapted from the U.S. Navy, called SBAR, in 2002.[49] The SBAR model standardizes information to be given and reduces communication variability, making reports concise, objective, and relevant (see Table 7.4). It has been widely adopted in critical care teams, in patient rounding, and in many other situations and is one of the most recommended effective health care communication mnemonic tools used for improving teamwork internationally as well.[60] Both Joint Commission and the Institute for Healthcare Improvement recommend this communication technique as a situational briefing model.

TeamSTEPPS—Team Strategies and Tools to Enhance Performance and Patient Safety

Team Strategies and Tools to Enhance Performance and Patient Safety (TeamSTEPPS) was developed jointly by the Department of Defense (DoD) and the Agency for Healthcare Research and Quality (AHRQ) to improve institutional collaboration and communication of HCPs for better patient safety and care and it was based in crew resource management (CRM). TeamSTEPPS 2.0, a recently released updated version, highlights the key principles and concepts of TeamSTEPPS and includes additional modules about measurement, coaching, and communication. Thousands of health care providers, in particular nurses, have been trained in this evidence-based system through regionally available courses, often using simulations. Complete and flexible set of training materials, including a series of videos, pocket guides and reminders, and tools for simulation training providing assessment and feedback, are available from the AHRQ Web site http://www.ahrq.gov/professionals/education/curriculum-tools/teamstepps/index.html.[50] Communication tools such as SBAR, callout, checkback as closed loop communication, and handoffs are included as part of the resources. The TeamSTEPPS curriculum, or its elements, can be successfully incorporated in CME/CPD curricula and activities in communication training of interprofessional teams. It can also be used very effectively when imbedded in a specific clinical context or a problem that is complex and where the successful management requires multifactorial training strategies or performance improvement type of interventions such as reducing sepsis rates and improving care across an entire hospital or a health care system.[61]

FUTURE DIRECTIONS

In this chapter, the focus has been on the critical importance that communication skills and competence hold in health care. Improving these skills with training of individual health care providers and clinical teams using evidence-based methods, frameworks, and communication tools has been shown to be very effective in many areas of health care. It is also important to remember that while for decades communication failures have been associated with critical errors and safety problems, the clinical educators and researchers in medical education have been studying, refining, and evaluating many of the training modalities that seem to hold the promise of fixing many, if not all, of the issues. These include patient adherence and relationship experience to providing safe, high-quality, efficient care every time, delivered by individual providers and diverse and interprofessional teams whose self-efficacy and job satisfaction all seem to be, at some important level, a function of communicative, relational, and, generally, social dimension of health care, a point that was lost in traditional education of health care professionals. And, while improvements are now being made by routinely incorporating evidence-based training, at least to some degree, in undergraduate and graduate curricula, much more needs to be done in the CPD arena.

In addition, there is danger in oversimplifying communication issues as just a result of poor transmission or lack of information exchange. Communication failures are much more complex and relate to vertical hierarchical differences, concerns with upward influence, conflicting roles and ambiguities, and struggles with interpersonal power and influence both providers and patients face as part of the health care systems. Sutcliffe and colleagues wrote about organizational communication culture and systemic relationship issues that need to be more carefully studied and understood.[62] We significantly underestimate the social, relational, and organizational factors in generating adverse medical events. The authors point out that "communication behaviors are imbedded in the structure of the organization and reside in the socially structured and culturally patterned behaviors of groups, subgroups, specialties, departments, and practices of the institution."

Overcoming these barriers to effective communication, therefore, needs to be addressed at the appropriate level. Continuing education programs in health care professions across all levels of training and professional organizations must start offering evidence-based training for improving communication skills of providers and health care teams at the appropriate level and using a comprehensive approach to address systemic as well as individual communicative barriers. These efforts will likely include a focus on interprofessional training and should be cognizant of the IOM recommendation that the "teams who work together should train together." Designing effective interventions to improve team communication will likely represent the next major advance in improving patient outcomes. These interventions should include teaching structured simulation-enabled methods for addressing handovers such as SBAR but also making sure that the teams are redefined from a collection of disciplines to a cohesive whole with common goals in which each member is valued and encouraged to communicate openly with others. As Weller and colleagues have pointed out, a critical part of the redesign toward a safer patient care must also include support system for the teams—implementation of protocols, procedures, checklists, IT briefs, and other system measures that encourage information sharing across the whole team and between teams as a whole.[63]

Greater attention must be paid to the role of assessments at all levels, individual professional skills, but also team-care metrics. These assessments should be normalized and imbedded in the work flow so that they are not seen as punitive and that they can drive specific communication training interventions and reminders in a CPD effort. A system that will accomplish this will also have to integrate and align the work that has traditionally been siloed in academic medical centers and health systems across CME, CNE and CPD, GME, faculty development, behavioral and assessment expertise, quality and safety and performance improvement departments, sim centers, IT, and implementation science and health economics research, where available.

Because longer, live courses that have been studied and described in the communication literature tend to be resource-intensive and often require prolonged time away from practice, future research and educational focus should extend to developing and studying effectiveness of technology-enabled self-study–targeted resources that may be combined with live experiential training. While there are some excellent examples of such on-demand communication modules,[64,65] there is a need for less expensive, shorter, and more focused educational blocs, ideally organized in curricula that would be readily available to learners across all areas of health care delivery. We can anticipate that use of simulation training methodologies will be further adapted for online delivery models and asynchronous training.

Another, currently largely untapped opportunity lies in clinical educational topics in CPD that could routinely reference communicative and relationship building guides as part of more traditional programming such as conferences, grand rounds, and clinical case conferences, when appropriate. Safety and performance improvement topics should incorporate elements of TeamSTEPPS training and similar strategies. In addition, communication training must become a part of leadership training at all levels of health care and professional administrative structures.

More studies about communicative training needs and effectiveness are needed in the outpatient setting that will not only focus on relationship building with patients and the care team but also address and legitimize current information sharing and learning that patients engage in online support groups and forums.

Finally, we need more studies that look at longitudinal outcomes of communication skills training and evaluate effectiveness from the patient experience and understanding, but also systems outcomes, such as effect on safety issues, true health outcomes metrics and changes associated with organizational and team culture.

Effective, empathic, and respectful communication as an individual skill must become a behavioral expectation and part of the professional identity of health care providers that is closely linked to the ethics and values of professional practice of individuals and clinical teams alike. This will require systems that fully support their health care providers and patient needs and enable open communication with education but also in other ways discussed.

REFERENCES

1. Gerteis M, Edgman-Levitan S, Daley J, et al., eds. *Through the Patient's Eyes: Understanding and Promoting Patient-Centered Care*. San Francisco, CA: Jossey-Bass; 1993.
2. Committee on Quality of Health Care in America: Institute of Medicine. *Crossing the Quality Chasm: A New Health System for the 21st Century*. Washington, DC: National Academies Press; 2001.
3. Barry MJ, Edgman-Levita S. Shared decision making—the pinnacle of patient-centered care. *N Engl J Med*. 2012;366:780–781.
4. Institute of Medicine. *Health Professions Education: A Bridge to Quality*. Washington, DC: National Academies Press; 2003.
5. Impact of Communication in Healthcare. *Institute for Healthcare Communication* [Internet]. 2011 July. [cited 2016 July 8]. http://healthcarecomm.org/about-us/impact-of-communication-in-healthcare/. Accessed July 16, 2016.
6. Haskard Zolnierek KB, DiMatteo MR. Physician communication and patient adherence to treatment: a meta-analysis. *Med Care*. 2009;47(8):826–834.
7. Lapane KL, Dub CE, Schneider KL, et al. Misperceptions of patients vs providers regarding medication-related communication issues. *Am J Manag Care*. 2007;13:613–618.
8. Goldberg AI, Cohen G, Rubin AH. Physician assessments of patient compliance with medical treatment. *Soc Sci Med*. 1998;47(11):1873–1876.
9. Boxer H, Snyder S. Five communication strategies to promote self-management of chronic illness. *Fam Pract Manag*. 2009;16(5):12–16.
10. Davis K, Schoenbaum SC, Collins KS, et al. *Room for Improvement: Patients Report on the Quality of Their Health Care*. Washington, DC: Commonwealth Fund; 2002.
11. Thiedke CC. What do we really know about patient satisfaction? *Fam Pract Manag*. 2007;14(1):33–36.
12. Society for Participatory Medicine Survey. *Patients Overwhelmingly Believe in Partnership with Their Clinicians to Improve Health [Internet]*. 2015 December [cited 2016 July 8]. http://participatorymedicine.org/patients-overwhelmingly-want-partnership-with-their-clinicians/. Accessed July 16, 2016.
13. Joint Commission Report. *Sentinel Event Data: Root Causes by Event Type 2004–2015* [cited 2016 July 8]. https://www.jointcommission.org/assets/1/18/Root_Causes_by_Event_Type_2004-2015.pdf. Accessed July 16, 2016.
14. Joint Commission International. *International Patient Safety Goals* [cited 2016 July 8]. http://www.jointcommissioninternational.org/improve/international-patient-safety-goals/. Accessed July 16, 2016.
15. Agarwal R, Sands DZ, Schneider JD. Quantifying the economic impact of communication inefficiencies in U.S. hospitals. *J Healthc Manag*. 2010;55(4):265–281.
16. Lein C, Wills CE. Using patient-centered interviewing skills to manage complex patient encounters in primary care. *J Am Acad Nurse Pract*. 2007;19(5):215–220.
17. American Board of Medical Specialties: Core Competencies. http://www.abms.org/board-certification/a-trusted-credential/based-on-core-competencies/. Accessed July 16, 2016.
18. The Royal College of Physicians and Surgeons of Canada. *CanMEDS 2005 Physician Competency Framework*. http://canmeds.royalcollege.ca/en/framework. Accessed July 16, 2016.
19. General Medical Council. *Good Medical Practice 2013*. http://www.gmc-uk.org/guidance/good_medical_practice.asp. Accessed July 16, 2016.
20. Combes JR, Arespacochaga E. *Continuing Medical Education as a Strategic Resource*. Chicago, IL: American Hospital Association's Physician Leadership Forum; September 2014. http://www.ahaphysicianforum.org/resources/leadership-development/CME/index.shtml. Accessed July 16, 2016.
21. Rotthoff T, Baehring T, David DM, et al. The value of training in communication skills for continuing medical education. *Patient Educ Couns*. 2011;84(2):170–175.
22. Bandura A. *Social Learning Theory*. New York: General Learning Press; 1977.

23. Heaven C, Clegg J, Maguire P. Transfer of communication skills training from workshop to workplace: the impact of clinical supervision. *Patient Educ Couns.* 2006;60(3):313–325.
24. Habermas J. *The Theory of Communicative Action.* McCarthy T. transl. Boston, MA: Beacon Press; 1973.
25. Martin C. To what end communication? Developing a conceptual framework for communication in medical education. *Acad Med.* 2011;86(12):1566–1570.
26. Simpson M, Buckman R, Stewart M, et al. Doctor-patient communication: the Toronto consensus statement. *BMJ.* 1991;303(6814):1385–1387.
27. Fox RD, Mazmanian PE, Putnam RW. *Changing and Learning in the Lives of Physicians.* New York: Praeger; 1989.
28. Davis DA, Galbraith R. Continuing medical education effect on practice performance: effectiveness of continuing medical education: American College of Chest Physicians evidence-based educational guidelines. *Chest.* 2009;135(suppl 3):42S–48S.
29. Moore DE, Green JS, Gallis HA. Achieving desired results and improved outcomes: integrating planning and assessment throughout learning activities. *J Contin Educ Health Prof.* 2009;29(1):1–15.
30. Smithson J, Bellingan M, Glass B, et al. Standardized patients in pharmacy education: an integrative literature review. *Curr Pharm Teach Learn.* 2015;7(6):851–863.
31. Lane C, Rollnick S. The use of simulated patients and role-play in communication skills training: a review of literature to August 2005. *Patient Educ Couns.* 2007;67:13–20.
32. Bosse HM, Schultz JH, Nickel M, et al. The effect of using standardized patients or peer role play on ratings of undergraduate communication training: a randomized control trial. *Patient Educ Couns.* 2012;87:300–306.
33. Tannenbaum SI, Cerasoli CP. Do team and individual debriefs enhance performance? A meta-analysis. *Hum Factors.* 2013;55(1):231–245.
34. Ventres WB, Frankel RM. Shared presence in physician-patient communication: a graphic representation. *Fam Syst Health.* 2015;33(3):270–279.
35. Nimmon L, Stenfors-Hayes T. The "handling" of power in the physician-patient encounter: perceptions from experienced physicians. *BMC Med Educ.* 2016;16:114, 1–9.
36. Smith RC. *Patient-Centered Interviewing: An Evidence-Based Method.* Philadelphia, PA: Lippincott Williams & Wilkins; 2002.
37. Steele D, Harrison J. *Challenging Physician Patient Interactions.* Leawood, KS: American Academy of Family Physicians; 2002.
38. Mastow C, Crosson J, Gordon S, et al. Treating and precepting with RESPECT: a relational model addressing race, ethnicity, and culture in medical training. *J Gen Intern Med.* 2010;25(suppl 2): 146–154.
39. Kostic M. Teaching and assessing communication skills: using simulation-based interprofessional interventions to improve communication skills of providers can enhance quality of care and patient outcomes in type 2 diabetes. *AMEE 2015 Conference Abstract Book #9AA09 (27865).* https://amee.org/getattachment/Conferences/AMEE-2015/AMEE-2015-App-Data/9AA-ePosters.pdf. Accessed July 24, 2016.
40. Middleton JF, McKinley RK, Gillies CL. Effect of patient completed agenda forms and doctors' education about the agenda on the outcome of consultations: randomized controlled trial. *BMJ.* 2006;332:1238–1242.
41. Makoul G. The SEGUE framework for teaching and assessing communication skills. *Patient Educ Couns.* 2001;45(1):23–34.
42. Kurtz S, Silverman J, Benson J, et al. Marrying content and process in clinical method teaching: enhancing the Calgary–Cambridge guides. *Acad Med.* 2003;78(8):802–809.
43. Silverman JD, Kurtz SM, Draper J. *Skills for Communicating with Patients,* 3rd ed. Boca Raton, London, New York: CRC Press, Taylor & Francis Group; 2013.
44. Frankel RM, Stein T. Getting the most of the clinical encounter: the four habits model. *J Med Pract Manage.* 2001;16:184–191.
45. Krupat E, Frankel R, Stein T, et al. The four habits coding scheme: validation of an instrument to assess clinicians' communication behavior. *Patient Educ Couns.* 2006;62:38–45.
46. Boissy A, Windover AK, Bokar D, et al. Communication skills training for physicians improves patient satisfaction. *J Gen Intern Med.* 2016;31(7):755–761.
47. Connolly M, Thomas JM, Orford JA, et al. The impact of SAGE & THYME foundation level workshop on factors influencing communication skills in health care professionals. *J Contin Educ Health Prof.* 2014;34(1):37–46.
48. Baile WF, Buckman R, Lenzi R, et al. SPIKES—a six-step protocol for delivering bad news: application to the patient with cancer. *Oncologist.* 2000;5:302–311.
49. Haig K, Sutton S, Whittington J. SBAR: a shared mental model for improving communication between clinicians. *Jt Comm J Qual Patient Saf.* 2006;32:167–175.

50. Agency for Healthcare Research and Quality (AHRQ). *TeamSTEPPS®: Strategies and Tools to Enhance Performance and Patient Safety* http://www.ahrq.gov/professionals/education/curriculum-tools/team-stepps/index.html. Accessed July 24, 2016.
51. Ammentorp J, Kofoed PE. Research in communication skill training translated into practice in a large organization: a proactive use of the RE-AIM framework. *Patient Educ Couns.* 2011;82:482–487.
52. Nørgard B, Ammentorp J, Kofoed PK, et al. Training improves inter-collegial communication. *Clin Teach.* 2012;9:173–177.
53. Jansen BF, Guldbransen P, Dahl FA, et al. Effectiveness of a short course in clinical communication skills for hospital doctors: results of a crossover randomized controlled trial. *Patient Educ Couns.* 2011;84:163–169.
54. Guldbransen P, Jansen BF, Finset A, et al. Long term effect of communication training on the relationship between physician's self-efficacy and performance. *Patient Educ Couns.* 2013;91(2):180–185.
55. Davis DA, Mazmanian PE, Fordis M, et al. Accuracy of physician self-assessment compared with observed measures of competence. A systematic review. *JAMA.* 2006;296:1094–1102.
56. MD Anderson Cancer Center. *Managing Difficult Communication [Internet].* https://www.mdanderson.org/education-and-research/resources-for-professionals/professional-educational-resources/i-care/complete-library-of-communication-videos/managing-difficult-communication.html. Accessed July 21, 2016.
57. Interprofessional Education Collaborative Expert Panel. *Core Competencies for Interprofessional Collaborative Practice: Report of an Expert Panel.* Washington, DC: Interprofessional Education Collaborative; 2011.
58. Suter E, Arndt J, Arthur N, et al. Role understanding and effective communication as core competencies for collaborative practice. *J Interprof Care.* 2009;23(1):41–51.
59. Abraham J, Nguyen V, Almoosa F, et al. Falling through the cracks: information breakdowns in critical care handoff communication. *AMIA Annu Symp Proc.* 2011;2011:28–37.
60. Riesenberg LA, Leitzsch J, Little BW. Systematic review of handoff mnemonics literature. *Am J Med Qual.* 2009;24(3):196–204.
61. Childs A, Jenson L, Kostic M, et al. Evaluating a performance improvement CME activity designed to improve early intervention and treatment of sepsis. Poster presented at AAMC Integrating Quality Meeting: Improving Value through Clinical Transformation, Education and Science, Rosemount, IL, June 2014.
62. Sutcliffe KM, Lewton E, Rosenthal MM. Communication failures: an insidious contributor to medical mishaps. *Acad Med.* 2004;79(2):186–194.
63. Weller J, Boyd M, Cumin D. Teams, tribes and patient safety: overcoming barriers to effective teamwork in healthcare. *Postgrad Med J.* 2014;90:149–154.
64. American Academy on Communication in Healthcare (AACH) Online Communication Curriculum. *DocCom [Internet].* http://www.aachonline.org/DocCom. Accessed August 22, 2016.
65. *Penn Medicine's Talking Diabetes with Your Patients: Practical Strategies for Overcoming Barriers and Improving Care with Effective Communication Strategies* [Internet]. http://www.talking-diabetes-cpd.upenn.edu. Accessed August 31, 2016.

Chapter 8

COLLABORATING INTERPROFESSIONALLY *for* TEAM-BASED CARE

Scott Reeves and Simon Kitto

Case

You meet with the chief quality officer of your academic medical center who has described a lack of teamwork on previous occasions. He appreciates your efforts in CE/CPD but still faces challenges in professional-to-professional communication and interprofessional collaboration. He points to several recent reports of incidents that highlight these problems. He believes the problem stems from a lack of basic training in the study of team science and preparation for interprofessional work, for example, in undergraduate education, residency, and even single-profession continuing education.

Questions

Isn't team-based care what we have been practicing for years? Do you agree that there are deficiencies in collaboration here? How can you learn more if improvement is necessary?

INTRODUCTION

Traditional approaches for delivering continuing education (CE) and continuing professional development (CPD) are evolving. In addition to profession-specific clinical competence, learners need other types of competences to work effectively within health care systems that have embraced team-based models of care to improve patient quality and safety. As a result, CE/CPD programs are increasingly offering activities to enhance skills, knowledge, and behaviors designed to promote effective interprofessional communication, teamwork, and collaboration. In this chapter, we explore pertinent issues relating to how health professionals can learn together to improve their abilities to collaborate, communicate, and coordinate their services to support the delivery of effective team-based care.

BACKGROUND

Definitions and Core Concepts

Learning together to deliver team-based care is an interactive CE/CPD activity. It involves different professionals coming together to learn how to improve the way they collaborate in order to enhance the patient care they deliver. Referred to as continuing interprofessional education (CIPE) or continuing interprofessional development (CIPD), these activities have been defined as an activity, "undertaken after initial qualification when members of two or more health and or social care professions learn with, from, and about each other to improve collaboration and the quality of care."[1] As such, CIPE/CIPD activities draw upon the well-established broader definition of interprofessional education (IPE) as "occasions when two or more professions learn with, from, and about each other to improve collaboration and the quality of care."[2]

Linked to these definitions are the following underlying core concepts. First, CIPE/CIPD activities are founded on promoting collaboration, not only between learners but between developers, facilitators, and patients. Second, in achieving collaboration, this form of learning is egalitarian in nature—a particularly important concept given the hierarchical division of labor that exists between the health professions.[3] Third, CIPE/CIPD activities are learner-led and team oriented. Fourth, drawing upon adult learning principles, this form of learning uses real-life clinical problems to develop its activities—an important element in generating learner motivation.[4] Finally, CIPE/CIPD activities use shared reflection to provide opportunities for learners to discuss and debrief the successes and challenges related to their collaborative learning experiences in order to use in their clinical work.

Evolution of Collaborative Continuing Education

Globally, for over three decades, health care policy makers have identified the key role of CIPE/CIPD in improving the organization of health care systems and outcomes.[5-8] The support for this type of collaborative learning is rooted in the complex and multifaceted nature of patients' needs which requires effective collaboration among different health professions to meet those care needs.

National health education policy documents have repeatedly called for the use of team-based learning to help improve the situation.[9-11] On an international level, the World Health Organization (WHO) has highlighted the importance of team-based learning in the development of the competencies needed to become part of a collaborative ready health workforce.[6] The WHO report outlines the importance of collaborative learning to improve fragmented health systems throughout the world to "optimize the skills of their members, share case management, and provide better health services to patients and the community. The resulting strengthened health system leads to improved health outcomes."[6]

Problems with communication and collaboration have been well documented in the international research literature, repeatedly demonstrating that such problems result in serious compromises in patient safety and quality of care.[12-14] Such research indicates that traditional (professionally isolated) approaches to delivering CE/CPD have failed to adequately support the development of abilities required to provide effective care.[15–17] As a result, the education and training of health professions, around the world, has refocused attention on providing interprofessional opportunities to develop the attitudes, knowledge, skills, and behaviors needed to work effectively together to deliver safe, high-quality care. Encouragingly, there have been an increasing number of CIPE/ CIPD programs delivered throughout the world, in countries such as Australia, Canada, Japan, UK, and United States,[1,4,13] with many of these programs incorporating a range of competencies from frameworks designed to support interprofessional collaboration and teamwork.[18,19]

LEARNING AND TEACHING APPROACHES

Learning Together on an Interprofessional Basis

The definition of CIPE/CIPD outlined previously stresses the need for explicit interprofessional interaction between participants, as it is argued that this interactivity promotes the development of the competencies required for effective collaboration.[4] Educational strategies that enable interactivity are therefore a requirement of team-based learning. Barr et al.[4] outline the different types of interactive learning methods than can be employed in this form of education (Table 8.1).

The interprofessional literature contains numerous examples of how these interactive learning activities have been adopted within specific team-based learning. For example, Freeth and colleagues report on a 1-day UK-based CIPE simulation-based program for obstetricians, obstetric anesthetists, and midwives to help improve interprofessional working in obstetric settings. The focus of the course was on improving communication processes involved in care and their influence on patient safety, and involved an initial orientation to the environment, simulation scenarios, and facilitated debriefings.[20] See Refs.[21,22] for other examples involving a range of interactive learning methods in their CIPE/CIPD studies.

When learners come together to undertake CIPE/CIPD activities, attention should be paid to the initial interactive processes of group formation. The use of an "ice-breaking" session may be considered helpful in facilitating group cohesion. Ice-breaker

TABLE 8.1
Different Team-Based Learning Methods

Learning Methods	Examples
Exchange-based learning	Seminar-based discussions
Observation-based learning	Joint visits to patients'/clients' homes
Action-based learning	Problem-based or case-based learning
Simulation-based learning	Simulating clinical practice
Practice-based learning	Interprofessional clinical placements
E-learning	Online discussions
Blended learning	Combining e-learning with other traditional methods

sessions allow learners to interactively focus on professional stereotyping or professional assumptions they bring to an interprofessional initiative. Such sessions can be advantageous in unpacking and exploring, for instance, issues of professionalism (e.g., boundary protectionism) that can affect interprofessional interactions.[23] They are also helpful in team building, especially when a group of learners has not previously worked together. For established interprofessional teams, these sessions can also be useful in allowing them to unpack issues linked to hierarchy and power differentials that surround their daily practice. Such existing problems with established teams can also impact the effectiveness of a CIPE/CIPD program.

Effective interprofessional interaction requires a balance of professions. An equal mix of members from each profession helps overcome a team skewed too heavily in favor of one profession, which may inhibit interaction, as the larger group can dominate.[24] Similarly, for effective collaborative learning to occur, team size should not be too large. Large teams of learners may encounter challenges related to poorer quality interactions. In general, team sizes of between five and ten help optimize interprofessional interaction.[25] Fiscal restraints, nevertheless, may cause difficulties in creating such small group learning formats.

Securing participation in CIPE/CIPD activities can be challenging for some professional groups. For example, a few studies have noted the challenges of physician participation in interprofessional programs and the need to ensure their presence given their key role in supporting changes in interprofessional collaboration.[26] Engaging in CIPE/CIPD activities are often affected by the demands of clinical work. For many professionals, CE/CPD credits may provide the needed status, and therefore incentive, to encourage their participation. Nevertheless, as CIPE/CIPD activities tend to be undertaken on a voluntary basis, the incentive for participation is mainly related to an individual's own professional development needs and/or a wish to enhance the coordination and delivery of care.

Opportunities for informal learning—when learners meet socially and discuss aspects of their formal education—are a useful approach for CIPE/CIPD activities. Informal learning can be helpful in allowing individuals to exchange ideas and obtain guidance from their peers, work colleagues, or managers. Informal learning activities can be explicitly built into an interprofessional program. For example, they can be used to provide opportunities to share time during breaks to informally discuss educational experiences.

In relation to the key outcomes related to CIPE/CIPD activities, Table 8.2 provides a typology that modified Kirkpatrick's original four-level model to a six-level model.[4]

A number of systematic reviews of IPE have employed this typology to help classify the range of outcomes that can be generated from collaborative learning.[27,28] This typology has also been employed in a newly developed conceptual model to help with the measurement of IPE including CIPE/CIPD activities.[8]

Team-Based Interprofessional Facilitation

Facilitating CIPE/CIPD activities can be challenging and requires skill, experience, and preparation to deal with the various responsibilities and demands involved. There are a range of attributes required for this type of work, some of which are outlined in Table 8.3.

TABLE 8.2
Key Collaborative Learning Outcomes

Outcome	Description
Level 1: reaction	Learners' views on the learning experience and its interprofessional nature
Level 2a: modification of attitudes/perceptions	Changes in reciprocal attitudes or perceptions between participant groups/teams
Level 2b: acquisition of knowledge/skills	Gains of knowledge and skills linked to interprofessional collaboration
Level 3: behavioral change	Individuals' transfer of interprofessional learning to their practice setting and their changed professional practice
Level 4a: change in organizational practice	Wider changes in the organization and delivery of care
Level 4b: benefits to patients	Improvements in health or well-being of patients

Similar to other small-group education, facilitators need to focus on team formation and team maintenance, create a nonthreatening environment, and enable all learners to participate equally. However, these aims are more challenging in an interprofessional context given the history of social and economic inequalities and friction that exist between the members of the health and social care professions.[3] For example, it has been argued that different professional cultures shape differing definitions of health, wellness, and treatment success, as well as power differences, which CIPE/CIPD needs to address to promote collaborative competence.[13,29]

Faculty development is needed for those involved in facilitating CIPE/CIPD. For most educators, teaching students how to learn about, from, and with each other is a new and challenging experience. Interprofessional faculty development may reduce feelings

TABLE 8.3
Key Attributes of Effective Team-Based Facilitators

Key Attribute	Details
Experience of interprofessional work	To draw upon prior experiences to provide real-life (meaningful) examples of collaboration issues
Commitment to collaboration and teamwork	To provide authenticity for facilitation processes
Understanding of interactive learning methods	To use to maximize interprofessional interaction between learners
Knowledge of group dynamics	To facilitate interaction and help overcome problematic group dynamics
Confidence in working with interprofessional groups	To ensure an engaging yet relaxed approach to facilitation
Flexibility	To creatively explore professional differences within interprofessional groups
Approachability	To be open and accessible to encourage discussion
Good sense of humor	To employ humor to resolve tensions between learners and encourage open dialogue

of isolation, develop a more collaborative approach to facilitation, as well as provide opportunities for faculty to share knowledge, experiences, and ideas.[30] Encouragingly, there has been a growing number of faculty development programs focusing on offering a range of preparatory activities, such as understanding the roles and responsibilities of the different professions, exploring issues of professionalism, and planning learning strategies for interprofessional groups. There is also a need for interprofessional faculty development programs to enable individuals to promote change at departmental and organizational levels, and thus these programs should target diverse stakeholders and involve institutional leaders.[31]

To ensure that faculty maintain their knowledge of interprofessional facilitation, they need ongoing faculty development opportunities. Often, it is useful to consider team teaching with more experienced colleagues to help develop the range of necessary skills, knowledge, and confidence that are vital for interprofessional facilitation. Regular opportunities for discussion and reflection can be a useful type of support for facilitators of CIPE/CIPD. Where formal training cannot be obtained, it is advisable to seek informal input from a colleague more experienced in this type of work. For CIPE/CIPD to be successfully embedded in curricula and training packages, the early experiences of staff must be positive. This will ensure continued involvement and a willingness to further develop the curriculum based on learner feedback.

IMPLEMENTING TEAM-BASED LEARNING

Organizational Issues

Organizational support is crucial to a successful CIPE/CIPD program and consists of various components. It is critical to have leadership with interest, knowledge, and experience to forward the interprofessional agenda, and an organization and faculty supportive of CIPE/CIPD activities are needed to instill within students a positive attitude to this type of learning.[32] Institutional policies and managerial commitment are also crucial given the resources required to develop and implement CIPE/CIPD. This form of leadership and "buy-in" is needed from all the participating organizations or departments within an organization. In addition, the issue of finance needs careful consideration during the planning of any interprofessional initiative. As the cost of this form of education tends to span a number of different professional or departmental budgets,[33] agreement over financial arrangements can often be a significant hurdle for CIPE/CIPD activities.

Planning the Learning

Developing CIPE/CIPD curricula is a complex process and may involve educators from different faculties, work settings, and locations. Indeed, involving faculty from the different programs involved in a CIPE/CIPD initiative is central in order to generate a sense of shared interprofessional ownership. This can be challenging with smaller faculty. Equal representation of professions ensures that no one group can dominate the planning process and skew the initiative in any one direction.

As developing CIPE/CIPD activities can take considerable time and energy, team members need to have dedication and enthusiasm. However, when CIPE/CIPD activities are dependent on the input of a few key enthusiasts, their long-term sustainability can be threatened when these individuals move to other organizations. For example, in an evaluation of work-based interprofessional initiative based in acute care, it was found that the sustained enthusiasm of steering group members was critical to overcoming various practical issues such as joint validation and the establishment of a pilot placement.[33] Without this type of group effort, collaborative learning activities cannot be successfully developed and implemented.

The election of an educational leader is important to coordinate CIPE/CIPD development activities and ensure that progress is achieved. Such leaders need to arrange regular meetings and consider all professional perspectives and ensure good levels of discussion and interaction.[34] Curricula developers need to share their aims and assumptions about the initiative to ensure that all members are working toward a common goal. Where differences are identified, these need to be discussed and resolved.

Sustaining CIPE/CIPD programs can be equally complex and requires good communication among participants, enthusiasm for the work being done, and a shared vision and understanding of the benefits of introducing or modifying curricula offerings for professional learners. Organizations need to regularly evaluate and revise their CIPE/CIPD (if needed) to ensure its long-term viability.

SCHOLARSHIP

The Evidence Base

During the past decade, a number of systematic reviews have been conducted to examine and summarize the international IPE evidence.[27,28,35] To generate a "meta-synthesis" of this growing evidence base, a review of reviews was undertaken.[36] Following a comprehensive search, six systematic reviews were identified. The following section reports the key results from this synthesis.

The six included reviews reported on the effects of over 200 IPE studies spanning over 40 years—with around 60% of the included studies reporting on CIPE/CIPD activities. It was found that these reviews shared similar definitions of IPE (as outlined above) and employed similar methodologically inclusive approaches to their inclusion criteria and a similar approach to recording learning outcomes (see Table 8.2).

The synthesis revealed that IPE was delivered in a variety of acute, primary, and community care settings and addressed a range of different clinical conditions (e.g., asthma, arthritis) or acute conditions (e.g., cardiac care). While different combinations of professional groups participated in the interprofessional programs, medicine and nursing were the core participants. The duration of IPE programs varied, ranging from 1- to 2-hour sessions to programs delivered over a period of months; yet most programs lasted between 1 and 5 days. IPE was most commonly delivered to professional learners in their workplaces. While IPE programs used a variety of different combinations of interactive learning methods, seminar-based discussions, group problem-solving, and/or role play activities were the most commonly employed. Quality improvement principles were often drawn upon within CIPE/CIPD programs.

In general, IPE programs used formative assessments of learning, typically using assessment techniques in the form of individual written assignments and/or joint/team presentations, which provided a collective account of learners' interprofessional experiences.[36]

There was a widespread use of nonvalidated instruments to detect the impact of IPE on learner and/or patient satisfaction. While the use of such tools can provide helpful data for local quality assurance issues, the quality of these data are limited as it is difficult to assess their validity or credibility. Measures to detect changes in individual behavior were poor, often relying on simple self-reported descriptive accounts of this form of change. Most change recorded in the studies was change that the learners reported themselves. This type of evidence is not regarded as robust, as it does not necessarily detect *actual change*; it can only report on a person's *perception of change*. In addition, most studies were undertaken in single-site studies, in isolation from other studies, limiting the generalizability of research.

Despite some weaknesses in the quality of evidence offered by the reviews, there were some encouraging quality issues. Most notably, there was a fairly common use of quasi-experimental research designs (e.g., before-and-after studies; before-during-and-after studies), which can provide some indication of change associated with the delivery of IPE, CIPE, and CIPD activities; most studies gathered two or more forms of data (typically survey and interviews); and there is a growing use of longitudinal studies to begin establishing the longer-term impact of IPE on organizations and patient care.[36]

The synthesis found that most studies reported that IPE can result in positive learner reactions, where the learners "enjoyed" their collaborative experiences. Such studies also reported positive changes in learner perceptions/attitudes in relation to views of other professional groups, changes in views of interprofessional collaboration, and/or changes in views of the value attached to working on a collaborative basis with other professions. In addition, these types of studies reported positive changes in learner knowledge and skills of interprofessional collaboration, usually related to an enhanced understanding of roles and responsibilities of other professional groups, improved knowledge of the nature of interprofessional collaboration, and/or the development of collaboration/communication skills. Fewer studies reported outcomes related to individual behavior, usually reported as practitioners' working in a more collaborative manner with their colleagues from other professional groups. Of those studies that did provide evidence at this level, positive change in individual practitioners' interactions was usually cited. A small number of studies reported positive changes to organizational practice resulting from the delivery of IPE. Outcomes used to report this type of impact usually focused on changes to interprofessional referral practices/working patterns or improved documentation (i.e., guidelines, protocols, use of shared records) related to the organization of care. A smaller amount of studies reported changes to the delivery of care to patients/clients. These studies typically recorded positive changes to clinical outcomes (e.g., infection rates, clinical error rates), patient satisfaction scores, and/or length of patient stay.

Recently, this work was updated and found eight additional IPE reviews.[37] Despite a growth of the international IPE evidence contained in this newer review of reviews, the key results in relation to use of learning activities, methods of evaluation, and reported outcomes described in the initial work[36] in essence remained unchanged. As a result, the evidence for the effects of IPE continues to rest upon a variety of different inter-professional programs (e.g., in terms of learning activities, duration, and professional mix) and study methods (experimental studies, mixed methods, qualitative designs) of variable quality. Nevertheless, this updated review of reviews revealed that IPE can nurture collaborative knowledge, skills, and attitudes. It also found more limited, but growing, evidence that IPE can help enhance collaborative practice and improve patient care. Mindful of these (and other) limitations to the IPE evidence base, Reeves and colleagues[38] recently published guidance for improving the quality of IPE studies to support evaluation teams, in their future work, to generate more rigorous interprofes-sional scholarship.

Theoretical Approaches

Social science theory can inform the development and evaluation team-based learning, yet to date, as noted above, while most IPE programs draw (implicitly) upon adult learn-ing principles, there is minimal explicit use of social science theory. Barr et al.[4] identified three interprofessional foci in which a number of social science theories could be situ-ated: (1) preparing individuals for collaborative practice, (2) cultivating collaboration in groups and teams, and (3) improving services and the quality of care. See Table 8.4 for a summary of the theories related to the different foci.

In relation to preparing individuals for collaborative practice, three theories (contact theory, social exchange theory, and negotiation theory) provide approaches to support effective interactions between different professional groups. First, contact theory is based on Allport's studies of prejudice between different social groups, and his conclusion that contact between members is the most effective way to reduce tension between groups.[39] Allport found though that simply bringing individuals from the different groups together was insufficient to effect change. He therefore identified three conditions that had to be addressed for prejudice to be reduced: equality of status between the groups, group members working toward common

TABLE 8.4
Key Theories for Team-Based Learning

Interprofessional Focus	Theory
Preparing individuals for collaborative practice	Contact theory (Allport)
	Social exchange theory (Challis et al.)
	Negotiation theory (Strauss)
Cultivating collaboration in teams	Work-group mentality theory (Bion)
	Team learning theory (Senge)
Improving services and the quality of care	Systems theory (Von Bertalanffy)
	Activity theory (Engestrom et al.)
	Discourse theory (Foucault)

goals, and cooperation during the contact. Such an approach can be applied to CIPE/ CIPD activities to help diminish negative stereotyping and promote positive interprofessional relations.

Second, social exchange theory explains social change and stability as a process of negotiated exchanges between parties.[40] According to this theory, all human relationships are formed according to a subjective cost–benefit analysis and the comparison of alternatives. This theory can be used to provide insight into the nature of relationships among different professionals during a CIPE/CIPD program and help in developing individuals' understandings of their relationships with others across workplace settings.[4] Third, negotiation theory was developed by Strauss to explain how formal roles are often transgressed by informal trade-offs between individuals' own goals and those of others.[41] This theory can be used to explain how negotiations shape the nature of interprofessional relations between health providers and also how negotiations affect the development and delivery of IPE.

In regard to cultivating group/team collaboration, two theories (work-group mentality and team learning) are offered to help understand how they can support interprofessional team learning.

First, workgroup mentality theory is based in a psychodynamic perspective that aims to explain the unconscious processes involved in a group unable to deal with its "primary task."[42] According to this theory, groups will often avoid making decisions to prevent members from addressing potentially difficult group issues. Stokes and colleagues[43] have extended this theory to interprofessional relations, suggesting that interprofessional team meetings can be frequently not productive as a false sense of collaboration prevents members from dealing with potentially difficult issues. CIPE/CIPD programs with a group dynamic format can enable learners to reflect on unconscious forces that shape interprofessional relations, with the aim of increasing their understanding of such forces in their clinical workplaces.

Second, the concept of the learning team, developed from organizational learning theory.[44] Team learning is an approach aimed to support the development of high performance teams. Typically, in a team, members do not necessarily trust one another and share collective goals, but if a learning team emerges, the members begin to develop a shared commitment, have mutually agreed goals, and share a concern for the well-being of the team. In relation to CIPE/CIPD, team learning can help transform a loosely affiliated work "group" of health care professionals into a more effective interprofessional "team" in which members trust one another and share a commitment to collective goals and welfare of their colleagues.[4]

In respect to improving services and the quality of care, the following three theories (systems theory, activity theory, and discourse theory) can be used in an interprofessional context to improve services and the quality of care. For Von Bertalanffy, the concept of "system" was developed as a response to the limitations of specialist disciplines in addressing complex problems.[45] Systems theory can be applied across disciplines from physics and biology to the social and behavioral sciences. It sees the whole as more than the sum of their parts, interactions between parties as purposeful, boundaries between them as permeable, and cause and effect as interdependent not linear. The underlying philosophy of systems theory is the unity of nature, governed by the same fundamental laws in all its realms. Intervention by one profession at one point in the system affects the whole in ways that can only be anticipated from multiple professional perspectives. Systems theory has multiple applications in CIPE/CIPD. It offers a framework within which all health professionals can relate person, family, community, and environment, one or more of which may be points of intervention interacting with a system. It can also be used to understand relationships within and between professions and between education and practice organizations.

Activity theory provides a means to understand and intervene in relations at micro and macro levels in order to effect change in interpersonal, interprofessional, and interagency relations.[46] An analysis of activity involves an understanding of individual relationships and how they relate to macro level of collective and community. An important component of this approach is the notion of "knotworking"—a concept that helps describe the nature of collaborative work in which individuals connect—through tying, untying, and retying separate threads of activity during their interactions. Such an approach can be used in CIPE/CIPD to understand the sometimes "fluid" nature of interprofessional relationships in the delivery of care.

According to Foucault, discourse helps to define a particular culture, its language and the behavior of individuals who belong to that culture.[47] Lessa has helpfully summarized Foucault's approach, as she stated that discourses are knowledge systems made up of ideas, attitudes, actions, beliefs, and practices that influence how individuals think, see, and speak.[48] Koppel used this approach to uncover prevalent discourses in CIPE/CIPD and demonstrated how three main discourses shaped the thinking and behavior of the main parties in the education field, namely, the discourses of management, professions, and education.[49]

FUTURE DIRECTIONS

As discussed in this chapter, CIPE/CIPD activities have expanded across the globe over the past few decades in response to failures of interprofessional collaboration that have resulted in compromises to patient quality and safety. Through this growth and its associated publications, we have developed a more informed understanding on collaborative learning. As previously presented, there is an important role for the use of social science theories to underpin the development and implementation of CIPE/CIPD activities. Future CIPE/CIPD programs should aim to draw more widely on these theories to strengthen the quality of collaborative learning opportunities. In addition, research has also provided a comprehensive set of insights into CIPE/CIPD. As noted above, systematic reviews have shown that this type of learning can have positive outcomes in relation to participants' reactions, attitudes, knowledge/skills, behaviors, and practice, as well as patient benefits. Moving forward, future investment in CIPE/CIPD must be based on the interprofessional evidence base, which is gradually accumulating. Indeed, further research can focus on addressing current gaps in knowledge relating to the longer-term impacts (costs/benefits) of CIPE/CIPD on behavior, organizational practice (e.g., avoiding duplication, avoiding hospitalization, reducing lengths of patient stays and unnecessary patient readmissions), as well as improvements to health care outcomes.

REFERENCES

1. Reeves S. An overview of continuing interprofessional education. *J Contin Educ Health Prof.* 2009;29: 142–146.
2. Centre for the Advancement of Interprofessional Education. *Interprofessional Education: A Definition.* Retrieved from: www.caipe.org.uk/about-us/defining-ipe
3. Reeves S, MacMillan K, van Soeren M. Leadership within interprofessional health and social care teams: a socio-historical overview of some key trials and tribulations. *J Nurs Manag.* 2010;18:258–264.
4. Barr H, Koppel I, Reeves S, et al. *Effective Interprofessional Education: Argument, Assumption and Evidence.* Oxford, UK: Blackwell; 2005.
5. World Health Organisation. *Continuing Education of Health Personnel.* Copenhagen, Denmark: WHO Regional Office for Europe; 1976.
6. World Health Organization. *Framework for Action on Interprofessional Education & Collaborative Practice.* Geneva, Switzerland: WHO; 2010.
7. Frenk J, Chen L, Bhutta Z, et al. Health professionals for a new century: transforming education to strengthen health systems in an interdependent world. *Lancet.* 2010;376(9756):1923–1958.
8. Institute of Medicine. *Measuring the Impact of Interprofessional Education (IPE) on Collaborative Practice and Patient Outcomes.* Washington, DC: National Academies Press; 2015.
9. Department of Health. *A Health Service of All the Talents: Developing the NHS Workforce.* London, UK: HMSO; 2000.
10. Health Canada. *Interprofessional Education for Collaborative Patient-Centred Practice.* Retrieved from http://www.hc-sc.gc.ca/hcs-sss/pubs/hhrhs/2006-iecps-fipccp-workatel/index-eng.php
11. Institute of Medicine. *Interprofessional Education for Collaboration: Learning How to Improve Health from Interprofessional Models Across the Continuum of Education to Practice.* Washington, DC: The National Academies; 2013.
12. Williams R, Silverman R, Schwind C, et al. Surgeon information transfer and communication: factors affecting quality and efficiency of inpatient care. *Ann Surg.* 2007;245(2):159–169.
13. Reeves S, Lewin S, Espin S, et al. *Interprofessional Teamwork for Health and Social Care.* Oxford, UK: Wiley-Blackwell; 2010.
14. The Joint Commission. *Sentinel Event Data—Root Causes by Event Type.* Retrieved from http://www.jointcommission.org/sentinel_event_statistics/
15. Kitto S, Bell M, Goldman J, et al. (Mis)perceptions of continuing education: Insights from knowledge translation, quality improvement and patient safety leaders. *J Contin Educ Health Prof.* 2013;33(2):81–88.
16. Kitto S, Bell M, Peller J, et al. Positioning continuing education: Boundaries and intersections between domains continuing education, knowledge translation, patient safety, and quality improvement. *Adv Health Sci Educ Theory Pract.* 2013;18(1):141–156.
17. Kitto S, Bell M, Goldman J, et al. Quality Improvement, patient safety and continuing education: a qualitative study of current boundaries and potential collaborations. *Acad Med.* 2015;90(2):240–245.
18. Canadian Interprofessional Health Collaborative. *A National Interprofessional Competency Framework.* Retrieved from www.cihc.ca/files/CIHC_IPCompetencies_Feb1210.pdf
19. Interprofessional Education Collaborative Expert Panel. *Core Competencies for Interprofessional Collaborative Practice: Report of an Expert Panel.* Washington, DC: Interprofessional Education Collaborative; 2011.
20. Freeth D, Ayida G, Berridge E, et al. Multidisciplinary obstetric simulated emergency scenarios (MOSES): promoting patient safety in obstetrics with teamwork-focused interprofessional simulations. *J Contin Educ Health Prof.* 2009;29(2):98–104.
21. Owen J, Brashers V, Littlewood K, et al. Designing and evaluating an effective theory-based continuing interprofessional education program to improve sepsis care by enhancing healthcare team collaboration. *J Interprof Care.* 2014;28:212–217.
22. Luetsch K, Rowettb D. Developing interprofessional communication skills for pharmacists to improve their ability to collaborate with other professions. *J Interprof Care.* 2016;30:458–465.
23. Baker L, Egan-Lee E, Martimianakis M, et al. Relationships of power: implications for interprofessional education. *J Interprof Care.* 2011;25:98–104.
24. Van Hoof T, Grant R, Sajdlowska J, et al. Society for Academic Continuing Medical Education Intervention Guideline Series: Guideline 4, Interprofessional Education. *J Contin Educ Health Prof.* 2015;35(suppl 2):S65–S69.
25. West M. *Effective Teamwork.* Leicester, UK: British Psychology Society Books; 1994.
26. Goldman J, Meuser J, Lawrie L, et al. Interprofessional primary care protocols: a strategy to promote an evidence-based approach to teamwork and the delivery of care. *J Interprof Care.* 2010;24:653–665

27. Hammick M, Freeth D, Koppel I, et al. A best evidence systematic review of interprofessional education. *Med Teach.* 2007;29:735–751.

28. Reeves S, Perrier L, Goldman J, et al. Interprofessional education: effects on professional practice and healthcare outcomes (update). *Cochrane Database Syst Rev.* 2013;(3):CD002213.

29. Pecukonis E, Doyle O, Bliss D. Reducing barriers to interprofessional training: promoting interprofessional cultural competence. *J Interprof Care.* 2008;22:417–428.

30. Silver I, Leslie K. Faculty development for continuing interprofessional education and collaborative practice. *J Contin Educ Health Prof.* 2009;29:172–177.

31. Leslie K, Baker L, Egan-Lee E, et al. Advancing faculty development in medical education: a systematic review. *Acad Med.* 2013;88:1038–1045.

32. Brewer M, Flavell H, Trede F, et al. A scoping review to understand leadership in interprofessional education and practice. *J Interprof Care.* 2016;30:408–415.

33. Reeves S. *Developing and Delivering Practice-Based Interprofessional Education.* Munich, Germany: VDM publications; 2008.

34. Howkins E, Bray J. *Preparing for Interprofessional Teaching: Theory and Practice.* Oxford, UK: Radcliffe Publishing; 2008.

35. Pauze E, Reeves S. Examining the effects of interprofessional education on mental health providers: findings from an updated systematic review. *J Ment Health.* 2010;19:259–271.

36. Reeves S, Goldman J, Sawatzky-Girling B, et al. A Synthesis of systematic reviews of interprofessional education. *J Allied Health.* 2010;39:S198–S203.

37. Reeves S, Palaganas J, Zierler B. Synthesis of interprofessional education reviews. In: Institute of Medicine. *Measuring the Impact of Interprofessional Education on Collaborative Practice and Patient Outcomes.* Washington, DC: The National Academies Press; 2015.

38. Reeves S, Boet S, Zierler B, et al. Interprofessional Education and Practice Guide No. 3: evaluating interprofessional education. *J Interprof Care.* 2015;29:305–312.

39. Allport G. *The Nature of Prejudice.* Reading, MA: Addison-Wesley; 1979.

40. Challis L, Fuller S, Henwood M, et al. *Joint Approaches to Social Policy.* Cambridge, UK: Cambridge University Press; 1988.

41. Strauss A. *Negotiations: Varieties, Contexts, Processes and Social Order.* San Francisco, CA: Jossey-Bass; 1978.

42. Bion WR. *Experiences in Groups and Other Papers.* London, UK: Tavistock Publications; 1961.

43. Stokes J. Problems in multidisciplinary teams: the unconscious at work. *J Soc Work Pract.* 1994;8:161–167.

44. Senge P. *The fifth Discipline the Art and Practice of the Learning Organization,* 1st ed. Doubleday/Currency: New York; 1990.

45. Von Bertalanffy L. *General Systems Theory.* London, UK: Allen Lane. The Penguin Press; 1971.

46. Engestrom Y, Engestrom R, Vahaaho T. When the center does not hold: the importance of knotworking. In: Chaklin S, Hedegaard M, Jensen U, eds. *Activity Theory and Social Practice.* Aarhus, Denmark: Aarhus University Press; 1999.

47. Foucault M. *The Archeology of Knowledge.* London, UK: Tavistock; 1972.

48. Lessa I. Discursive struggles within social welfare: restaging teen motherhood. *Br J Soc Work.* 2006;36:283–298.

49. Koppel I. *Autonomy Eroded? Changing Discourses in the Education of Health and Community Care Professionals.* Unpublished PhD Thesis. University of London, 2003.

Chapter 9

ACCESSING ONLINE INFORMATION RESOURCES *for* POINT *of* CARE (POC) LEARNING

Sarah Knox Morley and William F. Rayburn

Case

It is clear to the health system leadership that much of what their physicians learn is from direct patient care. In addition, their patients are asking more questions. Younger health professionals are very accustomed to using their computers for accessing medical information. As the CME/CPD director, you conclude that a system needs to be in place to facilitate learning at the point of care (POC).

Questions

What types of online information resources exist at your institution? Is there some framework to teach how to access this information? How can the best evidence be obtained most quickly? What challenges exist in using the computer or mobile devices for information seeking?

INTRODUCTION

Leaders in continuing professional development (CPD) appreciate that the learning of most physicians and health care professionals is directed by patient encounters in the clinical environment.[1] The reported number of clinical questions prompting additional information seeking has increased over the years.[2] This movement is likely due to better informed patients, more patient comfort in searching for this information, more peer-reviewed literature being published with resultant changes in diagnosis and management, and information being more accessible at the provider's and patient's fingertips.

Physicians differ in their information-seeking behaviors, as summarized by Salinas.[2] The physician's specialty, age, and recentness of training play some role. A pattern of information seeking is also shaped by convenience of access to resources, habits of the practitioner, and reliability, quality, and applicability of information. The sheer volume of medical literature bears witness to Internet (or online) searches as playing a major role to answer questions arising in clinical practice.

Patient-related information that we seek can be simply classified as resulting from either "background" or "foreground" questions. As described by Worster and Haynes, "background" questions are important for understanding the pathophysiology and epidemiology of a condition but are insufficient for dealing with specific patient's needs.[3] Answers to "background" questions can often be found in traditional textbooks (whether paper or electronic), while answers to "foreground" questions are best found in recent medical publications. Answers to "background" questions have not changed as rapidly as "foreground" questions (e.g., which is the best imaging study to rule in or exclude a disorder? What is the best therapy for this patient's disease?).

The subject of this chapter deals with accessing medical information from an online computer or a portable Wi-Fi (or mobile) device at the point of care (POC). Information from different online resources can often vary for the same topics, quality of evidence cited, cost, and credit for continuing education. Conscientious decision-making for individual patients is not merely from randomized trials and meta-analyses but from tracking the best evidence with which to answer a specific clinical question.

FRAMEWORK FOR LOCATING USEFUL INFORMATION

Many practitioners lack information management skills or time to navigate the evidence and, therefore, are overwhelmed by the volume of available information. Determining the applicability of results from peer-reviewed original research articles is beyond the time constraints of many busy clinicians. Although prior studies have examined the learning and reading behaviors of physicians in training, little is known about the drivers of resource selection at the POC and its effectiveness in obtaining answers.[1,3,4] Online searches for answering clinical questions, especially those related to diagnosis and treatment, can be challenging.

A framework is necessary in accessing POC evidence-based information to address clinical questions. Efficient and productive searching requires selecting the most appropriate information resources for the clinical question. An ideal resource should meet several criteria: (1) be evidence-based (trust), (2) cover the specific topic (relevant), (3) be easy to use (convenient), (4) be readily available (accessible), and (5) answer the question quickly (speed). These criteria that significantly influence resource selection (speed, trust, easy access) are based on a survey conducted by Duran-Nelson et al. of 167 internal medicine residents responding to a survey at three US medical schools.[5] While portability is not considered to be essential, it is valuable for accessing information at multiple locations.

Resources used in decision-making to meet these criteria are well organized in a framework originally described by Haynes and colleagues in 2006 and refined in 2016 as the "5S model for retrieving preappraised evidence."[6,7] These five levels consist of systems, synthesized summaries, systematically derived recommendations (guidelines), systematic reviews, and studies. The levels are shown in Figure 9.1 as an EBHC (evidence-based health care) pyramid. The highest level of evidence ("systems") is usually unavailable or most difficult to obtain. Health care providers can be trained to begin searching for evidence at the second level near the top of the pyramid ("synthesized summaries") and work their way down the pyramid (increasing the work necessary) to answer the clinical question. Following this

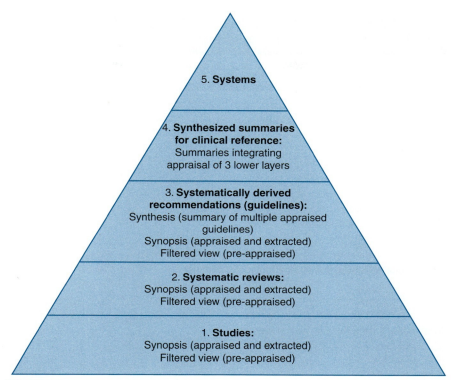

FIGURE 9.1.   The "5S" EBHC pyramid for accessing preappraised evidence and guidance in decision-making. (Reproduced from Alper BS, Haynes RB. EBHC pyramid 5.0 for accessing pre-appraised evidence and guidance. *Evid Based Med.* 2016;21(4):123–125, with permission from BMJ Publishing Group LTD.)

framework can increase the speed of clinical decision-making, as well as assuring confidence in the validity or trust of the evidence found.[8]

Experience will aid in determining what quality information is available (the resources themselves) and when to delve deeper into the pyramid or go directly to the studies. Many physicians use search engines such as Google/Google Scholar and sources like Wikipedia in the initial discovery phase to direct them to a different level of evidence in the information pyramid such as a specialty practice guideline or Cochrane Review.[5] Furthermore, Google can be used as a "system" to answer a particular question (e.g., How do I calculate a body mass index for a patient who is morbidly obese?).

ONLINE RESOURCES

Online medical resources for use at the POC may be categorized according to the 5S model of preappraised information. Examples of online medical resources are listed in Table 9.1, along with descriptions of cost, availability, and continuing medical education (CME) credit. Each level of the evidence pyramid adds to and builds on the ones below. Other hybrid products (e.g., AccessMedicine) provide information from

TABLE 9.1

Examples of Online Medical Resources, According to the Level of the EBHC Pyramid, for Locating Preappraised Evidence and Guidance

Resource	Cost	App (+) Wireless (W)	CME
Studies			
BioMed Central	Free	W	—
Medscape	Free	+	+
Online Databases	$	+	—
Public Library of Science (PLOS)	Free	+	—
PubMed/Medline	Free	+	—
CINAHL	$	+	—
Systematic Reviews			
ACP JournalWise	$	W	—
Cochrane Library	$	+	—
Essential Evidence Plus	$	W	+
Systematically Derived Recommendations (Guidelines)			
ACP	Free	W	—
AHRQ ePSS	Free	+	—
Guideline Central	$	+	—
Synthesized Summaries for Clinical Reference			
ACP Journal Club	$	W	+
BMJ Best Practice	$	+	+
BMJ Clinical Evidence	$	+	+
ClinicalKey for Nursing	$	+	+
CINAHL Evidence-based Care Sheets	$	+	—
DynaMed Plus	$	+	
Epocrates Plus	$	+	+
Essential Evidence Plus	$	W	+
Evidence Central	$	W	—
Micromedex Clinical Knowledge	$	+	—
NEJM Journal Watch	$	+	+
Nursing Reference Center	$	+	+
TRIP	Free	W	—
TRIP Pro	$	W	—
UpToDate	$	+	+

textbooks, journal articles, guidelines, and POC resources like calculators and quick diagnosis summaries. These products encompass the five levels found in the 5S model and are frequently consulted at the POC.

Studies

Throughout their training, health care providers are taught to search for primary literature using any number of online databases (i.e., CINAHL, Medline, and PsycINFO). Databases such as Medline, produced and maintained by the National Library of

Medicine (NLM), may be licensed to other online vendors (i.e., EBSCOhost or Ovid). The vendors develop retrieval software unique to their search platform, and their subscription fee may or may not include links to access full-text articles. Database subscription costs can be high and, therefore, not always available to individuals. The NLM makes its own Medline product (PubMed) available at no cost to anyone in the world with links to freely available articles through the PubMed Central (PMC) archive.

Many practitioners find database searching difficult due to the use of seemingly arcane subject headings and Boolean operators [AND, OR, NOT] necessary to build effective search strategies. Time to practice and perfect search skills is in short supply, and even when search results retrieve a manageable number of citations, the clinician must locate the full-text article and evaluate the evidence. In an attempt to lessen the burden on the busy clinician, the NLM created PubMed Clinical Queries, which employs a predetermined search strategy for locating study categories (i.e., therapy, diagnosis, etiology, and prognosis). The clinician types in a topic (e.g., pneumonia), chooses the study category of interest, and indicates either a broad (sensitivity) or narrow (specificity) focus. Based on the chosen filters, the PubMed search engine retrieves articles and systematic reviews from the Medline database. Although PubMed Clinical Queries streamlines the search process, it does not alleviate the need for locating and evaluating individual articles.

Bibliographic databases are excellent resources for locating primary literature. These databases are not a top choice for answering POC questions due to limitations in accessibility, convenience, and speed.

Systematic Reviews

Systematic reviews summarize research on a topic. Most highly regarded are systematic reviews that conduct a meta-analysis on numerical data from randomized clinical trials. The most widely used resource for finding these meta-analyses is the Cochrane Database of Systematic Reviews, which publishes full-text systematic reviews. Access to the full-text reviews is free to certain countries in Europe and Africa; otherwise, access to the abstract and the plain language summary is free, but a subscription is necessary to view the full-text review.

While systematic reviews are considered the gold standard for evidence-based practice, these reviews take years to develop, can be extraordinarily lengthy, and may not address the specific patient question the clinician wants to address. The Cochrane database is a trusted source but using systematic reviews at the POC fails the tests of accessibility, convenience, relevance, and speed. In addition, some articles found in resources other than Cochrane call themselves a "systematic review," which either may be a review of papers found in the literature using a systematic process (e.g., PRISMA criteria) or may be a review without a strict methodology, which is less evidence-based.

Systematically Derived Recommendations

Systematically derived recommendations consist of clinical and practice guidelines. Guideline synopses may be found in databases while resources such as Guideline Central provide summaries from worldwide medical associations. Subscription-based POC products often include guidelines. The freely available National Guideline Clearinghouse through the Agency for Healthcare Research and Quality (AHRQ) offers both association and locally developed guidelines. Full text is available as is a feature allowing a side-by-side summary comparison of several guidelines on a particular topic. Guideline accessibility is generally good; however, finding relevant guidelines and evaluating the material affects convenience and speed.

Synthesized Summaries for Clinical Reference

Synthesized summaries developed from current best evidence is the second highest level of resource available to providers. While evidence-based textbooks and guidelines are frequently mentioned in this category, currency may be an issue if publishers or organizations do not provide frequent online updates. Summaries used at the POC and for CPD or continuing education (CE) include licensed resources such as DynaMed Plus and UpToDate. These peer-reviewed summaries cover multiple topics from various specialties, are written by clinicians and updated regularly, and contain reference citations that sometimes lead to a full text of the article. Subscription-based access is available to individuals, while institutions pay considerably more when the pricing model is based on FTE equivalents. Other synthesized summary resources, such as BMJ Clinical Evidence, Essential Evidence Plus, and Evidence Central, are available by paid subscription, while ACP Journal Club is included in ACP association membership. While cost may be a negative factor, convenience, accessibility, speed, and trust all play into the popularity of these resources.

Systems

Infobuttons located within the electronic health record (EHR) provide links to online information resources to support POC decision-making.[9,10] These information resources, externally licensed or developed in-house, may include textbooks, government and patient education Web sites, guidelines, images, PubMed/Medline, and evidence-based synopses or syntheses. Some EHR systems also include infobuttons that generate requests to a librarian.[11] The practitioner may see a list of general information resources to choose from, or a more targeted set leading to patient or context specific information. To be considered at the top level of the evidence pyramid requires a computerized decision support systems (CDSS) that goes beyond the basic infobuttons. The CDSS relies on a knowledge base or repository wherein e-resource profiles are created that will accurately match resource content to answer specific clinical questions. The CDSS that extracts patient data elements from the EHR and then automatically queries and retrieves information from relevant evidence-based resources is not yet available to most clinicians.

BENEFITS AND LIMITATIONS OF MOBILE DEVICES

The desktop or laptop computer retains its superior position when compared with mobile or handheld devices in performing an effective literature search and in determining the best evidence.[12] Since the advent of personal digital assistants (PDAs), mobile devices (smartphones and tablet computers) have grown in acceptance by medical professionals.[13,14] These devices are rapidly becoming tools for accessing POC information.

Introduction of the iPhone, iPad, androids, and other smartphones and tablets has changed the type of information that can be easily accessed. These changes have been accompanied by an increase in published research in the medical and library literatures. Recent studies in the medical literature examined mobile device use for POC information among medical students and physicians. One study explored use of the devices among residents in the United States, another in medical education at the University of Alberta, and a third by medical students and junior physicians in the United Kingdom.[15–17] Boruff and Storie conducted an electronic survey of 1,210 medical students, residents, and faculty members about the widespread use of smartphones and tablets in clinical settings at four Canadian universities.[18] All four of the above investigations confirmed the frequent use of mobile devices as reference and information management tools in clinical practice and medical training, despite technological and intellectual barriers.

Friederichs and colleagues conducted a randomized controlled pilot study in Muenster, Germany, to assess the practicality of tablets, smartphones, and computers at the bedside.[12] Mobility of the tablet and smartphone was a significant advantage over the computer. However, for performing effective literature searches, the computer was rated superior to both tablet computers and smartphones. No significant differences were detected between tablets and smartphones, except the larger screen of the tablet was more appealing.

Other limitations, in addition to the smaller screen size, make the mobile devices less attractive for POC use. While a device increases the frequency of searching for answers, the quality of information can be inadequate or questioned.[15,19] Mobile versions of databases may not be optimized for doing an extensive search. Some applications are free and developed by unknown publishers that could influence or bias content. Other apps are expensive with limited opportunities to field-test in advance.[15]

SOCIAL MEDIA AS A SOURCE FOR ONLINE EDUCATION

The term social media covers an array of Web-based collaboration tools used for individual reasons as well as professional and education purposes. Use of social media to access medical information is in its infancy. Its value as a medical information resource has not been either fully realized or perceived as being useful and safe.[20] Without refinement of medical information in social media, any uptake by physicians will continue to be slow, especially at the POC.[21]

In reviewing data from several surveys, von Muhlen and Ohno-Machado reported that students are most likely to use social media, making it probable that we will see an increased adoption of social media for education and communication.[22] For that reason, it is reasonable to briefly review the types of social media that could eventually be used at the POC. Physicians and other health care professionals are reminded to use good judgment when posting or evaluating materials for their accuracy and relevance.[23]

Wikis are Web sites that allow collaborative editing of their content and structure by their users. Wikipedia, the most well-known wiki, is an open encyclopedia that anyone can access to add to or edit its content. Medical wikis may contain an open repository of easily accessible health-related materials, but adding or editing content is restricted to medical experts by the site owner. Wikipedia as a reference source for patients and health professionals is understandable due to its ease of use, yet troubling because it lacks peer review. Other health-related wikis may be reliable sources of information (from expert authors) but no longer current.

Facebook, an online social networking service, allows individuals to share and connect with family, friends, and others. Initially developed as a personal profile site, problems with posting unprofessional material content online is a recognized concern. Inappropriate comments or photos and violations of privacy have led to the development of professional standards and guidelines by major health care associations.[23,24]

Educational Web-based tools that are less social or communication oriented should be considered for either POC learning or continuing education. *Podcasts* are audio or video files downloaded to a device for use at a convenient time to enable self-directed learning.[25–28] The Science/Medicine category incorporates freely available podcasts from government agencies, journal publishers, professional associations, and universities.

YouTube, the video-sharing Web site, can be uploaded by individuals, corporations, universities, and media companies for viewing. While it contains many sites to access entertaining videos, there are educational videos that apply to medically related education and procedures. For example, Oxford University Medical School posts free, open access medical videos on YouTube (https://www.youtube.com/user/OxfordMedicalVideos/featured). Videos on Oxford Medical Education are produced by medical students under the supervision of faculty.

RSS (rapid syndication service) feeds use push technology in real time to deliver new information from Web sites of interest. One example to help keep clinicians up to date is the use of an RSS feed to automatically set up a journal table of contents. Ease of use depends on the service provider (database or journal publisher) but, once set up, enables routine access to new material without effort on the part of the clinician.

OTHER CONSIDERATIONS

Online Clinical Calculators and Multimedia Tools

Along with information from textbooks, journals, and guidelines, Web-based technology offers the capability to access clinical calculators and multimedia tools. These resources are often helpful before, during, or after the POC. Examples of online information resources for clinical calculators and multimedia tools are shown in Table 9.2. By way of example, clinical calculators used in obstetrics would be for calculating the estimated delivery date, determining the maternal body mass index, and estimating the fetal weight.

Multimedia tools include video libraries for learning about procedures (e.g., placement of nasogastric tubes, arterial line placement, arthrocentesis, and urethral catheterization), learning from simulations (e.g., interview techniques, communication with

TABLE 9.2
Examples of Online Resources Used as Clinical Calculators or Multimedia Tools

Resources	Cost	App
Clinical Calculators		
Epocrates MedTools	$	+
Dynamed Plus	$	+
MedCalc 3000	$	+
MedCalc 3000 EBM Stats	$	+
Medicine Toolkit for Academic Physicians	$	+
Medscape	Free	+
Qx Calculate	Free	+
Multimedia Tools		
ACCESS Medicine	$	–
NEJM Clinical Videos	$	–
Visual DX	$	+
Essential Evidence Plus	$	-
Medscape	Free	+

patients and other professionals), and improving in physical diagnosis and imaging interpretation (e.g., cardiac auscultation, dermatologic lesions, ultrasonography findings). One source of peer-reviewed procedural technique videos is the NEJM clinical videos series, which is available by subscription. Many medical specialty societies or associations offer access to their video libraries or forums for their members to post POC questions or cases for review and discussion.

Aid from Librarians in Accessing Online Information

Health sciences librarians, whether in the hospital or academic institution, play invaluable roles in providing information necessary for direct patient care, as well as education and research.[29] Titles and services of librarians are wide-ranging, as described in Table 9.3. A single librarian may provide many of the listed services within the library walls, at the

TABLE 9.3
Titles and Services of Health Science Librarians in Accessing Online Information Resources

Title	Service
Clinical librarian or informationist	Answer clinical questions at the point of care
Liaison librarian	Provide enhanced services to department or clinical units
Emerging technology librarian	Assist with Web site development and incorporate web 2.0 and social media tools
Scholarly communications librarian	Promote new avenues for sharing clinical and research findings

POC, and in the community. Using their knowledge and expertise, librarians evaluate and select relevant evidence-based material (books, journals, online resources) for their clientele, utilizing technologies to support the access to and dissemination of information. Instructing physicians and other health care professionals about the efficient use of these resources and technologies may take place either in person or online, in a formal or informal learning environment.

Instruction and training by health sciences librarians crosses all levels of learners from undergraduate and graduate to the practicing clinician within or outside the institution. Librarians play an integral role in teaching practice-based learning and improvement (PBLI). Acquiring these skills is particularly relevant at the POC in choosing the most appropriate resource for answering a specific question.

Electronic Health Record and Computerized Decision Support System

Given the medical problems encountered in the hospital and clinic and the rate at which new information is produced, there is a need to have updated literature to access from the health record. Infobuttons on EHRs provide easy access to many resources (e.g., UpToDate, PubMed, Dynamed) that can be time-saving. EHR vendors collaborate with librarians and health record companies in evaluating, selecting, and maintaining information resources embedded in the EHR.[9,11]

Understanding a patient's complaint can produce a list of differential diagnoses with links to diagnostic criteria and management information for each option. It requires a CDSS to be built for each specialty to support that information.[30,31] Construction of clinical decision pathways depends on evolving evidence, and CDSSs are designed to support rather than replace clinical decision-making processes. While CDSSs in several areas of medicine can be found at many hospitals and clinics, they often cover a limited range of topics and are not comprehensive. As demonstrated in randomized controlled trials, results indicate that current use of CDSSs alone is suboptimal in improving clinical solutions.[31]

Obtaining CME Credit for POC Learning

Continuing education credit is becoming more important in a physician's maintenance of certification and performance improvement. While cumbersome, CME credit can be obtained from self-directed online learning. An accredited CME provider can structure credit for practitioners undertaking online learning on topics relevant to POC practice. The process for obtaining CME credit incorporates a three-step cycle: (1) a reflective process in which the physician documents a clinical question, (2) a list of resources consulted, and (3) the application of resources to practice.[31]

To be certified for one-half (0.5) *AMA PRA Category 1 Credit*, each online cycle must meet all of the objectives listed in Table 9.4.[32] The accredited CME provider has responsibilities that include, but are not limited to, the appropriate selection and use of professional, peer-reviewed literature and some assurance that algorithms are unbiased. The CME provider must clearly instruct the physician on how to access the portal/database, which databases were vetted for use, how participation will be tracked, and

TABLE 9.4
Objectives to be Met by an Accredited CME Provider before Providing
***AMA PRA Category 1* Credit to a Physician**

- Meet all AMA core requirements for certifying an activity.
- Have an established process for the accredited CME provider to oversee content integrity.
- Provide clear instructions to the physician on how to access and use the portal/database.
- Verify physician participation by tracking the topics and sources searched.
- Provide some mechanism by which physicians can give feedback on overall system effectiveness.
- Establish a mechanism by which physicians may claim credit for this learning activity by completing and documenting the required three-step cycle.

From American Medical Association. *The Physician's Recognition Award and Credit System: Information for Accredited Providers and Physicians.* Chicago, IL: American Medical Association; 2010.

how credit will be awarded. Continuing education credit is offered through many POC resources as shown in Table 9.1. Credit is not provided by using apps for clinical calculations (Table 9.2).

Overlap in Content in POC Information and CME Offerings

There is likely a misalignment of topics warranting POC access to information resources and curricula of many CME courses. Bjerre and colleagues from the University of Ottawa highlighted differences between questions asked by physicians at the POC and the content of contemporaneous CME refresher courses as a means to identify gaps in CME offerings.[33] Implementing a system to collect POC questions from physicians should stimulate educational programs to be more relevant and serve as an efficient approach to guide professional and CME development. Clinical librarians have a deep understanding of these needs and can act collaboratively in curriculum and course design.[29]

Accessing Online Resources in Underserved Areas

Health care providers who are affiliated with well-funded institutions worldwide benefit from access to a variety of high-quality information resources to support their evidence-based practices. Clinicians not affiliated with such centers are more likely to have no or limited access to these same resources due to prohibitively high licensing costs. Not having access to easy-to-use, updated information can impair sound clinical decision-making and result in hospitalized patients being more vulnerable to a longer length of stay and a higher risk-adjusted mortality rate for prespecified conditions.[30,34,35] Conversely, online access can be of great utility to anyone anywhere. Academic health centers can serve as invaluable resources to clinicians in underserved areas, especially for those in rural, solo practice.

Primary health care practitioners who are not affiliated with academic centers, particularly those in underserved areas, often articulate a need for increased access to POC resources for speed and accuracy. For example, Eldredge et al. demonstrated the potential power of rigorous comparisons between information resources in rural New Mexico.[36] Health care providers increased their use of POC information resources when provided free access. Practitioners reported that greater use of PubMed/Medline increased satisfaction substantially in their practices. Those who used these free resources reported a reduced mean time to search for information and a higher percentage of successful searches. Lastly, providers reported a perceived change from having too little to having about the right amount of access to health-related resources.

FUTURE DIRECTIONS

Content in this chapter highlights how patient encounters generate clinical questions that occasionally require access to online resources. Leaders in CPD appreciate that more health-related information is becoming widely accessible, which should drive a greater use of online resources especially at the POC. Additional research will be directed toward how physicians access and use medical information and whether they are doing so effectively and efficiently.

Leaders in medical education and health care reform need to facilitate the strategic placement of online systems to promptly answer POC questions for better informed clinical decision-making. The future looks promising for clinical information specialists (e.g., clinical librarians, clinical informationists, bioinformationists) trained to filter and provide medical literature to aid in answering complex clinical questions. More support needs to be provided in measuring how updates in the medical literature impact patient care outcomes. Research will expand beyond documenting variations in user experience and satisfaction to examining how access to POC information resources influences quality of care and practitioner's performance improvement, health care costs, and patient experiences. These reports will apply worldwide, especially in less advanced or undeserved areas.

Advancements in technology of desk and laptop computers and mobile devices will provide greater and perhaps more user-friendly access to information for POC learning. Further research is needed to evaluate other ways of providing evidence-based practice at the bedside such as with mobile PCs on ward trolleys. Barriers to using mobile devices to find medical information will undoubtedly be less. How institutions support mobile users' clinical information needs will gain more attention.

Increases in seeking online information will need to be accompanied with greater ease in earning CME credits. Many continuing education units are not taking full advantage of the technological resources available for improving desirable learning and quality improvement. Experience from online access to medical information could also prove to be helpful in designing CME events, in encouraging more information-seeking for evidence-based practice, and in crediting practitioners for POC efforts to broaden or strengthen their knowledge.

Whether desirable or not, we also anticipate that efforts will be made to further refine and disseminate medical information in social media. Its role at the POC will likely not gain center attention but may be a source of developing questions by patients. Communication with patients will be more important, so health professionals will need to exercise judgment in interpreting relevance and accuracy of health-related information from social media.

Online technology formats for accessing medical information will gain acceptance and popularity as a means to receive "foreground" medical information. Such technology will be more widespread globally yet likely remain expensive. Therefore, effectiveness of information resources needs to be reviewed broadly from the perspective of benefitting health care systems and organizations. Mechanisms by which online resources support clinical practice will require complementary qualitative and mixed methods studies.

Finally, the role of online information resources should be to supplement and not replace clinical judgment. The growing body of accessible medical information needs cautious interpretation and applicability in decision-making. The contents and citations in POC information resources on a specific topic need continual surveillance. Critical evaluation about quality of the citations is essential for patient care to be more evidence-based. Leaders in CPD should encourage that standards be determined to minimize variation and reduce arbitrary designations in resource content for which diagnostic or management recommendations are made. Lastly, it would be helpful for such leaders to examine patient care outcomes from recommendations in answering POC questions where either information is minimal or differences are found in recommendations across resources.

REFERENCES

1. Edson RS, Beckman TJ, West CP, et al. A multi-institutional survey of internal medicine residents' learning habits. *Med Teach.* 2010;32:773–775.
2. Salinas GD. Trends in physician preferences for and use of sources of medical information in response to questions arising at the point of care: 2009–2013. *J Contin Educ Health Prof.* 2014;3:S11–S16.
3. Worster A, Haynes RB. How do I find a point-of-care answer to my clinical question? *CJEM.* 2012;14:31–35.
4. Lai CJ, Aagaard E, Brandenburg S, et al. Brief report: multi-program evaluation of reading habits of primary care internal medicine residents on ambulatory rotations. *J Gen Intern Med.* 2006;21: 486–489.
5. Duran-Nelson A, Gladding S, Beattie J, et al. Should we Google it? Resource use by internal medicine residents for point-of-care clinical decision making. *Acad Med.* 2013;88:788–794.
6. Haynes RB, Cotoi C, Holland J, et al.; McMaster Premium Literature Service (PLUS) Project. Second-order peer review of the medical literature for clinical practitioners. *JAMA.* 2006;295:1801–1808.
7. Alper BS, Haynes RB. EBHC pyramid 5.0 for accessing pre-appraised evidence and guidance. *Evid Based Med.* 2016;21(4):123–125.
8. DiCenso A, Bayley L, Haynes RB; ACP Journal Club. Editorial: accessing pre-appraised evidence: fine-tuning the 5S model into a 6S model. *Ann Intern Med.* 2009;151:JC 3-2–JC 3-3.
9. Cimino JJ. Infobuttons: anticipatory passive decision support. *AMIA Annu Symp Proc.* 2008;1203–1204.
10. Del Fiol G, Curtis C, Cimino JJ, et al. Disseminating context-specific access to online knowledge resources within electronic health record systems. *Stud Health Technol Inform.* 2013;192:672–676.
11. Fowler SA, Yaeger LH, Yu F, et al. Electronic health record: integrating evidence-based information at the point of clinical decision making. *J Med Libr Asso.* 2014;102:52–55.
12. Friederichs H, Marshall M, Weissenstein A. Practicing evidence based medicine at the bedside: a randomized controlled pilot study in undergraduate medical students assessing the practicality of tablets, smartphones, and computers in clinical life. *BMC Med Inform Decis Mak.* 2014;14:113–118.
13. Berger E. The iPad: gadget or medical godsend? *Ann Emerg Med.* 2010;56:21–22.
14. Jackson and Coker Research Associates. *Apps, Doctors, and Digital Devices* [Internet]. The Associates; 2011. http://www.jacksoncoker.com/physician-career-resources/newsletters/monthlymain/des/Apps.aspx. Accessed July 8, 2016.
15. Franko OI, Tirrell TF. Smartphone app use among medical providers in ACGME training programs. *J Med Syst.* 2012;36:3135–3139.
16. Wallace S, Clark M, White J. "It's on my iPhone": attitudes to the use of mobile computing devices in medical education, a mixed-methods study. *BMJ Open.* 2012;2:pii: e001099.
17. Payne KB, Wharrad H, Watts K. Smartphone and medical related app use among medical students and junior doctors in the United Kingdom (UK): a regional survey. *BMC Med Inform Decis Mak.* 2012;12:121–126.
18. Boruff JT, Storie D. Mobile devices in medicine: a survey of how medical students, residents, and faculty use smartphones and mobile devices to find information. *J Med Libr Assoc.* 2014;102:22–30.

19. Alper BS, White DS, Ge B. Physicians answer more clinical questions and change clinical decisions more often with synthesized evidence: a randomized trial in primary care. *Ann Fam Med.* 2005;3:507–513.

20. George DR. "Friending Facebook?"A minicourse on the use of social media by health professionals. *J Contin Educ Health Prof.* 2011;31:215–219.

21. McGowan BS, Wasko M, Vartabedian BS, et al. Understanding the factors that influence the adoption and meaningful use of social media by physicians to share medical information. *J Med Internet Res.* 2012;14:e117.

22. Von Muhlen M, Ohno-Machado L. Reviewing social media use by clinicians. *J Am Med Inform Assoc.* 2012;19(5):777–781.

23. American Society of Health-System Pharmacists (ASHP). ASHP statement on use of social media by pharmacy professionals: developed through the ASHP pharmacy student forum and the ASHP section of pharmacy informatics and technology and approved by the ASHP Board of Directors on April 13, 2012, and by the ASHP House of Delegates on June 10, 2012. *Am J Health Syst Pharm.* 2012;69(23):2095–2097.

24. American Medical Association. *Professionalism in the Use of Social Media* [Internet]; 2011 Jun [cited 2016 Jun 7]. p. 1. (AMA Code of Medical Ethics). Report No.: 9.124. http://www.ama-assn.org/ama/pub/physician-resources/medical-ethics/code-medical-ethics/opinion9124.page. Accessed July 9, 2016.

25. Wilson P, Petticrew M, Booth A. After the gold rush? A systematic and critical review of general medical podcasts. *J R Soc Med.* 2009;102(2):69–74.

26. Thapa MM, Richardson ML. Dissemination of radiological information using enhanced podcasts. *Acad Radiol.* 2010;17(3):387–391.

27. Matava CT, Rosen D, Siu E, et al. eLearning among Canadian anesthesia residents: a survey of podcast use and content needs. *BMC Med Educ.* 2013;13:59.

28. Marrocco GF, Kazer MW, Neal-Boylan L. Transformational learning in graduate nurse education through podcasting. *Nurs Educ Perspect.* 2014;35(1):49–53.

29. Marshall JG, Sollenberger J, Easterby-Gannett S, et al. The value of library and information services in patient care: results of a multisite study. *J Med Libr Assoc.* 2013;101(1):38–46.

30. Garg AX, Adhirkari N, McDonald H, et al. Effects of computerized clinical decision support systems on practitioner performance and patient outcomes: a systematic review. *JAMA.* 2005;293:1323–1338.

31. Sahota N, Lloyd R, Ramakrishna A, et al. Computerized clinical decision support systems for acute care management: a decision-maker-researcher partnership systematic review of effects on process of care and patient outcomes. *Implement Sci.* 2011;6:91–97.

32. American Medical Association. *The Physician's Recognition Award and Credit System: Information for Accredited Providers and Physicians.* Chicago, IL: American Medical Association; 2010.

33. Bjerre LM, Paterson NR, McGowan J, et al. Do continuing medical education (CME) events cover the content physicians want to know? A content analysis of CME offerings. *J Contin Educ Health Prof.* 2015;35:27–37.

34. Ely JW, Osheroff JA, Ebell MH, et al. Obstacles to answering doctors' questions about patient care with evidence: qualitative study. *BMJ.* 2002;324:710–716.

35. Isaac T, Zheng J, Jha A. Use of UpToDate and outcomes in US hospitals. *J Hosp Med.* 2012;7:85–90.

36. Eldredge JD, Hall LJ, McElfresh KR, et al. Rural providers' access to online resources: a randomized controlled trial. *J Med Libr Assoc.* 2016;104(1):33–41.

Chapter 10

SYSTEMS-BASED LEARNING *in* CONTINUING PROFESSIONAL DEVELOPMENT

Charles M. Kilo and George Mejicano

Case

Your CME committee chair, a wise and experienced family physician, says, "You know, I think we do a great job of developing CME and CPD, the kind that's directed at managing the individual patient. Diagnosing and treating heart disease in geriatrics, managing the diabetic patient—that sort of thing. What I don't think we do is teach our physicians and others about the system in which they work, how to manage it, how to improve it." He emphasizes the word "system" and then adds, "I'm not referring to understanding our health system organization and all of that, but rather how our clinical systems work, the literal systems in which we work day by day, in our clinics and in the hospital. We need to think about how we help our clinicians move toward more systems-based practice." The committee is struck by this and asks you to prepare a presentation for next month's meeting.

Questions

What is a system, and what does "systems-based practice" mean? How can you incorporate this concept into the content and mission of continuous professional development (CPD) and continuing medical education (CME)? How will thinking and planning in terms of systems help you deliver better care?

INTRODUCTION

Despite broad recognition that health care providers must embrace systems-based practices to improve outcomes, an understanding and adoption of systems competency in practice has been unfortunately slow.[1-3] In large part, this is the result of failures in training, both of new health care providers and of practicing providers, including residency program directors and faculty, through CME and CPD. This chapter explores these issues after taking a step back and answering a more fundamental question: What is a *system*?

That might not seem like a difficult or controversial question, but how one defines the word *system* serves as a lens through which systems-based practices operate. If that definition or lens is not clear, how one studies and implements systems will remain equally unclear. A clearly stated, concise definition is as follows: *A system is a set of interdependent parts that share a common purpose.*[4-7] This simple yet elegant definition has important implications for performance improvement, systems-based learning, systems-based practice, and continuing professional development (CPD). It serves as this chapter's cornerstone as it develops a deeper understanding of systems and performance improvement.

A historical context is valuable. Starting about 1990, health care transitioned from its historical focus on quality assurance to a focus on quality management and quality improvement. While this might seem like a simple change in words, it represented a paradigm shift that turned attention to understanding systems and system design, not individuals, as the determinant of outcomes—how systems work, how they are designed, and how one changes them. One phrase captured the new focus—all systems are perfectly designed to achieve the results they achieve. The conclusion should be obvious—if one wants a different "result" or outcome from the system, a change in the design of the system is necessary. Given that a system is a set of interdependent parts that share a common purpose, humans, perhaps especially, are some of those interdependent parts.

Quality assurance attempted to measure performance and hold individuals responsible, while q*uality management* acknowledged that outcomes are determined by system design with humans as parts of the system, most of whom are hardworking and well motivated. With quality management, performance improvement is not about individuals trying harder or being more motivated to succeed, but rather it is about system design and the continual improvement of these systems in which individuals work, in order that better, collective outcomes results, while simultaneously making it easier to do so.

In this definition then, the participatory role of individuals in the system is paramount: individuals make up some of the parts, and the individuals are interdependent on each other and on other inanimate parts of the system such as the electronic health record. In other words, in few if any circumstances do individuals work alone or in isolation to produce clinical outcomes. Even in a solo medical practice, physicians are interdependent with the pharmacy, the laboratory, or their staff, even if that staff comprises one medical assistant and their records and whether those records are paper based or electronic. Further, clinicians always operate in an interdependent fashion with the patient. Thus, we never really function in isolation; we always function in systems.

There are a few additional definitional items of note. Systems and processes are essentially the same thing. However, for clarity, the word "system" is employed almost exclusively. Systems are also nested within systems: for example, a large health care system may comprise many systems and several hospitals and clinics. Further, a hospital has a wide array of systems within it, and a laboratory contains many systems.

Many confuse the improvement of specific systems of work with larger, organizational discussion of how health systems themselves are designed. When it comes to performance improvement, the focus is generally on our specific systems of work, for example, the way a clinic as a system is planned, the way an accounting system is designed, or the way individuals work within an intensive care unit as a system. Larger health system design is of vital importance to societal-level outcomes, but is not as pertinent to, and for the most part not within the control of, most individuals interested in and driving continuous performance improvement.

SYSTEMS-BASED PRACTICE

The Accreditation Council for Graduate Medical Education (ACGME) in the United States further acknowledged the central importance of systems in 2001 when it included "systems-based practice" as one of its six newly described physician competencies.[8,9] ACGME intended that graduate medical education (GME) programs inculcate all six competencies into resident education. Yet more than 25 years since the shift to quality management and more than 15 years since the ACGME issued its six competencies, many health care professionals still lack a solid grounding in systems science and its application.

Systems science is the study and measurement of system function. It is the basis for quality management, quality improvement, performance improvement, systems-based practice, implementation and dissemination science, and others, all essentially synonyms. Methods used for systems improvement include the Plan–Do–Study–Act (PDSA) cycle (explored in detail in Chapter 4), which is essentially the scientific method of hypothesis testing, root cause analysis (RCA), failure modes and effects analysis (FMEA), Six Sigma, and Lean (the Toyota Production System improvement method).

The definition of a system (*a set of interdependent parts that share a common purpose*) has two primary components: a common purpose and interdependent parts. First, systems should share a common purpose. While a system and its interdependent parts should have a common purpose, that purpose is often assumed and not specified. The purpose is often not clearly articulated in a manner that orients and informs the interdependent parts. For instance, if asked, most medical practices can only provide vague notions of their common purpose. If asked the purpose, goals, or objective of a medical clinic, physicians and staff of the clinic would typically describe a general purpose such as "our purpose is to provide really great care," an expression without a clear definition or meaning. Similarly, if a physical therapy group states that its purpose is to provide the best possible customer service, it is also hard to know exactly what that means. Thus, while common purpose is critical to a system's design and performance, it is often not clearly and specifically stated.

Second, a system is made up of interdependent parts that intended to work toward the common purpose (i.e., objectives or goals). What about the *interdependent parts* of a system? As noted above, the parts may be animate (e.g., humans) such as physicians, nurses, medical assistants, pharmacists, physical therapists, laboratory technicians, administrators, and many others or inanimate items such as exam room, electrocardiograph machine, electronic health record, information technology network, pharmacy, and others.

These parts have to work together to generate the common purpose. They should preferably be intentionally designed to do so, with "intention" being much more specific a process than many may perceive. Intentionality here implies specific engineering. Just as a bridge is specifically engineered to carry a certain load of traffic, to be safe, to last for many decades, and to tolerate specific weather conditions, a medical clinic should be intentionally engineered or designed to serve a specific purpose—to care for patients in a way that produces a very specific outcomes, to create a specified patient experience, and to provide care at a particular cost level. All bridges are designed with these considerations in mind—that is, they are specifically engineered—but few medical clinics are designed in this manner. Instead, clinics, like other systems in health care, are designed based on a historical understanding of their design, not on specific engineering to produce specified results.

System planners and leaders tend to adopt historical design for reasons of familiarity using the common phrase, "That's the way we have always done things." Or, "We've always organized a clinic or an intensive care unit in this way." This design tends to lack intentionality, because most health care planners were never taught to think like engineers and to understand the work of planning as designers of specific systems to produce specific outcomes. Instead, our educational system tends to give the message that our work as individuals is to personally stay smart, work hard, and remain focused on patients. Those are good things, but they may not produce reliably better results that are sustained. Focusing on individual excellence is valuable, but individuals are parts of systems and the focus has to be on individuals as parts of the system, along with and in relationship with other parts of the system. In other words, the interdependency of the parts are as important, if not more important, than the individual parts themselves.

Bridges offer a useful analogy. A train bridge differs from a pedestrian bridge; bridges crossing a river valley differ from those which span a bay. To design an optimal bridge, architects and engineers work together with as much knowledge as possible about the purpose of the particular bridge including data traffic volumes, geological conditions, temperature variability, and much more.[10] The overall bridge is designed on paper and specifies all of the parts, their interactions, the specific construction materials, and more. The piers, foundations, cross girders, and expansion joints, for example, all have to work together to accomplish the common purpose—all are specifically designed to work together to achieve the common purpose. Each is a system unto itself that joins with the others to form the larger system of a bridge; the bridge itself is a part of a larger transportation system. If the engineers do not clearly understand what the purpose is (e.g., if they are told just to build a bridge but not that it will carry trains), there is a very good chance it will fail.

Engineers and architects think very structurally about systems. For a new system or one that is being renovated, they first develop clarity about the desired purpose and then create a design that specifies the various parts of the system and how the parts interact with each other. The common purpose of the system gives coherence to the interdependency of these components.

What lessons does bridge building have for health care? If every system is perfectly designed to achieve the result it achieves, and if health care systems tend to be more unintentionally designed based on historical concepts as opposed to specific intentional design with clear, specific outcomes in mind, systems will produce highly variable, not highly reliable, results. That is exactly what we have in health care. Poorly or highly variably performing systems are poorly designed systems. To change the outcomes, we must change the system's design.

If a system is not performing optimally, the problem might not even lie with any one specific part of the system. Every part can be well designed and meet its expectations, but how they all interact can be broken. In a health care setting, each person might be competent and well trained and have the tools he or she needs to do the job successfully, but if they are not designed to work well together, the broader system will fail. Each person in the system and each task or piece of work they do must be considered to achieve optimal outcomes. Only a carefully and intentionally designed system will achieve the desired purpose in the most efficient manner. Outcomes emerge from the interactions of interdependent parts.

SYSTEMS IMPROVEMENT

Improvement does not happen accidentally. It requires forethought, planning, and intention. Like most complex work, systems design and improvement requires training. Most people are good at picking out one or two problems within a system, usually those problems that affect them directly or annoy them most. Individuals with training in systems science will understand the "big picture"; they have a much better chance of seeing how even small changes in one part of a system can have widespread effects throughout the entire system. A system analyst will recognize not just one or two isolated problems, but also the ripples they cause throughout and the underlying design flaws potentially manifesting in seemingly disparate ways.

Variability is a natural part of system, particularly those that involve humans. Because humans behave in variable ways and because their interactions with each other are also variable (e.g., no individual and no relationship is absolutely consistent over time), the outcomes of the systems they are involved in are variable. A significant part of systems science is the study of variation and the influence of system design on variation in the system's output.

Studying system performance requires an appreciation of that variability so that a system can be monitored and improved intentionally. This is why systems science so strongly encourages standardization as a primary method of reducing variability and producing more consistently improved performance. Standardization is not about "dumbing down" the roles of health care professionals or creating "cookbook" medicine; it is about building knowledge into the system so that the system and those who work in it can more easily produce a higher-quality outcome. Standardization does not mean that everyone does everything exactly the same at all times. Rather, it means that work is done with shared, consistent practices that lead to better, reproducible results.[11]

Challenges are common to systems that have not been optimized and lack leadership that pushes systems thinking. Bergemann and Levi have described several of those challenges:[12]

- Lack of shared goals—Parts of the system focus on meeting their own goals without alignment to the broader system goals.
- Lack of shared visualization of the system—Parts of the system do not share a common view of what the system is and how it is structured.
- Lack of shared processes—Parts of the system do not share common practices, and the system lacks a way to resolve conflicts.
- Contradicting design features—Parts of the system are designed to achieve local goals but they do not integrate with other parts.

- Delayed feedback—A system does not understand and adapt to delayed outcomes of actions.
- Habits and culture—Parts of the system and perhaps the whole system resist change because of entrenched practices and organization.

Like most skills, systems science and performance improvement require training and practice. Educational programs (residency and faculty training in particular) must go beyond lectures and simple improvement projects to provide real-world experience at managing and improving systems in a strategic way that creates sustainable results. Once faculty and mentors have themselves been trained in systems-based practices, their job will be to embed those lessons in the daily experience of other learners such as residents, allowing them to see both how the system works and why that understanding is important to the routine functioning of our systems of care.

Being true systems designers and engineers, understanding how the parts of a system can be individually improved and their interactions can also be improved toward a common, shared, specified purpose(s) requires industrial-strength performance improvement methods and skills. It requires much more than an institution running a large number of nonstrategic, nonaligned, independent project. True performance improvement requires methods that involve leadership and that change the way leaders, staff, and clinicians work, think about their work, and improve their work.

Health care has been stuck in a PDSA project approach (see Chapter 4) to improvement since its inception. Instead, institutions really need methods and management system as contained within Lean to drive deep, sustained improvement. Methods such as Lean are as pertinent and applicable to and usable by small institutions such as a medical practice as they are to larger health care organizations.

FUTURE DIRECTIONS

Systems science, systems-based practice, and performance improvement all represent a discipline of understanding and managing systems geared toward consistently higher performance. Done right, they provide tools for analyzing systems and making recommendations to improve them. Improvement is not a linear path; it is not pure engineering like that of building a bridge because systems of care do contain human elements. Those trained in improvement science never know precisely which changes to the system will yield the desired outcome. Instead, trial and error over time moves a system closer to attaining desired outcomes. The goal is to make the trial and error as informed as possible.

When health care practitioners are trained in systems science, they are equipped to make informed proposals about how to improve a system. Systems science can help steer trials and suggest which changes might have the best chance to succeed. Excellence in performance requires several components: leadership, culture (mindset), infrastructure, methods, and measurement. A strategic approach to change, focusing on systems, is more meaningful than a project, nonstrategic approach over time. This concept is shown graphically in Figure 10.1.

Strategic systems planning is essential for improving health care systems and incorporating systems science. Strategic in this case means more than just making systems

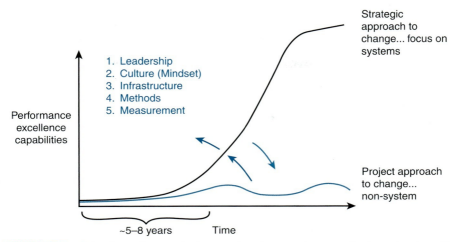

1. Leadership
2. Culture (Mindset)
3. Infrastructure
4. Methods
5. Measurement

Performance excellence capabilities

Strategic approach to change... focus on systems

Project approach to change... non-system

~5–8 years   Time

FIGURE 10.1.   Roles of strategic approaches (systems change) versus project approaches (nonsystem change) in capabilities of performance excellence.

science a priority. It must be woven into everything a health system or other organization does if excellence, clearly defined, is the goal. A large number of disconnected, isolated improvement projects rarely add up to a significant, sustainable, strategic change and excellence for an organization. Physicians and health care organizations must understand how a particular project integrates into a broader strategy to improve their work and health outcomes. Strategic planning is fundamentally about articulating the common purpose of the system, which is necessary to orient and direct the interdependent parts of the organization.

When a health system or any organization chooses the scattershot, project-based approach to improvement over strategic institutional approach, long-term improvement suffers. The earliest years of learning might not show marked difference under either a random or a strategic approach, but over time, the latter has a positive, cumulative effect. More random, project-based approaches often lead to a situation in which health professionals ultimately question why they bothered learning about something that did not become part of their daily practice.

Change requires strong leadership committed to systems science and other desired goals. Simply teaching or learning about systems-based practices without fully integrating it into the organization's daily work flow undercuts the goal. Physicians trained in systems science in undergraduate or graduate training or through CPD will be well equipped to fill those leadership roles and drive change toward this view of health care. They must begin to think of themselves not just as medical practitioners but also as managers of systems of care.

This is not a new notion; going back to the early 1990s, the idea of physicians as managers was being promulgated.[13,14] Adoption of the "physician as manager" approach, like that of systems science itself, has been slow in the medical community. If current leaders do not strategically incorporate systems science into their CPD priorities, few physicians will pursue it and become suitable managers who can improve the system. Breaking that circle requires early adopters who understand the importance of systems science and can serve as champions for it to become part of the organizational culture.

Just because current leaders are not trained in the tools of systems science does not mean they cannot be shown its value. Those early adopters who incorporate systems-based practice into the work of their teams can help educate the leadership of the broader system as to its importance. Not that success is guaranteed. In the early years of change, success often hinges on individual performance and willingness to try a new managerial structure. An example is described of a case study in a New Zealand hospital.[15]

If health care systems embrace a systems-based approach in line with the ACGME competencies, measurable changes will emerge in coming years. None of this will happen easily or immediately. Entrenched interests and individuals resistant to change will erect hurdles to what is seen as new or a deviation from the way things have been done. For this reason, the leaders of health care organizations must strategically internalize the change. They must make it a central priority that weaves through everything the organization does. If it is viewed as an isolated project, it will remain an afterthought. If it is viewed at all levels of the organization as the way to continually improve the organization based on everyone's engagement, using industrial-strength methods such as Lean, then it will help transform the organization and its results.

REFERENCES

1. Frenk J, Chen L, Bhutta ZA, et al. Health professionals for a new century: transforming education to strengthen health systems in an interdependent world. *Lancet*. 2010;376(9756):1923–1958.
2. Guralnick S, Ludwig S, Englander R. Domain of competence: systems-based practice. *Acad Pediatr*. 2010;14:S70–S79.
3. Bagian JP. The future of graduate medical education: a systems-based approach to ensure patient safety. *Acad Med*. 2015;90(9):1199–1202.
4. Institute of Medicine. *Crossing the Quality Chasm: A New Health System for the Twenty-first Century*. Washington, DC: National Academy Press; 2001.
5. Berwick DM. A primer on leading the improvement of systems. *BMJ*. 1996;312:619–622.
6. Langley GJ, Nolan KM, Nolan TW, et al. *The Improvement Guide: A Practical Approach to Enhancing Organizational Performance*. San Francisco, CA: Jossey-Bass; 1996.
7. Kilo CM, Bisognano M. Health care leadership and the improvement of care. In: Ransom SB, Pinsky WW, Tropman JE, eds. *Enhancing Physician Performance: Advanced Principles of Medical Management*. Tampa, FL: American College of Physician Executives; 2000.
8. Batalden P, Leach D, Swing S, et al. General competencies and accreditation in graduate medical education. *Health Aff (Millwood)*. 2002;21(5):103–111.
9. Dyne PL, Strauss RW, Rinnert S. Systems-based practice: the sixth core competency. *Acad Emerg Med*. 2002;9(11):1270–1277.
10. Wheeler DJ. *Understanding Variation: The Key to Managing Chaos*. Knoxville, TN: SPC Press, Inc.; 1993.
11. Bagian JP. The future of graduate medical education: a systems-based approach to ensure patient safety. *Acad Med*. 2005;90(9):1199–1202.
12. Bergemann E, Levi R. *Systems Thinking in Academic Medical Centers: Organizations as Complex Systems*. Boston, MA: MIT Sloan School of Management; 2013.
13. Hunter DJ. Doctors as managers: poachers turned gamekeepers? *Soc Sci Med*. 1992;35(4):557–566.
14. Goes JB, Zhan C. The effects of hospital-physician integration strategies on hospital financial performance. *Health Serv Res*. 1995;30(4):507.
15. Doolin B. Doctors as managers. New public management in a New Zealand hospital. *Public Manage Rev*. 2001;3(2):231–254.

Chapter 11

Meaningful Involvement *of* Patients, Families, *and* Caregivers *in* Continuing Professional Development

David Wiljer

Case

One of your CME committee members discloses that he has just been diagnosed with prostate cancer. He shares his story—an early diagnosis, the possibility of good outcomes, and reasonably good management on the part of his urologist, his oncologist, and their staff members. He does indicate, however, that there were gaps in communication, many times in which his emotional and some clinical needs were not met. He has, he says, become more of a patient advocate and less of a physician. He proposes that the CME committee—and perhaps all planning committees—incorporate using patients' input as a form of needs assessment. His comments strike home, but not all members agree.

Questions

What are the major issues in this case? Is there a role here for the committee? Do you think the committee should expand in its membership to include patients?

INTRODUCTION

Patients, families, and caregivers involved in meaningful ways in better continuous professional development have the potential to improve care, resulting in the best outcomes. The focus of this chapter will be on understanding the diverse ways patients can be involved and on exploring some particular considerations that may optimize meaningful involvement. Two key domains will be explored: (1) involving patients as partners and teachers in the continuing professional development (CPD) of health professionals and in the improvement of quality, evidence-based care and (2) improving the impact of CPD by activating patients through effective patient education.

In the era of patient-centered care, it is time to move beyond the often-asked question: do patients have a role in the continuing professional development of health professionals? Rather, this discussion will start from the assumption that patients and families should be involved in the lifelong learning cycle of health care professionals (HCPs).[1-6] As in the case study above, taking time to learn together with, for, and from patients and their families can enrich the clinical experience and professional growth. Working from this assumption, the discussion seeks to drive the conversation forward and ask the question, how do we meaningfully involve patients and families in the continuing professional development of health professionals to improve the quality of care that is delivered?[7]

The assumption that patients should be involved in CPD, of course, could be debated at great length. As the opening case study illustrates, there may be resistance when it is suggested that patients join any health care committee, especially in situations where this is not the cultural or organizational norm. This particular case study is interesting because it explores the notion that a patient joins a CPD committee to help inform the learning needs of health professionals. It is important to ask why not all members of a committee would agree that patients could help inform the needs assessment. It could simply be that some clinicians do not feel that patients fully understand their learning needs. In fact, there may be many health professionals who feel uncomfortable with patients and families being involved in continuing professional development or perhaps consider it unnecessary because of their daily clinical experiences with patients and families. In this context of daily and constant contact with patients and families, what value could be added by having patients involved in continuing professional development?

In order to explore this question, I would like to share a quick personal anecdote. Several years ago, my wife was pregnant with our second child. We were being seen in a high-risk clinic in a large academic health sciences center for several reasons including the concern that the baby had Rh disease. We were very interested in the issues around the Rh disease and had done some extensive research. We found a recent research study that seemed quite relevant to our situation. With a bit of hesitation, we decided to bring a copy of the article into the clinic. We were being seen by a medical trainee who listened as we described the study to her. A few minutes later, the attending physician came in, and as the resident was reporting status, she mentioned the paper we had brought in. What happened next had a profound impact on me personally and professionally. The attending physician asked to see a copy of the paper. As he read it, he asked us if we had a few minutes to meet with other members of the clinic, and when we said "yes," he went out and asked members of the team to come into the clinic room for a *knowledge exchange clinical huddle*. We all reviewed the paper together and then discussed the findings from a number of different interprofessional perspectives including the patient perspective. The rich discussion ultimately informed a better, evidence-informed decision. This kind of *knowledge exchange clinical huddle* involving patients certainly takes some time, but creates an invaluable *in situ* learning experience that may improve the quality of evidence-based care a patient receives.

It is important to acknowledge that the involvement of patients and families in health professions education has been part of the health professions practice and teaching for many decades.[8] The involvement, however, has not been consistent across health systems, organizations, or different health professions. Some countries and regions have promoted the idea of patient involvement. In the United Kingdom, for example, there are mandates and expectations for the involvement of patients and families in the "everyday practice in the National Health Service (NHS) and must lead to action for improvement," which includes the training of health professionals.[5] There are some professions, such as nursing, that have focused more on the involvement of patients than other professions.[9] In addition, much of the work that is being done to involve patients and families is initiated at the early stages of professional formation, such as the undergraduate, graduate, or postgraduate levels.[3,10]

There has been less focus on the involvement of patients and families in continuing professional development than in other areas of health professions education. In one systematic review of patient involvement in health professions education, 19 studies were identified that involved patients in undergraduate education, 7 studies in postgraduate education, and 2 in continuing professional development—both of these studies involved the education of family practitioners.[10] In another study, 41 studies were identified involving patients in health professions education: 30 focused on preregistration and 11 on postprofessional registration.[11]

In CPD, patients or patient advocacy groups do at times partner with HCPs in planning events together that address common goals and priorities. In one example, HCPs and cancer survivorship advocacy groups came together to establish common priorities and discuss professional development and educational opportunities.[12] Continued and sustained collaborations and partnerships between patient groups and HCPs could fundamentally alter how CPD events and activities reflect common and agreed-upon priorities that align with both professional and patient needs and values.

CPD providers also integrate patient experiences through the use of standardized patients (SPs). Standardized patients are trained actors who utilize predetermined patient scenarios in the education and assessment of HCPs. The majority of studies report the use of SPs in the training of medical and nursing students and trainees.[13] In the majority of studies, SPs have been employed in teaching and assessing communication and clinical skills.[13] In CPD, SPs have been integrated into the teaching and assessing of clinical skills, reflective practice, communication around sensitive or difficult issues, empathic responses, and the development of counseling skills.[14] Although there is growing evidence regarding the impact of SPs on HCPs, this is still an emergent practice. The use of SPs may be used to improve HCP skills, but this practice should not necessarily be seen as equivalent to involving patients themselves into CPD. Patient involvement in SPs could be achieved by including patients in the development of patient scenarios.

WE ARE ALL TEACHERS AND WE ARE ALL LEARNERS

The integration of learning and teaching experiences has the potential to create a positive, experiential, dynamic, interactive, bidirectional, engaging, and relevant approach to exchanging knowledge. The same notion creates a fundamental dissonance or, at least, some challenges to the training models of health professions that are based on professional standards and explicit and hidden curricula that lead to professional formation.[15] If we are all teachers and learners, when do we teach and when do we learn? How does this duality become actualized in the structures of education and providing care. Who are the teachers? Who are the learners? What is the role of the patient in the learning? What is the role of the patient in teaching? The earlier example of the *knowledge exchange clinical huddle* illustrates the power of the democratization of learning in the clinical context. At the same time, it raises important issues around who has power and who controls the learning agenda, who is the authority, and what is the source of "truth" in a clinical encounter in which roles, responsibilities, hierarchies, and decision-making accountabilities are often held sacred and perceived as immutable.

In the early part of the last century, William Osler articulated that "there should be no teaching without a patient for a text, and the best teaching is that taught by the patient himself."[16] In 2011, the UK-based Health Foundation issued a report asking: Can patients be teachers? *Involving Patients and Service Users in Health Professions Education.*[5] This report lays out a clear roadmap to the involvement of patients in health professions education and offers guidance in addressing barriers and optimizing facilitators for meaningful patient involvement. The report finds that "significant cultural change may be required within institutions as patient/user involvement becomes embedded"[5] despite finding numerous examples of excellent work and evidence of the potential impact of involving patients in health professions education. The reality is that despite a century of conversation about involving patients, the field of HCP education is still addressing basic and fundamental issues around what the role of patients should be in the education, formation, and continued professional growth and development of health professionals.

UNDERSTANDING THE ROLES OF PATIENTS IN HEALTH PROFESSIONS EDUCATION

Defining Terms

One of the first issues that often surfaces in involving patients in health professions education is nomenclature. Over the years, there have been many debates around how to refer to the individuals who receive service. A number of terms have been considered from patients to clients, consumers, service users, experts by experience, etc.[17] The shift in nomenclature to a certain extent reflects the changing attitudes and roles of individuals in health care over the last several decades: a shift from a more passive role to a more active one in self-management and in decision-making. The shifts in nomenclature also reflect the issues of different health care domains. The language used in one domain of health or in one profession does not necessarily capture the issues in other domains or professions. For example, the discourse and language used in mental health may not be appropriate or resonate in other areas such as oncology or cardiology. In addition, the language needs to reflect not only the individual receiving care, but the circle of carers, family members, or members of support systems who have important roles to play in delivery of health care. For the purposes of this discussion, the term patient will be used for those who receive care and those who support them. The language is intended to be inclusive and respectful, acknowledging that nomenclature requires conversation in interactions between providers and service users.[18]

The issue of nomenclature also raises questions around how to refer to patients who are involved in health professions education. There are a number of ways and degrees to which patients can be involved in education activities. As the involvement increases, the roles become more nuanced and overlapping. This may be especially true as partnerships develop and become more complex. Also, if a patient has a professional role in the health professions, such as is the situation with the case for this chapter, the lines between patient and health professional become blurred. In our case, the CPD member "has become more of a patient advocate and less of a physician." The intersection of personal and professional identify is key to consider within this context. Individuals will identify themselves in different ways in different situations. Some individuals will completely separate their professional and personal identities, some will choose to assume different roles at different points in the conversation, and others will simply recognize the complexity of their experiences, without differentiating roles. In achieving meaningful involvement, it is essential that the individuals have the autonomy to define their roles and to have discussions to address assumptions or preconceived notions. In the context of the case, it may be tempting for the committee to appoint this particular CME member as their patient representative. In this case, it would be important to have an open and transparent conversation about how that would impact the individual, the committee, and other patients who may want different types of representation on the committee.

In order to begin to address these complexities of patient involvement, it has been suggested that patient teaching roles be described, defined, formalized, and legitimized. Some studies have adapted the language of patient instructor,[3,19] patient teacher, or patient supervisor. Happell et al. have argued that *consumer academic positions* should be explored in order to further promote patient involvement.[6] At the minimum, it is recommended that, in developing a relationship with patients who are involved in teaching, ample time be spent discussing with patients how the roles should be described and what language is preferred in referring to the role. The roles should be negotiated in order to foster a true and equitable partnership.

From Tokenism to Meaningful Involvement

Many health professionals recognize the importance of involving patients in the education and training of HCPs, especially when it comes to students and trainees.[5] However, there are many issues in involving patients in a meaningful way (see Table 11.1). Involving patients in education activities does not follow a clearly defined pathway or process, but stems more from preexisting relationships, rather than an application or in-take process. Health professions educators may ask one or two patients to share their personal experience: this may be a patient that the clinician has known for a long period of time or a patient who has done well or has an inspired story. This experience can be very positive, but it also raises some challenges and runs the risk of being *tokenistic* either in perception or reality. Often, patients are chosen because they are recognized by conference organizers as good speakers or have very powerful or moving experiences to share with the group. In some cases, patients may express a very specific experience or focus on a particular

Stakeholders	Some Questions to Consider
	TABLE 11.1 **Reflective Questions to Consider in Involving Patients in Education Activities**
HCP educators	• How do you select or recruit patient teachers? • Should you recruit your own patients or patients you have seen in the past? • How do you compensate patient teachers appropriately? • In which type of teaching activities do you involve patient teachers? • How do you navigate and negotiate diverse views that may not reflect the teaching or values of the curricula?
Patient teachers	• How do you prepare patient teachers? • What are the competencies and accountabilities of the patient teachers? • How do you provide any required support before, during, or after the education activity? • How do you address ethical issues that may arise? • How do you manage clinical or therapeutic issues that may surface?
Learners	• How do you prepare students to optimize learning? • How do you cocreate and negotiate mutually agreed upon code of conduct? • How do you address ethical or support issues that may surface in from experiences shared by patient teachers?

issue. Focusing on one experience can leave learners with a very narrow perspective, especially if the topic is new for the learner. If only one patient will be included in the educational activity, the educators must reflect carefully on how the experience is presented, contextualized, and discussed by the learners. There are many approaches that can be employed to contextualize individual experiences. Other perspectives can be introduced through case-based discussions, videos of patients, social media, etc. in a respectful, deliberate, and meaningful manner.

Developing and Cocreating Productive Interactions

Involving patients in a meaningful way requires the development of collaborations and partnerships between the patients, health professions educators, and learners. Wagner identified the importance of productive interactions between patients and health care providers in the management of chronic diseases.[20] In describing his model for chronic care, Wagner argues that in order for better health outcomes to be realized, an engaged, activated, and informed patient must come together with a prepared, proactive provider to create a productive interaction.[20]

It is useful to think of a similar model for involving patients in a meaningful way in the education of HCPs. In both the care and educational settings, patients must be activated and informed so that they can relate their own personal experiences to the learning goals, objectives, curricula, and educational activities. Patients should have a clear idea of their role in the teaching and the intended outcomes of their involvement. The patient's perspectives may be very different from those of the HCPs, and if patients are properly informed, they can relate their own experiences and perspectives to address the learning objectives. At the same time, students should be prepared in advance for the experience and have the opportunity to debrief the experience. Studies involving patients in teaching have identified the importance of ensuring that learners are properly equipped to integrate the patient experience into their own learning.[3,6] This process requires proactive and prepared HCP educators who have the skills and self-efficacy to ensure that the patient involvement is properly integrated into the learning environment and evaluated to ensure that the intended results are being achieved.

Enabled and activated patients, prepared students, and proactive HCP educators can ensure a productive interaction and ideally one that is coconstructed or coproduced. The shift to cocreating and coproducing educational experiences both with the learners and with patients to establish equal learning partnerships has been an important trend in health care and medical education over the last several years. The notion of coproduction stems from a systems-level approach to improve the delivery of health services to meet the needs of the service users and has developed particular traction in some parts of the NHS in the United Kingdom. Within this context, cocreation has been defined as "delivering services in an equal and reciprocal relationship between professionals, people using services, their families and their neighbours. Where activities are coproduced in this way, both services and neighbourhoods become far more effective agents of change."[21] The concept of coproduction in the educational context is very similar. Coproduction connotes the development of relationships in which partners have equal and reciprocal roles with shared responsibilities and accountabilities (Fig. 11.1).[22] It fundamentally changes the flow of information and knowledge for learning and creates a bidirectional flow in which accountability for learning must be shared.

The educational experience can be coconstructed in many different ways: between the HCP educator and learner, the HCP educator and patient, or the patient and learner or between all three (Fig. 11.2). In the education context, this multifaceted concept has several layers of complexity to it that must be considered. Within this context, patients and HCP educators would work together to achieve an equal partnership. There are practical considerations that pose barriers to the formation of such partnerships. These barriers include time and resources, but they also include issues related to existing curriculum, competen-

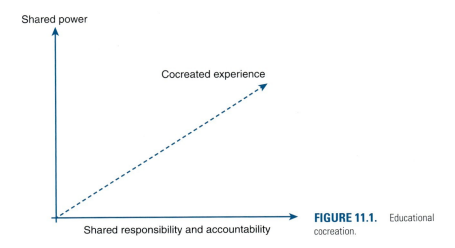

Shared power

Cocreated experience

Shared responsibility and accountability

FIGURE 11.1. Educational cocreation.

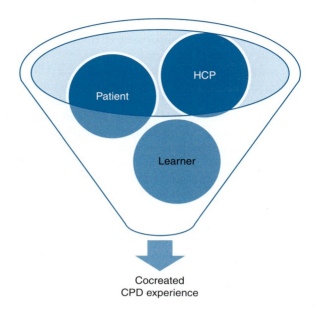

FIGURE 11.2. Potential cocreators.

Cocreated
CPD experience

cies set by regulating bodies, and issues related to assessment. These issues may be less of a barrier in CPD than in other contexts such as undergraduate and postgraduate educational settings. In fact, CPD offers a fertile environment to explore the idea of cocreation and the development of equal partnerships where HCPs and patients and their families can learn and teach together to improve the quality of care. This creation of equal partnerships does require the adoption of a framework or model in which power and control are shared and negotiated. This negotiation requires conversations and the building of relationships so that equal partnerships can develop in a healthy, respectful, and productive way.

Developing Equal Partnerships

The development of equal partnerships requires a transformational shift in the approach to health professions education: the shift of learning from patients to being taught by patients. As witnessed by Osler's famous quote, the idea of learning from patients is well rooted in the tradition of health professions education. The patient has been, in the words of Osler, the *text* from which lessons should be learned. In involving patients as teachers, the role fundamentally shifts to an active role in which patients impart and transfer knowledge. Embedded in our case for the chapter is the suggestion that the patient should inform the assessment of need. Developing the role of patient as teacher goes well beyond informing the needs assessment or providing input into what should be taught, although these are important steps along the way. By considering the role of patient as teachers, the spectrum of involvement could be much broader. In the example of the informal knowledge exchange huddle, all participants are learning together with the evidence, not the patient, as the text. Within this new paradigm, patients may actively drive, to varying degrees, the development of goals, objectives, curricula, delivery, and assessment. This new role for patients, their families and caregivers has significant implications for the future of CPD and the lifelong learning of health professionals in which they learn as much from patients as they learn for the benefit of their patients.

WHERE IS THE PATIENT VOICE IN MEDICAL EDUCATION?

The question has been asked, where is the *patient voice* in the health professions education? Involving patients in health professions education has not been the norm or the standard, although it is happening more and more. The question has been, at its core, more of a call to action that reflects a changing landscape of health care in which the movement toward patient-centered care and patients as partners have been reframing the discourse of health care and, to varying degrees, its delivery. This shift in care models has changed the role of patient as educator not only in the delivery model of health care but also in the training of health professionals. The notion of actively involving patients has developed significantly in undergraduate, graduate, and postgraduate training in several disciplines including nursing and medicine. The focus has been on involving patients in the formation of our next generation of HCPs.

The change in practice has been witnessed by the emergence of international conferences specifically devoted to the question of *Where Is the Patient Voice* in HCP education. One of the first conferences to address the question was held in 2005 in Vancouver[2] with a second held 10 years later in 2015 and giving rise to a number of similar forums around the world. This movement has served to bring together patients, family members, patient groups, students, health professions educators, administrators, and researchers from schools of medicine, nursing, pharmacy, occupational therapy, social work, and other related disciplines to accelerate the integration of patients and their families into the training of HCPs.[2]

Roles of Patients in CPD: Ladder of Involvement

The involvement of patients in the education of HCPs can vary widely. The type of activity can range both in the role that patients play in the education process and in the level of engagement they have in those activities (passive vs. active roles).[8,23,24] There are a number of ways in which patients can be involved in medical education: (1) introducing case-based approaches, (2) scripting clinical-based scenarios, (3) sharing personal experiences and relating personal or individual perspectives, (4) contributing to teaching or assessing, (5) coteaching and assessing, and (6) directing curricular development and shaping the overall educational experience. These roles have largely been developed in response to the experience of health professions students and trainees.

There are many potential avenues to expand the involvement of patients and their families in CPD: (1) informing needs assessments, (2) sitting on committees, (3) speaking about personal experiences, (4) assessing and providing feedback, (5) delivering and developing curricula, (6) contributing to accreditation, (7) directing education programs and setting standards, and (8) contributing to research. Each of these activities requires different levels of involvement and contributions. As our case suggests, there is an important opportunity for patients to contribute to the development of CPD activities, by informing needs assessments, identifying gaps in care, and providing unique perspectives through informal and/or formal mechanisms such as surveys, focus groups, or interviews and conversations. In addition, CPD providers can partner with patient groups to cocreate priorities and develop programs to address gaps or emerging needs. Patients, patient representatives, or family members can be invited in a more formal way to be part of CPD planning committees and provide feedback into program content and activities.

CPD programs may include various opportunities for patients to share their personal experiences. Patients are often invited to share experiences either in person or through video, and this may be the most common type of involvement.[3] Patients may be asked to be involved based on their ability to convey powerful messages that encourage HCPs to reflect on key aspects of care such as patient safety, patient experience, etc. or based on inspirational and powerful narratives that encourage HCPs to engage in reflective practice. Programs have also been developed to bring patients into the workplace. Kidd et al. developed an innovative program to bring former patients on inpatient psychiatry wards back to the units to share their narratives and experiences about what it was like to be on the unit.[25] The evaluation of the speaker series demonstrated an impact on the attitudes and knowledge of staff with respect to recovery-oriented mental health care.[25] The study also reported an increased sense of "hope for clients" as well as a sense of hope for the impact that the clinicians have on the recovery of the clients.[25] These types of interventions can have an important impact on the ongoing professional development of HCPs and raise awareness with respect to important issues and gaps in care that patients may experience.

Patient involvement can also extend to activities and roles that are more commonly filled by HCP educators. These types of roles, for example, can include providing feedback or assessing the skills of HCPs. Patients have been involved in teaching and in assessing general practitioners.[10] There are also opportunities to involve patients and family members in the ongoing assessment of clinical, psychotherapeutic, and communications skills. In preregistration education, there are several examples of patients participating in curriculum development.[6,26] In curricula in which patients participated, Happell et al. identified increased emphasis on interpersonal skills, acceptance of experience and difference, continuity of support, avoiding jargon, and openly sharing information.[6] The infusion of different perspectives at both the curriculum development and administrative levels through cocreated content, strategy, and policy could have meaningful impact on the relevance to clinical setting and the patient experience. Involving patients and family members in conducting, assessing, and peer-reviewing CPD research and evaluation and its impact in improving knowledge, attitudes, behaviors, and outcomes could significantly shape the research questions and focus of CPD research, leading to an evidence base for CPD that is closely aligned with patient priorities.

There are many benefits that have been identified in involving patients in the training of health professionals. The benefits for learners include a better understanding of the patient experiences and perspectives, an opportunity for feedback from patients themselves, a reduction in anxiety in working with patient populations, an improvement in attitudes toward patients, improved clinical skills, and an increase in respect for the patients that they are serving.[10] The benefits for patients have also been well documented in the literature. The benefits for patients include an opportunity to share their experiences in a positive context to make a difference in the attitudes and perceptions of health professionals, a sense of validation of personal experience, and an increase in knowledge and personal skills.[10] There can also be an improvement in the understanding of the health professional perspective and an opportunity to help future patients.[10]

Some studies have also explored the impact on the HCP educators. The benefits for the HCP educators include capacity building, the development of mutual understanding, the creation of new learning experiences, and the development of new advocates within the discipline.[27] While studies have explored the benefits of involving patients in health professions education, they have focused heavily on the experience of the learners, patients, or health professions trainers and changes in attitudes. There is very little evidence with respect to changes in behaviors and health outcomes at the individual, organizational, or systems level.[11]

One area that is particularly underdeveloped in the literature and CPD health professions education is the utilization of digital information and communication technologies. There are many opportunities to enhance the ability of patients to become involved in CPD and address barriers to participation by exploring technology solutions. Video is already frequently used to provide a vehicle for patients to share their personal experiences. Organizations like DIPEx International have created databases of patient narratives and developed research methods for better understanding the role of narrative in knowledge exchange and health professions research.[28–30] There are additional opportunities such as tele- and videoconferencing to reduce the need for patients to travel long distances to participate in CPD activities. Patients can become involved in CPD through participation in digital networks, discussion boards, and online communities of practice. There are opportunities to involve patients in online CPD activities as moderators and commentators, especially through the use of video. Social media also creates the opportunity for patients to become involved through participation in blogs and social interactions such as Twitter. There is, however, limited evidence in terms of how best to utilize technology to facilitate patient involvement in HCP CPD, and this is an area that should be explored in more depth through both CPD practice and research.

In fact, many questions do remain in terms of how best to involve patients in CPD. Regan de Bere and Nunn have attempted to address the complexity of involving patients in health professions education and have called for the development of a "pedagogy" of patient and public involvement in HCP education.[31,32] Addressing the complexity of involving patients and the public in HCP education requires the development of frameworks, tools, and practices that will promote systematic implementation and rigorous evaluation approaches. Tew et al. have developed a good practice guide by the NHS for the implementation of patients roles in teaching in the health professions entitled, *Learning from Experience: Involving Service Users and Carers in Mental Health Education*.[24] By further developing the pedagogy of patient involvement in HCP, this area will become its own domain with CPD much like course delivery, accreditation, and assessment. This new domain will form the basis for new directions in CPD and create new opportunities for intersectionality with clinical practice.

ROLE OF PATIENT AS TEACHER

Many patients or service users see education as an opportunity to make a difference, whether the desire is fuelled by a positive or negative experience in the health care system. Patients with a desire to make change through teaching health professionals may, however, face many challenges. Individuals may want to get involved and not know where to start. They might be approached by an HCP educator and be unsure about when to say yes to an opportunity and under which set of conditions. They may not feel comfortable teaching HCPs. Many programs do report developing formal or informal training opportunities to assist patient teachers.[3] There are some programs that have demonstrated positive training results with the addition of formally providing instruction on teaching.[3,6,19,26,33]

As Spencer et al. have pointed out, there is no "right way" to involve patients in HCP education,[5] but there are several issues that do need to be addressed. The chapter has already explored issues related to language and tokenism. Patients themselves may be concerned about being the sole patient voice and concerned that they are being asked to speak for all patients or represent a patient community that is not well defined. Clear and transparent approaches need to be developed to include patients in educational activities. Depending on the level of involvement, the issues that may arise include roles and responsibilities, reporting structures, accountabilities, and expectations for the roles. In addition, there are issues related to logistic, contractual issues, sustainability, and funding.[5,6] In some organizations or health care domains, patient involvement is perceived as a volunteer role and presented as an opportunity for patients to "give back" or to have an opportunity to share a different perspective that would lead to change in the delivery of care. Some patients may feel that if they are paid by an organization, they are giving up their autonomy or ability to be critically minded on sensitive issues or gaps in care. There are others, however, who advocate for the equitable acknowledgment of the commitment and expertise that patients bring to the role. From a CPD perspective, clear guidelines and sharing of best practices would help to remove uncertainty that often exists in involving patients in activities.

THE ROLE OF PATIENT EDUCATION IN CPD

The concept of patient education is not necessarily often associated with CPD in medicine or the health professions. Patient education is focused on ensuring that patients have the information, education tools, and support to understand and be involved in their own care if they so choose. Patient education is an essential element in ensuring productive interactions between providers and patients that is at the heart of Wagner's model of chronic care.[20] By providing patients with education and specifically addressing issues of health literacy, patients may be activated to become more engaged partners in their care. As patients become more knowledgeable and engaged, they may develop a sense of self-efficacy or confidence that they could make a valuable contribution to the formation and development of health professionals. Secondly, within the framework of the Wagner model, part of the potential impact of professional development is to promote the formation of proactive and prepared providers who can have productive interactions with activated patients. CPD therefore should focus not only on what a provider needs to know about a specific issue to change practice but also on supporting patients to acquire new knowledge and change their behaviors. In this approach, patients become potential agents of change in accelerating the translation of knowledge into practice.

Defining Patient Education

Patient education is the deliberate engagement and involvement of the patient and family in the process of care. Patient education has been framed as "any set of planned educational activities, using a combination of methods (teaching, counselling and behaviour modification), that is designed to improve patients' knowledge and health behaviours."[34] There is emerging evidence suggesting that patient education can have significant impacts on the patient experience and, in many cases, patient outcomes.[35,36] Having the right knowledge will transform the role of a patient from a passive one to an active one in which patients are better able to participate in all aspects of their care. The degree of participation varies greatly depending on the context and can change over time depending on health status, state of readiness, interest, motivation, etc.

An essential goal of patient education is to improve health literacy and change behaviors to improve health outcomes. The World Health Organization (WHO) defined health literacy to link it to knowledge as well as health behaviors, stating that it is "the cognitive and social skills which determine the motivation and ability of individuals to gain access to, understand and use information in ways which promote and maintain good health."[37-40] By focusing on patient education and health literacy, providers can enable and encourage patients to be more involved in their care and in the decision-making process. Involving patients through an equal partnership can result in shared decision-making. Shared decision-making is "an approach where clinicians and patients share the best available evidence when faced with the task of making decisions and where patients are supported to consider options, to achieve informed preferences."[41] There are many tools that can assist in the promotion of shared decision-making such as decision aids. Decisions aids provide "information interventions that help clients to understand the pros and cons of a medical decision and may also include exercises to help the client clarify their own values and preferences."[42] There are opportunities to build the education and engagement of patients into the scope of CPD to improve the ability of providers to participate in these activities. CPD activities could better equip HCPs to build the patient education, engagement, and shared decision-making into their practice as they acquire new knowledge and incorporate the new knowledge into their practice and care for their patients.

FUTURE DIRECTIONS

There are many benefits and opportunities for involving patients in CPD. The involvement of patients is evolving in medical and health professions education, but it is still a relatively new area in continuing professional development, and therefore, there are many opportunities in CPD. First, CPD should increase the involvement of patients in the development and delivery of educational activities as part of practice improvement, behavior change, and impact on patient outcomes. The case presented at the beginning of this chapter explores the idea of including patients on committees to identify learning needs. This is a very important first step in initiating the conversations around patient involvement. Including patients in planning committees could become a standard of CPD practice and create pathways for involving patients in the full range of education activities from identifying needs to developing and delivering curriculum and assessing outcomes.

In order to facilitate the integration of patient involvement into good CPD practice, guidelines should be developed. Guidelines could address ethical issues such as involving current and former patients, compensation, issues related to working with vulnerable populations, addressing trauma-informed approaches to working with patients, and understanding the importance of cultural competencies and cultural humility. These guidelines could help to normalize involvement so that patients can have a stronger voice in medical and health professions education.

Patient education and engagement should be built into the planning and delivery of CPD activities. As part of accrediting CPD activities, objectives and goals should be developed to ensure health care providers have the knowledge and skills to ensure productive interactions with their patients. CPD providers should extend the focus of activities to include what patients need to know as well as what providers need to know and better equip health care providers to engage and involve patients in the change process.

There are many remaining questions about how to meaningfully involve patients and their families in CPD activities. A gap in the literature as well as practical knowledge has been identified. There is a need to focus on developing better research and evaluation mechanisms that will guide CDP in the evolution of this field. Involving patients and their families in these new research and evaluation activities will be essential to the success of responding to the needs of both patients and providers. Developing productive interactions will enable the field of CPD to move beyond the question of whether patients should be involved and begin to examine how best to optimize the involvement of patients in all aspects of the continuing professional development of HCPs.

REFERENCES

1. Spencer J. Patients as teachers. *Clin Teach.* 2008;5(3):131–132.
2. Towle A. Where's the patient's voice in health professional education? *Nurse Educ Pract.* 2006;6(5):300–302.
3. Repper J, Breeze J. User and carer involvement in the training and education of health professionals: a review of the literature. *Int J Nurs Stud.* 2007;44:511–519.
4. Jha V, Quinton ND, Bekker HL, et al. Strategies and interventions for the involvement of real patients in medical education: a systematic review. *Med Educ.* 2009;43(1):10–20.
5. Spencer J, Godolphin W, Karpenko N, et al. *Can Patients be Teachers? Involving Patients and Service Users in Healthcare Professionals' Education.* London, UK: The Health Foundation; 2011.
6. Happell B, Byrne L, Mcallister M, et al. Consumer involvement in the tertiary-level education of mental health professionals: a systematic review. *Int J Ment Health Nurs.* 2014;23(1):3–16.
7. Ruitenberg CW, Towle A. "How to do things with words" in health professions education. *Adv Health Sci Educ Theory Pract.* 2015;20(4):857–872.
8. Towle A, Bainbridge L, Godolphin W, et al. Active patient involvement in the education of health professionals. *Med Educ.* 2010;44:64–74.
9. Renkert S, Nutbeam D. Opportunities to improve maternal health literacy through antenatal education: an exploratory study. *Health Promot Int.* 2001;16(4):381–388.
10. Wykurz G, Kelly D. Developing the role of patients as teachers: literature review. *BMJ.* 2002;325(7368):818–821.

11. Morgan A, Jones D. Perceptions of service user and carer involvement in healthcare education and impact on students' knowledge and practice: a literature review. *Med Teach.* 2009;31(2):82–95.
12. Bender JL, Wiljer D, Matthew A, et al. Fostering partnerships in survivorship care: report of the 2011 Canadian Genitourinary Cancers Survivorship Conference. *J Cancer Surviv.* 2012;6(3):296–304.
13. May W, Park JH, Lee JP. A ten-year review of the literature on the use of standardized patients in teaching and learning: 1996–2005. *Med Teach.* 2009;31(6):487–492.
14. Weaver M, Erby L. Standardized patients: a promising tool for health education and health promotion. *Health Promot Pract.* 2012;13(2):169–174.
15. Hafferty FW, O'Donnell JF. *The Hidden Curriculum in Health Professional Education.* Lebanon, NH: Dartmouth College Press; 2015.
16. Roter D, Hall JA. *Doctors Talking with Patients/Patients Talking with Doctors: Improving Communication in Medical Visits.* Westport, CT: Praeger; 2006.
17. McLaughlin H. What's in a name: 'Client', 'Patient', 'Customer', 'Consumer', 'Expert by Experience', 'Service User'-What's Next? *Br J Soc Work.* 2009;39(6):1101–1117.
18. Wing PC. Patient of client? If in doubt, ask. *CMAJ.* 1997;157(3):287–289.
19. Gall EP, Meredith KE, Stillman PL, et al. The use of trained patient instructors for teaching and assessing rheumatologic care. *Arthritis Rheum.* 1984;27(5):557–563.
20. Wagner EH. Chronic disease management: what will it take to improve care for chronic illness? *Eff Clin Pract.* 1997;1(1):2–4.
21. Boyle D, Harris M. *The Challenge of Co-production.* London, UK: New Economics Foundation; 2009
22. Hanson JL, Randall VF. Advancing a partnership: patients, families, and medical educators. *Teach Learn Med.* 2007;19(2):191–197.
23. Spencer J, Blackmore D, Heard S, et al. Patient-oriented learning: a review of the role of the patient in the education of medical students. *Med Educ.* 2000;34(10):851–857.
24. Tew J, Gell C, Foster S. *Learning from Experience: Involving Service Users and Carers in Mental Health Education and Training.* Nottingham, UK: Higher Education Academy/NIMHE/Trent Workforce Development Confederation; 2004.
25. Kidd SA, McKenzie K, Collins A, et al. Advancing the recovery orientation of hospital care through staff engagement with former clients of inpatient units. *Psychiatr Serv.* 2013;65(2):221–225.
26. Masters H, Forrest S, Harley A, et al. Involving mental health service users and carers in curriculum development: moving beyond 'classroom' involvement. *J Psychiatr Ment Health Nurs.* 2002;9(3):309–316.
27. Bandman BM, Bandman CE, Pennell N, et al. Patients as real time teachers. *J Cancer Educ.* 2007;22(2):131–133.
28. Herxheimer A, Ziebland S. The DIPEx project: collecting personal experiences of illness and health care. In: Hurwitz B, et al. *Narrative Research in Health and Illness.* Oxford, UK: Blackwell Publishing Ltd.; 2004:115–131.
29. Herxheimer A, Ziebland S. DIPEx: fresh insights for medical practice. *J R Soc Med.* 2003;96(5):209–210.
30. Ash JS, Cottrell E, Saxton L, et al. Patient narratives representing patient voices to inform research: a pilot qualitative study. *Stud Health Technol Inform.* 2015;208:55.
31. Anderson MB. Patient and public involvement in medical education: is a new pedagogy necessary? *Med Educ.* 2016;50(1):8–10.
32. Regan de Bere S, Nunn S. Towards a pedagogy for patient and public involvement in medical education. *Med Educ.* 2016;50(1):79–92.
33. Hanson B, Mitchell DP. Involving mental health service users in the classroom: a course of preparation. *Nurse Educ Pract.* 2001;1(3):120–126.
34. Friedman AJ, Cosby R, Boyko S, et al. Effective teaching strategies and methods of delivery for patient education: a systematic review and practice guideline recommendations. *J Cancer Educ.* 2011;26(1):12–21.
35. Bastable SB. *Essentials of Patient Education,* 2nd ed. Burlington, MA: Jones & Bartlett Learning; 2016.
36. Redman BK. *The Practice of Patient Education: A Case Study Approach.* St. Louis, MO: Mosby Elsevier; 2007.
37. Nutbeam D. Health literacy as a public health goal: a challenge for contemporary health education and communication strategies into the 21st century. *Health Promot Int.* 2000;15(3):259–267.
38. Nutbeam D. Advancing health literacy: a global challenge for the 21st century. *Health Promot Int.* 2000;15(3):183–184.
39. Nutbeam D. The evolving concept of health literacy. *Soc Sci Med* 2008;67(12):2072–2078.
40. Hoffman-Goetz L, Donelle L, Ahmed R. *Health Literacy in Canada: A Primer for Students.* Toronto, ON: Canadian Scholars' Press; 2014.
41. Elwyn G, Laitner S, Coulter A, et al. Implementing shared decision making in the NHS. *BMJ.* 2010;341(7780):971–973.
42. Adams JR, Drake RE. Shared decision-making and evidence-based practice. *Community Ment Health J.* 2006;42(1):87–105.

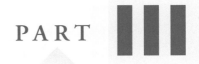

PART **III**

BETTER FACULTY, BETTER CONTENT, BETTER OUTCOMES

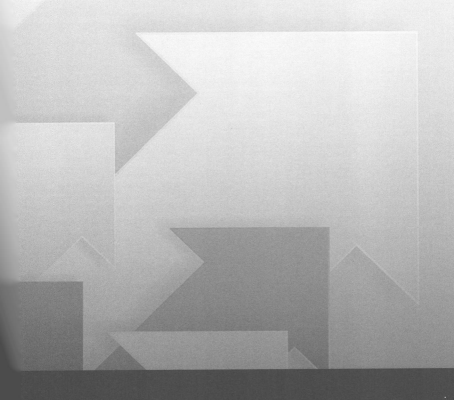

ENGAGING SCHOLARS *and* ADVANCING SCHOLARSHIP *in* CONTINUING PROFESSIONAL DEVELOPMENT

Tanya Horsley and Sharon Straus

Case

Your unit has recently sponsored a number of CME/CPD innovations, including new program formats and instructional techniques. Lessons from these changes have the potential to advance the science and practice of CPD (through knowledge translation into the clinical world and elsewhere). However, few, if any, of the faculty or staff in your unit feel that they have the time or expertise to design and conduct a study, evaluate outcomes, or write papers describing the results.

Questions

What can be done to enable and advance scholarship capacity of a unit? What strategies can be implemented to transition innovations into successful scholarship? How does scholarship relate to continuing professional development?

INTRODUCTION

Most educators would support the principles that scholarship contributes to building a strong scientific foundation and that it is imperative to integrate new discoveries into practice and policy. Scholarship as originally defined by Boyer includes four overlapping yet distinct types: (1) discovery (identifying new knowledge), (2) integration (connecting knowledge across disciplines), (3) application (bringing theory into practice), and (4) teaching (bridging teachers' knowledge and students' understanding).[1] For nearly three decades since, scholars have advocated to redefine the vocabulary of "scholarship" and the activities that define it. Boyer's framework has most notably been lauded for expanding and validating the career and academic options of educators.[2] Troubled by the lack of agreement for the meaning of "the scholarship of teaching" and the question of how the quality of scholarship should be measured, Glassick et al.[3] popularized six standards to be applied specifically to all four forms of scholarship proposed by Boyer. The standards were resultant from data collected from a diverse set of sources including granting agencies, scholarly press directors, and journal editors and include (1) clear goals, (2) adequate framework, (3) appropriate methods, (4) significant results, (5) effective presentation, and (6) reflective critique.[3]

Inspired by the original case example (turning practice into scholarship), this chapter presents common definitions of scholarship and describes the importance of scholarship for advancing the science and practice of continuing medical education/continuing professional development (CPD). Given the increasing entanglement of CPD and domains of knowledge translation (KT), patient safety (PS), and quality improvement (QI), this chapter also provides a very brief description for where each conceptually intersects. Recognizing that the act of "turning practice into scholarship" is easier said than done, strategies for enabling, promoting, and reinforcing the practice of scholarship are also provided. Finally, future needs and directions are proposed.

SCHOLARSHIP

As the discipline of medical education matures, conversations in its major publications characterize, challenge, and expand Boyer's original vision of the academy. One recent example extends Boyer's more traditional framework to include standards that document and evaluate faculty scholarship.[4] This conceptual framework includes six qualitative standards of a scholar's published work that include setting clear goals, ensuring adequate preparation, appropriate methods, significant results, effective presentation, and reflective critique.[4] Here, recommendations for faculty evaluation advocate for the inclusion of emerging genres of reporting such as a statement of responsibilities, a biographical sketch, and documented samples of the scholar's unpublished work (e.g., presentation abstracts).

Motivated by a desire to professionalize education scholarship for the purposes of promotion and academic advancement of clinical faculty, Van Melle and colleagues offered a highly inclusive definition of education scholarship to be "...an umbrella term...encompassing both research and innovation in health professions education. Quality in education scholarship is thus attained through work that is: peer-reviewed, publicly disseminated and provides a platform that others can build on."[5] This chapter is not categorical of any one definition, choosing instead to promote inclusivity that allows many forms of scholarship to be represented. What constitutes scholarship and the metrics in which individuals are subjected for promotion are often predicated by the policies and structures imposed by the institutions in which individuals are situated themselves.

SCHOLARSHIP AND CONTINUING PROFESSIONAL DEVELOPMENT

What could scholarship in CPD look like and what do you need to do to foster and develop it? Boyer is widely cited but often difficult to interpret; given this tension of familiarity and applicability, this section uses his four common pillars (discovery, integration, application, and teaching) to illuminate and provides examples for the multifaceted nature of CPD scholarship.

The *scholarship of discovery* aligns with more traditional activities of academia: generating knowledge that results in peer-reviewed publications, presentations at meetings, competitive awards and grants, and mentorship of junior faculty. The scholarship of discovery seeks to answer questions such as "What is not yet known?" As a result, publication often includes describing empirical research. However, beyond the more traditional forms of "research," the scholarship of discovery could also include methodological or historical activities, theory development or testing, and philosophical inquiry and analysis.[6] What does a methodological research paper look like? What is an example of the scholarship of discovery within CPD? Table 12.1 provides a select

TABLE 12.1
Examples of Scholarship for Each of Boyer's Four Domains

Scholarship Domain	Definition	Sample Citations
Discovery	The scholarship of discovery seeks to answer questions such as "What is not yet known?" and can include methodological or historical research, theory development or testing, and philosophical inquiry and analysis.	1. The effect of continuing professional development on public complaints: a case–control study (Wenghofer EF, Campbell C, Marlow B, et al. *Med Educ.* 2015;49(3):264–275)[7] 2. Smoking cessation: a community-based approach to continuing medical education (Shershneva M, Cohen A, Larrison C, et al. *Transl Behav Med.* 2014;4(4):391–397)[8]
Integration	The scholarship of integration is described as the synthesizing tradition and expects the scholar to fit localized innovations (isolated facts) into broader intellectual patterns and discourses to develop deeper, more authentic meanings of knowledge or data.	1. How to create conditions for adapting physicians' skills to new needs and lifelong learning (Horsley T, Grimshaw J, Campbell C. Ed: WHO Regional Office for Europe and European Observatory on Health Systems and Policies, 2010 Policy Brief 14)[9] 2. Dissemination of an innovative mastery learning curriculum grounded in implementation science principles: a case study (McGaghie WC, Barsuk JH, Cohen ER, et al. *Acad Med.* 2015;90(11):1487–1494)[10]
Application	Discovering of ways that new knowledge can be used to solve real-world problems	1. Continuing professional development and social accountability: a review of the literature (Fleet LJ, Kirby F, Cutler S, et al. *J Interprof Care.* 2008;22(suppl 1):15–29)[11] 2. The effects of aviation-style nontechnical skills training on technical performance and outcome in the operating theatre (McCulloch P, Mishra A, Handa A, et al. *Qual Saf Health Care.* 2009;18(2):109–115)[12]
Teaching	Scholarship of teaching seeks to innovate approaches and identify best practices to develop skills and disseminate knowledge. It could include informal/formal teaching, advising, and mentoring.	1. Fostering education scholarship: the mentored research group (Goldszmidt MA, Zibrowski EM, Watling CJ. *Med Educ.* 2009;43(11):1084–1085)[13] 2. Evolving curriculum design: a novel framework for continuous, timely, and relevant curriculum adaptation in faculty development (Lieff SJ. *Acad Med.* 2009;84(1):127–134)[14]

sample of previously published work for each form of scholarship and should serve to stimulate ideas.[7-14]

The *scholarship of integration* is frequently referred to as the synthesizing tradition and expects a scholar to fit localized innovations (isolated facts) into broader intellectual patterns and discourses to develop deeper, more authentic meanings of knowledge or data.[1] In this way, the scholarship of integration seeks to answer questions that ask "What do the findings mean?"[1] Given the intersection of CPD with multiple other disciplines, the scholarship of integration can materialize in the form of curricula, grant applications, technical reports, consensus documents, and media briefings among others. Areas of inquiry could explore questions pertaining to phenomena of inter- and intradisciplinary education programs, the completion of complex knowledge syntheses, or policy analysis.

Boyer describes the *scholarship of application* (also known as the scholarship of engagement) as a highly dynamic interaction between theory and practice and often seeks to answer questions that ask "How can new knowledge be responsibly applied to consequential problems?"[1] To this end, the scholarship of application produces policy or best practice that can be disseminated to influence change or be evaluated by peers. It differentiates good citizenship (attending committee meetings) from dynamic scholarly activities that deeply align with one's specialty of knowledge and as a result advance learning and ways of knowing reciprocally.[15,16]

Knowledge constructed through the act of teaching constitutes the *scholarship of teaching*.[1] In its simplest form, teaching can be thought of as a reflection of what the teacher knows; a transmission of knowledge, ideas, concepts, and processes intended to bridge the knowledge chasm between teacher and student–learner—a logical fallacy. At its best, teaching is a communal dialogue in which questions and ideas are exchanged, not transmitted, between teacher and student.[1] Successful teaching promotes innovation, extends opportunity for debate, and creates spaces where teachers become learners. Physicians, educators, and faculty are at the front lines of teaching innovation and curricular reform. They should be encouraged to seek and share novel teaching approaches that can be discussed and challenged through the review of peers. Stories of success, for example, should be presented locally or in environments external to their origins. Of the four forms of scholarship Boyer proposed, the scholarship of teaching is arguably the most contended, particularly as it has remained the most challenging to assess for quality standards.[17]

These multiple forms of scholarship expand the questions and outputs available to scholars. Within CPD specifically, scholarship has expanded beyond traditional hierarchical approaches that idolize a "gold standard" of knowledge production, for example, via a randomized approach. Contemporary thinking now seeks to identify and align scholarly approaches and questions to appropriate methods, assessments of feasibility, existing theories, best practices, and principles. These ideas become increasingly important when considering the complex and challenging questions scholars in CPD will be asking.

Implementation of wide-scale educational innovations like competency-based CPD makes the prospects of turning practice and innovations into scholarship highly compelling, particularly scholarship evaluating and monitoring CPD plans, recording and tracking conclusions from practice experiences, and practice- or workplace-based assessments.[18] Other areas of focus include inter- and intraprofessional/team-based learning and care, the use of practice data for identifying learning needs (audit and feedback for individuals, teams, and systems), innovative formats for delivering educational activities (e.g., the role of in situ simulation), and, in particular, patient outcomes and organizational and system-based change.

There are so many important questions to be asked and answered in CPD and many more theories to emerge; but any one discipline can only advance in so far as it is able to influence others beyond what is gleaned within the local learning environment.[17] This act of "giving back to the CPD" is powerful and further falsifies the expectation that only those seeking tenure, for example, can contribute to or advance a field.

CONCEPTUAL ENTANGLEMENT OF CPD, KNOWLEDGE TRANSLATION, QUALITY IMPROVEMENT, AND PATIENT SAFETY

Failures in health care are abundant, and improving quality of care and reducing adverse events are galvanizing forces for scholarship in CPD.[19] However, the goal of improving patient care, reducing adverse events, and applying knowledge to improve health and the health system is not exclusive to CPD. Conceptually CPD intersects, interacts, and relates to some extent with three other academic disciplines: KT, PS, and QI. Health professionals and educators are important connectors between scholarship and patient care. Thus, CPD can be seen as complementing and collaborating—even unifying these powerful discourses and disciplines to advance the health of all citizens.

CPD has been defined in many ways, but at its core, it embodies both professional learning and personal growth.[20] It incorporates much of the theory and practice of adult learning, self-directed learning, reflective practice, and other models. It also offers the possibility of embracing topics beyond those included in traditional medical education—for example, bioethics, business management, and communication skills—topics rarely included in continuing medical education (CME) programs.[19]

Numerous authors have expressed confusion about the concepts of KT, knowledge transfer, knowledge exchange, research utilization, implementation, diffusion, and dissemination.[21] Gaining wide acceptance is the definition proposed by the Canadian Institutes of Health Research that defines KT as "the exchange, synthesis and ethically-sound application of knowledge—within translation a complex system of interactions among researchers and users—to accelerate the capture of the benefits of research for Canadians through improved health, more effective services and products, and a strengthened health care system."[22] CPD shares several core values with KT, specifically a desire to narrow the knowledge gap of health care providers through distinctly evidence-based medicine traditions. Furthermore, as KT is less learner driven than CME and CPD, it permits a greater emphasis on initiatives to improve population health such as screening, early diagnosis, and preventive measures.[20]

Fundamentally, QI approaches consist of systematic and continuous actions that lead to measurable improvement in health care services and the health status of targeted patient groups. Said differently, it has been defined as "combined and unceasing efforts of everyone—healthcare professionals, patients and their families, researchers, payers, planners and educators—to make the changes that will lead to better patient outcomes (health), better system performance (care) and better professional development."[23]

Finally, PS has been defined and conceptualized in many ways.[24] While several influential definitions exist, the World Health Organization defines it as "the prevention of errors and adverse effects to patients associated with health care. While health care has become more effective it has also become more complex, with greater use of new technologies, medicines and treatments."[25]

CPD, KT, QI, and PS are distinct, but as each area matures and advances, they increasingly share common rhetorical and conceptual paradigms. The areas of conceptual intersection have been described previously and include (1) a shared mission (collaboration and patient care), (2) interdisciplinary stakeholders, (3) a shared change agenda with a focus on positivist research, and (4) a shared concern over sustainability and context specificity.[26]

Greater understanding of each specific area and how they relate will allow for greater clarity and dialogue among between scholars and promotes the likelihood that those concepts from one area will be integrated into other scholarly work and into practice (scholarship of integration). To operationalize this idea, an extract articulating these connections between CPD/CME and QI within the context of Maintenance of Certification (MOC) is provided:

> "MOC provides a powerful tool that the academic educational community can use to achieve its explicit goals of linking CME activities with QI activities. Connecting organizational education, quality, and community service goals with MOC support and credit will help ensure the quality of the MOC experience, achieve organizational goals, and provide a benefit for the faculty member. Activities performed in relationship to the ACGME Clinical Learning Environment Review Program and to the Association of American Medical Colleges' (AAMC's) Aligning & Educating for Quality program provide examples of work that could potentially link with the MOC program."[27]

INTENTIONAL SCHOLARSHIP IN CPD

The desire to increase the production of high-quality CPD scholarship amplifies the paucity of scholarly work in your environment. What strategies can engage and enable CPD scholarship and what role can leadership play? At the outset, it is important to acknowledge that turning CPD innovations into publishable scholarship requires intentionality and planning. CPD scholars commonly address an innovation or change in practice too distal (retrospectively) from the activity making it difficult, and sometimes impossible, to publish and disseminate. This "lack of planning" is a well-known issue, and busy faculty and staff who desire to be scholarly are encouraged to intentionally reflect, scan their environment (for patterns or phenomena), and think critically about what it is they do each day. Two core ideas that contribute to a culture of engaged scholarship include encouraging active scanning and creating a mentorship culture.

Active Scanning

Continuous scanning and reflection promote the identification of scholarly innovations more readily—particularly given the unique position physicians, educators, and other potential scholars have at the forefront of CPD and associated activities (e.g., audit and feedback, group learning, academic detailing). For example, every patient or trainee encounter is the opportunity to ask a question or to challenge assumptions about theories (Does this follow an expected pattern?). Some of these questions may already be answered within the literature and instead could lead to the scholarship of integration (using information generated within another discipline), implementation work, or identifying a need for a summary of current literature.

Useful steps for developing a scholarly question are readily available[28]; allow passion to be a guide—what about your practice or environment keeps you up at night? What drives you to "look something up" in the literature? Given the enormous time and resource demands scholarship requires, choosing something that you are deeply curious about contributes to the likelihood that you will sustain interest through to publication or dissemination. Here lies the importance of approaching scholarship with intention and reflection that then leads to an important next step—using theory or frameworks to refine your question (What scholarship domain am I inquiring within?) and then negotiating the most appropriate method. Those new to CPD scholarship can use the many reference guides available that outline the "how to" of scholarship as an initial step.[29–33]

Mentorship

Creating a mentorship culture is crucial for engaging and advancing scholarship; really good scholarship is rarely produced in complete isolation. For staff, particularly early career scholars, it is vitally important they seek and connect to a senior mentor to help guide scholarly developments.[34] One component of a mentorship culture involves understanding what a good mentorship relationship looks like. The authors of Medical Education Scholarship: An Introductory Guide (AMEE Guide No. 89) have carefully curated a series of "best practices" a mentee should consider, given the competing time demands placed on potential mentors[28] (Table 12.2). These best practices include (1) active listening and reflection (both mentor and mentee), (2) spending time on the relationship (developing mutual trust), (3) understanding the mentor role (differentiate between mentor and coach), (4) setting boundaries (it is not about finding a friend), (5) providing focus (identify a program of scholarship), (6) establishing support networks (engage mentors to build and foster networking opportunities), (7) understanding promotion and tenure requirements (what does success look like?), and (8) viewing mentoring as a journey not an absolute (mentorship is not a predefined role). Simple in their connotation, these best practices are often difficult to operationalize. Ask a busy clinician, educator, or researcher to recount the greatest barrier of academic productivity, and, not surprisingly, you will find that it universally relates to time management.[35–38]

TABLE 12.2 Suggested "Best Practices" and Mentorship[a]		
No.	**Best Practice**	**Information**
(1)	Listen	Key feature. Listening and reflection can help and contribute to guiding career direction. Mentors should be mindful that not all mentees will choose to follow their advice.
(2)	Spend time on the relationship	Increasingly challenging in academic climates. Identify and commit time to meet.
(3)	Understand the mentoring role	Coaching and mentoring are not analogous. Mentors provide longitudinal support across several pursuits. Schedule time, even without an obvious agenda.
(4)	Set boundaries	It is not about being "friends." Setting boundaries allows for needed feedback, which may be critical at times. Be explicit about roles and expectations (e.g., credit for scholarship).
(5)	Provide focus	A good mentor will help a mentee say "no" to projects that are not feasible or are a poor fit of the mentees long-term goals.
(6)	Establish support networks	Building research capacity through network building is important. Mentors can help identify other scholars and experts. Establishing networks allows the mentor to "fade the scaffolding" of support for the mentee.
(7)	Be mindful of promotion and tenure requirements	Mentor's advice for long-term success needs to account for short-term milestones. Mentors are essential to help navigate this journey.
(8)	Mentoring as a "journey"	Here, scholarly output is not prioritized; instead, the focus is on building a trustful relationship, sharing expertise, providing moral support, and knowing when to advance to independence.

[a]Information applicable from the perspective of the mentee and as adapted from AMEE Guide No. 89; recommendations derived from article authors' experiences and synthesis of qualitative information.[27]

CPD SCHOLARSHIP AS AN IMPERATIVE

Research and scholarship have had profound effects on the way CPD is modeled and delivered. There is agreement that initial certification obtained at the end of residency training is no longer adequate to sustain quality care across a physicians' career; the "once in, good for life"[39] model has been successfully challenged by longitudinal studies showing that physicians benefit from well-structured educational programs and approaches to their learning.[7,40,41] To this end, medical regulators now view participation in CPD as a professional obligation and the role of assessment to identify unperceived needs in light of convincing evidence demonstrating self-assessment is ineffective without feedback and observation.[42]

New knowledge, thus, challenges CPD to continuously reorganize and reinvent itself. The necessity to identify and attract clinically—and educationally—focused staff and faculty to CPD is met with greater importance and urgency. What can be done to build an extensive and sustainable base of CPD scholars? Cultivating a culture of scholarship locally is an important component of a complex solution.

TOWARD A CULTURE OF SCHOLARSHIP

There are no magic bullets or simple solutions that ensure scholarly productivity. Scholarship is a multifaceted, social activity with no one singular contributing factor. Without question, scholars themselves are the key ingredient in any successful scholarly pursuit; however, institutional factors can greatly influence and determine academic outputs. The complexity of environments in which scholarship is expected to occur further complicates matters; changing to a scholarly environment will be met with many significant barriers that will need to be prevailed.[43,44] These change management barriers aside, there are a number of key factors that have been identified as greatly influencing academic outputs: (1) establishing clear goals that serve as a coordinating function (set a plan in motion), (2) a distinctive culture of research emphasis with assertive participation, (3) frequent communication, (4) accessible resources, and (5) leadership with expertise in skill.[45,46]

Given the heterogeneity of departments and institutions in which CPD scholarship occurs, systematic solutions are not summarized; as an alternative, we highlight that many champions already exist and have been positive forces for change to great success.[47–51] While success is resultant of many interconnected factors, programs often share common values such as the existence of intramural funding support, mandated scholarship, mentorship programs of junior faculty, networking activities through a community of scholars, and, finally, formal systems for multiple forms of scholarship that includes recognition through awards and promotion tracks.[46]

Assessing Readiness for Scholarship

Transforming to a culture of scholarship requires asking important questions and developing solutions (e.g., who can I partner with in my department or faculty?) to advance to a (more) desirable state. Organizational readiness for change is considered a critical precursor to the successful implementation of complex changes.[52] What questions can you ask to assess the readiness for scholarship within your own unit? Using Bolman and Deal's "Four Frames" as an organizing strategy, Chan TM summarizes important questions that individuals could ask when assessing your environment and draws attention to key factors toward success.[53] Questions are categorized against four particular domains of inquiry: (1) structural (Does the organization structure support scholarship? Is there a Director, Education Scholarship?), (2) human resources (Do you have individuals with the appropriate level of expertise?), (3) political (Who holds the power to affect change?), or (4) symbolic (Is the scholarly mission of the department clear and consistent with other priorities?). These factors are however, not stable; examining and reexamining the environment should be a continuous exercise (e.g., when you renew or refresh your strategic plan) and is key.[53]

FUNDING SCHOLARSHIP IN CPD

Medical education scholarship is now globally recognized as a discipline unto itself with distinct scientific challenges than those in other biomedical sciences.[54–58] These scientific challenges become increasingly important for funding scholarship in CPD. First, CPD research projects historically fall outside the scope of calls from funding agencies targeted at health outcomes making funding opportunities, particularly for multisite or collaborative projects, difficult to identify and harness.[55] Second, given the influx of scholars into health professions education through newly minted health terminal-degree programs, direct funding opportunities for medical education research appear to be more competitive than some of the most hard-fought medical research grants.[58,59] As a result, seemingly low-quality medical education research is conducted and disseminated in the absence of sufficient funding.[60,61]

Given that the substantive cuts in federal funding for research have impacted most universities, realizing a sophisticated funding infrastructure for CPD scholarship will require novel partnerships, formidable energy, and resources at all levels.[62] In the interim, early findings examining the impact of intramural funding have demonstrated promising and important impacts. A relatively modest investment by institutions (perhaps $40,000) can lead to matched funding, catalyze applications for larger funding programs (e.g., National Institutes of Health), and result in presentation at conferences and publication in peer-reviewed journals.[63] Establishing an "in-house" or institutional funding mechanism to stimulate grant writing can also have important impacts beyond receiving the funding itself. The act of writing a grant is powerful for mobilizing researchers to seek collaborations, promotes experiential learning, strengthens the writing process, and is valuable for subjecting both the idea and approach to peer review.

These small seed grants also play an important role for making educational scholarship visible and can be seen as a surrogate measure of support from leadership to advance an institutions' mission. The impact of establishing funding as well as implementing it can foster a culture of scholarship among the administration as well. In a recent commentary, Albanese shares a powerful narrative concerning the diffusion of impact of grants across an environment "...*the Dean can cite a tangible program supporting faculty innovation in medical education, the hospital director can speak of a concrete way in which he is supporting innovation in residency education, and the (sic) Medical Foundation can point to ways it is supporting education.*"[63]

FUTURE DIRECTIONS

This chapter illuminates the variability under which the term scholarship is defined and provides information for how to engage and advance scholarship when there seems to be little interest or resources to do so. Many pathways to productivity exist, and the task for CPD scholars will be to provide the foundational insights needed to mentor and support successful scholarship not necessarily to define the right one.

To foster and promote a culture of scholarship, CPD directors and leaders should create strong change management strategies. A good strategy is two pronged and begins with assessing an environment's readiness for change. Assessing readiness involves raising and answering simple yet fundamental questions about available resources, stakeholders, and potential partners. The process of assessing readiness is not constrained to local perspectives; setting a national or international agenda for CPD scholarship would follow a similar process of stocktaking and resource identification. In this context, many stakeholders play a role in CPD scholarship, and through authentic partnership, these stakeholders could join to assess a countries' readiness for scholarship. The process would seek to identify and categorize resources and stakeholders, assess the political climate (who holds what power to effect change), and articulate a collaborative mission. This particular assessment is distinctly systems-based and could foster multi-institutional collaborations and data-sharing agreements, reduce redundancy, and establish a plan for national funding.

For the foreseeable future, the Holy Grail of CPD scholarship will continue to evaluate and estimate the effectiveness of maintaining physician competence and impacts on patient-related outcomes. CPD scholars are now also exploring emerging topics such as social accountability, systems-based learning, and health informatics. These areas of inquiry give credence to multiple forms of inquiry and approaches and are perceived to be highly complementary to more traditional experimental designs. As a community, CPD scholars have raised questions that expand the concept of CPD and challenge core assumptions in the field. These questions are increasingly complex and draw on multiple theories, perspectives, methods, and information.

Attracting staff and faculty who approach scholarship using varying theoretical paradigms, epistemologies, and methodologic approaches should be a priority. The diversity is an essential ingredient for examining underlying assumptions of CPD to unearth a deeper and more comprehensive understanding than could be provided by any one approach alone. These diverse approaches will stimulate new questions and challenge conventional wisdom. CPD has benefited from strong scholars; however, the discipline will be made richer when a critical mass of individuals (across institutions and countries) are committed to raising and answering diverse sets of questions that draw on multiple ways of knowing to advance the science and practice of CPD.

As staff and faculty produce new knowledge across journals (e.g., *Journal of Continuing Education in the Health Professions*), bibliographic databases (e.g., PubMed), and social media outlets (e.g., Twitter—#meded) for example, the role that networks of CPD scholars, associations, and international groups could have in identifying, conducting, and disseminating information comes into question.[64] Critical summaries of evidence afford scholars a unique vantage point for examining a body of literature deeply to, among other things, identify patterns in research, prioritize future research questions, and have the potential to influence policy and decision-making. With so few resources to support their production, leadership from all facets of CPD will need to come together to harness the unrealized potential of strategic partnerships. Global partners could include synthesis groups (e.g., Best Evidence Medical Education, Campbell Collaboration, and Cochrane Collaboration), associations (e.g., Association for Medical Education Europe, Canadian Associate for Medical Education, etc.), and both the private and public sector groups to establish priorities and reduce redundancy.

Creating a mentorship culture is crucial for engaging and advancing scholarship in any environment. This chapter has provided a set of factors that should be considered when establishing and engaging in a mentor/mentee relationship. With multiple competing priorities even when mentorship dyads are established, time becomes a hurdle not easily overcome. Linking senior faculty and full-time researchers with novice scholars is a challenge particularly in historically nonacademic environments. Providing recognition or awards for exemplary mentorship collaborations may be one mechanism to ignite interest. Future CPD programs will succeed when they leverage technologies that facilitate and promote opportunities to link senior faculty or educators with medical students, residents, or staff interested in raising and answering questions within the context of CPD. Scholars in isolated environments, away from resources and peers, are encouraged to build capacity beyond their local context by establishing or integrating into e-networks (e.g., MedEdWorld, Canadian Association for Medical Education [CAME], Society for Academic Continuing Medical Education [SACME]).

Geographic boundaries have disintegrated due to advances in digital technologies and social media that have given rise to virtual communities (e.g., chat rooms, mailing lists, Web sites). These virtual communities can be synchronous or asynchronous and are designed to establish new partnerships, translate and disseminate new knowledge, pilot test educational innovations and peer review (e.g., crowd sourcing), and extend dialogue across a community. These networks have the potential to reshape the landscape of scholarship in CPD of the future and could be used to develop relationships between regulators, service providers, scholars, and other members to provide education or shared work spaces for cocreated scholarship.

Protected time for scholarship has been identified as a key factor associated with scholarly productivity.[30] However, even when time is protected through grant funding, for example, a common complaint from our colleagues involves skepticism that protected time for CPD research will ever actually be a reality. This time-limited approach is impossibly difficult and may be contributing to the paucity of scholarship and research that gets presented at conferences yet never enters into mainstream literature.[65] To this end, alternative payment plans (APPs) will be important to consider in future. These APPs currently exist for faculty members in most settings globally, most often for those in group settings with the multifaceted requirements—teaching, research, administration, and clinical care. Derived from clinical practice remuneration sources, APPs are frequently augmented by contributions from deans' offices, health system leadership, research overage, and other sources. In most APPs, incentives are added for achievements considered desirable by the academic environment (e.g., publication). In the future, it is conceivable—in fact highly likely—that those incentives will be added to the payment model to reward activity that leads to health system improvements. The argument can be made that CPD research can lead to such outcomes and improvements.

Finally, the future holds greater promise when CPD scholars and policy makers work in tandem to develop strategic priorities and conduct scholarship to advance the science of CPD. An important step forward is to establish partnerships at all levels (local, regional, national, and international) to reduce silos and stimulate scholarly efficiencies to advance the discipline. For example, creating an environment that helps to connect full-time researchers (who often struggle to find pathways to connect to CPD faculty, students, or health professionals) and CPD professionals (at the front line of educational innovations) may be an important and academically profitable alliance. Further to this point, the chasm that exists between new knowledge and its use practice may actually be increasing. Organizations and associations can play a critical role in bridging this divide by engaging scholars through engagement and cocreation (integrated KT). Leadership within organizations must take an active role in identifying individuals and networks of scholars to work in authentic partnership to define research priorities in CPD, cocreate scholarship, and establish a sophisticated dissemination model that leverages the various intersections of influence and points of entry into systems for which they can act as champions and true levers for change.

REFERENCES

1. Boyer EL. *Scholarship Reconsidered: Priorities of the Professoriate*. Princeton, NJ: Carnegie Foundation for the Advancement of Teaching; 1990.
2. Sherbino J. Education scholarship and its impact on emergency medicine education. *West J Emerg Med*. 2015;16(6):804–809.
3. Glassick CE. Boyer's expanded definitions of scholarship, the standards for assessing scholarship, and the elusiveness of the scholarship of teaching. *Acad Med*. 2000;75(9):877–880.
4. Glassick CE, Huber MR, Maeroff GI. *Scholarship Assessed: Evaluation of the Professoriate. Special Report*. San Francisco, CA: Jossey-Bass; 1997.
5. Van Melle E, Curran V, Goldszmidt M, et al. *Toward a Common Understanding: Advancing Education Scholarship for Clinical Faculty in Canadian Medical Schools. A Position Paper*. Ottawa, ON: Canadian Association for Medical Education; 2012.
6. American Association of Colleges of Nursing. *Defining Scholarship for the Discipline of Nursing*. 1999. http://www.aacn.nche.edu/publications/position/defining-scholarship. Accessed June 19, 2016.
7. Wenghofer EF, Campbell C, Marlow B, et al. The effect of continuing professional development on public complaints: a case–control study. *Med Educ*. 2015;49(3):264–275.
8. Shershneva M, Cohen A, Larrison C, et al. Smoking cessation: a community-based approach to continuing medical education. *Transl Behav Med*. 2014;4(4):391–397.
9. Horsley T, Grimshaw J, Campbell C. *How to Create Conditions for Adapting Physicians' Skills to New Needs and Lifelong Learning*. Report No.: 14. 2010.
10. McGaghie WC, Barsuk JH, Cohen ER, et al. Dissemination of an innovative mastery learning curriculum grounded in implementation science principles: a case study. *Acad Med*. 2015;90(11):1487–1494.
11. Fleet LJ, Kirby F, Cutler S, et al. Continuing professional development and social accountability: a review of the literature. *J Interprof Care*. 2008;22(suppl 1):15–29.
12. McCulloch P, Mishra A, Handa A, et al. The effects of aviation-style non-technical skills training on technical performance and outcome in the operating theatre. *Qual Saf Health Care*. 2009;18(2):109–115.
13. Goldszmidt MA, Zibrowski EM, Watling CJ. Fostering education scholarship: the mentored research group. *Med Educ*. 2009;43(11):1084–1085.
14. Lieff SJ. Evolving curriculum design: a novel framework for continuous, timely, and relevant curriculum adaptation in faculty development. *Acad Med*. 2009;84(1):127–134.
15. Hofmeyer A, Newton M, Scott C. Valuing the scholarship of integration and the scholarship of application in the academy for health sciences scholars: recommended methods. *Health Res Policy Syst*. 2007;5:5.
16. Calleson DC, Jordan C, Seifer SD. Community-engaged scholarship: is faculty work in communities a true academic enterprise? *Acad Med*. 2005;80(4):317–321.
17. Ruth-Marie EF, Work JA. Perspectives on the scholarship of teaching. *Med Educ*. 2006;40(4):293–295.
18. Campbell C, Silver I, Sherbino J, et al. Competency-based continuing professional development. *Med Teach*. 2010;32(8):657–662.
19. Institute of Medicine of the National Academies. *Redesigning Continuing Education in the Health Professions*. Washington, DC: The National Academies Press; 2010.
20. Davis D, Evans M, Jadad A, et al. The case for knowledge translation: shortening the journey from evidence to effect. *BMJ*. 2003;327(7405):33–35.
21. Graham ID, Logan J, Harrison MB, et al. Lost in knowledge translation: time for a map? *J Contin Educ Health Prof*. 2006;26(1):13–24.
22. Canadian Institute of Health Research KT. *Knowledge Translation—Definition*. http://www.cihr-irsc.gc.ca/e/29418.html. 2016. Accessed June 8, 2016.
23. Batalden PB, Davidoff F. What is "quality improvement" and how can it transform healthcare? *Qual Saf Health Care*. 2007;16(1):2–3.
24. Mitchell PH. Defining safety and quality care. In: Hughes RG, ed. *Patient Safety and Quality: An Evidence-Based Handbook for Nurses*. Rockville, MD: AHRQ Publication No. 08-0043; 2008:1–5.
25. World Health Organization. *Patient Safety*. 2016. http://www.euro.who.int/en/health-topics/Health-systems/patient-safety. Accessed June 8, 2016.

26. Kitto S, Bell M, Peller J, et al. Positioning continuing education: boundaries and intersections between the domains continuing education, knowledge translation, patient safety and quality improvement. *Adv Health Sci Educ Theory Pract.* 2013;18(1):141–156.

27. Nora LM, Pouwels MV, Irons M. Expanding educators' contributions to continuous quality improvement of American Board of Medical Specialties maintenance of certification. *Acad Med.* 2016;91(1):16–19.

28. Crites GE, Gaines JK, Cottrell S, et al. Medical education scholarship: an introductory guide: AMEE Guide No. 89. *Med Teach.* 2014;36(8):657–674.

29. Gusic M, Amiel J, Baldwin C, et al. Using the AAMC toolbox for evaluating educators: you be the judge! *MedEdPORTAL Publications.* 2013;9:9313.

30. Ahmed R, Farooq A, Storie D, et al. Building capacity for education research among clinical educators in the health professions: a BEME (Best Evidence Medical Education) systematic review of the outcomes of interventions: BEME Guide No. 34. *Med Teach.* 2016;38(2):123–136.

31. Hautz SC, Hautz WE, Feufel MA, et al. What makes a doctor a scholar: a systematic review and content analysis of outcome frameworks. *BMC Med Educ.* 2016;16(1):119.

32. Royal College of Physicians and Surgeons of Canada. *CanMEDS 2015 Physician Competency Framework.* 2016. http://canmeds.royalcollege.ca/en/framework. Accessed June 8, 2016.

33. Bhanji F, Cheng A, Frank JR, et al. Education scholarship in emergency medicine, part 3: a "how-to" guide. *CJEM.* 2014;16(suppl 1):S13–S18.

34. Sambunjak D, Strauss SE, Marusic A. What makes a good mentor-mentee relationship? *J Gen Intern Med.* 2010;25:72–78.

35. Gill S, Levin A, Djurdjev O, et al. Obstacles to residents' conducting research and predictors of publication. *Acad Med.* 2001;76(5):477.

36. Alghanim SA, Alhamali RM. Research productivity among faculty members at medical and health schools in Saudi Arabia. Prevalence, obstacles, and associated factors. *Saudi Med J.* 2011;32(12):1297–1303.

37. Bakken S, Lantigua RA, Busacca LV, et al. Barriers, enablers, and incentives for research participation: a report from the Ambulatory Care Research Network (ACRN). *J Am Board Fam Med.* 2009;22(4):436–445.

38. Sabzwari S, Kauser S, Khuwaja AK. Experiences, attitudes and barriers towards research amongst junior faculty of Pakistani medical universities. *BMC Med Educ.* 2009;9:68.

39. Klass D. A performance-based conception of competence is changing the regulation of physicians' professional behavior. *Acad Med.* 2007;82(6):529–535.

40. Goulet F, Hudon E, Gagnon R, et al. Effects of continuing professional development on clinical performance: results of a study involving family practitioners in Quebec. *Can Fam Physician.* 2013;59(5):518–525.

41. Wenghofer EF, Marlow B, Campbell C, et al. The relationship between physician participation in continuing professional development programs and physician in-practice peer assessments. *Acad Med.* 2014;89(6):920–927.

42. Eva KW, Regehr G. Self-assessment in the health professions: a reformulation and research agenda. *Acad Med.* 2005;80(suppl 10):S46–S54.

43. Kezar A, Eckel PD. The effect of institutional culture on change strategies in higher education: universal principles or culturally responsive concepts? *J High Educ.* 2002;73(4):435–460.

44. Ovseiko PV, Buchan AM. Organizational culture in an academic health center: an exploratory study using a competing values framework. *Acad Med.* 2012;87(6):709–718.

45. Bland CJ, Hitchcock MA, Anderson WA, et al. Faculty development fellowship programs in family medicine. *J Med Educ.* 1987;62(8):632–641.

46. Bland CJ, Ruffin MT. Characteristics of a productive research environment: literature review. *Acad Med.* 1992;67(6):385–397.

47. Forbes M, White JH. Using Boyer to create a culture of scholarship: outcomes from a faculty development program. *J Nurs Educ Pract.* 2012;2(3):54–65.

48. Cash PA. Fostering scholarship capacity: the experience of nurse educators. *Can J Scholarship Teach Learn.* 2012;3(1):1–22.

49. Kennedy RH, Gubbins PO, Luer M, et al. Developing and sustaining a culture of scholarship. *Am J Pharm Educ.* 2003;67(3):Article 92.

50. Bandiera G, Leblanc C, Regehr G, et al. Education scholarship in emergency medicine, part 2: supporting and developing scholars. *CJEM.* 2014;16(suppl 1):S6–S12.

51. Association of American Medical Colleges (AAMC). *Medical Education Research Certificate (MERC) Program.* 2016. https://www.aamc.org/members/gea/merc/. Accessed August 6, 2016.

52. Weiner BJ. A theory of organizational readiness for change. *Implement Sci.* 2009;4:67.

53. Chan TM, Luckett-Gatopoulos S, Thoma B. Commentary on competency-based medical education and scholarship: creating an active academic culture during residency. *Perspect Med Educ.* 2015;4(5):214–217.

54. Ellaway RH. Challenges of synthesizing medical education research. *BMC Med.* 2014;12:193.
55. Irby DM, Wilkerson L. Educational innovations in academic medicine and environmental trends. *J Gen Intern Med.* 2003;18(5):370–376.
56. El-Sawi NI, Sharp GF, Gruppen LD. A small grants program improves medical education research productivity. *Acad Med.* 2009;84(10 suppl):S105–S108.
57. Archer J, McManus C, Woolf K, et al. Without proper research funding, how can medical education be evidence based? *BMJ.* 2015;350:h3445.
58. Gruppen LD, Durning SJ. Needles and haystacks: finding funding for medical education research. *Acad Med.* 2016;91(4):480–484.
59. Durning SJ, Gruppen LD. Learning and instruction: the world inside the head or the head inside the world? *Med Educ.* 2015;49(4):351–352.
60. Reed DA, Kern DE, Levine RB, et al. Costs and funding for published medical education research. *JAMA.* 2005;294(9):1052–1057.
61. Reed DA, Cook DA, Beckman TJ, et al. Association between funding and quality of published medical education research. *JAMA.* 2007;298(9):1002–1009.
62. Wartman SA, O'Sullivan PS. The case for a national center for health professions education research. *Acad Med.* 1989;64(6):295–299.
63. Albanese M, Horowitz S, Moss R, et al. An institutionally funded program for educational research and development grants: it makes dollars and sense. *Acad Med.* 1998;73(7):756–761.
64. Doja A, Horsley T, Sampson M. Productivity in medical education research: an examination of countries of origin. *BMC Med Educ.* 2014;14:243.
65. Walsh CM, Fung M, Ginsburg S. Publication of results of abstracts presented at medical education conferences. *JAMA.* 2013;310(21):2307–2309.

Chapter 13

MAINTENANCE *of* BOARD CERTIFICATION, CONTINUING PROFESSIONAL DEVELOPMENT, *and* PERFORMANCE IMPROVEMENT

David W. Price

Case

A senior staff physician drops by your office, concerned about the changing and more extensive process for maintaining his specialty board certification. He realizes that this is important for his hospital privileges but says, "This takes me away from what I do best—practice medicine." You agree that the recertification or revalidation system in his specialty isn't perfect, but believe that it is directed at maintaining and improving the competence of practicing physicians.

Questions

How do you address his concerns? What do you know about the history and future directions of Specialty Certification?

INTRODUCTION

The American Board of Medical Specialties (ABMS) is a federated, umbrella organization of 24 independent nonprofit allopathic medical boards (Table 13.1) comprising 37 specialties and 124 subspecialties. Founded on the principles of professional self-regulation,[1] ABMS' mission is to serve the public and the medical profession by improving the quality of health care through setting professional standards for lifelong certification in partnership with Member Boards.[2] More than 850,000 practicing physicians in the United States are certified by one or more of the 24 ABMS Member Boards.

Specialty Board Certification indicates to the public that a physician has exceeded minimum requirements for licensure and the undifferentiated practice of medicine and possesses the competencies to provide high-quality care in a defined specialty domain. While there are several certifying boards in the United States (American Osteopathic Association Specialty Certifying Boards, among others), this chapter focuses on the

TABLE 13.1
Incorporation of the 24 Member Boards of the American Board of Medical Specialties

ABMS Board	Incorporated
Allergy and Immunology	1971
Anesthesiology	1938
Colon and Rectal Surgery	1935
Dermatology[a]	1932
Emergency Medicine	1976
Family Medicine	1969
Internal Medicine	1936
Medical Genetics and Genomics	1980
Neurological Surgery	1940
Nuclear Medicine	1971
Obstetrics and Gynecology[a]	1930
Ophthalmology[a]	1917
Orthopedic Surgery	1934
Otolaryngology[a]	1924
Pathology	1936
Pediatrics	1933
Physical Medicine and Rehabilitation	1947
Plastic Surgery	1937
Preventive Medicine	1948
Psychiatry and Neurology	1934
Radiology	1934
Surgery	1937
Thoracic Surgery	1948
Urology	1935

[a]Founding Member.

ABMS certification system and the evolution of its standards of assessment, continuing professional development (CPD), and improvement.

THE EVOLUTION OF BOARD CERTIFICATION

Certification

"…when we require students to qualify by years of study in general medicine or by a year or two of experience as an interne in a general hospital and then, after a sufficiently long time of service in an ophthalmic institution in America or abroad, he should be permitted to appear before a proper examining board, similar to any State Board of Examinations and Registration, for examination, and if he is found competent let him then be permitted and licensed to practice ophthalmology"[3]

—Derrick T. Vail, Sr., MD, 1908

At the beginning of the 20th century, few standards existed for medical professionalism, organized medical practice, or medical education in the United States. A wide variety of individuals claimed to be "physicians" and "surgeons." As medical knowledge and the requisite skills to practice medicine began to expand, physician leaders became concerned that regulation of medical practice by nonphysicians would be difficult. In response, Derrick T. Vail, Sr., MD, proposed the concept of Specialty Board Certification as a form of professional self-regulation during his 1908 presidential address to the American Academy of Ophthalmology and Otolaryngology.[3] Furthered by the work of ophthalmologist and previous American Academy of Ophthalmology and Otolaryngology president Edward M. Jackson, MD,[4] creation of the certification system began in 1917 with the incorporation of the American Board of Ophthalmology. It was designed as a system of exam administration upon completion of specialty training to ensure that a physician entering practice had the requisite knowledge to be deemed a specialist. The first four specialty boards (Ophthalmology, Otolaryngology, Obstetrics and Gynecology, and Dermatology) established the Advisory Board of Medical Specialties in 1933 as a convener and coordinating umbrella organization for the growing Boards community; it was renamed and reorganized as ABMS in 1970.

Recertification

Certification remained a one-time event with lifelong duration until 1969 when the newly formed American Board of Family Medicine (ABFM) and the American Board of Internal Medicine proposed a system for recertification. In 1970, ABFM became the first Member Board to issue time-limited certificates (requiring periodic reexamination). By the mid-1980s, most ABMS Member Boards were administering secure, psychometrically validated recertification exams as the standard to assess knowledge in their specialty area. By 1995, all Member Boards were administering recertification examinations at intervals ranging from 6 to 10 years. With the exception of ABFM and the American Board of Emergency Medicine (established in 1976), diplomates who were initially certified before the onset of a Member Board's reexamination continued to hold time-unlimited certification status. As of 2015, approximately two-thirds of the physicians certified by a Member Board have time-limited certificates; that number is projected to exceed 90% by 2020.

Competencies

In 1999, ABMS and the Accreditation Council for Graduate Medical Education (ACGME) developed a framework of six general competencies for training and physician professional practice (Table 13.2).[5] The inclusion of competencies beyond medical knowledge, particularly Practice-based Learning and Improvement and Systems-based Practice, had important implications, stimulating the move to a more continuous process for specialty Board Certification.

Maintenance of Certification

In 2000, the Member Boards Community adopted the concept of the ABMS Program for Maintenance of Certification (ABMS MOC), incorporating the six ABMS/ACGME competencies into four parts: professionalism, periodic self-assessment, cognitive expertise, and practice-based learning and improvement. Each ABMS Member Board

TABLE 13.2
American Board of Medical Specialties/Accreditation Council for Graduate Medical Education Competencies

Practice-based Learning and Improvement:
   Show an ability to investigate and evaluate patient care practices, appraise and assimilate scientific evidence, and improve the practice of medicine.
Patient Care and Procedural Skills:
   Provide care that is compassionate, appropriate, and effective treatment for health problems and to promote health.
Systems-based Practice:
   Demonstrate awareness of and responsibility to the larger context and systems of health care
   Be able to call on system resources to provide optimal care (e.g., coordinating care across sites or serving as the primary case manager when care involves multiple specialties, professions, or sites)
Medical Knowledge:
   Demonstrate knowledge about established and evolving biomedical, clinical, and cognate sciences and their application in patient care
Interpersonal and Communication Skills:
   Demonstrate skills that result in effective information exchange and teaming with patients, their families, and professional associates (e.g., fostering a therapeutic relationship that is ethically sound; using effective listening skills with nonverbal and verbal communication; working as both a team member and at times as a leader)
Professionalism:
   Demonstrate a commitment to carrying out professional responsibilities, adherence to ethical principles, and sensitivity to diverse patient populations

From http://www.abms.org/board-certification/a-trusted-credential/based-on-core-competencies/. Accessed May 5, 2016.

developed a specialty-specific Program for MOC including all four parts, but with variations across boards for how the requirements within each area would be met. Each Member Board MOC program was presented for review, feedback, and approval by the Member Boards community. By 2006, all Member Boards had received approval for their MOC programs; by 2010, all Member Boards had fully implemented their MOC programs. Consistent with ABMS' accountability, public reporting of physician participation in MOC began in 2011.

MOC was designed to be an evolving and dynamic process. During 2012 and 2013, ABMS and its Member Boards reviewed the overall Program for MOC and proposed updated standards, which included gaining input from multiple constituencies and seeking public comment. These standards, which were adopted in 2014 and became effective in 2015,[6] were designed to be responsive to physician concerns about perceived relevance to practice and burden of completing MOC activities[7] and continued the transformation of Board Certification from a single early career event to an ongoing program for continuing learning and assessment and outlined a relevant and meaningful mechanism for CPD for diplomates while helping support the social compact between the public and the profession. The updated standards were designed to:

- Help diplomates remain current in an increasingly complex practice environment
- Help improve patient care through practice improvement activities
- Align with other quality improvement (QI), educational, and regulatory activities in which diplomates engage

TABLE 13.3
Components of the American Board of Medical Specialties Program for Maintenance of Certification (ABMS MOC), 2015

Part I: Professionalism and Professional Standing
 Behave in a professional manner
 Act in the patients' best interest
 Hold a valid, unrestricted medical license
Part II: Lifelong Learning and Self-Assessment
 Participate in high-quality, unbiased educational and self-assessment activities determined by each Member
  Board
Part III: Assessment of Knowledge, Judgment, and Skills
 Pass a written examination and other evaluations
Part IV: Improvement in Medical Practice
 Engage in ongoing assessment and improvement activities to improve patient outcomes
 Demonstrate use of evidence and best practices compared to peers and national benchmarks

From http://www.abms.org/board-certification/a-trusted-credential/assessed-through-a-four-part-framework/. Accessed May 5, 2016.

In addition, the components of MOC were renamed to be more reflective of the updated standards (Table 13.3).[8] The 2015 standards also called for an increased emphasis on professionalism, patient experience of care, a reduction in care-related harm, flexibility in examination delivery, and feedback from exams to be used to guide self-assessment and individual professional development. The standards call on the Member Boards to increase the value of their MOC programs for their diplomates, while reinforcing the role of MOC in ongoing improvement of patient care, team-based QI, and patient care systems. There were over 850,000 ABMS board-certified physicians as of spring 2016; more than 530,000 (including some physicians with lifetime certification status by virtue of receiving initial certification before the advent of the recertification process) were participating in MOC.

The Multispecialty Portfolio Program

One initiative that illustrates the evolution of the MOC standards on Improvement in Medical Practice is the ABMS Multi-Specialty Portfolio Approval Program (Portfolio Program). Started as a pilot in 2010 by the American Boards of Family Medicine, Internal Medicine, and Pediatrics as well as the Mayo Clinic, the Portfolio Program is designed to provide a mechanism for physicians to receive Improvement in Medical Practice MOC credit for meaningful participation in improvement of activities of organizations with mature quality/performance improvement programs.[9] Transitioned to ABMS in April 2014, the Portfolio Program continues to grow. As of spring 2016, 21 of the 24 Member Boards and over 70 organizations (academic medical centers, hospitals, health systems, societies, and others) are participating in the Portfolio Program, which provides diplomates practice-relevant ways of examining and improving their practices that are aligned with the goals and priorities of their organizations, using the support and resources of their organizations while receiving MOC credit. As of December 2016, more than 9,300 physicians have received MOC credit for nearly 13,000 instances of improvement in more than

1,800 approved improvement activities. Many improvement activities have been disease specific (hypertension control, depression screening, diabetes control), while others have focused on preventive measures such as improving immunization rates. Many of these activities involve improvements focused on patient safety, including reduction of Central-Line Associated Blood Stream Infection, improving hand hygiene, Ventilator-Associated Pneumonia prevention, Adverse Drug Event reduction, and Surgical Site Infection reduction. Others have focused on improving transitions of care for patients between care settings (emergency room to inpatient, inpatient to outpatient, discharge from skilled nursing facilities), improving communication between physicians and patients, and other patient perceptions of the care experience. Continued evolution of the Portfolio Program is designed to engage more and different types of organizations, allowing more physicians to participate in these efforts that leverage multiple competing requirements for the benefit of their patients.

FROM "MOC" TO AN INTEGRATED CYCLE OF CONTINUOUS CERTIFICATION CONTRIBUTING TO ONGOING PROFESSIONAL DEVELOPMENT AND IMPROVEMENT

Table 13.4 shows how the components of MOC, as updated in the 2015 standards, align with three major outcomes frameworks for CPD: Moore's Outcomes Hierarchy (from participation to community health),[11] Miller's Pyramid (knows, knows how, shows how, does),[10] and Kirkpatrick's Evaluation Levels (reaction, learning, behavior,

TABLE 13.4
Alignment of the Components of ABMS MOC with Other Outcomes Frameworks for Continuing Professional Development

Component of ABMS Maintenance of Certification 2015[7]	Miller's Pyramid[10]	Moore's Outcomes, Modified[11,12]		Kirkpatrick Levels[13]
Evaluation of improvement in medical practice		7	Community health	Results
		6	Patient health	
(Participation in) improvement in medical practice	Does applies/ shows how	5	Performance	Behavior (transfer)
Lifelong learning and self-assessment	Knows how	4	Competence (shows how)	
	Knows	3C	Conditional knowledge (knows when)	Learning
		3B	Procedural knowledge (knows how)	
		3A	Declarative knowledge (knows what)	
Assessment of knowledge, judgment, and skills		2	Satisfaction	Reaction
		1	Participation	

results).[13] The initial conceptualization of MOC in "parts" makes historical sense because most physicians and Member Boards had little experience with the competencies in Board Certification. One of the goals of the evolution of Board Certification articulated in the 2015 standards is a closer integration of the parts into a more integrated framework of continuous certification. CPD has been posited to be a cycle of continuous professional improvement[14]; an integrated framework of continuous certification and professional improvement could overlay a PSDA (Plan, Do, Study, Act) cycle.[15] Figure 13.1 illustrates how such a cycle might look. Starting at the "study" part of a PDSA cycle, the need for improvement in one's professional practice can be identified from one or more sources, including quality process or outcome metrics measured by a health system, payor, or the Centers for Medicare and Medicaid Services, peer or patient surveys (linking to the professionalism aspects of MOC), and adverse events, or derived from a physician's performance on his/her Board examination assessing knowledge, judgment, and skills. If improvement opportunities are identified, causes of the gap between current and desired performance could be explored ("act"). Strategies for addressing the gap can be developed ("plan"). One could identify a need for improvement of knowledge ("knows what to do"), competence ("knows how to do"), or conditional knowledge ("knows when to do").[12,13] These can be addressed by a Lifelong Learning and Self-Assessment activity that could be certified for continuing

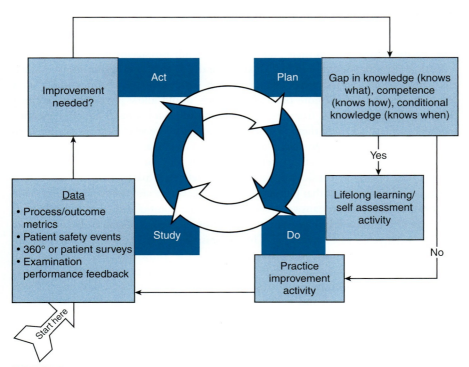

FIGURE 13.1.   An integrated cycle of the components of continuing certification. (Copyright © 2016 American Board of Medical Specialties Research and Education Foundation. Used with permission.)

medical education (CME) credit coupled with a guided, follow-up self-assessment to see if the desired level of learning has occurred ("do"). This step could be followed by an Improvement in Medical Practice activity whereby the physician applies his/her learning in practice over time, corresponding to Performance" in Moore's outcomes hierarchy,[13] "Does" on Miller's Pyramid,[14] or "Behavior" in Kirkpatrick's schema[15] (see Table 13.4). Alternatively, an analysis of the differences in current versus ideal performance might not find any gaps in knowledge, only the need to do things differently—in which case the physician can proceed directly to the Improvement in Medical Practice activity. In either case, the activity would include an analysis of successes and barriers to closing the gap over time ("study"). The cycle could continue until the desired improvements in practice and on patient and population outcomes are achieved and sustained.

FUTURE DIRECTIONS

"A little knowledge that acts is worth infinitely more than much knowledge that is idle."

—Khalil Gibran

New Methods of Assessing Knowledge, Judgment, and Skills

Consistent with the 2015 MOC standards, several Member Boards have started to provide specific feedback from their examination to guide physicians' self-assessment and individual learning. Several Member Boards are developing and beginning to evaluate alternatives to the every-6-to-10-year secure, test-center–delivered examinations. Some boards are considering remote proctoring, which would allow physicians to securely complete these assessments from their home computer. More boards are implementing modular formats, allowing them to continue to assess a core level of knowledge in their specialty, while allowing physicians to somewhat tailor assessments to their practice, given that a physician's practice often differentiates and focuses over the course of a career. Other boards are considering limited use of reference material during these assessments, based on feedback that physicians have increasing access to reference material in practice and can search for answers to questions at the point of care.

Several Boards will be exploring the use of smaller longitudinal, frequent, spaced, computer-delivered assessments.[16,17] These assessments can also allow some customization to a physician's practice while covering basic knowledge that every specialist in a field should have. Immediate feedback and critiques can be provided after answering each question, and physicians can receive a customized dashboard showing their areas of strength and knowledge gaps. Physicians can use this dashboard to guide their professional development; the physician education community can serve as a resource to guide physicians to learning opportunities to address their knowledge gaps. Subsequent questions can be delivered to each diplomate to follow up or probe in areas of weaker knowledge. These Boards will be exploring how this longitudinal assessment can contribute to a summative assessment of physician knowledge, judgment, and skills.

Decreasing Variation in MOC Requirements across the Member Boards

As noted earlier, while each Member Board's MOC program contains each of the MOC components, the activities and requirements for fulfilling each component varies across the boards.[18,19] Some of this variation is reflective of differences between the specialties. Other types of variation, such as differences in the number or duration of practice improvement activities, may not be as important. Over the next several years, the ABMS and its Member Boards will be examining the differences in requirements within each component of the MOC framework, in an attempt to create more consistency between the boards, while continuing to recognize important and necessary variations in the requirements.

Studying MOC: Research and Evaluation for Improvement

Meaningful engagement in CPD requires physicians to evaluate their current knowledge, skills, and performance in order to improve. Similarly, MOC should be evaluated in order to improve the program. The ABMS Research and Education Foundation (REF) has developed frameworks for studying the MOC process. Figure 13.2 depicts

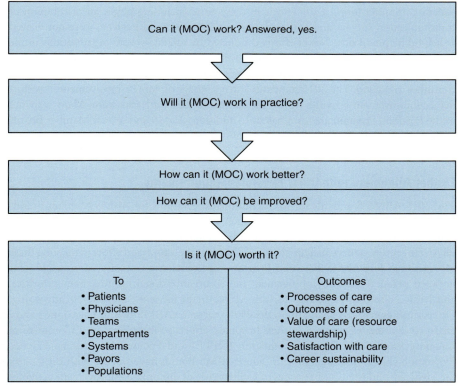

FIGURE 13.2. A framework for the study of Maintenance of Certification (MOC). (Modified from Cochrane AL. *Effectiveness and Efficiency: Random Reflection on Health Services.* London, UK: Nuffield Provincial Hospitals Trust; 1972. Copyright © 2016 American Board of Medical Specialties Research and Education Foundation. Used with permission.)

a framework for the study of MOC modified from Cochrane's aphorisms: Can it work? Will it work in practice? Is it worth it?[20] REF contends that "Can it (MOC) work?" has been largely addressed and answered by others, as MOC is a combination of components (CME, QI) that have been shown to be effective under the correct conditions.[21] "Will MOC work in practice?" can be examined by evaluating the effectiveness of how the different components of MOC are used, similar to the framework presented in Figure 13.1. REF has added "How can MOC be improved?" to the framework to look at the potential incremental effect of new methods of MOC (such as frequent, longitudinal formative assessments) on the current methods of MOC. "Is MOC worth it?" can be evaluated from the perspective of several different stakeholders (patients, physicians, teams, systems, payors, and populations). Ultimately, the goal is, in the realist evaluation framework, to determine "what works for whom under what circumstances.[22]"

Increasing Emphasis on Patient Safety, Communication Skills, Team-Based Care

The 2015 ABMS Standards for MOC call for Member Boards to increase the emphasis on patient safety/harm reduction, and reemphasize the importance of physician–patient communication.[6] Early efforts in these areas, including physician distribution of communication surveys and completion of modules on hand hygiene, were not viewed as helpful by physicians. Newer efforts conducted by several sponsor organizations in the ABMS Multispecialty Portfolio Program have been viewed as more relevant to practice. Additional systems-relevant opportunities are expected to emerge as the Portfolio Program continues to expand. The 2015 standards also encourage diplomate involvement in performance improvement activities within the context of the health care team. Many activities in the Portfolio Program are team based. In addition, ABMS and several Member Boards will be exploring the potential for inclusion of simulation areas in their programs for MOC.

Further Alignment with Other Physician Requirements

The 2015 ABMS Standards for MOC outline expectations for ABMS Member Boards to "enhance the value and relevance of their MOC programs for their diplomates by being sensitive to time, administrative burden, and cost."[6,23] Aligning MOC with other physician requirements can help physicians leverage their time and effort in meeting these expectations. The ABMS Portfolio Program represents one way of creating alignment between practice-relevant improvement needs, organizational improvement priorities, and MOC, allowing physicians to earn MOC credit for work they are already doing. Opportunities exist to expand upon the work that some ABMS Boards have done to give credit to diplomates engaged in their hospitals' efforts to meet The Joint Commission Ongoing Professional Practice Evaluation (OPPE) and Focused Professional Practice Evaluation (FPPE) requirements.[24,25] Some ABMS Boards have worked with the Center for Medicare and Medicaid Services to facilitate use of diplomate improvement activities as a means of meeting quality reporting requirements.[26] Over the next few years, Member Boards will be exploring how their MOC requirements can better align with reporting requirements of the Merit-Based Incentive Payment System (MIPS, now known as the Quality Payment Program [QPP]) and Alternative Payment Models (APMs) requirements in the Medicare Access and CHIP Reauthorization Act of 2015 (MACRA).[27]

During the last century, ABMS Board Certification has evolved from a singular, capstone, diploma-like event at the completion of training to an ongoing, continuous, renewing credential that not only assesses knowledge but reinforces implementation of knowledge and the evaluation of its effect in support of "Continuing Professional Development and Improvement"[12] throughout a physician's career. Feedback from ABMS diplomates and partnerships with specialty societies, CPD providers for physicians, other members of the health care team, QI and safety science experts, health services and educational researchers, patients, and others will be critical for Board Certification to continue to evolve and be patient centered and physician sensitive, in order to meet its obligations to the public and the medical profession.

ACKNOWLEDGEMENT

The author would like to thank Ruth Carol for her helpful editorial assistance with this chapter.

REFERENCES

1. Cruess SR, Cruess RL. The medical profession and self-regulation: a current challenge. *Virtual Mentor.* 2005;7(4):pii: virtualmentor.2005.7.4.oped1-0504. doi:10.1001/virtualmentor.2005.7.4.oped1-0504.
2. *ABMS Mission Statement.* http://www.abms.org/about-abms/governance/abms-mission-statement. Accessed December 28, 2015.
3. Vail DT. The limitations of ophthalmic practice. *Trans Am Acad Ophthalmol Otolaryngol.* 1908;13: 1–6.
4. O'Day DM, Ladden MR. The Influence of Derrick T. Vail Sr, MD, and Edward M. Jackson, MD, on the Creation of the American Board of Ophthalmology and the Specialist Board System in the United States. *Arch Ophthalmol.* 2012;130(2):224–232.
5. http://www.abms.org/board-certification/a-trusted-credential/based-on-core-competencies/. Accessed May 5, 2016.
6. http://www.abms.org/media/1109/standards-for-the-abms-program-for-moc-final.pdf. Accessed May 5, 2016.
7. Cook DA, Holmboe ES, Sorensen KJ, et al. Getting maintenance of certification to work: a grounded theory study of physicians' perceptions. *JAMA Intern Med.* 2015;175(1):35–42. doi:10.1001/jamainternmed.2014.5437.
8. http://www.abms.org/board-certification/a-trusted-credential/assessed-through-a-four-part-framework/. Accessed May 5, 2016.
9. *Multi-Specialty Portfolio Approval Program.* http://www.mocportfolioprogram.org. Accessed December 28, 2015.
10. Miller GE. The assessment of clinical skills/competence/performance. *Acad Med.* 1990;65(9 suppl):S63–S67.
11. Moore DE Jr, Green JS, Gallis HA. Achieving desired results and improved outcomes: integrating planning and assessment throughout learning activities. *J Contin Educ Health Prof.* 2009 Winter;29(1):1–15. doi:10.1002/chp.20001.
12. Bruning RH, Schraw GJ, Norby MN, et al. Ch. 2: Sensory, short term and working memory. pp. 14–35 and Ch. 3: Long term memory: structures and models. pp. 36–64. *Cognitive Psychology and Instruction.* Upper Saddle River, NJ: Pearson/Merrill/Prentice Hall; 2004.
13. Kirkpatrick DL, Kirkpatrick JD. *Transferring Learning to Behavior: Using the Four Levels to Improve Performance.* San Francisco, CA: Berrett-Koehler Publishers; 2005.

14. Price D, Havens C, Bell M. Continuing professional development and improvement to meet current and future continuing medical education needs of physicians. In: Wentz DK, ed. *Continuing Medical Education: Looking Back, Planning Ahead.* Hanover, NH: Dartmouth University Press; 2011.

15. Berwick DM. Developing and testing changes in delivery of care. *Ann Intern Med.* 1998;128(8):651–656.

16. Karpicke JD, Roediger HL III. The critical importance of retrieval for learning. *Science.* 2008;319(5865):966–968.

17. Larsen DP, Butler AC. Test-enhanced learning. In: Walsh K, ed. *Oxford Textbook of Medical Education.* Oxford, UK: Oxford University Press; 2013:443–452.

18. http://www.abms.org/media/84748/abms_memberboardsrequirementsproject_moc_partii.pdf. Accessed May 7, 2016.

19. http://www.abms.org/media/84747/abms_memberboardsrequirementsproject_moc_partiv.pdf. Accessed May 7, 2016.

20. Cochrane AL. *Effectiveness and Efficiency: Random Reflection on Health Services.* London, UK: Nuffield Provincial Hospitals Trust; 1972.

21. Hawkins RE, Lipner RS, Ham HP, et al. American Board of Medical Specialties Maintenance of Certification: theory and evidence regarding the current framework. *J Contin Educ Health Prof.* 2013 Fall;33(suppl 1):S7–S19. doi:10.1002/chp.21201.

22. Pawson R, Tilley N. *Realistic Evaluation.* London, UK: SAGE; 1997.

23. Irons MB, Nora LM. Maintenance of certification 2.0—strong start, continued evolution. *N Engl J Med.* 2015;372(2):104–106.

24. https://www.jointcommission.org/jc_physician_blog/oppe_fppe_tools_privileging_decisions/. Accessed May 13, 2016.

25. https://www.jointcommission.org/jc_physician_blog/using_oppe_as_a_performance_improvement_tool/. Accessed May 13, 2016.

26. https://www.theabfm.org/moc/pqrs.aspx. Accessed May 13, 2016.

27. https://www.cms.gov/Medicare/Quality-Initiatives-Patient-Assessment-Instruments/Value-Based-Programs/MACRA-MIPS-and-APMs/MACRA-MIPS-and-APMs.html. Accessed May 13, 2016.

Chapter 14

COMPARING *and* CONTRASTING: FACULTY DEVELOPMENT *and* CONTINUING PROFESSIONAL DEVELOPMENT

Ivan Silver and Karen Leslie

Case

It appears that there is a need for clarity about the distinctions and overlap between faculty development (FD) and continuing professional development (CPD). While the content is different (learning related to academic roles such as teaching, mentorship, and leadership in FD and learning related to clinical roles in CPD), many of the methods, needs assessments, evaluation strategies, motivation, and program logistics appear to be very similar.

Questions

Should and could faculty development (FD) and continuing professional development (CPD) operate in closer alignment? How has each field evolved, and what elements do they have common? What distinguishes FD from CPD? How might they be linked? Are there shared challenges and opportunities?

INTRODUCTION

Health care professionals have numerous roles relating to their scope of their "practice" and the setting and contexts in which they practice. The scope of practice for many physicians and other health care professionals may include patient care and education, teaching and supervision of students at various levels, engagement in various forms of scholarship, and holding leadership roles in health care organizations, the university, or both. Practice settings can be community and/or university based, in urban and rural contexts. As one progresses through formal training to professional practices, one's learning needs relating to one's role evolve, and thus, various types of professional learning are required, specific to these needs. Learning needs can be identified and informed by the individual health professional, as well as the organizational settings in which they work.[1]

Continuing professional development (CPD) and faculty development (FD) both focus on continuing and lifelong learning for health professionals with the traditional distinction being that CPD focuses on the clinician role and FD on the academic role, with an emphasis on the teacher role. In recent years, there has been an expansion of the areas in which CPD and FD have developed such that there is now overlap. This has led to confusion about how individuals and organizations understand these two very important entities and how they might be resourced, supported, and developed in our health care communities.

This chapter will begin with some definitions of CPD and FD followed by a brief historical review of the evolution of both areas. Subsequently, it will outline for readers the shared elements and distinguishing features for CPD and FD. It will conclude with a discussion about shared challenges and opportunities, in addition to some thoughts and ideas for future directions.

DEFINITIONS

Faculty Development

Faculty development has been defined as a broad range of activities that institutions use to renew or assist faculty, supervisors, preceptors, field instructors, and clinical educators, in their roles. These activities are designed to improve an individual's knowledge and skills in teaching, education, administration, leadership, and research.[2,3] Implicit in this definition is that the desired outcomes are at both the individual and organization level; this then influences how needs are determined, the systems of support for the development, delivery, and evaluation of faculty development, as well as how faculty development is conceptualized as both an organizational practice and an academic field of study.

Continuing Professional Development

CPD has been defined by the World Federation of Medical Education (WFME) as "including all activities that doctors (health professionals) undertake formally and informally in order to maintain, update, develop and enhance their knowledge, skills and attitudes in response to the needs of their patients."[4] Implicit in this definition is the motivation required by health professionals for continuous professional lifelong learning and the desire to provide high-quality care. The scope of CPD is wide and includes all of the professional competencies outlined by CanMEDS and the ACGME.[5,6] Using the CanMEDS framework, FD activities would support, maintain, and update the CanMEDS competencies primarily within the Scholar and Leader (formerly Manager) roles.[6]

HISTORICAL PERSPECTIVE

The field and practice of FD and CPD have evolved from distinct origins to their current orientations in the academic medical culture and the practice of medicine. Faculty development has its origins in higher education[7,8] and has moved through "stages" described by Sorcinelli from the Age of the Scholar (mid 1950 to early 1960) where the focus of faculty development was on research success; the Age of the Teacher (1970s); the Age of the Developer (1980s); the Age of the Learner (1990s) where teaching approaches moved toward being learner based, as opposed to teacher centered; and finally to the Age of Networker (current times) where he states that we need to "preserve, clarify, and enhance the purpose of faculty development, and to network with faculty and institutional leaders to respond to institutional problems and propose constructive solutions as we meet the challenge of the new century."[8]

The Professional and Organizational Development (POD) Network, beginning in 1976, was one of the first organizations that promoted the scholarship of FD in higher education.[9] Subsequently, the concept of faculty development was taken up by medical education and, in the past decade, the health professions more broadly.[2,3]

Wilkerson and Irby wrote one of the most widely cited papers in which they described the scope of faculty development as it aligns with faculty members' academic roles and responsibilities.[10] They identified four broad areas for which faculty development could play a role: instructional development, professional/career development, leadership development, and organizational development. They described a comprehensive model for faculty development that builds as faculty progress in their careers from involvement in teaching, to educational development and scholarship, to educational leadership. They also identified the importance of assessing outcomes for faculty development and cite literature (including Davis' 1995 meta-analysis of outcomes of CME programs) that reinforced formats such as series of workshops with opportunities to practice and receive feedback and reminders as being more effective.[11]

Over the past 20 years, the field and practice of faculty development has evolved substantially, with several organizations including the American Association of Medical Colleges (AAMC) holding annual meetings that demonstrate some of the innovative and scholarly FD work taking place at North American medical schools. The AAMC Group on Education Affairs National Grant encourages submissions for innovations in faculty development. In Canada, the Association of Faculties of Medicine of Canada (AFMC) created a special committee on Faculty Development that has evolved in the past few years to be a standing committee, representing faculty development offices and centers from all 17 Canadian medical schools. In 2011, the first International Conference on Faculty Development in the Health Professions was held in Toronto, Canada, bringing faculty developers from over 28 countries to share best practices and showcase faculty development research and scholarship. Subsequent to this inaugural conference, there have been 2 additional international conferences, with a fourth being planned for 2017 in conjunction with the Association for Medical Education in Europe (AMEE) conference. In additional to these national and international groups and conferences, faculty development is represented in the medical and health professions education literature with empirical work, as well as systematic reviews on faculty development literature.[11,12] Recently, the first book on Faculty Development in the Health Professions was published, with contributions from faculty development leaders from around the world, including Australia, the United Kingdom, the Netherlands, and South Africa, as well as North America.[13]

As the boundaries of the concept of a "faculty" member have expanded, so has the need to understand health professionals' diverse practice settings and roles. The expansion of medical schools into community and rural settings has resulted in many physicians who would never have considered themselves as "faculty" acquiring faculty appointments in order to supervise and assess undergraduate and (post)graduate trainees. Teams of health professionals working in both outpatient and inpatient settings are engaged with learners from numerous professions and disciplines. More recently, there has been work done to better understand the role that faculty development plays in the knowledge translation (KT) or mobilization of best evidence and practice in health professional education.[14] Faculty development has been identified as assisting medical educators in being able to use the medical education literature in their practices as curriculum developers and course directors.[15] Further study is needed to explore if and how current KT models can apply to medical education and faculty development.[16]

Unlike faculty development, CPD had a much earlier origin within each health discipline and was not originally informed by studies and scholarship in higher education.[4] Within medicine, in the early part of the 20th century, medical societies offered lectures and other activities focusing mainly on the medical expert role. In the 1940s and 1950s, medical schools began to create offices for continuing medical education (CME), which provided primarily lecture-based updates to physicians at the university and in the community. Pharmaceutical companies also became active providers of CME until significant concerns about influence and bias reduced their collaboration with universities in the past 10 years. Unlike faculty development, CME standards have been regulated by accreditation bodies both in the United States by the Accreditation Council for Continuing Medical Education (ACCME) and in Canada by the Committee on Accreditation of Continuing Medical Education (CACME) since the early 1980s.[17] Global interest in CME has been enhanced by the establishment of the Global Alliance for Medical Education in 1995, the European Accreditation Council for Continuing Medical Education (EACCME) in 1999, and other similar accreditation bodies in Australia and New Zealand.[18,19] The scholarship and study of CME accelerated with the establishment of two organizations—the Alliance for Continuing Medical Education and the Society of Medical College Directors of Continuing Medical Education (SMCDCME) in 1976, later changing its name to the Society for Academic Continuing Medical Education (SACME) in 1998.[20] The establishment of the Journal of Continuing Education in the Health Professions Journal in 1980 helped to consolidate scholarship and best practices in this field. The term CME has gradually evolved to the concept of CPD for two key reasons: (1) our understanding of professional competencies has expanded beyond the role of the medical expert with the creation of the CanMEDS and ACGME competencies for residents and medical students, and (2) the expansion of pedagogical approaches to educating practicing health professionals has evolved from lecture-based methods to more evidence-based and practice- and work-based approaches including performance improvement CME, academic detailing, clinical audits with feedback, communities of practice, the use of reminders, and more recently the use of simulation including virtual reality and massive online open courses.[21–27] This transition of CME to CPD is reflected in the fact that some medical schools in Canada have changed the names of their offices from "Office of Continuing Medical Education" to "Office of Continuing Professional Development" to better reflect the diversification of education delivery methods and broader target audiences including team-based and continuing interprofessional education.[28]

Academic CME became attached to the field of knowledge translation (KT) and implementation science in the 1990s when evidence accumulated that continuing education is a significant factor in changing physician behavior and influencing patient outcomes.[29,30] Prominent CME educators also realized that putting research knowledge into practice not only requires educating health professionals, it also requires bringing together health policymakers, health researchers, administrators, and other stakeholders.[30] Most recently, through the leadership of the AAMC, quality improvement (Aligning and Educating for Quality—AE4Q) has become another important framework aligned to CPD.[31] Comparing and contrasting the fields of CPD, knowledge translation, and quality improvement have also been further elucidated.[32]

SHARED ELEMENTS

The Learner and Groups of Learners

Health professionals who are practicing clinicians in an academic context (or have an academic affiliation) are participants in both FD and CPD. These individuals have diverse learning needs relating to the various roles they play as clinicians, teachers, leaders, and scholars. FD and CPD can be delivered to uniprofessional and to multiprofessional groups of learners. Both FD and CPD develop and deliver focused education for targeted learners (cycle of developing learning needs, formatting content and process for specific audiences, and common evaluation frameworks). For example, clinicians who are teaching using a particular method such as problem-based learning or clinicians who are learning a novel technique in diagnostic imaging will benefit from education from similar education planning frameworks. Learners come with a range of internal and external motivators. They may participate in FD and CPD activities at their own initiative, as part of the expectations of a new role or position or as part of a mandated program for those who have been identified as performing below expectations in one or more of their clinical or academic roles. The case below illustrates a typical faculty learner with both FD and CPD needs:

Case 1. Dr. Gold is an internist in his first 3 years of an academic appointment. He spends 4 months a year on the clinical teaching unit of his hospital and supervises medical students, nurse practitioner students, and residents in family medicine and internal medicine. He also teaches a seminar to the 2nd year students on ethics. He attends his annual specialty society meeting and his departmental grand rounds. He has recently been considering an opportunity to take on a leadership role that will require him to reduce his clinical teaching time significantly. He wonders how he will keep up his clinical skills if this happens.

Questions to consider about Dr. Gold:

- What skills might he need for this leadership role that he does not currently have?
- How might be acquire these skills?
- How might he monitor his clinical skills and ongoing learning needs relating to his clinical and teaching practices?

Best Practices in Teaching and Learning

Both FD and CPD utilize best evidence and practices from the research base on teaching and learning to inform the development, delivery, and evaluation of their programs. Both are focused on outcomes-based paradigms such as Kirkpatrick's four levels and Moore's six levels of outcome evaluation.[33,34] The fields of FD and CPD share an interest in learner satisfaction (Kirkpatrick level 1) and improvement in learner competencies (level 2). At Kirkpatrick's level 3, faculty development outcomes may measure teaching skill improvement in practice and other academic achievements. Level 4 may include changes in student learning and behavior. In contrast, CPD outcomes at level 3 may focus on changes in the clinician's practices and level 4, improvement in their patients' outcomes. Moore added an additional two levels on either end of the scale, to account for assessment of the demographics of the learner population (level 1) and changes in community health (level 6). The relationship between practice-based assessments (whether be it patient-related practice, teaching practice [e.g., peer assessment and teaching evaluations], feedback on leadership skills, or acceptance rates of grant and publication submissions) is that all are used in various ways to assess the impact and outcomes of learning (the extent to which learning has resulted in practice change).

Both fields are also informed by the cognitive science related to self-assessment, reflection, and feedback. For example, education planners in both areas of education development will note that it is often the learner who least requires the education that will show up for their respective education activities.[35,36] Learners who are more competent in a particular domain will have more awareness of their personal learning gaps and thus are more likely to participate in professional development. Faculty and clinicians who are less competent in any of the professional competencies will have less awareness and likelihood of participating in learning activities that they might require.[35,37] Addressing this self-awareness gap can be a challenge for education planners. Multisource feedback can inform learners in both areas of professional development including the use of new evidence-based models of feedback that incorporate novel strategies for increasing motivation to accept feedback and to stimulate learning and change.[38]

Formats for Learning

Both FD and CPD are offered in many different formats. Traditionally, FD has taken the form of workshops, whereas CME and later CPD have maintained the didactic lecture as the key format. However, in recent years, interactive methods and workplace-based learning and online learning have all made their way into both FD and CPD. Despite this, the majority of FD remains as face to face single or longitudinal sessions, often over months or one to two years, whereas CPD conference and meetings are held over 1 to 4 days that include large group "plenaries", panel and poster presentations, workshops, seminars, and audience response systems.[39,40] There are also differently framed models for understanding the scope and impact of FD and CPD formats (see Table 14.1 and Fig. 14.1). Each of these

TABLE 14.1
Models for Understanding the Scope and Impact of Faculty Development and Continuing Professional Development Formats

Methods/ Stages	Awareness	Agreement	Adoption	Adherence
Predisposing	Distribution of educational materials Conferences (live and online) Grand rounds E-mail Mass (social) media	Practice audit with feedback		
Enabling		Local opinion leaders M and M rounds Interactive workshops Interprofessional education	Interactive workshops Simulation-based learning Algorithms/flow charts Education outreach Performance improvement CPD Mentor (coach) Interprofessional education	
Reinforcing			Communities of practice	Reminders Multifaceted interventions

Adapted from BMJ Publishing Group Limited[30] and Pathman-PRECEED model for knowledge translation,[43] with permission.

is a dominant discourse in their respective fields.[30,41-43] They mirror differences in process and content, with the emphasis in CPD on indelibly changing the behavior of clinicians and sustaining this change. Looking closely at each framework, it is clear that each could inform the other. The fields of CPD and FD in fact are at different stages of development in terms of evidence of impact. For example, there are several Cochrane reviews of CPD formats and additional systematic reviews of the impact of CPD on physician behavior and patient outcomes that include many randomized controlled trials dating back to the 1970s.[44-46] Currently, there are no Cochrane reviews and just three systematic reviews of FD outcomes in the past 10 years.[12,39,47]

A second case illustrates a community-based practitioner's needs and questions about effective FD and CPD:

Case 2. Dr. Scott is a family practitioner working in a small community about 60 miles from a large university. She has been approached by the Department of Family

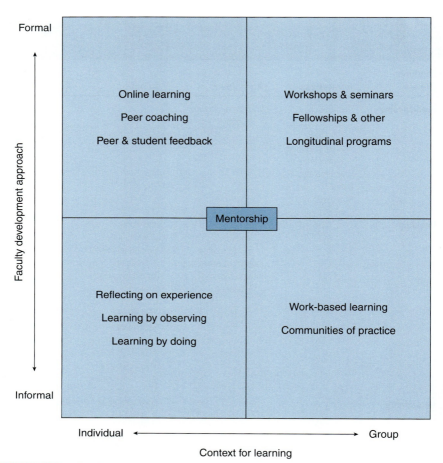

Formal

Faculty development approach

Online learning

Peer coaching

Peer & student feedback

Workshops & seminars

Fellowships & other

Longitudinal programs

Mentorship

Reflecting on experience

Learning by observing

Learning by doing

Work-based learning

Communities of practice

Informal

Individual ◄——————————————————► Group

Context for learning

FIGURE 14.1. The role of mentorship in the context of faculty development and learning. From workshops to communities of practice. (Reprinted from Ende J. *Theory and Practice of Teaching Medicine.* Philadelphia, PA: American College of Physicians; 2010, Fig. 1, with permission.)

Practice to become a preceptor to first-year family medicine residents and to supervise a resident for a three-month rotation in her office practice twice a year. Since she qualified 10 years ago, Dr. Scott has not done any teaching and wonders (1) if there is any guidance and/or support provided about what her role should be with these learners and (2) if her clinical practice is up-to-date enough to be able to "teach" these learners what they need to know about family medicine.

Questions to consider about Dr. Scott's ongoing learning needs include:

- How does Dr. Scott determine if her clinical practice is up-to-date?
- What types of CPD has Dr. Scott undertaken since she qualified 10 years ago?
- Does she attend her specialty society annual meetings or any other event in her region?
- How might Dr. Scott access learning relating to her anticipated role as a teacher/supervisor of a graduate/postgraduate learner?

- What formats are available for her to access this learning? Which are most effective?
- Will she have to travel to the university to attend supervisor training?
- Will she receive feedback on her teaching in order to see what additional skill development she might pursue?

DISTINGUISHING FEATURES

In addition to the similarities and differences in approaches and formats discussed in previous sections of this chapter, several key points can be identified that serve to distinguish FD and CPD from each other:

- FD is focused on enhancing the academic aspects of professional development with an emphasis on enhancement of teaching and education knowledge and skills.
- CPD is linked more closely to knowledge translation, quality improvement, patient safety, and physician competencies relating to clinical care as outlined in CanMEDs and ACGME frameworks.
- CPD is a mandatory requirement for health professionals in most countries; FD is not mandated at most medical schools, although some countries now have faculty development for teachers as a mandatory requirement for program accreditation.[7,48,49]
- Distinct areas of learning content between CPD and FD (as well as some that are shared) are listed in Table 14.2.

HOW FD AND CPD CAN BE LINKED

FD and CPD can be linked in various ways and this alignment and linkage can take place at the individual faculty, programming, and governance/administrative levels.

Faculty Development for CPD

Faculty developers and CPD educators share professional development as a field. Research in the best methods to change behavior that would have the most impact on

---

TABLE 14.2
Comparison of CPD and FD Areas of Focus

Continuing Professional Development	Faculty Development
Learning related to one's professional roles	Learning related to one's academic roles
Clinical expert/patient care	Teaching of learners, colleagues
Patient education	Development of curriculum
	Program evaluation, learner assessment
Collaborative care	Research and scholarship skills
Health care leadership	Academic leadership
Career development, coaching, mentoring, professionalism, quality improvement, knowledge mobilization/ translation	

patient care and student learning and behavior could be more collaborative and strategic. Continuing education providers can benefit from specific faculty development in evidence-based learning formats unique to CPD including academic detailing, performance improvement, audit with feedback, simulation formats, and the use of reminders. However, there will need to be more alignment of continuing educators and faculty developers for this to occur. Faculty developers may not be skilled in CPD approaches to education, and so mutual capacity building will need to be more collaborative. It is likely that faculty developers would benefit from learning about CPD approaches like academic detailing, performance improvement, and audit with feedback that could be uniquely applied to improving teaching and other academic skills. Similarly, CPD educators could benefit from applying faculty development models of changing behavior that are individual or group focused including peer observation and coaching and communities of practice.[41]

Programming that Blends or Combines FD and CPD Learning

Identifying opportunities to integrate selected CPD and FD activities can have several advantages. Faculty developers and CPD educators can collaborate to provide joint continuing education to targeted learners where clinical practice updates and teaching skills training are both relevant to the learners. Busy health professionals in academic settings will appreciate the efficiency of updating their knowledge and skills in a particular domain and at the same time practice their teaching of these new skills and knowledge, keeping in mind the specific target audience.[50,51] There is some evidence from cognitive psychology that teaching medical content along with the specific recommended teaching methods for specific students can consolidate knowledge acquisition and recall, for example, a workshop that offers an update on assessment of ankle injuries and inclusion of how to teach the ankle examination to medical students.[52]

There is evidence that contextualizing teaching content for specific target audiences of students and residents, practicing and rehearsing these teaching behaviors in front of peers and faculty developers, and receiving feedback from this audience can improve teaching performance and student learning.[14] There is also evidence that enabling faculty (through faculty development) to design mini-CEX (short structured clinical assessment) examinations for students can stimulate new learning of medical knowledge and be an unintended source of efficient CPD.[53] Similarly, mentoring medical students has been shown to enhance the CPD of the mentors.[54] Continuing interprofessional education can be enhanced through a systematic program of faculty development.[55]

Governance and Administrative Structures

Administratively, many medical schools have linked their CPD and FD programs either through oversight by a single Associate Dean or close programmatic connections. According to the most recently available SACME survey of CME units in North America, ~90% of academic CME units have some meaningful programmatic connection with their FD counterparts.[56] There may be certain advantages to facilitate the above joint programming. It is however important to distinguish between the administrative structures and procedural aspects of shared governance and/or administration, with the idea that program development and scholarship might not necessarily be fully (or even partially) integrated. Alternatively, to preserve the unique professional identity of CPD and FD educators and their respective fields of education, separating them provides the necessary autonomy to stimulate innovation in both fields. What has not been sufficiently enunciated in the literature is the evidence for linking these two related areas of professional development, and to what extent this linkage might facilitate or impede either field.

SHARED CHALLENGES AND OPPORTUNITIES

Individual versus System Needs

One of the areas for discussion in the faculty development literature relates to how faculty development can be aligned with the needs of the organization, with the idea being that outcomes are both for the individual faculty member as well as resulting in change at the organizational level. Bligh proposed that the goals of faculty development are to improve practice in teaching, research, and other areas of organization practice and also to "manage change by enhancing individual strengths and abilities as well as organizational capacities and the overall culture."[57] In a similar vein, for CPD, this continuum of outcomes can be outlined for the individual practitioner, their patients, and the health system.[58] The challenge inherent in these broader outcomes from individual learning is in being able to evaluate this impact.[59,60] A model has been suggested to reframe outcomes research in less of a linear and more of a systems framework.[61] The opportunity for CPD and FD in positioning professional learning and development as a change strategy is that organizational (university and health care) resources can be leveraged in ways that learning and development selected to meet individual learning needs may not be.

FUTURE DIRECTIONS

FD and CPD should retain their individual identities. These two areas of professional learning, although related, are both individually broad enough to warrant distinct fields with the generation of new knowledge and practice. Close alignment and opportunities for collaboration should be promoted and supported within and between schools and could subsequently inform how structures and processes are oriented to achieve the desired individual and system outcomes. This will look differently depending on the contexts and cultures of each institution. The future might include the following directions.

Synergistic Scholarship and Research

With the advent of new social media, and simulation learning strategies including virtual reality, joint research programs to establish the evidence of efficacy of these new approaches would be helpful to each field. It will be important to also foster opportunities for shared dialogue about scholarship. It is unusual to see faculty development scholarship presented at national and international CME meetings that could promote synergies between these two fields. Alternatively, these CME organizations could explicitly establish an faculty development paper/poster section and/or workshops at each conference. The Journal of Continuing Education in the Health Professions could also consider publishing a biannual special supplement on faculty development in the health professions. Similarly, the journal Medical Teacher that frequently features faculty development scholarship could feature a special supplement on continuing professional development. The Association of American Medical Colleges (AAMC) annual conference, the Canadian Conference on Medical Education (CCME), the Association of Medical Education in Europe (AMEE) conference, and the Asia Pacific Medical Education (APMEC) conference offer opportunities for faculty developers and CPD educators to present their scholarly work, currently in separate symposia. These educators should consider some shared sessions explicitly labeled as such, to explore the synergies and opportunities for joint scholarship.

Additionally, the AAMC or AMEE could consider sponsoring a new Journal of Faculty Development in the Health Professions that would provide international academic leadership in this field. There is also room for a new journal of Professional Development in the Health Professions that deliberately crosses the health professions in its scope, fosters a global perspective, supports the integration of all forms of professional development, and focuses on innovations and best practices in the integration of CPD and FD.

Governance and Standard Setting

From an international organizational point of view, the Accreditation Council for Continuing Medical (ACCME) in the United States and the Canadian Accreditation for Continuing Medical Education (CACME) in Canada accredit CPD offices. This provides a uniform standard setting that also fosters the academic development of the field and helps develop the individual careers of its leaders and scholars. Almost all the regulatory bodies in countries where CPD is mandatory have developed standards and guidelines on the use of CPD.[48,49] For example, the Medical Council of New Zealand requires nonspecialist doctors to form collegial relationships and take part in CME, clinical audit, and peer review. In contrast, there are no formal accreditation standards for faculty development offices at medical schools currently. For example, undergraduate and postgraduate accreditation standards in both the United States and Canada require that FD is provided to faculty but does not specify the degree or the quality standards. There have been standards in place for several years in the United Kingdom by the General Medical Council in this regard.[62] Consideration to the establishment of accreditation criteria for faculty development of offices or centers could facilitate more explicit identification of the core content and scope of curriculum for faculty and their organizations. Some movement in this area had been made recently with the addition of a Faculty Development award in the Association of Medical Education Europe ASPIRE awards process.[61]

Utilizing Clinical and Academic Practice Data to Inform Learning Needs

We practice in an era of data and performance management. Attention to the relationship between "practice" data and learning needs and outcomes has relevance for both CPD and FD for several reasons. As mentioned earlier in the chapter, individuals tend to select their learning informed by their own perceived learning needs. There is compelling literature on self-assessment that demonstrates that using this as the only way to identify learning needs has major limitations. However, simply bringing in data that might illuminate unperceived needs (such as patient data from a clinician's practice) is also not sufficient,[37,38] and others are exploring ways that coaching and other relational approaches can enhance the incorporation of practice/performance data to "drive" CPD learning.

Similarly, faculty tend to choose faculty development topics and learning that they self-identify as being of interest to them or may be directed to certain programs by their medical school leaders. At the organizational level, there is much interest in the use of "Big Data" and how this might be used to inform CPD and practice change. Smaller in scale but similar in focus, some faculty development programs are linked to the teacher evaluation units at their schools and so may develop program in response to areas in which are identified as being less well taught.[63] Further exploration and development of ways in which individual and pooled data about practices and performance are an area of great opportunity for both CPD and FD and may benefit from shared infrastructure such as databases that can populate individual and group learning plans.

Assessment of "Competence"

Undergraduate and graduate/postgraduate medical education training programs are now focused on "competence" as the basis for curriculum development and outcomes of learning.[64] It follows that the assessment of competence might also be applied to postlicensure health professionals.[65] For CPD and FD, key questions arise about how competence is assessed once an individual is an independent practitioner and engaged in academic practices such as teaching. Several areas have emerged that will need further consideration by CPD and FD leaders. These include how faculty who are identified as performing below expectations in areas such as teaching and research are both identified and assisted with whatever type of professional learning and assessment might be required for them to be deemed competent to continue or resume their duties with learners. Similar issues present with clinical performance and patient care (with a range of minor to egregious events). The other very murky area of competence relates to late career physicians for whom decisions about retirement are being considered by themselves and/or by others working with them. The role of CPD and faculty developers in the assessment of competence at these various points in the careers of physicians and other health professionals is not clear and thus an opportunity for further exploration.

Busy health professionals of the future will benefit from the planning that can now be done to ensure robust growth of both fields of professional development in addition to new approaches to closer alignment of these fields. Health systems and their patients will be the ultimate beneficiaries of this creative planning and development.

REFERENCES

1. Simpson D, Marcdante K, Morzinski J, et al. Fifteen years of aligning faculty development with primary care clinician-educator roles and academic advancement at the Medical College of Wisconsin. *Acad Med.* 2006;81(11):945–953.
2. Centra JA. Types of faculty development programs. *J Higher Educ.* 1978;49(2):151–162.
3. Sheets KJ, Schwenk TL. Faculty development for family medicine educators: an agenda for future activities. *Teach Learn Med.* 1990;2(3):141–148.
4. Wentz D, ed. *Continuing Medical Education: Looking Back, Looking Ahead.* Hanover, NH: Dartmouth College Press; 2011.
5. *ACGME Core Competencies* [Internet]. Accreditation Council for Graduate Medical Education; c2000-2016 [Last accessed July 10, 2016]. Available from: http://www.acgme.org/Specialties/Program-Requirements-and-FAQs-and-Applications
6. *CanMEDS 2015 Physician Competency Framework.* Ottawa, ON: Royal College of Physicians and Surgeons of Canada; 2015.
7. McLean M, Cilliers F, Van Wyk JM. Faculty development: yesterday, today and tomorrow. *Med Teach.* 2008;30(6):555–584.
8. Sorcinelli M, Austin A, Eddy P, et al. *Creating the Future of Faculty Development: Learning From the Past, Understanding the Present.* Bolton, MA: Anker; 2006.
9. *Professional Organizational Development in Higher Education (POD) Homepage* [Internet]. c2007-2016 [Last accessed July 13, 2016]. Available from: http://podnetwork.org/.
10. Wilkerson L, Irby DM. Strategies for improving teaching practices: a comprehensive approach to faculty development. *Acad Med.* 1998;73(4):387–396.
11. Davis DA, Thomson MA, Oxman AD, et al. Changing physician performance. a systematic review of the effect of continuing medical education strategies. *JAMA.* 1995;274(9):700–705.
12. Steinert Y, Mann K, Anderson B, et al. A systematic review of faculty development initiatives designed to enhance teaching effectiveness: a 10-year update: BEME Guide No. 40. *Med Teach.* 2016;38(8):769–786.
13. Steinert Y, ed. *Faculty Development in the Health Professions: A Focus on Research and Practice.* New York: Springer; 2014.
14. Irby DM. Excellence in clinical teaching: knowledge transformation and development required. *Med Educ.* 2014;48(8):776–784.
15. Onyura B, Ng SL, Baker LR, et al. A mandala of faculty development: using theory-based evaluation to explore contexts, mechanisms and outcomes. *Adv Health Sci Educ Theory Pract.* 2016. [Epub ahead of print].
16. Steinert Y, Thomas A. When I say … literature reviews. *Med Educ.* 2016;50(4):398–399.
17. Partin C, Kushner HI, Horton ME. A tale of Congress, continuing medical education, and the history of medicine. *Proc (BAYL Univ Med Cent).* 2014;27(2):156–160.
18. *UEMS Activities: The European Accreditation Council for CME (EACCME®)* [Internet]. Union Européenne des Médecins Spécialistes (UEMS)/The European Union of Medical Specialists; c2013 [Last accessed July 10, 2016].
19. *Global Alliance for Medical Education (GAME) Homepage* [Internet]. Global Alliance for Medical Education; c2016 [Last accessed July 10, 2016]. Available from: http://game-cme.org
20. *A Brief History of SACME* [Internet]. Society for Academic Continuing Medical Education (SACME); c2015 [Last accessed July 10, 2016]. Available from: http://www.sacme.org/History
21. Arditi C, Rege-Walther M, Wyatt JC, et al. Computer-generated reminders delivered on paper to healthcare professionals; effects on professional practice and health care outcomes. *Cochrane Database Syst Rev.* 2012;(12):CD001175.
22. Barwick MA, Peters J, Boydell K. Getting to uptake: do communities of practice support the implementation of evidence-based practice? *J Can Acad Child Adolesc Psychiatr [Journal de l'Academie canadienne de psychiatrie de l'enfant et de l'adolescent].* 2009;18(1):16–29.
23. Ivers N, Jamtvedt G, Flottorp S, et al. Audit and feedback: effects on professional practice and healthcare outcomes. *Cochrane Database Syst Rev.* 2012;(6):CD000259.
24. McFadden P, Crim A. Comparison of the effectiveness of interactive didactic lecture versus online simulation-based CME programs directed at improving the diagnostic capabilities of primary care practitioners. *J Contin Educ Health Prof.* 2016;36(1):32–37.
25. O'Brien MA, Rogers S, Jamtvedt G, et al. Educational outreach visits: effects on professional practice and health care outcomes. *Cochrane Database Syst Rev.* 2007;(4):CD000409.
26. Rosen MA, Hunt EA, Pronovost PJ, et al. In situ simulation in continuing education for the health care professions: a systematic review. *J Contin Educ Health Prof.* 2012;32(4):243–254.

27. Vakani FS, O'Beirne R. Performance improvement CME for quality: challenges inherent to the process. *Int J Health Care Qual Assur.* 2015;28(7):746–750.
28. Reeves S. An overview of continuing interprofessional education. *J Contin Educ Health Prof.* 2009;29(3):142–146.
29. Davis D. Continuing education, guideline implementation, and the emerging transdisciplinary field of knowledge translation. *J Contin Educ Health Prof.* 2006;26(1):5–12.
30. Davis D, Evans M, Jadad A, et al. The case for knowledge translation: shortening the journey from evidence to effect. *BMJ.* 2003;327(7405):33–35.
31. Davis NL, Davis DA, Johnson NM, et al. Aligning academic continuing medical education with quality improvement: a model for the 21st century. *Acad Med.* 2013;88(10):1437–1441.
32. Kitto SC, Bell M, Goldman J, et al. (Mis)perceptions of continuing education: insights from knowledge translation, quality improvement, and patient safety leaders. *J Contin Educ Health Prof.* 2013;33(2):81–88.
33. Kirkpatrick D. *Evaluating Training Programs: The Four Levels,* 2nd ed. San Francisco, CA: Berrett-Koehler; 1998.
34. Moore D. A framework for outcomes evaluation in the continuing professional development of physicians. In: Davis D, Barnes BE, Fox R, eds. *The Continuing Professional Development of Physicians: From Research to Practice.* Chicago, IL: American Medical Association Press; 2003:249–274.
35. Davis DA, Mazmanian PE, Fordis M, et al. Accuracy of physician self-assessment compared with observed measures of competence: a systematic review. *JAMA.* 2006;296(9):1094–1102.
36. Steinert Y, Macdonald ME, Boillat M, et al. Faculty development: if you build it, they will come. *Med Educ.* 2010;44(9):900–907.
37. Eva KW, Regehr G. Self-assessment in the health professions: a reformulation and research agenda. *Acad Med.* 2005;80(10 suppl):S46–S54.
38. Sargeant J, Lockyer J, Mann K, et al. Facilitated reflective performance feedback: developing an evidence- and theory-based model that builds relationship, explores reactions and content, and coaches for performance change (R2C2). *Acad Med.* 2015;90(12):1698–1706.
39. Leslie K, Baker L, Egan-Lee E, et al. Advancing faculty development in medical education: a systematic review. *Acad Med.* 2013;88(7):1038–1045.
40. Smith H, Brown H, Khanna J. *Continuing Education Meetings and Workshops: Effects on Professional Practice and Health-care Outcomes: RHL Commentary.* Geneva: World Health Organization; 2009 [last revised: 1 October, 2009].
41. Steinert Y. Faculty development: from workshops to communities of practice. *Med Teach.* 2010;32(5):425–428.
42. Steinert Y. Becoming a better teacher: from intuition to intent. In: Ende J, ed. *Theory and Practice of Teaching Medicine.* Philadelphia, PA: American College of Physicians; 2010:73–93.
43. Pathman DE, Konrad TR, Freed GL, et al. The awareness-to-adherence model of the steps to clinical guideline compliance. The case of pediatric vaccine recommendations. *Med Care.* 1996;34(9):873–889.
44. Davis D, Galbraith R. Continuing medical education effect on practice performance: effectiveness of continuing medical education: American College of Chest Physicians Evidence-Based Educational Guidelines. *Chest.* 2009;135(3 suppl):42s–48s.
45. Forsetlund L, Bjorndal A, Rashidian A, et al. Continuing education meetings and workshops: effects on professional practice and health care outcomes. *Cochrane Database Syst Rev.* 2009;(2):CD003030.
46. Marinopoulos SS, Dorman T, Ratanawongsa N, et al. Effectiveness of continuing medical education. *Evid Rep Technol Assess (Full Rep).* 2007;(149):1–69.
47. Steinert Y, Mann K, Centeno A, et al. A systematic review of faculty development initiatives designed to improve teaching effectiveness in medical education: BEME Guide No. 8. *Med Teach.* 2006;28(6):497–526.
48. Horsley T, Lockyer J, Cogo E, et al. National programmes for validating physician competence and fitness for practice: a scoping review. *BMJ Open.* 2016;6(4):e010368.
49. Murgatroyd GB. *Continuing Professional Development: The International Perspective.* General Medical Council; July 2011. Available from: http://www.gmc-uk.org/static/documents/content/CPD___The_International_Perspective_Jul_11.pdf_44810902.pdf
50. Green ML, Gross CP, Kernan WN, et al. Integrating teaching skills and clinical content in a faculty development workshop. *J Gen Intern Med.* 2003;18(6):468–474.
51. Karg A, Boendermaker PM, Brand PL, et al. Integrating continuing medical education and faculty development into a single course: effects on participants' behaviour. *Med Teach.* 2013;35(11):e1594–e1597.
52. Knowles MS, Holton EF, Swanson RA. *The Adult Learner.* Woburn, MA: Butterworth-Heinemann; 1998.
53. Chen W, Lai MM, Li TC, et al. Professional development is enhanced by serving as a mini-CEX preceptor. *J Contin Educ Health Prof.* 2011;31(4):225–230.

54. Stenfors-Hayes T, Kalen S, Hult H, et al. Being a mentor for undergraduate medical students enhances personal and professional development. *Med Teach.* 2010;32(2):148–153.
55. Silver IL, Leslie K. Faculty development for continuing interprofessional education and collaborative practice. *J Contin Educ Health Prof.* 2009;29(3):172–177.
56. *Academic CME in the United States and Canada: The 2013 AAMC/SACME Harrison Survey* [Internet]. Available from: http://www.sacme.org/Resources/Documents/SurveyResults/2013_survey_report.pdf
57. Bligh J. Faculty development. *Med Educ.* 2005;39(2):120–121.
58. Van Harrison R. Systems-based framework for continuing medical education and improvements in translating new knowledge into physicians' practices. *J Contin Educ Health Prof.* 2004;24(suppl 1):S50–S62.
59. Moore DE Jr, Green JS, Gallis HA. Achieving desired results and improved outcomes: integrating planning and assessment throughout learning activities. *J Contin Educ Health Prof.* 2009;29(1):1–15.
60. Onyura B, Legare F, Baker L, et al. Affordances of knowledge translation in medical education: a qualitative exploration of empirical knowledge use among medical educators. *Acad Med.* 2015;90(4):518–524.
61. O'Sullivan PS, Irby DM. Reframing research on faculty development. *Acad Med.* 2011;86(4):421–428.
62. *Recognition and Approval of Trainers* [Internet]. General Medical Council; c2016 [Last accessed July 27, 2016].
63. van der Leeuw RM, Slootweg IA, Heineman MJ, et al. Explaining how faculty members act upon residents' feedback to improve their teaching performance. *Med Educ.* 2013;47(11):1089–1098.
64. Carraccio C, Englander R, Van Melle E, et al. Advancing competency-based medical education: a charter for clinician-educators. *Acad Med.* 2016;91(5):645–649.
65. Campbell C, Silver I, Sherbino J, et al. Competency-based continuing professional development. *Med Teach.* 2010;32(8):657–662.

Chapter 15

FACULTY DEVELOPMENT *for* PRACTICING *and* TEACHING QUALITY IMPROVEMENT *and* PATIENT SAFETY

Karyn D. Baum and Nancy L. Davis

Case

Increasingly, national and local reports call for better preparation of undergraduate health professional students and resident physicians in the science of health care improvement. Preparation is both at the basic, cognitive level (delivered by lectures or online methods) and, more importantly, at the experiential level (undertaking quality improvement projects, engaging in patient safety reporting, etc.). As the Chief Academic Officer of a large urban health system, you acknowledge the importance of the reports but have a problem: few if any of your clinical faculty are trained in quality improvement and patient safety (QI/PS). They are excellent clinicians but unable to teach, role model, or coach learners in the science of quality and safety.

Questions

How can you develop a critical mass of clinicians with these skills? What should be taught to health care professionals to ensure they acquire these skills? How can their skills be best utilized at your institution?

INTRODUCTION

Since the publication of *To Err Is Human* in 1999, there has been an explosion of efforts to make health care safer and of higher quality. The 2016 article citing medical errors as the third leading cause of death in the United States has only spurred this work.[1] As noted in Chapter 1, essential to the support of improved care outcomes is faculty commitment to learn and teach about quality improvement and patient safety (QI/PS) across the continuum. An early and ongoing challenge has been the lack of providers trained in QI/PS and the science of improvement.[2,3]

One barrier is the ongoing argument over what the content areas within this emerging science should contain and which of those are crucial for providers to master. One of the most influential models was the one proposed by the Institute of Medicine (IOM) in 2001 with the following six aims[4]:

- Safe
- Timely
- Effective
- Efficient
- Equitable
- Patient centered

These six aims, often referred to as the STEEEP goals, have changed slightly over time; for example, the final term is sometimes altered to "patient and family centered," but they have otherwise stood the test of time. Value, defined as quality divided by cost, is a new and rising term; however, timeliness and efficiency encompass similar concepts. Agreement on the boundaries of this emerging science is only the first step. From there, we must assure that our current and emerging professionals are able to engage in, role model, and teach these competencies at a time of great change in health care throughout the world.

QUALITY IMPROVEMENT AND PATIENT SAFETY EDUCATION AND SKILLS FOR CLINICIANS

The most commonly taught QI/PS skills include defining aims, measurement, identifying waste, process mapping, and conducting root cause analyses. While there is not sufficient opportunity within this text to review the full breadth of knowledge, skills, and attitudes required to participate or lead QI/PS efforts, the use of an improvement model will guide providers as they seek to understand the outcomes they see and the data they review. We are not advocating any particular model such as Six Sigma, focusing on reliability; Lean/Define, Measure, Analyze, Improve, Control (DMAIC), focusing on reduction of waste; or the Nolan model of improvement, rather that providers and faculty use a consistent model as a construct for the improvement work they engage in and teach.[5,6] Ideally, this model should be the one used by the health system that they practice within.

It is also essential to recognize that these traditional skills and the ability to list the six IOM aims are not adequate preparation for faculty to engage in and teach QI/PS. The ability to operationalize improvement efforts, while less often taught, is in many ways more essential for physicians looking to successfully be part of, or run, improvement efforts. This increasing acknowledgment of the importance of both technical and nontechnical skills is similar to that seen in medical practice.

Essential nontechnical skills for engaging in QI include stakeholder analysis, project management, working in teams, and displaying results. Many improvement projects that fail do so for lack of project management reasons, rather than lack of interest in the topic.[7] However, many training programs for physicians concentrate on technical improvement skills rather than these management-focused skills, often to the detriment of those looking to utilize these skills in daily practice.[8]

Stakeholder analysis and involvement are often overlooked during improvement efforts but can make a significant difference to long-term success.[9] Health care providers, like most adults, are much more interested in having things done with them rather than to them and care deeply about the care they deliver. Consideration up front of stakeholder groups and assuring their continual involvement throughout planning and implementation will lead to a more robust effort that is more likely to succeed.[10]

The Project Management Institute defines project management as the "application of knowledge, skills, tools, and techniques to project activities to meet the project requirements."[11] The processes within it consist of initiating, planning, executing, monitoring and controlling, and closing projects. These processes, while similar to those mentioned in DMAIC and other QI models, require additional specific tools and skills often missing in QI/PS methodology. Examples include effectively running meetings, creating and meeting deadlines, and communication among large teams and organizations. QI/PS work requires execution skills, not simply will and a good idea.

Likewise, leading and working in teams is integral to QI/PS work yet is often overlooked in QI education.[12,13] While these skills overlap those of project management, they deserve special mention, especially when applied to an interprofessional health care context. The powerful hierarchy that still exists within health care can overpower even the most important QI project unless members can recognize and respond to the cultural issues at play.

Measurement and displaying results are subtly different yet equally crucial in improvement work. Knowing what and how to measure improvement efforts, from the concepts of process and outcome measures to utilization of statistical process control charts or qualitative analysis, are necessary but not sufficient in improvement work. Equally important is being able to take what are often large amounts of information and turn it into useable, readable, actionable data.[14]

No training in QI/PS would be complete without examining the vital role of context.[15] Context is why a checklist might produce astounding results in one hospital (or unit) while making no difference in another. Several models have recently been developed to help leaders understand the specific aspects of context at play in QI/PS work.[16–18] Common contextual factors cited in the literature include organizational culture, data availability, and leadership.[14] Preparing those involved in QI/PS to address and consider these factors will hopefully better arm them for this often-challenging work.

Two contextual components that deserve explicit attention when preparing faculty of all professions to engage in and teach QI/PS are organizational context and the interprofessional setting. As already noted, the larger organizational context is a key component that can influence the success of these efforts. Failing to align project to the organizational priorities is an all too common error, especially for those first starting out in the field. On the other hand, careful alignment can help ensure access to much-needed resources.[19] The interprofessional nature of QI/PS is also worth calling out. Unfortunately, most health providers were trained in silos; QI/PS requires us to work in teams, as noted in Chapters 9 and 20. Interprofessional teamwork also requires careful management of the unspoken power gradients still at play in health care.[20,21] Physicians in particular must be sensitive to these issues, as they tend to rate team cultures higher than other professions.[22,23]

The field of QI/PS itself is also continuing to expand, making any developed curriculum potentially outdated within a short period of time. Emergent concepts within this area include diagnostic errors (including bias) and value-based care. The original 1999 IOM report estimated that the impact of medical errors included those generated from clinical reasoning errors, which often lead to diagnostic errors or delays. The IOM has estimated that nearly all Americans will suffer one of these at least once in their lifetime, and in one study, they were the leading type of paid malpractice claims.[24,25] Educators are just beginning to work to reduce the frequency of these errors, and these efforts are likely to grow significantly. One example is the diagnostic error curriculum initiated by the University of Pennsylvania.[26]

The shift in health care from volume to value-based payments has spurred health systems, medical training programs, and national groups to consider better training for health care providers in this area.[27,28] Many studies have shown that providers have little to no understanding of health care costs, yet they control a large percentage of the spending.[29,30] Educational interventions are now springing up to address this gap at all levels, from undergraduate medical education to continuing professional development.[31] Accordingly, as CPD is developed in the QI/PS sphere, including cost issues will be increasingly critical.

Faculty development for QI/PS has taken on many forms, and there is not sufficient space within this chapter to review them all. However, a few themes have emerged. First, faculty need time to learn and practice this material. QI/PS is not well taught solely in the lecture hall. Second, linking project work to faculty clinical settings so that they can solve real problems that matter to them is essential. On the flip side, aligning their work with institutional priorities and data is essential. Faculty must also be rewarded, whether it be financially or from an academic standpoint, for engaging in improvement work in a scholarly manner.[32] Finally, longitudinal learning (such as a yearlong improvement fellowship), particularly those in interprofessional settings such as the Veterans Affairs Quality Scholars program, seems to be predictive of positive results.[33,34]

It is within this context of health care QI/PS that we address the needs of the Chief Academic Officer (CAO) in our case. Only through a thoughtful, systematic process for training and providing an effective clinical learning environment will our CAO be able to develop a critical mass of clinicians and interprofessional staff with the skills to ensure continuous QI/PS.

KNOWING THE LEARNER

Regardless of the context of teaching health care QI/PS, it is important to have an understanding of learners and their level of competence. A popular model, often modified, is that of Dreyfus and Dreyfus, shown in Table 15.1, which defines the learner as Novice, Proficient, Expert, or Master.[35]

In addition to knowing learners' level of competence, it is important to know their stage of learning. Donald Pathman developed a model of learner stages through which most learners must proceed in order for learning to stick.[36] Learners must first become aware of a new concept. Once aware, they must agree with the concept and be willing

TABLE 15.1 Dreyfus Model of Adult Skill Acquisition	
Competence Level	**Characteristics**
Novice	Rules based
Advanced Beginner	Meaningful aspects of the concept
Competent	Devise a plan and perspective
Proficient	Situational discrimination
Expert	Able to achieve the goal

to try it. After trying and accepting the new concept, they must adopt it into their regular practice. Finally, following successful adoption, adherence ensures that the new concept becomes routine. Different teaching strategies are more effective for each stage. Pathman's stages and corresponding teaching strategies are shown in Table 15.2.

Often in medical education, lecture is used to raise awareness for our learners, but the other stages are skipped and yet learners are expected to reach adherence to and sustain a new practice. Once aware, it is important to ensure learners are in agreement and have the resources to adopt and adhere to a new concept in practice.

Just as in all educational development, it is essential to plan the teaching of QI/PS concepts using sound educational theory. Once learners' level of competence and stage of learning are identified, effective learning objectives can be crafted. Sometimes viewed as a pointless exercise to satisfy accreditors, developing learning objectives provides a systematic way to think about the educational activity.

SMART LEARNING OBJECTIVES

A useful acronym for effective learning objectives is SMART: Specific, Measurable, Achievable, Relevant, and Time-bound.[37] Specific means detailed, focused, and clear. Measurable means quantifiable and able to show results. Achievable means the learner has the skills and resources needed to complete the activity. Relevant implies the learner's role and need for the content. Finally, time-bound gives a specific timeline and end point. These elements will produce specific and effective learning objectives that can be used to develop the learning activity.

TABLE 15.2 Pathman Model of Stages of Learning	
Stage of Learning	**Effective Teaching Strategies**
Awareness	Lecture, reading
Agreement	Champions, small groups
Adoption	Demonstrations, simulation
Adherence	Audit/feedback, reminders

Action verbs are used in learning objectives and are selected based on the level of cognitive dimension desired. Cognitive dimensions are based on Bloom's Taxonomy of Educational Objectives.[38] Effective action verbs are selected based on desired learner outcomes and level of cognitive processing in order to design the educational activity to that level. See Table 15.3 for appropriate action verbs for each of Bloom's levels.

Learning objectives have a standard format—a stem that defines the time frame and an action verb followed by the actual product, process, or outcome. Here are some examples:

Knowledge: By the end of the 50-minute lecture, learners will be able to list the components of a fishbone diagram.

Comprehension: By the end of the 30-minute discussion, learners will be able to describe the appropriate use of a fishbone diagram.

Application: By the end of the 30-minute exercise, learners will be able to illustrate the elements of a fishbone diagram.

Analysis: By the end of the 30-minute case discussion, the learners will be able to draw the fishbone using elements from the case.

Synthesis: By the end of the 30-minute case discussion, the learners will be able to formulate solutions to the problems posed by the fishbone diagram.

Evaluation: By the end of the 30-minute case discussion, the learners will be able to evaluate whether the fishbone diagram was the most useful tool to address the problem posed in the case.

Goals and objectives for the educational activity itself are slightly different. In addition to specific learner objectives, the course or other activity has a more global

---

TABLE 15.3
Action Verbs Based on Bloom's Taxonomy of Learning Objectives

Cognitive Dimension	Example Action Verbs
Knowledge *Learners will "know" something new.*	Define, list, record
Comprehension *Learners will be able to "convey" their new knowledge.*	Describe, discuss, explain, identify, recognize
Application *Learners will be able to "do" something based on new knowledge.*	Apply, demonstrate, illustrate, interpret
Analysis *Learners will be able to "analyze and interpret" new information.*	Analyze, calculate, compare, contrast, diagram
Synthesis *Learners will be able to formulate new models based on what they have learned.*	Arrange, collect, compose, construct, design, formulate
Evaluation *Learners will be able to "evaluate" situations or concepts based on what they have learned.*	Appraise, assess, choose, evaluate, measure, revise

objective. For example, for one of the learning activities listed above, the objective might be as follows: "By the end of this six-week course, learners will be able to implement a fishbone diagram in order to perform a root cause analysis of a quality issue described in a case."

DECIDING WHAT TO TEACH

Quality improvement principles are best taught in practice. Basic principles can be taught in the classroom, but only experience in clinical settings will provide the desired higher levels of learning. These principles must be learned in the context of systems thinking and organizational quality and safety priorities. Observing problems and gaps in practice will lead to effective aim statements and design of quality and safety initiatives that are relevant to the learner and the organization.

In developing a QI/PS curriculum, basic concepts should be considered including

- Quality improvement models such as Plan, Do, Study, Act (PDSA); LEAN; Define, Measure, Analyze, Improve, Control (DMAIC); and Six Sigma
- Literature review and assessment of current evidence
- Measures: types and how they are developed and endorsed
- Data collection and analysis techniques
- Quality improvement tools such as:
  - Flowchart (process analysis)
  - Brainstorming (identification of problems/gaps)
  - Five Whys (root cause analysis)
  - Fishbone/Ishikawa diagram (root cause analysis)
  - Pareto chart (rank order by importance)
  - Control chart (performance over time)
- Teamwork and communication skills
- Error identification and reporting
- Transformational change management (improvement requires change)
- Dissemination of findings (presentations and publications)

SELECTING TEACHING STRATEGIES AND FORMATS

Teaching strategies and formats are selected based on learning objectives and expected learner outcomes. While a lecture might work well to raise awareness and teach basic concepts that are new to the learner, it will not be effective in reaching higher cognitive dimensions. QI/PS principles, in particular, are content areas where learners must learn to use new tools, implement them into clinical practice, and be able to analyze changes based on implementation of new interventions. A lecture should only be used to introduce novice learners to new concepts, and then, they should be allowed to apply concepts right away in order to become proficient. Cases, small group discussion and exercises, team-based learning, demonstrations, and simulations will progress learners to higher levels of understanding and performance.

QUALITY IMPROVEMENT PROJECTS FOR LEARNERS

While traditional classroom and clinical teaching can and should be used for teaching quality improvement principles, the QI project can be very effective for giving learners the knowledge and experience they need to put QI into practice. There is some controversy as to how projects are used in teaching. If learners identify projects based on their limited experience, they may be more inclined to be interested and see them as relevant, but the project may lack rigor or connection to the quality improvement priorities of the clinical enterprise. Quality initiatives identified by the organization may be useful, but learners lack buy-in or, often, the ability to engage in a meaningful way due to time constraints, lack of understanding of concepts, and lack of interest in the area. Most educators concede that in order to teach learners basic skills, they should be encouraged to identify fairly simple projects that can be completed in a short time and are of interest to the learners. Using a simple PDSA cycle, faculty can walk learners through the process allowing them to first learn the concepts and then experience the cycle of improvement. A simple project design is as follows:

1. Identify a problem or gap.
2. Develop a clear AIM statement.
3. Review literature regarding the problem/gap.
4. Identify existing measures if available.
5. Identify benchmarks if available.
6. Identify target outcomes.
7. Determine data source(s).
8. Collect data.
9. Analyze data.
10. Implement intervention(s) for improvement.
11. Remeasure.
12. Repeat as time and resources allow.

Having learners work in teams and engaged in every step is the best way for them to learn the concepts, processes, and relevance to practice. Showing them that consideration of this process should be a part of routine practice will set the stage for their career.

LINKING QI/PS TO THE ACGME CORE COMPETENCIES AND THE CLINICAL LEARNING ENVIRONMENT

The Accreditation Council for Graduate Medical Education (ACGME) and American Board of Medical Specialties (ABMS) have endorsed the following core competencies to ensure learners are well prepared[39,40]:

- *Patient Care*: Identify, respect, and care about patients' differences, values, preferences, and expressed needs; listen to, clearly inform, communicate with, and educate patients; share decision-making and management; and continuously advocate disease prevention, wellness, and promotion of healthy lifestyles, including a focus on population health.

- *Medical Knowledge*: Established and evolving biomedical, clinical, and cognate (e.g., epidemiological and social behavioral) sciences and the application of knowledge to patient care.
- *Practice-based Learning and Improvement*: Involves investigation and evaluation of one's own patient care, appraisal and assimilation of scientific evidence, and improvements in patient care.
- *Interpersonal and Communication Skills*: Effective information exchange and teaming with patients, their families, and other health professionals.
- *Professionalism*: Commitment to carrying out professional responsibilities, adherence to ethical principles, and sensitivity to a diverse patient population.
- *Systems-based Practice*: Actions that demonstrate an awareness of and responsiveness to the larger context and system of health care and the ability to effectively call on system resources to provide care that is of optimal value.

While all six core competencies are important in teaching about QI/PS, those most relevant are Practice-based Learning and Improvement, Interpersonal and Communication Skills, and Systems-based Practice. These competencies focus on the systems thinking required for ongoing QI/PS. Communication skills are essential for team dynamics and error prevention.

In 2014, ACGME introduced its Clinical Learning Environment Review (CLER) to encourage engagement of trainees into their systems' QI/PS efforts.[41] Four of the six CLER focus areas are centered in health care quality improvement, including QI, Patient Safety, Disparities in care, and Transitions of Care. This new initiative led to much more emphasis on teaching QI principles and requiring resident trainees to participate in clinical QI/PS activities.

The Accreditation Council for Continuing Medical Education (ACCME) was an early adopter of QI/PS content in medical education. In 2006, it modified its Standards for Continuing Medical Education (CME) by including criteria for identification of practice gaps and using resources, particularly quality improvement, outside the CME office. In 2005, criteria for Performance Improvement CME (PI CME) were introduced to allow for value-added CME credit for physicians participating in performance improvement in practice. The American Academy of Family Physicians (AAFP) and the American Osteopathic Association (AOA) created parallel opportunities in their CME credit systems.[42-44]

Undergraduate medical education now includes QI/PS content in the curriculum for medical students, and in recent years, the National Board of Medical Education (NBME) has added questions to the United States Medical Licensing Exam (USMLE) germane to QI/PS concepts.[45]

ASSESSMENT OF LEARNERS IN QUALITY IMPROVEMENT

For novice learners, didactic teaching around basic principles will be necessary to raise awareness and comprehension of new concepts. Written quizzes and exams are effective methods for assessing this level of knowledge and skill acquisition.

Direct observation is required to assess learners' ability to apply, synthesize, and analyze new concepts. It is important that peer and/or faculty assessors have adequate training in observation methods as well as a standardized instrument to ensure fair and equitable assessment of learners. Solid learning objectives are required in order to determine what to assess relative to expected learner outcomes. Without measurable objectives, it is impossible to know how to measure.

PROGRAM EVALUATION

An important, but often overlooked, element of educational development is program evaluation. In order to assess whether an educational activity has had impact, all aspects of it must be evaluated. Certainly, learner success, including testing, observance of desired performance levels, and satisfaction metrics are important. But there are other metrics to consider. Who are the stakeholders and what are their expectations for this activity? Is there to be financial solvency? Are outcomes measurable and reportable and to whom? These are some of the questions to be considered in evaluating the overall success of the program.

A logic model can be useful in analyzing and reporting program outcomes.[46] A simple logic model includes Inputs, Outputs, and Outcomes. A more complex logic model might describe these elements in short-, medium-, and long-term categories as shown in Table 15.4.

Educational development in QI/PS is similar in many ways to that in any other content area, but its uniqueness in language, processes, and clinical application require new skill sets in teaching and practice. Today's medical education faculty must acquire these skills in order to support the learners they serve.

FUTURE DIRECTIONS

According the Association of American Medical College's Teaching for Quality report, it is essential to develop a critical mass of faculty able to engage in, teach, and model QI/PS.[2] Preparing faculty at every health professions school can seem like a daunting task, especially given a recent consensus paper noting the continued lack of local expertise to train those faculty.[47] Fortunately, new models are making headway, many of which are interprofessional in nature. Successful programs will likely utilize QI concepts for their own improvement purposes, thus allowing a real-time demonstration of the utility of these methods.

As payment models, especially those in the United States, continue to shift dramatically from volume to value, health systems have a growing incentive to engage their staff in QI/PS efforts. This incentive will likely lead to increased system efforts to train

TABLE 15.4
Simple Logic Model

Inputs	Outputs	Outcomes
Staff	Workshops	New knowledge
Funding	Projects	Improved learner performance
Materials/equipment	Web sites	Improved patient care

all members to become change agents and part of high reliability organizations. The increasing transparency in outcomes has the same impact. One striking aspect of the transition to value has been the shift toward population health and the inclusion of public health concepts in the daily work of many new professionals. It will be fascinating to see whether the line between public health and acute care continue to blur in the future. One thing is clear: health care professionals will be required to be integral parts of whole systems and continuous quality improvement will be essential to better outcomes, efficiencies, and cost-effectiveness.

However, it is still unclear what types of QI/PS education are most effective for whom, and under what circumstances, leaving much work for researchers in the near future. What should prelicensure students learn, as compared to those in practice? Must QI/PS be learned in an experiential manner, or would didactics suffice? Which topics are required and which ones are optional? Can asynchronous online learning be effective? Finally, is interprofessional education more effective?

By clearly defining the essential skills, taking full advantage of educational learning theory, trialing new processes such as co-learning, and rewarding faculty for this important work, organizations are making significant strides in developing health care professionals willing and able to add QI/PS to their daily work.[3,32,48] It will continue to be important to integrate faculty development and continuing professional development for our clinical faculty to ensure their expertise in QI/PS. However, with the current expansion of this study at the student, graduate, and continuing professional development levels, it is likely our health care professionals will only need ongoing maintenance of their skills rather than the need for learning basic skills today.

As improvement science becomes more sound and prevalent, there will no doubt be growth of new research and dissemination of new concepts, tools, and processes to continue the improvement of health care delivery. Concurrently, there will be new research in the methodologies for teaching and assessing learners in this field. Rather than the trial and error in much of today's quality improvement education, there will be sound principles to test and larger learning laboratories for implementing new strategies.

The CAO in our case has every reason to be optimistic as the pipeline of clinicians with QI/PS skills is increasing in volume every year. Not only are medical school, nursing school, pharmacy programs, and residency program curricula putting more emphasis on QI/PS, but CPD is playing a crucial role in these efforts and should always consider how they work the support will impact the health of the community.

REFERENCES

1. Makary M, Daniel M. Medical error—the third leading cause of death in the US. *BMJ*. 2016;353:i2139.
2. Association of American Medical Colleges. *Integrating Quality Improvement and Patient Safety across the Continuum of Medical Education*. 2013. https://members.aamc.org/eweb/upload/Teaching%20for%20 Quality%20Report.pdf. Accessed July 2, 2016.
3. Lannon CM, Levy FH, Moyer VA. The need to build capability and capacity in quality improvement and patient safety. *Pediatrics*. 2015;135(6):e1371–e1373.
4. Institute of Medicine (IOM). *Crossing the Quality Chasm: A New Health System for the 21st Century*. Washington, DC: National Academies Press; 2001.
5. Holweg M. The genealogy of lean production. *J Oper Manag*. 2007;25(2):420–437.
6. Langley GL, Nolan KM, Nolan TW, et al. *The Improvement Guide: A Practical Approach to Enhancing Organizational Performance*, 2nd ed. San Francisco, CA: Jossey Bass; 2009.

7. McLean R, Antony J. Why continuous improvement initiatives fail in manufacturing environments? A systematic review of the evidence. *Int J Prod Perf Manag.* 2013;63(3):370–376.

8. Karasick AS, Nash DB. Training in quality improvement and patient safety: the current landscape. *Am J Med Qual.* 2015;30(6):526–538.

9. Kirchner JE, Parker LE, Bonner LM, et al. The role of managers, frontline staff, and local champions in implementing quality improvement: stakeholders' perspectives. *J Eval Clin Pract.* 2012;18:63–69.

10. Tomoaia-Cotisel A, Scammon DL, Waitzman NJ, et al. Context matters: the experience of 14 research teams in systematically reporting contextual factors important for practice change. *Ann Fam Med.* 2013;11(suppl 1):S115–S123.

11. Project Management Institute. *What Is Project Management?* 2016. http://www.pmi.org/en/About-Us/About-Us-What-is-Project-Management.aspx. Accessed July 2, 2016.

12. Dietz AS, Pronovost PJ, Mendez-Tellez PA, et al. A systematic review of teamwork in the intensive care unit: what do we know about teamwork, team tasks, and improvement strategies? *J Crit Care.* 2014;29(6):908–914.

13. Brock D, Abu-Rish E, Chiu CR, et al. Interprofessional education in team communication: working together to improve patient safety. *BMJ Qual Saf.* 2013;22(5):414.

14. Dixon-Woods M, McNicol S, Martin G. Ten challenges in improving quality in healthcare: lessons from the Health Foundation's programme evaluations and relevant literature. *BMJ Qual Saf.* 2012;21:876–884.

15. Bataldan PB, Davidoff F. What is quality improvement and how can it transform healthcare? *Qual Saf Health Care.* 2007;16:2–3. doi:10.1136/qshc.2006.022046.

16. Kaplan HC, Brady PW, Dritz MC, et al. The influence of context on quality improvement success in health care: a systematic review of the literature. *Milbank Q.* 2010;88(4):500–559.

17. Kaplan HC, Provost LP, Froehle CM, et al. The model for understanding success in quality (MUSIQ): building a theory of context in healthcare quality. *BMJ Qual Saf.* 2012;21:13–20.

18. Headrick LA, Ogrinc G, Hoffman KG, et al. Exemplary care and learning sites: a model for improvement in care and learning in the clinical setting. *Acad Med.* 2016;91(3):354–359.

19. Tess A, Vidyarthi A, Yang J, et al. Bridging the gap: a framework and strategies for integrating the quality and safety mission of teaching hospitals and graduate medical education. *Acad Med.* 2015;90(9):1251–1257.

20. Cosby K, Croskerry P. Profiles in patient safety: authority gradients in medical error. *Acad Emerg Med.* 2004;11(12):1341–1345.

21. Friedman Z, Hayter MA, Everett TC, et al. Power and conflict: the effect of a superior's interpersonal behaviour on trainees' ability to challenge authority during a simulated airway emergency. *Anaesthesia.* 2015;70:1119–1129.

22. Brasaite I, Kaunonen M, Martinkenas A, et al. Health care professionals' attitudes regarding patient safety: cross-sectional survey. *BMC Res Notes.* 2016;9:177.

23. Henkin A, Chon TY, Christopherson ML, et al. Improving nurse-physician teamwork through interprofessional bedside rounding. *J Multdiscip Healthc.* 2016;9:201–205.

24. Institute of Medicine (IOM). *Improving Diagnosis in Healthcare.* Washington, DC: National Academies Press; 2015.

25. Tehrani ASS, Lee HE, Matthews SC, et al. 25-Year summary of US malpractice claims for diagnostic errors 1986–2010: an analysis from the National Practitioner Data Bank. *BMJ Qual Saf.* 2013;22(8):672–680.

26. Reilly JB, Ogdie AR, Von Feldt JM, et al. Teaching about how doctors think: a longitudinal curriculum in cognitive bias and diagnostic error for residents. *BMJ Qual Saf.* 2013;22:1044–1050.

27. Smith CD, Alliance for Academic Internal Medicine–American College of Physicians High Value; Cost-Conscious Care Curriculum Development Committee. Teaching high value, cost-conscious care to residents: The Alliance for Academic Internal Medicine–American College of Physicians Curriculum. *Ann Intern Med.* 2012;157:284–286.

28. Huang GC, Tibbles CD, Newman LR, et al. Consensus of the Millennium Conference on teaching high value care. *Teach Learn Med.* 2016;28(1):97–104.

29. Long T, Silvestri MT, Dashevsky M, et al. Exit survey of senior residents: cost conscious but uninformed. *J Grad Med Educ.* 2016;8(2):248–251.

30. Wang A, Dybul SL, Patel PJ, et al. A cross-sectional survey of interventional radiologists and vascular surgeons regarding the cost and reimbursement of common devices and procedures. *J Vasc Interv Radiol.* 2016;27:210–218.

31. Stammen LA, Stalmeijer RE, Paternotte E, et al. Training physicians to provide high-value, cost-conscious care: a systematic review. *JAMA.* 2015;314(22):2384–2400.

32. Shojania KG, Levinson W. Clinicians in quality improvement: a new career pathway in academic medicine. *JAMA.* 2009;301(7):766–768.

33. Splaine ME, Ogrinc G, Gilman SC, et al. The Department of Veterans Affairs National Quality Scholars Fellowship Program: experience from 10 years of training quality scholars. *Acad Med.* 2009; 84:1741–1748.

34. Kaminski GM, Britto MT, Schoettker PJ, et al. Developing capable quality improvement leaders. *BMJ Qual Saf.* 2012;21(11):903–911.
35. Dreyfus SE. The five-stage model of adult skill acquisition. *Bull Sci Technol Soc.* 2004;24(3):177–181.
36. Pathman DE, et al. The awareness-to-adherence model of the steps to clinical guideline compliance. *Med Care.* 1996;34(9):873–889.
37. College of Nurses of Ontario. *Developing SMART Learning Goals.* Pub. No. 44047.2014. http://www.cno.org/globalassets/docs/qa/developingsmartgoals.pdf. Accessed December 27, 2016.
38. Bloom BS, ed. *Taxonomy of Educational Objectives: The Classification of Educational Goals in Handbook 1: Cognitive Domain.* New York: David McKay; 1956.
39. Accreditation Council for Graduate Medical Education. *Common Program Requirements.* http://www.acgme.org/What-We-Do/Accreditation/Common-Program-Requirements. Accessed July 25, 2016.
40. American Board of Medical Specialties. *Board Certification Based on Core Competencies.* http://www.abms.org/board-certification/a-trusted-credential/based-on-core-competencies/. Accessed July 9, 2016.
41. Accreditation Council for Graduate Medical Education. *Clinical Learning Environment Review (CLER).* http://www.acgme.org/What-We-Do/Initiatives/Clinical-Learning-Environment-Review-CLER. Accessed July 9, 2016.
42. Accreditation Council for Continuing Medical Education. *ACCME Accreditation Requirements.* http://www.accme.org/sites/default/files/626_20160211_Accreditation_Requirements_Document.pdf. Accessed July 9, 2016.
43. American Academy of Family Physicians. *AAFP Credit Eligibility Requirements.* http://www.aafp.org/cme/creditsys/about/eligibility.html. Accessed July 9, 2016.
44. American Osteopathic Association. *CME Guide.* http://www.osteopathic.org/inside-aoa/development/continuing-medical-education/Pages/category-1-a-credit.aspx. Accessed July 9, 2016.
45. National Board of Medical Education. *Health System Reform Policies.* http://www.nbme.org/about/health-system-reform-policies/policy-2.html. Accessed July 9, 2016.
46. Millar A, Simeone RS, Carnevale JT. Logic models: a systems tool for performance management. *Eval Program Plann.* 2001;24:73–81.
47. Gonzalo JD, Baxley E, Borkan J, et al. Priority areas and potential solutions for successful integration and sustainment of health systems science in undergraduate medical education. *Acad Med.* 2016;91(8):1–7.
48. Wong BM, Giguen J, Shojania K. Building capacity for quality: a pilot co-learning curriculum in quality improvement for faculty and resident learners. *J Grad Med Educ.* 2013;5(4):689–693.

PART IV

CREATING BETTER LEARNERS AT ALL LEVELS

CREATING *the* PRACTICE-BASED LEARNER: ADVANCES *in* UNDERGRADUATE MEDICAL EDUCATION

Linda A. Headrick

Case

Years ago, a wise CME director said, "It's not our fault that CME doesn't always produce good results. They throw them in the river upstream before they can swim!" By "the river," he meant the long trajectory of practice, and by "swimming," he meant the ability to detect practice problems. Acquiring skills such as how to effectively and efficiently improve clinical practices is not routine or explicitly taught in medical school or residency. You sit with the senior associate dean for education on a small committee that oversees the full continuum of medical and health professional education in your medical center.

Questions

The dean asks the group, "If we did teach these skills, what would the educational experiences look like? How would we design the curricula? How would we determine the effectiveness of the educational effort?"

INTRODUCTION

The 1990s witnessed new applications of quality improvement (QI) in health care, with increasing evidence of benefits to patients.[1,2] In parallel, faculty began to develop and test ways in which improvement science could become part of undergraduate medical education, with an emphasis on interprofessional education.[3,4] In 1999 and 2001, landmark reports from the Institute of Medicine (IOM) established patient safety and QI as key to achieving health care that is patient centered, timely, effective, efficient, and equitable.[5,6] Identifying change in health professional education as a "bridge to quality," the IOM in 2003 wrote that "All health professionals should be educated to deliver patient-centered care as members of an interdisciplinary team, emphasizing evidence-based practice, quality improvement approaches, and informatics."[7] Influential bodies in other parts of the world have published similar conclusions.[8,9]

In 2010, the Carnegie Foundation for the Advancement of Teaching sponsored *Educating Physicians: A Call for Reform of Medical School and Residency* to mark the 100th anniversary of the Flexner Report, *Medical Education in the US and Canada*.[10,11] The authors described improving care for patients as part of physicians' professional responsibility, writing, "Encouraging learners to seek improvement in their own performance as well as the performance of the groups, teams, and systems in which they work must begin early in medical school and must be reinforced in residency and beyond." The AAMC Medical School Objectives Project Report V: Quality of Care identified specific learning goals for undergraduate medical education, recommending that by graduation, a medical student should be able to[12]:

1. Critically evaluate the knowledge base supporting good patient care.
2. Demonstrate understanding of the gap between prevailing practices and best practices, and the steps necessary to close that gap.
3. Contribute to closing the gap between prevailing and best practices.

Each of these landmark reports speaks to the creation of the QI-focused, continuing professional development (CPD)-proficient learner in the scenario presented at the beginning of this chapter. They also raise the question: After 20-plus years of work, how well are we preparing medical school graduates to improve care as part of their routine professional practice? Unfortunately, progress is limited. In the United States at least, both the Accreditation Council for Graduate Medical Education (ACGME) and the Accrediting Council for Continuing Medical Education (ACCME), respectively, require education for physicians at the graduate and continuing professional education levels to include health care improvement. In contrast, the same is not true for the Liaison Committee for Medical Education, which accredits undergraduate medical education in the United States and Canada.[13–15]

Despite the requirement that practice-based learning and improvement be taught as core competencies during residency, the ACGME's report of the first year of Clinical Learning Environment Review (CLER) visits found that many residents and fellows appeared to have a limited knowledge of QI concepts and the specific methods and approaches to QI employed by the organization in which they were training. While most residents and fellows reported involvement in QI projects, there was only limited participation in interprofessional QI teams.[16] There are similarly disappointing results at the medical student level. While 94% of recent medical school graduates surveyed by the Association of American Medical Colleges (AAMC) reported having "basic skills in clinical decision making and the application of evidence based information to medical practice" (also a core CPD competency), only 71.4% felt that they received an appropriate amount of training in health care QI.[17]

WHAT SHOULD WE TEACH MEDICAL STUDENTS ABOUT HEALTH CARE IMPROVEMENT?

There have been recent calls for an international consensus process to establish a common set of core competencies for health care improvement.[18] There is strong support for practice-based learning and improvement as a fundamental building block in physician training as a key driver of each physician's CPD. This includes both (1) the ability to execute required observable behaviors (e.g., write a "SMART" aim statement, construct and analyze a run chart) and (2) the professional motivation to engage in improvement as a core professional practice (e.g., review data because of desire to learn rather than in response to external reminders).

There are some helpful resources available now. For example, the AAMC's 2013 *Teaching for Quality* report identified the following competencies pertinent to health care improvement[19]:

- Practice-based learning and improvement
  - Critically evaluate and apply current health care information and scientific evidence for patient care.
  - Systematically analyze practice using QI methods and demonstrate improvements in practice.
  - Incorporate formative evaluation feedback into daily practice.
  - Use information technology to optimize learning and care delivery.
- Systems-based practice
  - Work effectively in various health care delivery settings and systems relevant to one's clinical specialty, including identifying systems' issues and improving them.
  - Incorporate considerations of cost awareness and risk–benefit analysis in patient and/or population-based care.
  - Participate in identifying system errors and implementing potential system solutions.
- Collaboration
  - Work in interprofessional teams to enhance patient safety and improve patient care quality.

An additional resource, *Fundamentals of Healthcare Improvement, second edition*, is a textbook for health professional students written by an interprofessional team of authors.[20] It presents specific learning objectives in practice-based learning and improvement, systems-based practice, and interprofessional teamwork (see Table 16.1). These map well to the Teaching for Quality competencies and might reasonably be used to guide medical student education.

HOW SHOULD WE TEACH MEDICAL STUDENTS ABOUT HEALTH CARE IMPROVEMENT?

As with other complex professional competencies, those related to health care improvement are built over time and best grounded in clinical practice. Educators can build a continuum of education starting with foundation concepts, skills, and

TABLE 16.1
Health Care Improvement Core Learning Objectives for Medical and Other Health Professional Students[20]

1. The Gap Between What We Know and What We Do
   a. Identify gaps in the quality of health care.
   b. Recognize the difference between making decisions for one patient's care and making decisions for a system of care.
   c. Describe how the Model for Improvement is used to help close the quality gap.
2. Finding Scientific Evidence to Apply for Clinical Improvement
   a. Describe the link between the best evidence and the context of care.
   b. Recognize the range and depth of questions that should be asked to find supporting evidence for the improvement of care.
   c. Recognize the relative strength of research evidence and the difference between filtered and unfiltered evidence.
   d. Identify the proper use of resources—including electronic resources and reference librarians—to find evidence for health care improvement.
3. Working in Interprofessional Teams for the Improvement of Patient Care
   a. Identify the criteria for effective teamwork and the outcomes of a successful team.
   b. Recognize the characteristics of the professionals who work together to provide safe and effective care to patients.
   c. Describe factors that influence team functioning and how to assess them.
   d. Choose members to be part of an interprofessional health care improvement team.
4. Targeting an Improvement Effort
   a. Identify areas of a system that need to be improved, informed by knowledge of the needs of the people to be served.
   b. State ways to narrow the focus of improvement work.
   c. Write an aim statement for improvement that is specific, measurable, attainable, and reasonable and has a time frame (S.M.A.R.T.)
5. Process Literacy
   a. Recognize the importance of describing the process of care that is being studied.
   b. Identify how the process of care is related to the context of care.
   c. Select from a variety of process modeling methods to describe patient care scenarios, including brainstorming and using cause-and-effect diagrams, flow diagrams, deployment flowcharts, and workflow diagrams.
6. Measurement Part 1: Data Analysis for Improvement
   a. Explain why data are necessary for the improvement of health care.
   b. Describe the differences between data used for research, for accountability, and for improvement.
   c. Define the concept of a balanced set of measures for improvement work.
   d. Describe one model—the clinical value compass—for identifying measures for improvement.
7. Measurement Part 2: Using Run Charts and Statistical Process Control Charts to Gain Insight into Systems
   a. Recognize the value of analyzing data over time by using run charts and statistical process control charts.
   b. Describe the difference between common cause variation and special cause variation.
   c. Interpret run charts and statistical process control charts.
8. Understanding and Making Changes in a System
   a. Recognize that systems change occurs in a complex—not linear—fashion.
   b. Identify the basic elements of a complex adaptive system.
   c. Appropriately use Everett Rogers' description of adoption of innovation to target an intervention.
   d. Identify barriers to change and how to address those barriers.
   e. Describe the role and utility of the Plan–Do–Study–Act (PDSA) cycle methodology for testing small changes and for building knowledge about a system.
9. Spreading Improvements
   a. Identify effective strategies for sustaining and spreading change.
   b. Follow a step-by-step approach to planning spread efforts.
   c. Avoid common mistakes and plan for success.

© Joint Commission Resources: Ogrinc G, Headrick LA, Moore S, et al. *Fundamentals of Health Care Improvement: A Guide to Improving Your Patients' Care*, 2nd ed. Chicago, IL: Joint Commission and the Institute for Healthcare Improvement; 2012:(1, 15, 29, 43, 57, 75, 97, 121, 145), adapted with permission.

values for beginning medical students, extending through clinical applications for advanced medical students, and continuing into demonstrations of basic competency for residents.

Armstrong and colleagues[21] suggest the following general principles for educational experiences in health care improvement: (1) create a learning experience with a combination of didactic and project-based work; (2) link with health system improvement efforts; (3) assess education outcomes; and (4) model QI in education processes.

Combining didactic and experiential learning in a continuum over time allows learners to start with basic content through Web-based modules, explore core concepts in the classroom, acquire basic skills in the simulation center, and practice with feedback in the clinical setting. Education programs that rely solely on classroom- or Web-based experiences may be effective for introducing basic concepts and relatively easy to implement, but are unlikely to result in behavior change.[22] Improvement education based in clinical practice creates an opportunity to demonstrate both change in the behavior of the learner and benefits to patients.[23]

Linking improvement education to health system improvement efforts echoes core education experiences in which students are embedded in the work of health care teams. There are considerable advantages: the time of clinical staff and other resources are already committed to the improvement effort; health system improvement professionals often are willing to teach in the context of work they are currently doing; and student learning is stimulated through authentic professional activities in collaboration with others.[24] The obvious challenge is the complexity of creating such experiences for more than a select number of learners.

Assessing education outcomes in a way that is visible and meaningful to the learners sends the message that the content is important. Otherwise, students may dismiss the learning experiences as a distraction to what "counts" (as in a course grade or a certification exam) and fail to engage. Strategies for assessment are discussed in the next section.

Modeling QI in education processes demonstrates the faculty's commitment to improvement as a professional practice. The result is improved education practice.[25] While obviously no substitute for experiences in clinical improvement, student engagement as partners in education improvement is another opportunity for experiential learning. Students will see direct benefits to their education that parallel the benefits patients will experience through clinical improvement efforts.

HOW SHOULD WE EVALUATE HEALTH CARE IMPROVEMENT EDUCATION PROGRAMS?

While there are many approaches to the evaluation of educational programs, the Kirkpatrick typology is a helpful approach to evaluating health care improvement education programs, capturing modifications in learners, changes in organizations, and benefits to patients.[26,27] Table 16.2 displays the typology and provides examples from improvement education programs. The Quality and Safety Education for Nursing Web site contains additional tools.[30] Using this approach, educators can build an evaluation strategy in accordance with the questions they wish to answer.

TABLE 16.2
Kirkpatrick Typology for Evaluation of Education in Health Care Improvement with Examples

Kirkpatrick Category	Examples in Health Care Improvement Education
1. Learner reaction	• Learner attendance • Learner feedback, quantitative (Likert-type rating scale) and qualitative (comments, reflections), e.g., Minute Paper[28]
2.a. Learner modification of attitudes/perceptions	• Readiness for Interprofessional Learning Scale[29] • Self-assessed attitudes[30,31]
2.b. Learner acquisition of knowledge/skills	• Quality Improvement Knowledge Application Test Revised (QI-KAT-R)[32] • Checklist-driven faculty ratings of student performance, e.g., QI project presentation[3] • Self-assessed knowledge and skills[30,31]
3. Learner behavioral change	• Checklist-driven faculty ratings of student performance during simulations[33] • Self-reported changes in behavior[34]
4.a. Change in organizational practice	• Learner observations/assessments leading to improved health care processes[23,35]
4.b. Benefits to patients/clients	• Improvements in patient experience or outcomes documented by patient interview or chart audit[23,36]

To this point, this chapter has described content, learning strategies, and evaluation systems that answer the dean's questions in the opening case. Graduating medical students with the ability to identify best practice, analyze current practice, and participate in efforts to close any gaps will require collaboration between the full continuum of education and clinical system leaders. In fact, graduating *all* medical students ready to take the next step in a continuum of learning in health care improvement likely will require conceptualizing education and clinical systems as one system, not two.

FUTURE DIRECTIONS

Given the broad consensus of QI as a core professional competency, why has change been so slow over the past 20-plus years? Supporting progress have been clinical results demonstrating clear improvements in clinical outcomes,[37,38] regulatory requirements from the ACCME and ACGME, payment systems that reward quality,[39] and academic health center investments in patient safety and QI.[40] Despite those investments, however, there are too few faculty—with experience and competence in improvement science and, in most clinical learning environments, a lack of timely actionable data to support improvement efforts.[19] Many faculty have found it difficult to construct meaningful, practice-based experiential learning opportunities for large numbers of learners. The most progress has occurred at the graduate medical education level, but many of these efforts use a "project on the side" model, with a requirement that learners complete one or more improvement projects in addition to their more typical clinical duties. While this model has helped faculty discover how to support learning efforts in QI, it may lead to the learners' sense that improving care is an "extra," a burdensome set of additional tasks that distracts from the core work of patient care. This, in turn, results in low learner buy-in, significantly limiting the benefit both to the learners and to their future patients. The impediment of unengaged faculty is a clear call to CPD providers to engage in faculty development activities supporting the future training and integration of clinical teachers into QI and patient safety initiatives and programs.

The path forward likely will also be to explicitly link improvement in care and improvement in education.[41] That is, to integrate both improvement work and improvement education into routine clinical activities. Such an approach has potential benefits for patients, in that it treats the clinical learning environment as one system encompassing both care and education, which is how our patients experience it. Routinely involving learners (medical students, residents, and other health professional trainees) in clinical improvement work likely also will benefit patients, as they are frontline personnel whose insights may be essential to the improvement of care.[42] For society as a whole, integrating care delivery and professional learning can improve health care outcomes and lower costs.[41]

For learners, there are multiple benefits to future attempts to link improvement in care and improvement in education. Already noted in this chapter is the power of learning in the context of meaningful professional practice; for medical students, clinically based education is usually more powerful than that which is classroom or even simulation based. Learning activities that are integrated and thus aligned with organizational improvement priorities more likely will attract partners and other resources. Focusing on the needs of patients can create and sustain meaningful interprofessional team experiences, setting the context for competency development in interprofessional teamwork. Similarly, high-quality team experiences can improve satisfaction and decrease burnout.[43]

The Exemplary Care and Learning Site (ECLS) model presents one approach to linking improvement in care and education.[44] At the core of the model are the "linked aims of improvement" proposed by Batalden and Davidoff[45]: better patient (and population outcomes), better system performance, and better professional development. Patient and population outcomes address both clinical results and the patient experience; system performance includes the value of health care; and professional development targets everyone, across the spectrum of professional life. The ECLS study group asked how health care and education leaders (and their teams) might come together to achieve such results. An iterative, interactive process between the study group and six clinical learning environments in the United States and Sweden identified five key elements that appear to support the continuous improvement of both care and learning:

- Leaders knowing, valuing, and practicing improvement
- Data transforming into useful information
- Health care professionals competently engaging in care improvement and teaching about care improvement
- Trainees engaging both in care and in the improvement of care
- Patients and families informing process changes

So far, the study group has published a three-part feasibility study in which the sites' clinical and education leaders reported that the ECLS model helped them take a systematic approach toward their improvement goals. The next step will be application of the model to a broader set of clinical environments with leaders, health professionals, learners, data, and patient and families all working together toward common goals.

ACKNOWLEDGMENT

The author would like to acknowledge Jane Mandel for her help in preparing this chapter.

REFERENCES

1. Berwick DM, Godfrey AB. *Curing Health Care: New Strategies for Quality Improvement.* San Francisco, CA: John Wiley & Sons, Inc.; 1990.
2. O'Connor GT, Plume SK, Olmstead EM, et al. A regional intervention to improve the hospital mortality associated with coronary artery bypass graft surgery. The Northern New England Cardiovascular Disease Study Group. *JAMA.* 1996;275:841–846.
3. Moore SM, Alemi F, Headrick LA, et al. Using learning cycles to build an interdisciplinary curriculum in continuous improvement for health professions students in Cleveland. *Jt Comm J Qual Improv.* 1996;22:165–171.
4. Baker GR, Gelmon S, Headrick LA, et al. Collaborating for improvement in health professions education. *Q Manag Health Care.* 1998;6(2):1–11.
5. Kohn LT, Corrigan J, Donaldson MS. *To Err Is Human: Building a Safer Health System.* Washington, DC: National Academy Press; 2000.
6. Institute of Medicine (U.S.). *Crossing the Quality Chasm: A New Health System for the 21st Century.* Washington, DC: National Academy Press; 2001.
7. Greiner A, Knebel E. *Health Professions Education: A Bridge to Quality.* Washington, DC: National Academies Press; 2003.
8. Australian Commission on Safety and Quality in Health Care (ACSQHC). Vital signs 2015. *The State of Safety and Quality in Australian Health Care.* Sydney: ACSQHC; 2015. www.safetyandquality.gov.au/wp-content/uploads/2015/11/Vital-Signs-2015.docx. Accessed July 8, 2016.
9. Ham C, Berwick D, Dixon J. *Improving Quality in the English NHS: A Strategy for Action.* London, UK: The King's Fund; 2016. http://www.kingsfund.org.uk/publications/quality-improvement. Accessed July 8, 2016.
10. Cooke M, Irby DM, O'Brien BC, et al. *Educating Physicians: A Call for Reform of Medical School and Residency.* San Francisco, CA: Jossey-Bass; 2010.
11. Flexner A. *Medical Education in the United States and Canada: A Report to the Carnegie Foundation for the Advancement of Teaching.* Boston, MA: D.B. Updike, The Merrymount Press; 1910.
12. Association of American Medical Colleges (AAMC) Medical School Objectives Project. *Report V Contemporary Issues in Medicine: Quality of Care.* Washington, DC: AAMC; 2001. https://members.aamc.org/eweb/upload/Contemporary%20Issues%20in%20Med%20Quality%20of%20Care%20Report%20V%20.pdf. Accessed July 6, 2016.
13. The Accreditation Requirements and Descriptions of the Accreditation Council for Continuing Medical Education (ACCME). Chicago, IL: ACCME; 2016. http://www.accme.org/sites/default/files/626_20160929_Accreditation_Requirements_Document_1.pdf. Accessed January 11, 2017.
14. Accreditation Council for Graduate Medical Education (ACGME). *ACGME Common Program Requirements.* Chicago, IL: ACGME; 2016. http://www.acgme.org/Portals/0/PFAssets/Program Requirements/CPRs_07012016.pdf. Accessed January 11, 2017.
15. Liaison Committee on Medical Education (LCME). *Functions and Structure of a Medical School: Standards for Accreditation of Medical Education Programs Leading to the MD Degree.* Chicago, IL and Washington, DC: LCME; 2016. http://lcme.org/publications/. Accessed July 6, 2016.
16. Weiss KB, Bagian JP, on behalf of the CLER Evaluation Committee. Challenges and opportunities in the six focus areas: CLER National Report of Findings 2016. *J Grad Med Educ.* 2016;8(2 suppl 1):26–35.

17. Association of American Medical Colleges. *Medical School Graduation Questionnaire: 2013 All Schools Summary Report.* Washington, DC: AAMC; 2013. https://www.aamc.org/download/350998/data/2013g qallschoolssummaryreport.pdf. Accessed July 6, 2016.
18. Moran KM, Harris IB, Valenta AL. Competencies for patient safety and quality improvement: a synthesis of recommendations in influential position papers. *Jt Comm J Qual Patient Saf* 2016;42:162–169.
19. Association of American Medical Colleges. *Teaching for Quality: Integrating Quality Improvement and Patient Safety across the Continuum of Medical Education, Report of an Expert Panel.* Washington, DC; Association of American Medical Colleges: 2013. https://members.aamc.org/eweb/upload/Teaching%20 for%20Quality%20Report.pdf. Accessed July 6, 2016.
20. Ogrinc G, Headrick LA, Moore S, et al. *Fundamentals of Health Care Improvement: A Guide to Improving Your Patients' Care,* 2nd ed. Chicago, IL: Joint Commission and the Institute for Healthcare Improvement; 2012.
21. Armstrong G, Headrick LA, Madigosky W, et al. Designing education to improve care. *Jt Comm J Qual Patient Saf.* 2012;38(12):5–14.
22. Wong BM, Levinson W, Shojania KG. Quality improvement in medical education: current state and future directions. *Med Educ.* 2012;46:107–119.
23. Headrick LA, Barton AJ, Ogrinc G, et al. Results of an effort to integrate quality and safety into medical and nursing school curricula and foster joint learning. *Health Aff (Millwood).* 2012;31:2669–2680.
24. Eraut E. Informal learning in the workplace: evidence on the real value of work-based learning (WBL). *Dev Learn Organ.* 2011;25(5):8–12.
25. Hoffman KG, Brown RMA, Gay J, et al. How an educational improvement project improved the summative evaluation of medical students. *Qual Saf Health Care.* 2009;18:283–287.
26. Kirkpatrick DL, Kirkpatrick JD. *Evaluating Training Programs: The Four Levels,* 3rd ed. San Francisco, CA: Berrett-Koehler Publishers, Inc.; 2006.
27. Barr H, Koppel I, Reeves S, et al. *Effective Interprofessional Education: Argument, Assumption & Evidence.* Oxford, UK: Blackwell Publishing; 2005:43.
28. Singh MK, Lawrence R, Headrick LA. Expanding educator's medical curriculum tool chest: Minute papers as an underutilized option for obtaining immediate feedback. *J Grad Med Educ.* 2011:3(2);239–242.
29. Parsell G, Bligh J. The development of a questionnaire to assess the readiness of health care students for interprofessional learning (RIPLS). *Med Educ.* 1999;33(2):95–100.
30. Ducore SE. *A Review of Literature for the Quality and Safety Education for Nurses (QSEN) Institute: Identifying Tools for Evaluating QI Competencies.* Cleveland, OH: Case Western Reserve University; 2013. http://qsen.org/faculty-resources/evaluation-tools/. Accessed July 6, 2016.
31. Vyas D, McCulloh R, Dyer C, et al. An interprofessional course using human patient simulation to teach patient safety and teamwork skills. *Am J Pharm Educ.* 2012;76(4):Article 71, 1–9.
32. Singh MK, Ogrinc G, Cox K, et al. Quality Improvement Knowledge Application Tool Revised (QIKAT-R). *Acad Med.* 2014;89(10):1386–1391.
33. Jensen AM, Sanders C, Doty J, et al. Characterizing information decay in patient handoffs. *J Surg Educ.* 2014;71:480–485.
34. Wong B, Etchells E, Kuper A, et al. Teaching quality improvement and patient safety to trainees: a systematic review. *Acad Med.* 2010;85:1425–1439.
35. Hall LW, Headrick LA, Cox KR, et al. Linking health professional learners and health care workers on action-based improvement teams. *Qual Manag Health Care.* 2009;18:194–201.
36. Adeola O, Ruthmann N, Boshard B, et al. *Patients identified as low risk may be safely discharged from the emergency department after presentation with chest pain.* Abstract presented at the American Heart Association Scientific Sessions, Orlando, 2015.
37. Crandall WV, Margolis PA, Kappelman MD, et al. Improved outcomes in a quality improvement collaborative for pediatric inflammatory bowel disease. *Pediatrics.* 2012;129:e1030–e1041.
38. Nelson EC, Dixon-Woods M, Batalden PB, et al. Patient focused registries can improve health, care, and science. *BMJ.* 2016;354:i3319.
39. Centers for Medicare & Medicaid Services. *Quality Payment Program: Delivery System Reform, Medicare Payment Reform, & MACRA.* CMS.gov. https://www.cms.gov/Medicare/Quality-Initiatives-Patient-Assessment-Instruments/Value-Based-Programs/MACRA-MIPS-and-APMs/MACRA-MIPS-and-APMs.html. Accessed July 6, 2016.
40. Cosgrove DM, Fisher M, Gabow P, et al. Ten strategies to lower costs, improve quality, and engage patients: the view from leading health system CEOs. *Health Aff.* 2013;32:321–327.

41. Cox M, Naylor M. *Transforming Patient Care: Aligning Interprofessional Education with Clinical Practice Redesign.* Proceedings of a Conference sponsored by the Josiah Macy Jr. Foundation in January 2013. New York: Josiah Macy Jr. Foundation; 2013. http://macyfoundation.org/docs/macy_pubs/JMF_TransformingPatientCare_Jan2013Conference_fin_Web.pdf. Accessed July 6, 2016.
42. Hall LW, Scott SD, Cox KR, et al. Effectiveness of patient safety training in equipping medical students to recognise safety hazards and propose robust interventions. *Qual Saf Health Care.* 2010;19:3–8.
43. Reid RJ, Coleman K, Johnson EA, et al. The group health medical home at year two: cost savings, higher patient satisfaction, and less burnout for providers. *Health Aff (Millwood).* 2010;29:835–843.
44. Headrick LA, Ogrinc G, Hoffman KG, et al. Exemplary care and learning sites: a model for achieving continual improvement in care and learning in the clinical setting. *Acad Med.* 2016;91(3):354–359.
45. Batalden PB, Davidoff F. What is "quality improvement" and how can it transform healthcare? *Qual Saf Health Care.* 2007;16:2–3.

Chapter 17

Reforming UME *and* GME *by* Implementing Competencies *to* Meet Public *and* Health System Needs

Brian M. Wong and Eric S. Holmboe

Case

Your institution has just placed a Vice Dean for education over all of its educational programs, from undergraduate to graduate medical education and including your continuing professional development (CPD) office. She has begun weekly meetings, some of which are logistical in nature, but some focus on one topic of importance across the continuum. The topic is "competency-based learning and assessment," a topic you might have thought would have little to do with CPD. You read a bit to prepare yourself but are stumped by certain terms.

Questions

What do competency, milestones, and entrustable professional activities mean? How might you apply these concepts in CPD to meet public and health system needs? Is co-learning a potential solution?

INTRODUCTION

The scenario above is becoming an increasingly common one as both educators and policy makers recognize the importance of integrating competencies across the continuum of education and practice. Competencies arose in recognition of growing concerns of deficiencies in medical education and clinical practice.[1,2] Core physician competencies, such as the six core competencies of the Accreditation Council for Graduate Medical Education (ACGME) and the American Board of Medical Specialties (ABMS), are defined as observable abilities that enable physicians, when done well, to effectively care for patients and populations. Competencies can form the foundational link between undergraduate medical education (UME), graduate medical education (GME), and continuing professional development (CPD) by defining the specific and essential abilities for modern clinical practice. They form the building blocks of competency-based medical education (CBME), a growing movement in physician training that offers the opportunity of a true continuum of learning.[3]

COMPETENCY, MILESTONES, AND ENTRUSTABLE PROFESSIONAL ACTIVITIES

CBME has been promoted as an approach to support a better focus on the ultimate goal of meeting public and health system needs. This is not a new concept in medicine. In fact, the World Health Organization (WHO) first highlighted this goal for CBME in a *1978* report entitled "Competency-based Curriculum Development for Medical Education"[4] as the following: "The intended output of a competency-based programme is a health professional who can practice medicine at a defined level of proficiency, in accord with local conditions, to *meet local needs*." Yet nearly 40 years later, questions remain about how best to achieve this aim and how best to practically implement competencies. Enter milestones and entrustable professional activities (EPAs).[5]

Milestones serve as the functional realization of competencies by clearly defining stages of professional development in narrative terms. In general terms, a milestone is simply a significant point in development. In the United States, the milestones in GME provide narrative descriptors of the competencies and subcompetencies along a developmental continuum with varying degrees of granularity.[6] They lay out a framework of observable behaviors and other attributes associated with a resident's or fellow's development as a physician.[7] Milestones also enable educators to develop shared mental models of how competence should look in education and practice.

Milestones are also different from many other assessment rubrics in that there is an opportunity for the learner to demonstrate the attainment of aspirational levels of the subcompetency within the training program. In essence, this aspirational level defines, at a minimum, goals for the early years of clinical practice and by extension CPD. Milestones can serve as a guide for the Vice Dean to examine what her medical students should be able to do at graduation (early milestone levels),[8] what the residents and fellows should be able to do at transition to practice (higher milestone levels), and what the faculty may also need to acquire as new competencies they were likely not taught in their training. Therefore, evolving conversations about competencies and milestones are of critical importance to the CPD community.

Potentially complicating matters is the introduction of the concept of entrustable professional activities, or EPAs. EPAs are measurable units of observable work that physicians perform by integrating multiple competencies.[9] Taken together, EPAs represent the broad range of activities that make up a particular specialty in medicine. This concept is gaining favor in the assessment field as a useful framework to guide assessment decisions, in particular because it introduces the idea of entrustment—that is, when can the learner be entrusted to perform a particular activity in unsupervised practice?

However, competencies, milestones, and EPAs are quite complementary and can often overlap. Competencies define the *abilities* needed by a health professional in order to effectively and safety perform the *activity*, or EPA. Thus, the competencies, described through milestone narratives, provide the substrate, or building blocks, for EPAs.[3,9] It is important to note that many key skills can be described as both an ability and activity, such as medical interviewing and informed decision-making. Both require a set of knowledge, skills, and attitudes (i.e., abilities) in order to actually perform them with patients (i.e., the activity). A good example of this intersection is the Core Entrustable Professional Activities for Entering Residency (CEPAERs) that guide the transition from UME to GME.[8]

USING CBME TO ADDRESS PUBLIC AND HEALTH SYSTEM NEEDS

In 1999, the Institute of Medicine published the seminal *To Err is Human* report, which estimated that 44,000 to 98,000 lives were lost every year in the United States as a result of medical errors and preventable adverse events.[10] Major adverse event studies in numerous countries, including Canada,[11] the United Kingdom,[12] and Australia,[13] reported similar rates of patient safety incidents. Despite significant investments in patient safety solutions in the 15 years following the publication of *To Err Is Human*, patients in our current health systems unfortunately still experience unacceptably high rates of preventable health care–associated harm.[14,15]

They receive suboptimal quality of care and the essential elements of care inconsistently. Two large-scale studies in the United States, the first involving adults and a similar follow-up study involving children, demonstrated that for a given diagnosis, patients receive evidence-based care ~50% of the time.[16,17] On top of underuse challenges, we are also seeing examples of gross overuse of unnecessary tests and treatments (with estimates of 30% of health care costs being wasteful),[18] to the extent that the costs of health care delivery are being driven to unsustainable levels.[19] Given the critical role that physicians need to play to close these widening gaps in quality and safety, the question then becomes: *what* should physicians be able to do to meet public and health system needs? And what is the role that CBME can and should play?

There have been numerous attempts in multiple jurisdictions (i.e., Institute of Medicine, ACGME, CanMEDS, Good Medical Practice, World Health Organization) to define *newer* competencies that allow physicians to deliver high-quality, safe, patient-centered care.[1,20–22] Beyond medicine, other professions have taken similar steps; most notably, the Quality and Safety Education for Nurses (QSEN) institute defines prelicensure and graduate quality and safety competencies for nursing education.[23] These fall within the domains of patient safety, quality improvement (QI), stewardship and cost consciousness, care coordination, interprofessional teamwork, shared decision-making, and use of health information technology and data. While there is no "gold standard" document that one can cite as having a "complete list" of these competencies, recent efforts to synthesize influential position papers provide greater clarity as to the types of abilities that typically appear across these varied sources (Table 17.1).[24] As these concepts have traditionally not been seen as core physician competencies and have not been emphasized in UME or GME until recently, the CPD community will be called upon to play a critical role in establishing these *newer* competencies among practicing physicians to support the continuum of learning in these critical domains.

TABLE 17.1
Synthesis of Patient Safety and Quality Improvement Competencies

Basic Proficiency	Expert Proficiency
Coordination and Transitions of Care • General concepts include *risks associated with transitions of care, coordination of care,* and *transmission of information.*	**Creating a Culture of Safety** • General concepts include *environments that promote safety.*
Effective Communication Skills • General concepts include *basic written and verbal communication skills, the impact of good or bad communication, communicating with patients and families, communicating with other health professionals, electronic health record (EHR) handoffs,* and *the benefits and limitations of communication technology.*	**Evidence-Based Practice** • General concepts include *changing policies and procedures to reflect evidence* and *evidence-based methods for quality improvement.*
Ethics and Legal Issues • General concepts include *ethical principles* and *managing ethical dilemmas.*	**Implementing and Sustaining Quality Initiatives** • General concepts include *integrating quality improvement projects* and *minimizing workflow disruption.*
Evidence-Based Practice • General concepts include *evaluating the literature, incorporating evidence into practice, guideline development,* and *combining evidence-based knowledge with patient preferences.*	**Interdisciplinary Teamwork and Collaboration** • General concepts include *promotion of interdisciplinary learning and training.*
Interdisciplinary Teamwork and Collaboration • General concepts include *teamwork, components of successful teams, interdisciplinary collaboration, trusting team relationships, interprofessional development, communication strategies, role definition, active listening, conflict resolution, negotiation, team leadership,* and *barriers to teamwork.*	**Management of Adverse Events** • General concepts include *guidelines for open disclosure* and *educating staff on effective disclosure.*
Management of Adverse Events • General concepts include *disclosure of adverse events to patients and families.*	**Motivating and Strategizing for Change** • General concepts include *stakeholder involvement.*
Organizational Knowledge and System Approach to Quality • General concepts include *appreciating health care as a system.*	**Organizational Knowledge and System Approach to Quality** • General concepts include *health care complexities* and *systems approach to improvement.*
Patient-Centered Focus • General concepts include *incorporating the patient/family in care management, patient–provider relationships, open communication, respect, empathy, patient privacy, identifying barriers for patient access, prioritizing patient preferences, cultural competence,* and *patient empowerment.*	**Population-Based Care and Preventative Health** • General concepts include *systems failures for population health problems* and *community education projects.*
Personal and Professional Accountability for Quality • General concepts include *acknowledging personal limitations* and *commitment to lifelong learning.*	**Quality Improvement** • General concepts include *quality processes and strategies, designing and testing improvement interventions,* and *creating safe and reliable systems.*

TABLE 17.1
Synthesis of Patient Safety and Quality Improvement Competencies (*Continued*)

Basic Proficiency	Expert Proficiency
Population-Based Care and Preventative Health • General concepts include *the economic, social, and cultural determinants of health, common population health problems,* and *disease prevention and health promotion.* **Quality and Safety Best Practices** • General concepts include *vigilance, monitoring outcomes,* and *using checklists.* **Quality and Safety Principles** • General concepts include *understanding safety risks, types of error, adverse outcomes, medication safety principles, human factors,* and *culture of safety.* **Quality Improvement** • General concepts include *contributing to approaches for improving quality and safety.* **Quality Measurement and Process Evaluation** • General concepts include *understanding types of quality measures, participating in outcomes monitoring, performance measurement,* and *care processes.* **Reporting Systems and Error Evaluation** • General concepts include *assessing and monitoring errors* and *using reporting systems.* **Risk Management** • General *concepts include managing errors, near misses,* and *adverse events.* **Utilization and Improvement of Health Information Technology** • General concepts include *information technology skills* and *use of the EHR*	**Quality Measurement and Process Evaluation** • General concepts include *process mapping, identifying improvement opportunities,* and *coordination of outcome and performance measurement.* **Reporting Systems and Error Evaluation** • General concepts include *nonpunitive reporting systems* and *tools for evaluating and monitoring errors.* **Staff Support** • General concepts include *supporting staff after an error* and *minimizing workplace fatigue.* **Utilization and Improvement of Health Information Technology** • General concepts include *integrating new technology, change management, usability assessment, staff training,* and *using technology to guide health care delivery improvements.*

THE EDUCATIONAL CHALLENGE AND ITS IMPLICATIONS

The Vice Dean will need to attend to four significant challenges:

1. Assist the faculty in acquiring and applying the newer competencies to improve their own clinical practice and teaching. This will require new approaches to faculty development (i.e., CPD!) that integrate education and clinical practice.[25,26]
2. Assist the surrounding community of health professionals to acquire and apply new competencies and approaches to practice through competency-based CPD approaches.[27] This is an important aspect of the social mission of the academic institution.
3. Ensure the UME and GME program's curriculum and assessment programs effectively prepare the learners for the next stage of their career. These transitions can be viewed as "launch points" that can enable or impede future trajectories of performance.[28–32]

4. Create meaningful, longitudinal feedback loops between UME, GME, and CPD to continuously inform necessary changes in all aspects of the continuum. Milestones and EPAs can assist in creating and informing these feedback loops.[3,33]

The move in medical education toward implementing CBME necessitates a careful examination of how learners progress through stages of training and eventually into practice (and ideally also how they progress once in practice). However, with respect to these newer competencies, there remains considerable debate as to how physicians should progress toward competence.[24] In other words, *when* should physicians be competent in the areas of applying patient safety and QI science for example? Defining milestones for these *newer* competencies is in evolution and continues to be hotly debated. Should junior residents be expected to have the ability to carry out QI initiatives when they have had limited exposure to the clinical processes that they are expected to improve? At what stage of training are residents expected to be able to disclose medical errors?

Despite the numerous potential advantages conferred by the use of milestones and EPAs, introducing these frameworks and using entrustment to make decisions about professional development and progression creates additional challenges.[34] Take the example of disclosing medical errors. Even if we could agree that residents at a certain stage of training should have the ability to disclose a medical error to a patient and family, how do we determine when a resident can perform this activity without direct supervision? What if the medical error resulted in severe harm—should the level of harm experienced by the patient influence the entrustment decision? Clearly, these are nuanced decisions without simple answers, and determining the "launch point" is particularly relevant to the CPD conversation.

Further complicating matters is the fact that, as mentioned earlier, faculty responsible for making entrustment decisions around these newer competencies may not be well suited to do so. For example, what if a faculty member or practicing physician is found to be dyscompetent in those same disclosure skills? Research clearly shows that many of our faculty and practicing physicians lack these types of specific competencies.[35–37] How then could that same faculty member determine whether the learner has achieved competence related to disclosure? This once again raises the importance of CPD in addressing the challenge of getting our faculty and practicing physicians up to speed in these newer competencies that are essential for 21st century practice.

Ten Cate and colleagues have also argued for the need of expiration dates for EPAs.[34] A good example here is procedural skills that require ongoing practice and assessment. Again, this represents a major opportunity for the CPD community to leverage the concepts of milestones and EPAs to guide an informed self-assessment by faculty and practicing physicians around their clinical activities (i.e., EPAs) using the competency milestones (needed abilities).

ENVIRONMENT AND INSTITUTIONAL SUPPORT MATTERS

The ACGME Clinical Learning Environment Review (CLER) program recently published its findings from ~300 organizational visits and found that most trainees and faculty still engage infrequently in organizational patient safety and QI practices.[38,39] Therefore, it would be unrealistic to expect, given the current state of physician training and the degree to which these *newer* competencies are taught and assessed, that physicians entering practice will have achieved more than a basic level of proficiency in these areas. In fact, just getting practicing physicians and new graduates of residency training programs to the level of proficiency is no small feat and will require a significant investment in curriculum, faculty development, and organizational leadership.[40]

This is another important issue for our Vice Dean. The experiential curriculum is by far the most impactful on learning and professional development. However, the concern about graduating physicians entering practice unprepared has broader implications. There is mounting evidence that the learning environment, and the quality and safety outcomes achieved in those environments, strongly influences the care provided by graduates of those environments. For example, Asch and colleagues found a correlation between the rate of major obstetrical complications among practicing physicians and the rate of complications at the hospital where they trained, an association that persisted over 15 years.[29] Therefore, there needs to be a better experience for trainees within the learning environment, which is largely influenced by the faculty and practicing physicians working in those environments. There needs to be good CPD *within* institutions to address these clinical environment issues and overall institutional performance. In other words, the Vice Dean will need to engage institutional leadership to ensure that the clinical and CPD experiences of medical students, residents, fellows, faculty, and community physicians are fully integrated into quality and safety initiatives and activities within the learning environment. The CPD activities and experiences will also need to be interprofessional; you cannot truly develop competence in interprofessional teamwork if you do not learn and practice in high-functioning interprofessional environments.

This only serves to heighten the importance of CPD with respect to these *newer* competencies, as over time, we should expect that physicians will need to continue to build on what was learned in practice. So, in order to meet population and health system needs, current and future training need to evolve in two important ways. First, as has been discussed, physician training must make these *newer* competencies a core focus across the learning continuum, from UME to GME to CPD. Within CPD specifically, there have been frameworks proposed that indicate how CPD and QI might intersect, align, and ultimately complement one another.[41] Second, there needs to be equal emphasis at the UME and GME level to equip learners with the foundational competencies needed to effectively engage in lifelong learning. These include self-regulated learning, reflection and mindful practice, self-directed assessment, informed self-assessment, and attention to wellness, to name a few.

CO-LEARNING AS A POTENTIAL SOLUTION

Beyond traditional approaches to CPD, there may be new approaches to engage faculty and practicing physicians in acquiring these newer competencies. One potential solution is to treat faculty and practicing physicians as "co-learners" with residents and medical students.[42] Why might this work?

- For many of these newer concepts, practicing physicians and physicians in training are developmentally and functionally the same, and so, learning activities primarily designed to teach residents and students could extend to include faculty and practicing physicians as co-learners.
- We have a major need to train learners *now* and cannot continue to wait for faculty and practicing physicians to get up to speed on these newer competencies, and a co-learning approach could accelerate the capacity-building process.
- Bringing faculty and practicing physicians into the learning activity, whether it is a patient safety morbidity and mortality conference or a faculty-resident team-based QI curriculum, models to learners the importance of these newer competencies as concepts that are core to physician learning and practice. It also allows faculty and practicing physicians to role model continuous learning and professional development.
- Faculty and practicing physicians have a wealth of clinical experience and awareness of "how things work" in the clinical environment and can help learners overcome some of the institutional and organizational barriers that can make learning about concepts such as patient safety and QI more challenging.
- Over time, faculty participants can acquire teaching and mentorship skills, which can allow them to contribute to ongoing development of peers and learners, a critical trickle-down effect of the co-learning approach.

Of course, co-learning is by no means a panacea, nor can it be the sole solution. Traditional faculty development approaches,[40,43] CPD approaches that integrate QI principles,[41,44] and ongoing efforts to train experts through certificate and graduate programs will all surely contribute to advancing the cause. But it may represent an innovative approach that has the potential to rapidly engage a larger number of practicing physicians in developing basic proficiency in these newer competencies. Co-learning can also occur within an interprofessional context as many other health care disciplines are struggling with many of the same newer competencies.

FUTURE DIRECTIONS

In order to fully realize the benefits of the reforms now occurring in UME and GME, with its strong focus on the implementation of CBME as a key driver of change to address public and health system needs, graduates must enter a highly functioning health care system strongly supported by an equally effective CPD system. Thus, we propose the following implications for CPD.

CPD Should Contribute to Ongoing CBME Conversations Regarding Milestones and EPAs

If CBME is to realize its goal of achieving a true continuum of learning from UME to GME and into practice, CPD must examine the final stages of progression as learners prepare for practice and establish the launch point as physicians enter into practice. For those abilities that are expected to be fully formed and established upon completing GME training, CPD plays a central role in ongoing maintenance of competence (which also includes identifying practices that have changed sufficiently such that they are no longer relevant). For other competencies, in particular the newer systems-based competencies, where exiting GME represents a launch point with an expected trajectory of ongoing development, CPD must ensure that physicians continue to progress through their careers toward even greater expertise. Indeed, GME competency frameworks already factor heavily in the organization of maintenance of certification (MOC) programs in the United States and recertification programs in Canada and the United Kingdom.[22,45,46] Thus, structures exist already that can facilitate the evolution toward a model of competency-based CPD.[27]

CPD Must Help Physicians Establish Competence in Newer System-Based Competencies

As mentioned earlier, most physicians did not train in an era when concepts such as patient safety, QI, and cost consciousness were emphasized. Therefore, CPD plays a critical role in helping physicians develop a basic level of proficiency in these newer competencies such that they can contribute as individuals and members of teams to address public and health system needs. A framework that integrates CPD with QI provides a useful set of guiding principles that could guide future CPD efforts in this regard.[41]

The most basic level of integration involves highlighting clinical areas with quality problems in a traditional CPD activity. For example, a grand rounds presentation on heart failure might include a focus on the challenge of avoidable readmissions involving heart failure patients and present local data regarding institutional readmission rates for heart failure patients. The next level of integration explicitly adds QI content in CPD on specific clinical topics. Here, the same grand rounds presentation might review the evidence surrounding evidence-based system-level interventions that have successfully prevented readmission to hospital or introduce participants to QI tools (e.g., a fishbone diagram that identifies various contributing factors that might result in an avoidable readmission) that could be used to further characterize the QI problem.

One level up would supplement a CPD activity with postevent deliverables. Here, participants might be encouraged to conduct an audit of their own practices to assess the quality of care in a certain clinical area. Some tools exist to support such activities. For example, the ABMS multispecialty portfolio program enables faculty to get MOC credit for meaningful participation in institutional QI and patient safety initiatives and many of these activities are interprofessional.[47]

The Notion of Competency-Based CPD Should Be Further Explored

This framing of CPD, as proposed by Campbell and colleagues,[27] is especially important given the first two recommendations and the recognized need for ongoing professional development beyond GME for these newer systems-based competencies. A competency-based model of CPD does not view competence as a static state to be achieved at the completion of GME. Instead, it is based on the premise that physicians must work to maintain and build upon core competencies and develop new abilities over the course of their professional careers.

Implicit in this model is the need to equip physicians with foundational competencies as they enter practice to engage effectively in lifelong learning. Campbell and colleagues suggest that these learning competencies fall into the following domains: (1) knowing one's practice, (2) scanning the environment, (3) managing learning in practice, (4) raising and answering questions, and (5) practice assessment and enhancement. Therefore, in such a model, CPD must loop back into the UME and GME environment and work with educators to ensure that these abilities are established to enable the lifelong learning that needs to occur within a competency-based CPD paradigm.

CPD, through Faculty Development, Must Prepare Academic Teaching Faculty to Contribute to Learner Assessment Activities

One of the central challenges to the implementation of CBME is the need for faculty members to actively participate in assessment activities in the workplace. For many faculty members, there are numerous barriers, including individual factors such as time constraints and intrinsic motivation to participate in assessment activities.[48] For the newer systems-based competencies, an additional challenge exists in that faculty members may lack the knowledge and skills themselves and so may not feel adequately prepared to assess abilities in others (thus the need for CPD for faculty members to establish knowledge and skills in these domains).

Perhaps underappreciated though are the structural barriers that exist that contribute to this challenge for faculty. Particularly for the newer systems-based competencies, faculty must situate themselves within the clinical care environment and observe interactions between learners, patients, and the clinical microsystem. Unfortunately, our traditional models of GME often separate faculty–learner interactions around teaching and assessment from the clinical environment (Fig. 17.1A), which limits the opportunity for faculty to observe learners engaging in systems-based activities.[26]

We have proposed a transformation of the academic faculty perspective, which necessarily requires greater interaction between faculty, learner, training program, and clinical microsystem, all centered around the *patient* (Fig. 17.1B). Not only does this bring into greater alignment clinical and educational outcomes, but also we believe that this structural reconfiguration is critical to promote academic faculty's ability to perform assessments and deliver feedback that is understandable, relevant, aligned with patient and practice needs, and, most importantly, actionable.

There Needs to Be CPD within Institutions to Enhance Systems of Care within Learning Environments

As mentioned earlier, the learning environment, and the quality and safety outcomes achieved in those environments, appears to strongly influence the care provided by graduates of those environments.[29] To address this problem, CPD must be an active and willing partner. In fact, Batalden and Davidoff's framework for better patient and population outcomes proposes that *everyone* (in this case academic faculty, practicing

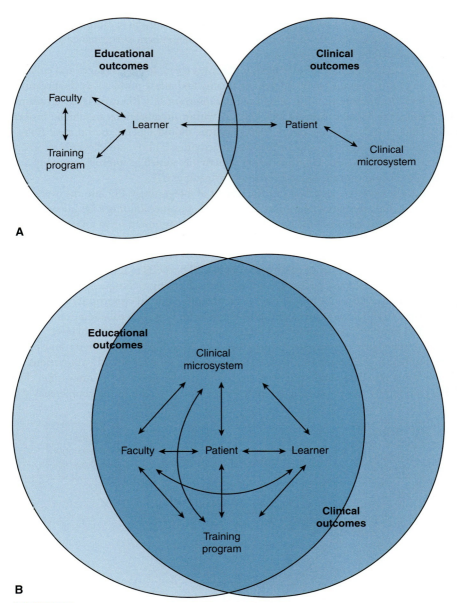

FIGURE 17.1.   The traditional academic faculty perspective **(A)** considers educational outcomes as separate from clinical outcomes, and focuses primarily on the dyad between learner and training program in their educational activities and the patient and the clinical microsystem in their clinical activities. This model places greater emphasis on the learner needs at the center from the academic faculty's perspective when engaging in educational activities. The proposed renewed academic faculty perspective **(B)** places the patient at the center and recognizes the interconnected relationships between faculty, learner, training program, and clinical microsystem. This perspective also brings a natural alignment between educational and clinical outcomes, centered on the patient. (Reprinted with permission from Wong BM, Holmboe ES. Transforming the academic faculty perspective in graduate medical education to better align educational and clinical outcomes. *Acad Med [Internet]*. 2016;91(4):473–479.)

physicians, and other health care professionals within the clinical learning environment) must pursue and contribute to the dual goals of better system performance and better professional development (Fig. 17.2).[25]

How might CPD contribute? First, CPD must create formal linkages and collaborate with groups responsible for addressing quality and safety problems at the organizational level. At a minimum, this would require insertion of CPD experts on QI teams. But ideally, the siloes between CPD and QI within organizations should be broken down, and models of integrated CPD/QI offices should emerge as the ideal framework to optimize organizational improvement activities. This would allow QI efforts to become part of a broader, coordinated set of activities aimed at improving quality and safety outcomes within the clinical learning environment.

Concrete examples that illustrate the benefit of integrating CPD into the overall QI approach include the use of education to raise awareness surrounding a QI initiative and to ensure that the rationale for change is clearly communicated or to engage frontline clinicians in conversations about the design and implementation of changes and allow for cocreation of interventions that respect the needs and preferences of the end user. Traditionally, QI teams have not partnered with CPD experts to take advantage of their ability to harness effective pedagogy and interactive learning techniques to optimize the educational experience. We believe that this represents a missed opportunity for CPD to play a part and should prompt careful consideration for how such collaboration could be fostered to improve upon quality and safety outcomes at an organizational level.

A number of the proposed future directions have direct applicability and could conceivably receive attention in the near term. Indeed, a number of CPD innovations are already being tested and evaluated, with examples available for others to draw upon. The CPD community can impact change early by beginning to address the competency gap

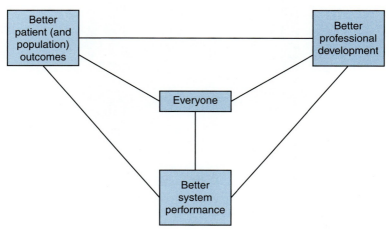

FIGURE 17.2. Linked aims of improvement. Batalden and Davidoff's definition of quality improvement (QI) proposes that everyone—health care professionals, patients and caregivers, payers, and educators—must work together to make changes that will result in better patient outcomes, better system performance, and better professional development. These linked aims of improvement are critical and must become an intrinsic part of everyone's job. (Reproduced from Batalden P, Davidoff F. What is "quality improvement" and how can it transform healthcare? *Qual Saf Health Care.* 2007;16(1):2–3, with permission from BMJ Publishing Group Ltd.)

among practicing physicians that exists with respect to the newer systems-based competencies. However, our other recommendations, such as the need for a competency-based CPD model, better integration of CPD into organizational QI efforts, and shifting the academic faculty's perspective with respect to education around these newer competencies, will take more time, as there are fewer examples for what works. But it is incumbent upon the CPD community to explore, innovate, test, and eventually evaluate interventions that can demonstrate how best to achieve these longer-term goals.

REFERENCES

1. Batalden P, Leach D, Swing S, et al. General competencies and accreditation in graduate medical education. *Health Aff.* 2002;21(5):103–111.
2. Carraccio C, Wolfsthal SD, Englander R, et al. Shifting paradigms: from Flexner to competencies. *Acad Med.* 2002;77(5):361–367.
3. Carraccio C, Englander R, Gilhooly J, et al. Building a framework of entrustable professional activities, supported by competencies and milestones, to bridge the educational continuum. *Acad Med.* 2016, March 8. [Epub ahead of print].
4. McGaghie WC, Sajid AW, Miller GE, et al. Competency-based curriculum development in medical education: an introduction. *Public Health Pap.* 1978;(68):11–91.
5. Carraccio C, Englander R, Holmboe ES, et al. Driving care quality: aligning trainee assessment and supervision through practical application of entrustable professional activities, competencies, and milestones. *Acad Med.* 2016;91(2):199–203.
6. Nasca TJ, Philibert I, Brigham T, et al. The Next GME accreditation system—rationale and benefits. *N Engl J Med.* 2012;366(11):1051–1056.
7. Green ML, Aagaard EM, Caverzagie KJ, et al. Charting the road to competence: developmental milestones for internal medicine residency training. *J Grad Med Educ.* 2009;1(1):5–20.
8. Englander R, Flynn T, Call S, et al. Toward defining the foundation of the MD Degree: core entrustable professional activities for entering residency. *Acad Med.* 2016;91(10):1352–1358.
9. Ten Cate O, Chen HC, Hoff RG, et al. Curriculum development for the workplace using entrustable professional activities (EPAs): AMEE Guide No. 99. *Med Teach.* 2015;37(11):983–1002.
10. Institute of Medicine; Kohn LT, Corrigan JM, Donaldson M, et al. *To Err Is Human: Building a Safer Health System.* Washington, DC: National Academies Press (US); 2000.
11. Baker GR, Norton PG, Flintoft V, et al. The Canadian Adverse Events Study: the incidence of adverse events among hospital patients in Canada. *CMAJ.* 2004;170(11):1678–1686.
12. Hogan H, Healey F, Neale G, et al. Preventable deaths due to problems in care in English acute hospitals: a retrospective case record review study. *BMJ Qual Saf.* 2012;21(9):737–745.
13. Wilson RM, Harrison BT, Gibberd RW, et al. An analysis of the causes of adverse events from the Quality in Australian Health Care Study. *Med J Aust.* 1999;170(9):411–415.
14. *Free from Harm: Accelerating Patient Safety Improvement Fifteen Years after To Err Is Human.* Boston, MA: National Patient Safety Foundation; 2016.
15. Landrigan CP, Parry GJ, Bones CB, et al. Temporal trends in rates of patient harm resulting from medical care—with comments. *N Engl J Med.* 2010;363(22):2124–2134.
16. Mangione-Smith R, DeCristofaro AH, Setodji CM, et al. The quality of ambulatory care delivered to children in the United States. *N Engl J Med.* 2007;357(15):1515–1523.
17. McGlynn EA, Asch SM, Adams J, et al. The quality of health care delivered to adults in the United States. *N Engl J Med.* 2003;348(26):2635–2645.
18. Berwick DM, Hackbarth AD. Eliminating waste in US health care. *JAMA.* 2012;307(14):1513–1516.
19. Levinson W, Kallewaard M, Bhatia RS, et al. "Choosing Wisely": a growing international campaign. *BMJ Qual Saf.* 2015;24(2):167–174.
20. Greiner A, Knebel E. *Health Professions Education: A Bridge to Quality.* 2003:192.
21. Frank JR, Snell LS, Sherbino J. The draft CanMEDS 2015 physician competency framework. *Can Fam Physician.* 2015.
22. GMC. *Good Medical Practice: Duties of a doctor. Good Medical Practice.* 2013. Available from http://www.gmc-uk.org/guidance/good_medical_practice/duties_of_a_doctor.asp. Accessed July 27, 2016.
23. Cronenwett L, Sherwood G, Gelmon SB. Improving quality and safety education: the QSEN Learning Collaborative. *Nurs Outlook.* 2009;57(6):304–312.
24. Moran KM, Harris IB, Valenta AL. Competencies for patient safety and quality improvement: a synthesis of recommendations in influential position papers. *Jt Comm J Qual Patient Saf.* 2016;42(4):162–169.

25. Batalden P, Davidoff F. What is "quality improvement" and how can it transform healthcare? *Qual Saf Health Care.* 2007;16(1):2–3.

26. Wong BM, Holmboe ES. Transforming the academic faculty perspective in graduate medical education to better align educational and clinical outcomes. *Acad Med [Internet].* 2016;91(4):473–479.

27. Campbell C, Silver I, Sherbino J, et al. Competency-based continuing professional development. *Med Teach.* 2010;32(8):657–662.

28. Asch DA, Nicholson S, Srinivas SK, et al. How do you deliver a good obstetrician? Outcome-based evaluation of medical education. *Acad Med.* 2014;89(1):24–26.

29. Asch DA, Nicholson S, Srinivas S, et al. Evaluating obstetrical residency programs using patient outcomes. *JAMA.* 2009;302(12):1277–1283.

30. Sirovich BE, Lipner RS, Johnston M, et al. The association between residency training and internists' ability to practice conservatively. *JAMA Intern Med.* 2014;174(10):1640–1648.

31. Chen C, Petterson S, Phillips R, et al. Spending patterns in region of residency training and subsequent expenditures for care provided by practicing physicians for Medicare beneficiaries. *JAMA.* 2014;312(22):2385–2393.

32. Bansal N, Simmons KD, Epstein AJ, et al. Using patient outcomes to evaluate general surgery residency program performance. *JAMA Surg.* 2015;19104(2):1–9.

33. Aschenbrener CA, Kirch DG. Graduate medical education: its role in achieving a true medical education continuum. *Acad Med.* 2015;90(9):1203–1209.

34. Ten Cate O, Hart D, Ankel F, et al. Entrustment decision making in clinical training. *Acad Med.* 2015;91(2):1.

35. Marvel MK, Epstein RM, Flowers K, et al. Soliciting the patient's agenda: have we improved? *JAMA.* 1999;281(3):283–287.

36. Braddock CHI, Edwards KA, Hasenberg NM, et al. Informed decision making in outpatient practice: time to get back to basics. *JAMA.* 1999;282(24):2313–2320.

37. Kogan JR, Conforti LN, Iobst WF, et al. Reconceptualizing variable rater assessments as both an educational and clinical care problem. *Acad Med.* 2014;89(5):721–727.

38. Wagner R, Patow C, Newton R, et al. The overview of the CLER program: CLER National Report of Findings 2016. *J Grad Med Educ.* 2016;8(2s1):11–13.

39. Bagian JB, Weiss KB. The overarching themes from the CLER National Report of Findings 2016. *J Grad Med Educ.* 2016;8(2s1):21–23.

40. Headrick LA, Baron RB, Pingleton SK, et al. *Teaching for Quality: Integrating Quality Improvement and Patient Safety across the Continuum of Medical Education.* Washington, DC: Association of American Medical Colleges; 2012.

41. Shojania KG, Silver I, Levinson W. Continuing medical education and quality improvement: a match made in heaven? *Ann Intern Med.* 2012;156(4):305–308.

42. Wong BM, Goguen J, Goguen J, et al. Faculty-Resident 'Co-learning': a longitudinal exploration of an innovative model for faculty development in quality improvement. *Acad Med.* 2016, Dec 13. [Epub ahead of print].

43. Ahmed M, Arora S, Baker P, et al. Building capacity and capability for patient safety education: a train-the-trainers programme for senior doctors. *BMJ Qual Saf.* 2013;22(8):618–625.

44. Davis NL, Davis DA, Johnson NM, et al. Aligning academic continuing medical education with quality improvement: a model for the 21st century. *Acad Med.* 2013;88(10):1437–1441.

45. Miller SH. American Board of Medical Specialties and repositioning for excellence in lifelong learning: maintenance of certification. *J Contin Educ Health Prof.* 2005;25(3):151–156.

46. Federation of Medical Regulatory Authorities of Canada. *Physician Practice Improvement.* 2016. Available from http://fmrac.ca/wp-content/uploads/2016/04/PPI-System_ENG.pdf. Accessed July 27, 2016.

47. American Board of Medical Specialties. *Multi-specialty Portfolio Program.* http://mocportfolioprogram.org/wp-content/uploads/2016/05/MSPPBrochure.pdf. Accessed July 27, 2016.

48. Hauer KE, Holmboe ES, Kogan JR. Twelve tips for implementing tools for direct observation of medical trainees' clinical skills during patient encounters. *Med Teach.* 2011;33(1):27–33.

Chapter 18

Advancing **CME** *and* **CPD**: Evolution, Innovation, Accreditation, *and* Alignment

Graham T. McMahon

Case

A working group has been convened to create a strategic vision for the future of CPD and its role in the evolving health care environment. Physicians and other health care professionals are facing enormous pressure in the rapidly changing health care environment, and look to the education community to help them stay current with advances in medicine and provide optimal care. Clinicians expect high-quality, relevant, and effective education that is independent of commercial bias and expect that when possible their participation meets the variety of expectations of the state licensing boards, specialty certification, hospital credentialing, and other regulatory requirements.

Questions

How can the various stakeholders—accreditors and other regulatory bodies in medicine, health systems and institutions, educators, and learners—collaborate to meet the needs of emerging generations of health care professionals in the United States and around the world? How can CPD fulfill its potential as a strategic partner in health care improvement?

INTRODUCTION

Continuing professional development (CPD) is a key asset in our efforts to create an effective, accessible, and affordable health care system. CPD is part of the health care community and the community at large. All the stakeholders—learners, educators, accreditors, health care systems, and institutions—share responsibility for advancing CPD so that it effectively meets the needs of emerging generations of clinicians in the United States and around the world and fulfills its potential as a strategic partner in health care improvement.

The primary currency of education used to be information. In today's digital age, information is ubiquitous and learners can access most of the information they need within seconds using handheld devices. The role of educators thus has been evolving, from purveyors of information to creators of educational experiences. That transition is challenging, since it requires a frame shift in the identity and skills of our educational community.

Clinicians today are responsive to activities that are practice-relevant, efficient, effective, rewarding, and personalized. Since many of today's practitioners have a task orientation, they respond to pragmatic information and cognitive or technical skills that they can apply immediately and that reward them with appropriate credits and credentials. They will readily abandon activities that feel inefficient, since they are sensitive to time utilization. They are astutely aware of when they are actually learning, and welcome that feeling. Health care practitioners, particularly earlier generation clinicians, are especially responsive to material that is personalized and targeted specifically to address their evolving personal needs and areas for growth.

CORE PRINCIPLES AND THE ACCREDITATION MODEL

Accreditation standards for CPD reflect the community's values about what matters for CPD and what works in continuing medical education (CME). In many systems across the world, these standards are based on educational principles that have been proven effective in motivating and sustaining changes in learners' competence, performance, and patient outcomes (see Fig. 18.1). Accreditation standards are intended to facilitate the development of educational experiences that uphold core standards: CME providers are expected to develop activities that address the learners' real needs and practice gaps

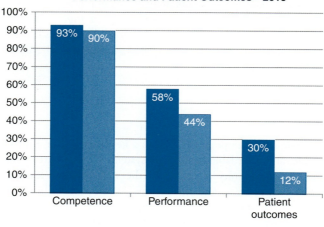

**CME Presented by Providers Accredited in the ACCME System
Rate of Activities Designed and Analyzed for Competence,
Performance and Patient Outcomes—2015**

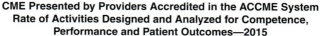

FIGURE 18.1. Accreditation standards require CME providers to design and evaluate activities for changes in learners' competence, performance, or patient outcomes. (From: Accreditation Council for Continuing Medical Education [ACCME®] 2015 Annual Report.)

TABLE 18.1
Shared Principles of International Accreditation Systems

CPD accreditation systems must ensure:
1. Learning activities are developed to address the needs and professional practice gaps of members of the target audience.
2. The content is informed by evidence and bias is minimized.
3. Learning activities are designed to efficiently maximize educational impact.
4. Learning activities are planned and managed to ensure independence from external interests.
5. There is a rigorous evaluation of educational outcomes including how education has impacted knowledge, competence, performance, and health outcomes.
6. The accreditation standards and processes are consistently and fairly applied and continuously enhanced.

CPD accreditors around the world collaborated to develop a shared set of values and principles.

From McMahon GT, Aboulsoud S, Gordon J, et al. Evolving alignment in international continuing professional development accreditation. *J Contin Educ Health Prof.* 2016;36:S22.

and are independent of commercial influences, evidence based, and evaluated to determine their effectiveness and outcomes (see Table 18.1).

EVOLUTION OF EDUCATIONAL PROVIDERS

The role of CPD accreditors is not only to establish core standards, expressing the community's shared values, but is also to design accreditation standards that serve as a guidepost for the future of CPD. These aspirational standards, such as ACCME's commendation criteria, can reward CPD provider organizations for implementing best practices in pedagogy, engagement, evaluation, and change management and for focusing on generating meaningful educational and clinical outcomes. The standards of accreditation endeavor to advance CPD's role in the changing health environment by recognizing the achievements of educational programs that support interprofessional collaborative practice (IPCP); address priorities in patient safety, public health, and population health; collaborate with health systems and communities; participate in regional, national, and international health initiatives; and contribute to measurable improvements in health care professionals' practice and patient care (see Figs. 18.2 and 18.3).

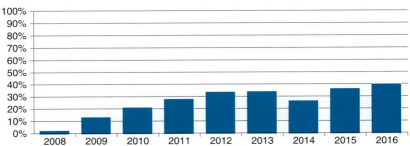

Percentage of Accreditation with Commendation Decisions for ACCME-Accredited Providers (*n* = 349)

FIGURE 18.2. CME providers demonstrated strong responsiveness to and engagement in ACCME's first set of commendation criteria, demonstrating—among other attributes—that they integrate CME into the process for improving professional practice and act as strategic partners in quality initiatives through collaborative alliances.

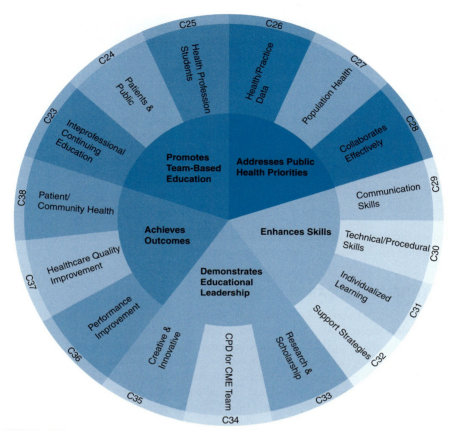

FIGURE 18.3. In 2016, the ACCME evolved the commendation criteria to reflect best practices and the CPD community's higher aspirations and to respond to the changing health care environment. These criteria are designed to serve as guideposts for the future of CME.

Providers who meet these higher expectations can be incented by extending their accreditation interval or by using an identifying mark that communicates the value of their programs to their leadership, stakeholders, and learners.

INNOVATION FOR EDUCATORS

Educators, for their part, can evolve their approach to create more powerful and active learning environments. Research shows that CME is most effective in changing physician performance and patient health outcomes if it is interactive, uses a variety of pedagogical methods, and involves multiple exposures to the same or related material.[1] To facilitate learning, educators need to shift from a teacher-centric to learner-centric focus. Educators create curiosity in learners by connecting the education to gaps that learners themselves recognize and by creating longitudinal relationships so that practitioners receive relevant, individualized learning with personalized feedback that

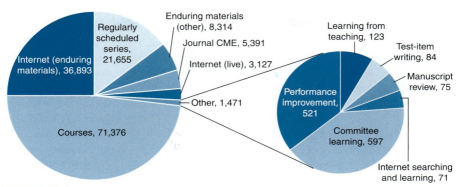

FIGURE 18.4. CME providers offer education in a range of synchronous and asynchronous formats. (From: Accreditation Council for Continuing Medical Education [ACCME®] 2015 Annual Report.)

enables them to create practical action plans for achieving their goals.[2] The personalized education, designed to close the individual's professional practice gaps over time, will serve to nurture and sustain long-term relationships between learners and educators. Thus, CPD providers create educational "homes" that help clinicians navigate their continuing growth—so that education is intertwined with practice throughout their careers.

There also needs to be continued evolution in educational delivery. As technology has developed and accredited CME has evolved, the range and diversity of activity types have evolved considerably (see Fig. 18.4). Educators now use a range of synchronous, asynchronous, and blended formats to achieve their mission—from simulation, bedside workplace learning, and digital education, to courses and collaborative learning sessions.

LEARNERS AS ACTIVE PARTICIPANTS

The profession of medicine entails a commitment to lifelong learning—to make this commitment meaningful, practitioners need to be active participants in their own learning. Clinicians can only really evolve if they take ownership of their own learning agenda. A key element of that evolution is self-awareness: professionals who know their own strengths and weaknesses are most likely to have a productive experience when they identify the types of activities that help them grow and then actively participate in them. There are many ways to increase self-awareness, such as taking a self-assessment quiz, asking a colleague to observe one's practice and provide feedback, asking patients or staff for suggestions, and reviewing patient charts. To become self-aware, clinicians have to step out of the protective cocoon of self-confidence and become humble and open enough to assess both how we can best maintain what's working and how they can grow further.[3]

ALIGNMENT TO PROMOTE TEAMWORK

Increasingly, health care is delivered by teams and those teams need to learn together. Interprofessional continuing education (IPCE) gives clinicians opportunities to learn from, with, and about their colleagues in other health professions to enable effective collaboration and improve health outcomes. In their governance role, CPD accreditors have the responsibility to facilitate team-based learning (see Fig. 18.5). Barriers between accreditation systems and professions must be overcome to achieve this shared mission.[4] The CE accrediting organizations in medicine (the ACCME), pharmacy, (the Accreditation Council for Pharmacy Education), and nursing (the American Nurses Credentialing Center) collaborated to develop the Joint Accreditation for Interprofessional Continuing Education, the first joint accreditation system to facilitate IPCE, a process that can improve alignment between education and health systems.[5] This alignment supports professionalism and reduces burnout. Jointly accredited providers have substantially increased the number of interprofessional educational activities they offer to health professionals.[6]

CME WITH PATIENTS AS GUIDES

Patients help keep clinicians grounded and pragmatic; including patients in CME can engage clinicians' hearts as well as minds and reinforce why their work matters. As part of the health care team, patients need to be included in CME activities, not only as

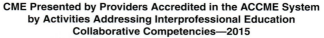

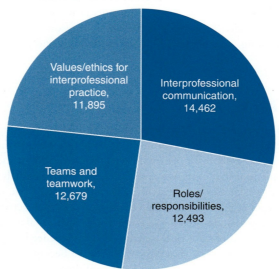

CME Presented by Providers Accredited in the ACCME System by Activities Addressing Interprofessional Education Collaborative Competencies—2015

Values/ethics for interprofessional practice, 11,895

Interprofessional communication, 14,462

Teams and teamwork, 12,679

Roles/ responsibilities, 12,493

FIGURE 18.5. To advance team-based care, CME providers design activities to address competencies such as those identified by the Interprofessional Education Collaborative. (From: Accreditation Council for Continuing Medical Education [ACCME®] 2015 Annual Report.)

participants where they can, for example, present at grand rounds to share their experiences with the health care system, but also as planners and teachers so they can guide educators and clinicians on anticipating and meeting their needs. Patients should be asked, "What would you like the health care community to know about your experience?" Education should reflect the priorities patients identify.

EVOLUTION OF HEALTH CARE LEADERS

Health institution leaders who appreciate the strategic power of education to maintain and improve quality within their organizations derive great benefit from their investment. Hospital and health system leaders report that investment in CME has helped them improve physician performance, patient outcomes, and care coordination; drive and manage change, including behavioral and cultural change; improve teamwork and collegiality as well as leadership skills; and reduce burnout and turnover.[7] Of the ~1,900 accredited CME programs in the ACCME system, approximately two thirds participate in quality improvement initiatives within their health systems and institutions. Yet, quality improvement and education offices are still sometimes separate and misaligned. Health care leaders need to recognize accredited CME as a partner in quality improvement and use education as a strategic resource to drive improvement and change.

To optimize the value of education in supporting strategic goals, health care leadership needs to ensure that their clinicians have the time and resources to engage in CME. Within our institutions and systems, our teachers and mentors must be celebrated, promoted, and remunerated for the value they bring in advancing care quality. By creating and funding the position of chief learning officer or the equivalent, health leaders will more effectively leverage educational resources to meet institutional needs and goals.[8] Chief learning officers can connect education across the continuum, overseeing the curricula for the lifespan of clinicians.

INNOVATION AND ALIGNMENT ACROSS THE CONTINUUM

Undergraduate medical education and graduate medical education serve essential roles, helping to nurture the development of the medical professional. Following these comparatively few years in intense formative development, the CPD community inherits these learners and is responsible for meeting their needs for the rest of their careers.

GME and CME can bring their spheres closer together, sharing needs data and reflecting together about how their systems can adopt their curricula to ease learners' transition from graduate medical education to CE and better meet health care challenges. For example, as resident physicians begin to have milestone data,[9] they could bring those data into practice and engage with the CPD system to help them learn and improve. GME and CME both have shared needs for faculty and faculty development, a key challenge in a time of increased pressure on the practitioner. CME programs can offer the expertise and resources to support rapid progress improvement initiatives in response to these identified needs for learners and faculty, and pass back needs data to the GME community (see Fig. 18.6 for an example of how CME aligns with the competencies established by the Accreditation Council for Graduate Medical Education [ACGME] and the American Board of Medical Specialties [ABMS]).

EVOLUTION AND ALIGNMENT AMONG REGULATORS

When regulatory authorities recognize the value of education in driving clinical practice and quality improvement and allow educational activities to count for multiple requirements, they can reduce the burden on physicians and other health professionals and promote lifelong learning (see Fig. 18.6).

For example, in response to physician requests, the ACCME and the American Board of Internal Medicine (ABIM) collaborated to simplify the integration of MOC and CME, giving physicians more options for receiving MOC credit through participation in accredited CME, which they already use to meet licensure and other professional

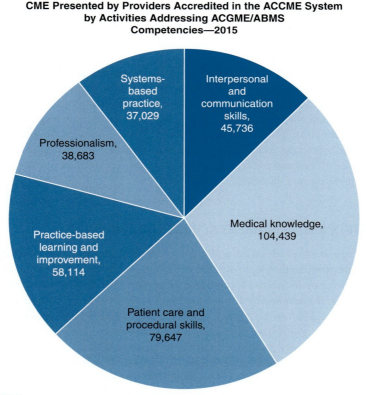

CME Presented by Providers Accredited in the ACCME System by Activities Addressing ACGME/ABMS Competencies—2015

- Systems-based practice, 37,029
- Interpersonal and communication skills, 45,736
- Professionalism, 38,683
- Medical knowledge, 104,439
- Practice-based learning and improvement, 58,114
- Patient care and procedural skills, 79,647

FIGURE 18.6.   Accreditation standards reflect the community's values about what matters in professional development. To meet the expectations of accreditation standards, CME providers design activities to address competencies such as those identified by the Accreditation Council for Graduate Medical Education/American Board of Medical Specialties. (From: Accreditation Council for Continuing Medical Education [ACCME®] 2015 Annual Report.)

obligations. Accredited CME providers can register their activities for both MOC and CME using the same system, physicians can find activities via an online search tool and receive MOC and CME credit at the same event, and diplomates' completion records are reported seamlessly to their certifying board. Building on that foundation, the ACCME has formed similar collaborations with other certifying boards.

Accreditors will be most effective at supporting the evolution of CPD if they focus on educational outcomes, rather than the educational process or the time the learner spends in a particular activity. By relinquishing the fixed structural requirements for health education and instead focusing on educational outcomes or achievements, rather than process and time spent, accreditors can create the right conditions for maximizing educators' flexibility and promoting innovation.

INTERNATIONAL EVOLUTION AND ALIGNMENT

CPD accreditors around the world are engaged in long-standing efforts to guide the enhancement of CPD accreditation systems at various stages of development and define the basis for mutual recognition of CPD accreditation systems. The substantial equivalency framework, created in 2002 by the ACCME and its colleague accreditors in Canada, is defined as a relationship between CME accreditors based on shared principles and values, while recognizing and accepting differences. The purpose of substantial equivalency is to foster international collaboration among CME accreditors, facilitate continuous improvement in accreditation, and expand opportunities for physicians and teams to participate in high-quality CME around the world. It is intended to support the mobility of learners in accessing accredited learning activities that are recognized by various CPD accreditation systems in a manner that maximizes the value of those accreditation systems while minimizing the burden of adhering to their requirements.[10]

EVOLUTION AND ALIGNMENT IN PUBLIC AND POPULATION HEALTH

The CPD community has demonstrated its capacity to collaborate with public and population health initiatives in institutions, systems, and communities. The government has recognized the value of CE in supporting patient safety and quality priorities. For example, the FDA leveraged the accredited CE community to deliver the prescriber education component of the Risk Evaluation and Mitigation Strategy (REMS) for extended-release and long-acting opioids. This was the first REMS to incorporate accredited CE; the FDA and the CE community are identifying other ways to work together to advance public health. As the CPD community continues to innovate, there will be more opportunities for strategic partnerships with organizations who focus on public health needs.

FUTURE DIRECTIONS

The accredited CPD community has the capacity to expand its contributions to performance and quality improvement, collegiality, and public health. To fulfill its potential, the following future short- and long-term priorities will need to be addressed:

Leadership and engagement: CPD needs the engagement of health care leaders, educators, and learners; it will not be successful until the systems, organizations, and institutions involved in health care recognize the strategic value of education to drive change and make a decision to support and invest in CPD professionals and educators.

A national research agenda: Research has demonstrated that CME effectively improves attitude, knowledge, skills, and performance.[1] However, much more research is needed about how to optimize the effectiveness of education and to demonstrate its contributions to improving patient health outcomes. By investing in educational research, we will be able to determine the most effective and efficient approaches for improving physician competence, performance, and patient care.

Freedom to innovate: CPD accreditation standards that facilitate choice and accommodate differences will enable educators to meet the diverse and changing needs of their learners. Accreditation standards should inspire—not constrain—CPD provider organizations from, for example, deploying new information and communication technologies, using simulation centers, games, blended learning, social media, and other applications. As new technologies emerge, as well as new research about educational effectiveness, CPD provider organizations need the freedom and flexibility to develop new learning methods. Fulfilling the role of coaches and leaders, rather than enforcement authorities, CPD accreditors can support the CPD of educators, provide services that respond to educators' concerns and needs, and create an environment where they can share best practices.

Longer-Term Priorities

Harmonization across professions: The harmonization of CPD accreditation standards and credits across professions and disciplines will facilitate team-based education that improves the quality and safety of health care delivery. Through these efforts, regulatory bodies themselves will learn how to engage in IPCP and, together with IPCE providers, demonstrate leadership and create communities of practice that advance health care education of, by, and for the team.

Harmonization across borders: CPD accreditors and credit systems across borders need to work together to align international CPD accreditation around a set of principles that can be demonstrated by any CPD accreditation system. This approach to harmonization will enable CPD educators to address the learning needs of clinicians across borders, cultures, generations, and professions and to collaborate with colleagues around the world to respond nimbly to emerging health priorities. It will assure learners that regardless of where they live, work, and practice, they have access to quality education that meets a common set of high standards. In addition, if more international medical regulatory authorities, such as licensing and certification bodies, allow educational activities to count for multiple requirements in multiple countries, they can not only significantly reduce the burden on practitioners but also motivate collaboration among practitioners across nations and cultures.

By focusing on collaboration, creativity, flexibility and mutual respect, the community of health care leaders, CPD accreditors, educators, and learners can evolve together to achieve its shared strategic vision of leveraging the power of education to improve health care quality for the patients we all serve.

REFERENCES

1. Cervero RM, Gaines J. The impact of CME on physician performance and patient health outcomes: an updated synthesis of systematic reviews. *J Contin Educ Health Prof.* 2015;35(2):131–137.
2. Vaughn LM, Baker RC. Psychological size and distance: emphasising the interpersonal relationship as a pathway to optimal teaching and learning conditions. *Med Educ.* 2004;38(10):1053–1060.
3. McMahon GT. What do I need to learn today?—The evolution of CME. *N Engl J Med.* 2016;374(15):1403–1406. doi:10.1056/NEJMp1515202.
4. McMahon GT. Advancing continuing medical education. *JAMA.* 2015;314(6):561–562.
5. Institute of Medicine. *Measuring the Impact of Interprofessional Education and Collaborative Practice and Patient Outcomes.* Washington, DC; Institute of Medicine: 2015. https://www.iom.edu/Reports/2015/Impact-of-IPE.aspx
6. Robert Wood Johnson Foundation. *Push for Interprofessional Education Picks Up Steam: Health Professions Accreditors Take Steps to Ensure Educational Programs Prepare Students to Participate in Team-Based Care.* Princeton, NJ: Robert Wood Johnson Foundation; 2013. http://www.rwjf.org/en/library/articles-and-news/2013/11/push-for-interprofessional-education-picks-up-steam.html
7. Combes JR, Arespacochaga E. *Continuing Medical Education as a Strategic Resource.* Chicago, IL: American Hospital Association's Physician Leadership Forum; September 2014.
8. Steinert Y, Naismith L, Mann K. Faculty development initiatives designed to promote leadership in medical education. A BEME systematic review: BEME Guide No. 19. *Med Teach.* 2012;34(6):483–503.
9. Accreditation Council for Graduate Medical Education. *Milestones.* http://www.acgme.org/acgmeweb/tabid/430/ProgramandInstitutionalAccreditation/NextAccreditationSystem/Milestones.aspx. Accessed July 1, 2016.
10. McMahon GT, Aboulsoud S, Gordon J, et al. Evolving alignment in international continuing professional development accreditation. *J Contin Educ Health Prof.* 2016;36:S22.

Chapter 19

OVERCOMING CHALLENGES *to* INTERPROFESSIONAL EDUCATION *in the* WORKPLACE

Mary A. Dolansky and Ellen Luebbers

Case

The chief quality officer at your academic medical center frequently points to a lack of teamwork, poor professional-to-professional communication, and inadequate interprofessional collaboration as key elements contributing to poor patient outcomes. In particular, he notes poor collaborative efforts between medicine and nursing, though many other examples exist. You believe that your continuing professional development (CPD) unit is positioned to meet these needs, and it has in fact offered several programs to multiprofessional audiences. You are prepared to move forward in this area and have had preliminary conversations with educational leaders in nursing, pharmacy, allied health, and social work.

Questions

What do you need to know to develop a thorough understanding and to develop and implement a full plan? How do you think CPD can help professionals in your system overcome the barriers to learning within teams and across professions?

INTRODUCTION

Continuing professional development (CPD) is an opportunity to learn interprofessional collaboration. The redesign from profession-specific continuing education (CE) to continuing interprofessional education (CIPE) requires an understanding of the current state of interprofessional education (IPE) and consideration of potential facilitators and barriers. A major challenge is addressing the attitudes of faculty and learners by highlighting the relevance and importance of moving from CE to CIPE. The purpose of this chapter is to present the steps necessary to develop and implement CIPE and to discuss facilitators and barriers associated with this process.

THE IMPERATIVE OF INTERPROFESSIONAL COLLABORATION

Health care is becoming increasingly complex due to rapidly advancing medical technology and increased patient longevity, resulting in the challenge of managing multiple chronic illnesses in these patients. The management of multiple chronic illnesses demands collaboration and expertise from many disciplines. In addition, the cost of health care is rising, and errors in patient care, although declining, still point to the need for improvement in both safety and quality.[1-3]

It has become clear that no single discipline can solve the complex patient needs of health care today. What is needed are health care professionals who are competent in interprofessional collaboration and who strive to improve the quality and safety of the care they deliver.[4] Working together on interprofessional teams and using the expertise of all health care professionals result in (1) health care professionals who are fully engaged and dedicated to the systems in which they work, (2) patient satisfaction, and (3) the achievement of the Quadruple Aim of health care.[5,6] The Quadruple Aim is (1) improving the health of populations, (2) enhancing the patient experience of care, (3) reducing the per capita cost of care, and (4) improving the work life of health care professionals and staff, which reflects the connection between satisfied workers and quality outcomes.[7] This fourth goal of the Quadruple Aim can be achieved through interprofessional collaboration and respecting the views of different disciplinary perspectives.

Incorporating interprofessional collaboration content has become a focal point of many professions' continuing professional development (CPD departments. The expansion of traditional continuing medical education (CME) and continuing nursing education (CNE) programs, to CIPE, is facilitated by the awareness of the limitations in disciplinary silos and that these education programs can effect practice change[8,9] to meet the growing need to improve quality and safety of care delivery.[10] In addition, IPE was identified as a critical element in all professional education in the Institute of Medicine (IOM) report on *Health Professions Education: A Bridge to Quality and Safety*[11] and in CPD in the report on *Redesigning Continuing Education in the Health Professions.*[12]

In prelicensure health professions education, interprofessional collaborative competencies are integrated into curricula, and students are given the opportunity to work with other professions, generally in classroom and community settings. At Case Western Reserve University, students from medicine, nursing, social work, and dentistry gather for a didactic class where they learn different disciplines' roles and responsibilities and the principles of communication. Students then are able to take this knowledge and apply it in a local student-run free clinic.[13] The need for clinical education models is evident; however, a growing challenge is the lack of faculty with experience and expertise to precept or facilitate interprofessional learning. CPD leaders have an opportunity to influence faculty development in this area by offering CIPE activities not only to health care professionals but also to their faculty.

In 2007, leaders in nursing developed and disseminated the Quality and Safety Education for Nurses (QSEN) competencies.[14] The competencies were modeled after the IOM competencies[15] and are patient-centered care, teamwork and collaboration, safety, evidence-based practice, quality improvement, and information technology. The mission of QSEN was to ensure that nurses have the resources to continually improve the care they deliver. In medicine, competencies were developed by the Accreditation

Council for Graduate Medical Education (ACGME), and these competencies include professionalism, practice-based learning and improvement, interpersonal communication, and systems-based practice.[16] In addition, the American Board of Medical Specialties (ABMS) adopted maintenance of certification (MOC) processes that require physicians to engage in quality improvement and demonstrate that they can assess the quality of care that they provide, compare their performance to their peers, and improve the care they deliver.[17] The World Health Organization (WHO) has endorsed IPE and is calling on nations to implement IPE and integrate IPE into CE. The WHO has developed a Framework for Action that links IPE, collaboration, and improved outcomes.[18] This framework has facilitated the integration of IPE across the world.

Discipline-specific competencies are necessary to contribute to improved patient safety and quality, but are not by themselves sufficient. Members of a team must learn collaborative skills together in the team setting to effectively achieve the Quadruple Aim. CIPE is defined as occasions when two or more professions learn with, from, and about each other to improve collaboration and the quality of care.[19] IPE emphasizes that persons in each discipline must share their disciplinary knowledge and that all of these individuals are valued as experts.

Essential interprofessional collaboration skills are listening to the views of others, sharing your views, and being willing to negotiate a plan of action. This is similar to the skill presented in teaching patient-centered cultural competency through the LEARN model,[20] and in fact, the LEARN model can also be used to assist with interprofessional collaboration. The acronym "LEARN" stands for <u>L</u>isten with understanding and respect to the expertise of the other's view, <u>E</u>xplain your perspective by providing the data and detail, <u>A</u>cknowledge and discuss the differences and similarities, <u>R</u>ecommend solutions, and <u>N</u>egotiate a next step.[20]

The IOM report, *Measuring the Impact of Interprofessional Education on Collaborative Practice and Patient Outcomes*, recognized the importance of interprofessional learning across the continuum of health profession education, including CPD, and the need to positively affect both learner objectives and patient outcomes.[21] The interprofessional learning continuum (IPLC) model is displayed in Figure 19.1. The model includes learning outcomes of reaction, attitude, knowledge, collaborative behavior, and performance in practice. The learning outcomes are influenced by the work of Kirkpatrick, who published an evaluation framework with these components that is used widely in IPE evaluation.[22]

A goal in CPD is to reach the highest level of the Kirkpatrick model, improving the performance in practice. To reach this goal, CPD must move from individual competencies to collective or team competencies.[23] It is not sufficient to have individuals on a team who are competent without having the collective competence of the team. For example, during a surgery, a competent surgeon and circulating nurse working independently does not result in a successful outcome. The surgical team must have collective competence in order to ensure quality and safety. With this in mind, it must be the goal of CIPE to improve not only individual learning but also team learning (collective competence). The IPLC model also includes systems outcomes for both the health of our patients (at the individual and population level) and organizational change (e.g., systems efficiencies and cost-effectiveness). Health and systems outcomes reflect the Quadruple

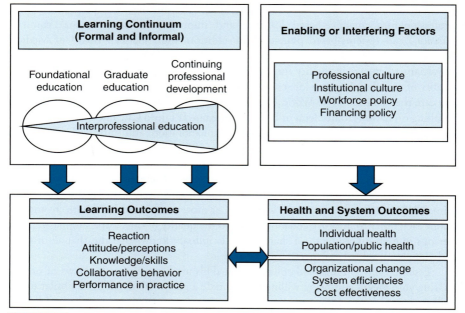

FIGURE 19.1. The interprofessional learning continuum (IPLC) model. *Note.* For this model, "graduate educa-tion" encompasses any advanced formal or supervised health professions training taking place between completion of foundational education and entry into unsupervised practice. Republished from Institute of Medicine. *Measuring the Impact of Interprofessional Education on Collaborative Practice and Patient Outcomes.* Washington, DC: National Academies Press; 2015; with permission of National Academies Press, permission conveyed through Copyright Clearance Center, Inc.

Aim (population health, better health care, lower costs, and work life of health care professionals and staff). Thus, CIPE has the potential to impact our complex, dynamic health care system through collective competence and health care system improvements in quality and safety.

DETAILS OF DEVELOPING CONTINUING INTERPROFESSIONAL EDUCATION

In the case study presented in this chapter, the CPD leaders have an opportunity to expand traditional CME, including multidisciplinary programs, to CIPE. These pro-grams by definition bring professionals of multiple disciplines together to learn using adult learning principles. The CPD leaders can expand the traditional CE model to include "learning from and about each other" using experiential learning activities. To accomplish this goal, they must include both adult learning and social learning theories.[24] Traditional CME includes Adult Learning Theory principles; however, the addition of Social Learning Theory broadens the scope of the CE activity by adding interactive and experiential activities. This requires an additional step that is often perceived as too time-consuming and unnecessary by most learners and CPD faculty.

One way to deliver interactive and experiential learning is through *simulation.* There are many examples of effective simulation activities published in the literature.[25] Another more promising pedagogy is *workplace learning*, a practitioner-centered approach that focuses on problem-solving of day-to-day challenges.[26] Workplace learning takes into consideration the context that includes the environment and the relationships among the staff. It also ensures that the CIPE is outcome oriented and demonstrates the added value of the educational activity. The integration of workplace learning into CIPE requires a redesign of CPD departments. CPD leaders from different departments will need to move CE activities from didactic and simulation sessions to education that takes place in the health care professional's environment. This redesign will require creative scheduling solutions to give health care professionals the time for learning and will require that managers have the tools and resources to accommodate these workplace learning activities.

Owen and Schmitt developed steps for integrating IPE into a CME program that includes designing, implementing, and evaluating continual educational activity.[27] Table 19.1 displays the defined steps for both programmatic and educational activities and the application to CIPE. An essential component of the redesign from CE to CIPE is the establishment of an interdisciplinary CPD leadership team. This team works together on the steps from the model.

TABLE 19.1
Planning Process for a Continuing Interprofessional Education Program (CIPE)

Activity Planning Component	Profession-Specific CE	CIPE	Application to CIPE
Systems Level: CE Program Development			
Step 1: Support the program mission.	Focus on profession-specific knowledge and skills to improve patient outcomes.	Focus on interprofessional knowledge and skills to improve patient care and outcomes relevant to team-based care.	CE coleaders review and integrate CIPE into existing program mission statements; seek interprofessional and institutional input to create a shared vision.
Step 2: Analyze practice gaps.	Profession-specific gap analysis and practice guidelines.	Interprofessional shared, pooled gap analysis. Performance data of clinical teams are utilized.	Representatives from interprofessional target audience conduct gap analysis (team-based care practice behaviors).
Step 3: Identify barriers.	Address anticipated barriers that could impede practice changes (e.g., insurance does not reimburse, patient compliance, systems issues).	Address anticipated barriers that could impede teamwork practice changes (e.g., poor communication and limited awareness of each other's knowledge, skills, and role relevant to team-based practice).	Course directors and CE educators identify interprofessional barriers at the individual, team, and organizational levels through literature reviews and focus groups.

(Continued)

TABLE 19.1
Planning Process for a Continuing Interprofessional Education Program (CIPE) (*Continued*)

Activity Planning Component	Profession-Specific CE	CIPE	Application to CIPE
Step 4: Articulate goals and objectives.	Focus on transfer of new clinical knowledge and profession-specific competencies. Describe changes in individual knowledge, competence, or performance.	Focus on the delivery process. Develop interprofessional competencies. Describe changes in team-based practice performance.	Write outcome-oriented goals and objectives that describe changes in interprofessional individual and team-based practice and clinical performance.
Activity Planning CIPE	Profession-Specific CE	CIPE	Application to Component
Activity Design, Implementation, and Evaluation			
Step 5: Design and implement educational activities.	Build on what learners know; give ownership in their learning. Use multiple modalities to aid learning transfer.	Facilitate interactive learning (i.e., learning about, from, and with other health professionals). Recognize the influence of professional identity on collaborative practice, facilitate reflective leaning, and encourage team member viewpoint.	CE faculty serve as IPE facilitators who give didactic presentations, engage learners in interactive, reflective learning opportunities, and role model collaborative practice; the educational setting resembles the practice situation; opportunities are available to apply new knowledge and skills in collaborative care.
Step 6: Evaluate the educational activity.	Measure changes in profession-specific knowledge, competence, and/or performance and patient outcomes.	Measure changes in individual interprofessional and team-based knowledge, competence, and/or performance and patient outcomes.	Modified from the four-level Kirkpatrick model to guide the assessment of CIPE outcomes.

Adapted and used from Owen JA, Schmitt MH. Integrating interprofessional education into continuing education: a planning process for continuing interprofessional education programs. *J Contin Educ Health Prof.* 2013;33(2):109–117, with permission.

The first step in the Owen and Schmitt is to support CIPE in all of the CPD department's mission statement to integrate an interprofessional component to the purpose, content areas, target audience, type of activity, and expected results. It is crucial that interprofessional CPD directors work together on a joint mission statement that can be added to all departmental CE programs. The second step is for the CPD department staff to analyze the overall local practice gaps that need to be addressed. This step is context specific, as local relevance adds meaning and purpose for the learners. The importance of providing meaning and relevance has been identified as key in IPE.[28,29]

For CIPE, it is essential to form an interprofessional CPD leadership team to work collaboratively and address barriers and understand credit requirements from all the involved professions' perspectives. The third step is for the CPD leadership team to identify program barriers. For CIPE, many barriers exist, and working through them as an interprofessional team is essential. During this step, the interprofessional CPD leadership team will benefit by using the LEARN model described previously. This includes respecting the needs and understanding the expertise of the other professionals. The fourth step in overall program planning is to articulate the educational goals and objectives of the redesign of the program from CE to CIPE. It is essential that interprofessional competencies be used to guide the selection of the program competencies. The interprofessional collaborative practice competencies are listed in Table 19.2.

TABLE 19.2
Interprofessional Collaborative Practice Competency Domains

Domain	Specific Competencies
Values/ethics for interprofessional practice	1. Place the interest of patient and populations at the center of interprofessional health care delivery 2. Respect the dignity and privacy of patient while maintaining confidentiality in the delivery of team-based care 3. Embrace the cultural diversity and individual differences that characterize patients, populations, and the health care team 4. Respect the unique cultures, values, roles/responsibilities, and expertise of other health professions 5. Work in cooperation with those who receive care, those who provide care, and others who contribute to or support the delivery of prevention and health services 6. Develop a trusting relationship with patients, families, and other team members 7. Demonstrate high standards of ethical conduct and quality of care in one's contributions to team-based care 8. Manage ethical dilemmas specific to interprofessional patient-/population-centered care situation 9. Act with honesty and integrity in relationships with patients, families, and other team members 10. Maintain competence in one's own profession appropriate to scope of practice
Roles and responsibilities	1. Communicate one's role and responsibilities clearly to patients, families, and other professionals 2. Recognize one's limitations in skills, knowledge, and abilities 3. Engage diverse health care professionals who complement one's own professional expertise, as well as associated resources, to develop strategies to meet specific patient care needs 4. Explain the roles and responsibilities of other care providers and how the team work together to provider care 5. Use the full scope of knowledge, skills, and abilities of available health professionals and health care workers to provide that is safe, timely, efficient, effective, and equitable 6. Communicate with team members to clarify each member's responsibility in executing components of a treatment plan or public health intervention

(Continued)

TABLE 19.2 Interprofessional Collaborative Practice Competency Domains (*Continued*)	
Domain	**Specific Competencies**
	7. Forge interdependent relationships with other professions to improve care and advance learning
	8. Engage in continuous professional and interprofessional development to enhance team performance
	9. Use unique and complementary abilities of all members of the team to optimize care
Interprofessional communication	1. Choose effective communication tools and techniques, including information systems and communication technologies to facilitate discussions and interactions that enhance team function
	2. Organize and communicate information with patients, families, and health care team members in a form that is understandable, avoiding discipline-specific terminology when possible
	3. Express one's knowledge and opinions to team members involved in patient care with confidence, clarity, and respect working to ensure common understanding of information and treatment and care decisions
	4. Listen actively, and encourage ideas and options of other team members
	5. Give timely, sensitive, instructive feedback to others about their performance on the team, responding respectfully as a team member to feedback from others
	6. Use respectful language appropriate for a given difficult situation, crucial conversation or interprofessional conflict
	7. Recognize how one's uniqueness, including experience level, expertise, culture, power, and hierarchy within the health care team, contributes to effective communication, conflict resolution, and positive interprofessional working relationship
	8. Communicate consistently the importance of teamwork in patient-centered and community-focused care
Teams and teamwork	1. Describe the process of team development and the roles and practices of effective teams
	2. Develop consensus on the ethical principles to guide all aspects of patient care and team work
	3. Engage other health professionals—appropriate to the specific care situation—in shared patient-centered problem-solving
	4. Integrate the knowledge and experience of other professions—appropriate to the specific care situation—to inform care decisions while respecting patient and community values and priorities/preferences for care
	5. Apply leadership practices that support collaborative practice and team effectiveness
	6. Engage self and others to constructively manage disagreement about values, roles, goals, and actions that arise among health care professionals and with patients and families
	7. Share accountability with other professions, patients, and communities for outcomes relevant to prevention and health care
	8. Reflect on individual and team performance for individual, as well as team, performance improvement
	9. Use process improvement strategies to increase the effectiveness of interprofessional teamwork and team-based care
	10. Use available evidence to inform effective teamwork and team-based practices
	11. Perform effectively on team and in different team roles in a variety of settings

Note: Reprint from Interprofessional Education Collaborative Expert Panel. *Core Competencies for Interprofessional Collaborative Practices: Report of an Expert Panel.* Washington, DC: Interprofessional Education Collaborative; 2016. https://ipecollaborative.org/uploads/IPEC-2016-Updated-Core-Competencies-Report__final_release_.PDF.

A key to the success of the interprofessional CPD leadership team is to incorporate a check in at each of these four steps.[27] This can be done by having each member assess the use of the interprofessional collaboration components. Specific components to assess include interprofessional member attendance, level of perceived opportunity to share their professional perspectives, perception that their disciplinary perspectives were respected, and assessment of process to make decisions. The interprofessional CPD leadership team's use of an IPE check in ensures that interprofessional collaboration is evident in the CIPE program.

The last steps for the interprofessional CPD team to consider are related specifically to the educational activity design, implementation, and evaluation (Table 19.1). The planning of the specific educational activity must be done with participation with the frontline learners. Workplace learning is context specific, which adds complexity but creates meaning for the learners. Use of adult learning principles and social learning principles are essential at this step.[24] Health educators are experienced in the principles of adult learning, and workplace learning is experiential, satisfying a major component of adult learning. The inclusion of reflection and feedback is important for effective adult learning. Social learning theories contribute the essential interprofessional components as they provide how people learn, not just together, but from and with each other as well. This social learning perspective is addressed in the IPE competencies, but must always be kept at the forefront during the planning of CIPE activities. Evaluation should be based on the Kirkpatrick model as described earlier.[22]

FACILITATORS OF CONTINUING INTERPROFESSIONAL EDUCATION: COMPETENCIES AND ACCREDITATION

In 2010, the movement for expanding CE to include CIPE was facilitated by the IOM report, *Redesigning Continuing Education in the Health Professions*, which called for CE to bring health care professionals together to learn collaborative skills in the health care setting.[12] In addition, in 2010, the Canadian Interprofessional Health Collaborative published competency standards to guide education,[30] and in 2011, the United States followed with the publication of competencies (recently updated).[31] The US competencies are organized into four domains: (1) values/ethics, (2) roles and responsibilities, (3) interprofessional communication, and (4) teams and teamwork (Table 19.2). The interprofessional competencies serve to target attitudes, knowledge, and behaviors to achieve individual competency. The competencies have created a common framework that guides educators at all levels from prelicensure education to CE.

Another facilitator for the interprofessional CPD leadership team to consider is the addition of CIPE in the formal processes for accrediting providers. The Accreditation Council for CME (ACCME), the American Nurses Credentialing Center (ANCC), and the Accreditation Council for Pharmacy Education now have a joint accreditation process for team-based, outcome-focused education.[32] The Alliance for Continuing Education in the Health Professions has a mission to increase IPE (acehp.org). These groups have agreed that CIPE must include (1) a decreased focus on didactic learning, (2) an increased focus on workplace learning, (3) demonstration of CE impact on improving outcome-linked performance in the clinical setting, and (4) emphasis on lifelong learning skills.[8]

OPPORTUNITIES TO OVERCOME BARRIERS AT THE SYSTEMS LEVEL: CIPE PROGRAM DEVELOPMENT

The Owen and Schmitt[27] planning framework that addresses CIPE program development provides an opportunity to address barriers and opportunities for improvement at each of four steps (Table 19.3). A systematic review of the barriers related to IPE identified 10 common themes: curriculum (content, integration, time, schedule), leadership (poor planning, lack of coordination, lack of support), resources (lack of funding), stereotypes and attitudes (physician seen as dominant professional, preference to own profession), learner diversity (different learning needs and knowledge levels), interprofessional collaboration (definition and expectations vary across professions), teaching (challenges with larger class sizes and lack of faculty IPE skill), lack of enthusiasm (not understanding reason for IPE), professional jargon (overuse of disciplinary terminology), and lack of IPE accreditation.[33] The interprofessional CPD leadership team will achieve success by anticipating these barriers and addressing them with a continuous quality improvement philosophy.

TABLE 19.3
Barriers and Potential Solutions for Systems Level CIPE Program Development (Steps 1–4)

Barrier	Potential Solutions
Step 1: Focus of the program mission statement. CIPE requires collaboration with the schools of medicine and nursing and other disciplines, organizational leaders, and academic partners. In systems when directives are top-down and leadership does not support the expansion, altering the mission statement is challenging.	• Meet with leadership and use data and evidence to demonstrate impact of interprofessional collaboration. • Interprofessional CPD leadership team with monthly meetings and ground rules for attendance
Step 2: Analyzing the practice gaps to identify content areas is often completed in siloes and is dominated by medicine's goals.	• Implement a process for interprofessional CPD leadership team consensus on identifying gaps and CIPE content. • Solicit information from the frontline professionals as to what the practice gaps are and the disciplinary learning opportunities.
Step 3: Identify program barriers. Equitable distribution of funds and resources is difficult to establish. Resistance may come from discipline-specific leadership and diverse perspectives on what a CPD leadership team constitutes.	• Establish buy-in from all departments, academic partners, and organizational leaders to share costs and resources. • Clarify at the beginning the ground rules for team function.
Step 4: Articulating program goals and objectives is difficult to accomplish, specifically, meeting the knowledge content and competencies of each discipline. For example, diagnostic reasoning might be good for physicians, but not good for nurses.	• Use the interprofessional competencies as mandatory for program objectives (values/ethics, roles and responsibilities, interprofessional communication, teams and teamwork). Look beyond content to systems perspectives that are common to all disciplines.

As the interprofessional CPD leadership team works together to align their departments, a guiding principle for success is to use the cultural competency LEARN technique and to integrate the interprofessional collaboration competencies. Working as an interprofessional team will provide the opportunity to experience what it takes to work with each other. A second guiding principle for the interprofessional CPD leadership team is to seek the views of their learners and codevelop the program mission and goals. Another strategy is to continually evaluate the process. Evaluating the process includes collecting data during the CIPE program development. Using a "minute paper," a brief survey used for immediate feedback, will provide a way to ensure that the interprofessional CPD leadership team is employing the principles of interprofessional collaboration in developing the program.[34] A minute paper that includes questions on interprofessional collaboration components—such as (1) "Did all members have an opportunity to share their views?"; (2) "Were all disciplines' views respected?"; (3) "Was negotiation carried out in a fair manner?"; and (4) "Did all team members attend?"—would help to facilitate ongoing quality improvement.

OVERCOMING BARRIERS AT THE ACTIVITY LEVEL: DESIGN, IMPLEMENTATION, AND EVALUATION

After the overall CIPE program is established, it is time for the interprofessional CPD leaders to design, implement, and evaluate CIPE activities. Using the Owen and Schmidt CIPE planning framework for steps 5 and 6 has identifiable barriers and potential solutions (Table 19.4). An essential approach is to create workplace learning that gives the learners meaning and includes the coproduction of the activity, including the views of the health care professionals. One example of workplace learning is coached quality improvement projects. A quality improvement project creates a place to practice the IPE competencies as individuals while simultaneously practicing collaborative competence. Evaluation can then include improvement in the interprofessional competencies as well as the improvement of clinical outcomes of the quality improvement project. Evaluation can include both process evaluation, such as the minute paper previously mentioned, and IPE individual learning, as well as the measurable clinical or systems outcomes of the team-based quality improvement project. Resources are available to overcome barriers, and examples of successful models have been published (Table 19.5).

To date, the majority of IPE assessments have been limited to self-report of attitudes and beliefs. The National Center for Interprofessional Practice has assembled a Web-based collection of existing IPE measurement instruments (https://nexusipe.org/measurement-instruments). An IPE evaluation guide was developed by Reeves and colleagues[44] that provides the following suggestions: (1) think about evaluation first and be clear with the purpose of the evaluation, (2) consider the outcomes, (3) use models and theoretical perspectives, (4) carefully select an evaluation design using both qualitative and quantitative methods, and (5) provide ideas about disseminating evaluation results to the broader IPE community.

TABLE 19.4
Barriers and Potential Solutions for CIPE Activity Level: Design, Implementation, and Evaluation (Steps 5 and 6)

Barrier	Potential Solutions
Step 5: Design and Implement educational activities	
Faculty traditionally use didactic pedagogy and are not familiar with workplace learning.	Faculty development to increase the skill of the faculty[35]
Faculty default to "disciplinary content" and avoid the integration of interprofessional competencies.	
Structure of the setting to work collaboratively and scheduling the interprofessional time together[36]	Have a clear commitment from the leadership to designate time for these activities as high priority and to use learning while doing improvement work. Using this model, the administrators have a win–win situation as quality metrics are met and processes improved.
Challenges to IPE attitude, including professional narcissism, arrogance, and acquisitiveness[37]	Debrief and reflect on the role of all professions and the expertise of each member.
The importance of IPE is undervalued due to insufficient support and unreasonable expectations of success.[37]	Use trained faculty with deep understanding of collaborative care and workplace learning.
Lack of knowledge about each other's backgrounds and strengths[36]	Ensure that each activity includes an opportunity to learn about disciplinary role, background, and strength.
Lack of understanding of how to work collaboratively.	Use coaches who understand what collaborative work means. Use IPE competencies as an explicit way of teaching about attitudes and skills for collaborative care.
Tensions among staff and relationships not established	Schedule interprofessional enrichment activities.
Step 6: Evaluate the Educational Activity	
Difficulty collecting survey data on IPE concepts and clinical outcomes	Use experts in electronic medical record to obtain clinical outcomes.
Lack of reliable and valid methods to evaluate IPE	Use a combination of different tools to measure specific learning and incorporate measurement of clinical, population, or systems outcomes.[34]

FUTURE DIRECTIONS

Interprofessional CPD leadership teams can develop and implement a CIPE program and design, implement, and evaluate workplace learning activities. These activities have the potential to impact professional-to-professional communication and interprofessional collaboration. More important, these initiatives have the potential to impact quality outcomes. Keys to success of CIPE are the CPD leadership team's use of the same interprofessional competencies (i.e., team skills, communication, values, and roles and responsibilities) and the adherence to cultural competency and continual evaluation of the process. Also key is engaging health care professionals in the development of the activities and using workplace learning as the pedagogy.

TABLE 19.5
Resources and Examples of Continuing Interprofessional Workplace Learning Education Activities

Resources

Patient Self-Management Support of Chronic Conditions: Framework for Clinicians Seeking Recertification Credit (MOC Part IV & PI-CME). June 2016. Agency for Healthcare Research and Quality, Rockville, MD[38]	Free, self-contained framework for clinicians to design their own QI project. Using this module, clinicians can improve how they support their patients' ability to self-manage chronic conditions—physicians, nurse practitioners, and PAs select chronic condition of interest to them and enhance their skills for helping patients with chronic conditions while improving the patient experience.
Take the Lead on Healthcare Improvement. Massive Open Online Course through Coursera[39]	Free massive open online course for clinicians to work together on a quality improvement project. Ten modules take the learners from problem identification to a cycle of change and completion of a quality improvement story board.

Examples

Project and Organization	Details of Program
COMPAS, the collective for best practices and improvement in health care and services in family practice in Quebec's Monteregie region[40]	A program to engage primary care practitioners in quality improvement: making explicit the program theory of an interprofessional education intervention
Health Services Management Centre, University of Birmingham, Edgbaston, Birmingham, UK[41]	An integrated care development program for continuing interprofessional education that is a partnership between the university and workplace-based learning activity
University of Western Sydney, Parramatta Australia, School of Business[42]	A proposed program that uses citizen social science that involves clinicians as coresearchers in the systematic examination of social phenomena using computers and smartphones. The program provides ways to improve and sustain workplace learning.
University of Colorado Institute for Healthcare Quality, Safety and Efficiency (IHQSE). IHQSE is a partnership between the University of Colorado School of Medicine, University of Colorado College of Nursing, University Physicians, Inc., Children's Hospital Colorado, and the University of Colorado Hospital[43]	A 12-month Certificate Training Program (CTP) for interprofessional teams of clinicians. The goal is to create a capable workforce to improve and create innovative models of care to transform our entire clinical enterprise.

Future directions include educating CPD faculty to coach workplace learning activities such as quality improvement projects and safety rounds. The CPD faculty coach can ensure that health care professionals overcome the barriers to learning within teams and across professions by integrating interprofessional competencies into workplace learning activities. The future of CIPE includes a focus on collective interprofessional competence and the improvement of measurement of clinical outcomes as a result of this IPE.

REFERENCES

1. James JT. A new, evidence-based estimate of patient harms associated with hospital care. *J Patient Saf.* 2013;9(3):122–128.
2. Kronick R, Arnold S, Brady J, et al. Improving safety for hospitalized patients. *JAMA.* 2016;315(17):1831–1832.
3. Makary MA, Daniel M. Medical error-the third leading cause of death in the US. *BMJ.* 2016;353:i2139. http://www.ncbi.nlm.nih.gov/pubmed/27143499. Accessed July 8, 2016.
4. Lutfiyya MN, Brandt BF, Cerra F. Reflections from the intersection of health professions education and clinical practice: the state of the science of interprofessional education and collaborative practice. *Acad Med.* 2016;91(6):766–771.
5. Sikka R, Morath JM, Leape L. The quadruple aim: care, health, cost and meaning in work. *BMJ Qual Saf.* 2015;24(10):608–610.
6. Whittington JW, Nolan K, Lewis N, et al. Pursuing the triple aim: the first 7 years. *Milbank Q.* 2015;93(2):263–300.
7. Bodenheimer T, Sinsky C. From triple to quadruple aim: care of the patient requires care of the provider. *Ann Fam Med.* 2014;12(6):573–576.
8. American Association of Colleges of Nursing and the Association of American Medical Colleges (AAMC). *Lifelong Learning in Medicine and Nursing.* 2010. http://www.aacn.nche.edu/education-resources/MacyReport.pdf. Accessed July 9, 2016.
9. Hager M, Russell S, Fletcher SW. *Continuing Education in the Health Professions: Improving Healthcare through Lifelong Learning.* Proceedings of a conference sponsored by the Josiah Macy, Jr. Foundation; 2007, 2008. http://macyfoundation.org/publications/publication/conference-proceedings-continuing-education-in-the-health-professions. Accessed December 19, 2016.
10. Institute of Medicine (US) Committee on Quality of Health Care in America. In: Kohn LT, Corrigan JM, Donaldson MS, eds. *To Err Is Human.* National Academies Press (US); 2000. http://www.ncbi.nlm.nih.gov/pubmed/25077248. Accessed July 9, 2016.
11. Institute of Medicine. *Health Professions Education.* Washington, DC: National Academies Press; 2003. doi:10.17226/10681.
12. *Redesigning Continuing Education in the Health Professions.* Washington, DC: National Academies Press; 2010. doi:10.17226/12704.
13. Lawrence D, Bryant T, Nobel T, et al. A comparative evaluation of patient satisfaction outcomes in an interprofessional student run free clinic. *J Interprof Care.* 2015;29(5):445–450. PMID: 25700220.
14. Cronenwett L, Sherwood G, Barnsteiner J, et al. Quality and safety education for nurses. *Nurs Outlook.* 2007;55(3):122–131.
15. Chasm Q, Committee C, Care H, et al. *Crossing the Quality Chasm: A New Health System for the 21st Century.* Washington, DC: National Academies Press; 2001.
16. Balmer JT. The transformation of continuing medical education (CME) in the United States. *Adv Med Educ Pract.* 2013;4:171–182.
17. Hawkins RE, Lipner RS, Ham HP, et al. American Board of Medical Specialties Maintenance of Certification: theory and evidence regarding the current framework. *J Contin Educ Health Prof.* 2013;33(suppl 1):S7–S19.
18. WHO. *Framework for Action on Interprofessional Education and Collaborative Practice.* Geneva, Switzerland: World Health Organization; 2010.
19. Reeves S. An overview of continuing interprofessional education. *J Contin Educ Health Prof.* 2009;29(3):142–146.
20. Berlin EA, Fowkes WC. A teaching framework for cross-cultural health care. Application in family practice. *West J Med.* 1983;139(6):934–938.
21. Institute of Medicine. *Measuring the Impact of Interprofessional Education on Collaborative Practice and Patient Outcomes.* Washington, DC: National Academies Press; 2015.
22. Kirkpatrick DL, Kirkpatrick JD. *Evaluating Training Programs: The Four Levels.* San Francisco, CA: Berrett-Koehler; 2006.
23. Lingard L. What we see and don't see when we look at competence: notes on a god term. *Adv Health Sci Educ Theory Pract.* 2009;14(5):625–628.
24. Sargeant J. Theories to aid understanding and implementation of interprofessional education. *J Contin Educ Health Prof.* 2009;29(3):178–184.
25. Murdoch NL, Bottorff JL, McCullough D. Simulation education approaches to enhance collaborative healthcare: a best practices review. *Int J Nurs Educ Scholarsh.* 2014;10(1):307–321.
26. Kitto S, Goldman J, Schmitt MH, et al. Examining the intersections between continuing education, interprofessional education and workplace learning. *J Interprof Care.* 2014;28(3):183–185.

27. Owen JA, Schmitt MH. Integrating interprofessional education into continuing education: a planning process for continuing interprofessional education programs. *J Contin Educ Health Prof.* 2013;33(2):109–117.
28. Matthews RL, Pockett BR, Nisbet G, et al. Building capacity in Australian interprofessional health education: perspectives from key health and higher education stakeholders. *Aust Health Rev.* 2011;35(2):136–140.
29. Gilligan C, Outram S, Levett-Jones T. Recommendations from recent graduates in medicine, nursing and pharmacy on improving interprofessional education in university programs: a qualitative study. *BMC Med Educ.* 2014;14:52.
30. Canadian Interprofessional Health Collaborative. *A National Interprofessional Competency Framework 2010.* http://www.cihc.ca/files/CIHC_IPCompetencies_Feb1210.pdf. Accessed December 19, 2016.
31. Interprofessional Education Collaborative Expert Panel. *Core Competencies for Interprofessional Collaborative Practices: Report of an Expert Panel.* Washington, DC: Interprofessional Education Collaborative; 2016. https://ipecollaborative.org/uploads/IPEC-2016-Updated-Core-Competencies-Report__final_release_.PDF
32. Continuing Education Accreditors in Nursing, Pharmacy, and Medicine Joint Accreditation. http://www.jointaccreditation.org/. Accessed July 9, 2016.
33. Sunguya BF, Hinthong W, Jimba M, Yasuoka J. Interprofessional education for whom?—Challenges and lessons learned from its implementation in developed countries and their application to developing countries: a systematic review. *PLoS One.* 2014;9(5):e96724.
34. Singh MK, Lawrence R, Headrick L. Expanding educators' medical curriculum tool chest: minute papers as an underutilized option for obtaining immediate feedback. *J Grad Med Educ.* 2011;3(2):239–242.
35. Hall LW, Zierler BK. Interprofessional Education and Practice Guide No. 1: developing faculty to effectively facilitate interprofessional education. *J Interprof Care.* 2015;29(1):3–7.
36. Headrick LA, Barton AJ, Ogrinc G, et al. Results of an effort to integrate quality and safety into medical and nursing school curricula and foster joint learning. *Health Aff (Millwood).* 2012;31(12):2669–2680.
37. Clark PG. Examining the interface between interprofessional practice and education: lessons learned from Norway for promoting teamwork. *J Interprof Care.* 2011;25(1):26–32.
38. Agency for Healthcare Research and Quality. *Patient Self-Management Support of Chronic Conditions: Framework for Clinicians Seeking Recertification Credit (MOC Part IV & PI-CME).* Rockville, MD: Agency for Healthcare Research and Quality; 2016. http://www.ahrq.gov/professionals/education/continuing-ed/moc-sms/index.html
39. Dolansky MA, Moore SM, Singh MK. (2014, 2015). Take the lead on quality improvement. *Massive Open Online Course.* https://www.coursera.org/course/hcqualityimprovement
40. Vachon B, Désorcy B, Camirand M, et al. Engaging primary care practitioners in quality improvement: making explicit the program theory of an interprofessional education intervention. *BMC Health Serv Res.* 2013;13:106. http://doi.org/10.1186/1472-6963-13-106
41. Miller R, Combes G, Brown H, et al. Interprofessional workplace learning: a catalyst for strategic change? *J Interprof Care.* 2014;28(3):186–193. http://doi.org/10.3109/13561820.2013.877428
42. Dadich A. Citizen social science: a methodology to facilitate and evaluate workplace learning in continuing interprofessional education. *J Interprof Care.* 2014;28(3):194–199. http://doi.org/10.3109/1356182 0.2013.874982
43. Dolansky MA, Leubbers E, Singh M, et al. Interprofessional approaches to quality and safety education. In: Sherwood G, Barnsteiner J, eds. *Quality and Safety in Nursing: A Competency Approach to Improving Outcomes,* 2nd ed. Ames, IA: Wiley Blackwell; 2017.
44. Reeves S, Boet S, Zierler B, et al. Interprofessional Education and Practice Guide No. 3: evaluating interprofessional education. *J Interprof Care.* 2015;29(4):305–312.

Chapter 20

ASSESSING *and* REMEDIATING *the* STRUGGLING PHYSICIAN

Betsy White Williams

Case

The physician medical licensing body in your jurisdiction has asked you to review the findings of two primary care physicians in the last 2 years. Further, your local academic medical center has asked you to review notes on one surgeon and two internists who have, in the hospital's opinion, delivered "suboptimal care." These files reveal a range of issues, from poor note-keeping, making it unable to judge what the clinician actually did, to one case in which an unfortunate event occurred, entirely unlike the physician's previous practices, to a clinician who appeared to practice consistently below the standards established by the medical community.

Questions

How would you assess these physicians to determine their needs in professional development? What do you know about "remedial CME/CPD," especially the impact of those programs? What are the challenges that these cases present?

INTRODUCTION

Dyscompetence is defined as a failure to maintain acceptable standards in one or more areas of professional practice,[1] while incompetence is a lack of the requisite abilities and qualities (cognitive, noncognitive, and communicative) to perform effectively in the scope of professional physician practice. Underperformance is a broader category than dyscompetence and includes those practitioners with a decline in performance and/or whose performance is significantly lower than that of his or her peers.[1] Physicians are key members of a health care team. Society relies on physicians to remain current and to consistently perform at the highest level. Unfortunately, physician performance failures are not rare; yet, the safety of patients depends, among other things, on the quality of care delivered by health care providers.[2]

A small, but significant, minority of practicing physicians are identified as dyscompetent. The literature suggests that 6% to 12% of practicing physicians may be dyscompetent.[3] Based on the number of physicians with active licenses in the United States in 2014,[4] somewhere between 54,975 and 109,951 practicing physicians would be anticipated to be dyscompetent. The need to recognize and remediate dyscompetent and underperforming physicians is clear. Yet, such tasks are challenging for many reasons. Difficulties exist in the definition, detection, and remediation of dyscompetent and/or underperforming practitioners. There is a lack of resources available for physicians with competency issues.[2] A final challenge is the lack of research to guide "best practices" in the assessment and remediation of these practitioners.[5]

CONSEQUENCE OF DYSCOMPETENCE

A recent study by Makary and Daniel (2016) suggests that medical error is the third most common cause of death in the United States with at least 250,000 deaths attributed to medical error.[6] Since medical errors are not coded on death certificates, these data likely represent an underestimate. Rosenstein[7] summarized financial costs associated with medical errors. These include 950,000 patient safety events and 99,000 deaths over a 3-year period, with a total of nearly $9 billion in additional health care costs. Likewise, he reported nearly 15 million annual instances of medical harm at a cost of between $17 billion and $29 billion a year in health care expenses, lost productivity, lost income, and disability, with another 20% to 30% of additional costs estimated in the postdischarge sector. He reported that an estimated 1.5 million preventable drug events occur each year with the cost of an adverse drug event ranging from $2,000 to $5,800 per hospitalization and an increased length of hospital stay of 2.2 to 4.6 days. The average cost of a medical error–based claim was $521,560.[7] Poor interpersonal and communication skills can contribute to increased errors, decreased patient and staff satisfaction, and increased malpractice liability for themselves and team members.[8] A critical role that CPD professionals can play is in increasing health care professionals' awareness of the many costs that are associated with dyscompetence.

IDENTIFICATION OF PERFORMANCE ISSUES

Underperformance occurs in medical students, trainees, and practicing physicians. Identification of performance issues becomes increasingly more difficult further along in the educational continuum. Historically in the United States, dyscompetent/underperforming physicians have been most typically identified through a peer review or regulatory (licensure board) process. It would be desirable if performance concerns were voiced early and when first observed. However, it is difficult for physicians to approach and report quality concerns about peers,[9,10] and few hospitals respond to physician performance failures promptly or effectively.[2] Additionally, underperforming physicians may not attract complaints if they communicate well.[11] A recent review of peer assessment instruments indicates that only three published instruments were found to have an appropriate scientific basis, thus raising concerns about the peer review process.[12] Perhaps of most concern, if a peer review or a regulatory process has been used to identify the practitioner, patient harm may have already occurred.

Patient safety concerns have led to suggestions about the need for routine screening of physicians in practice. Three levels of performance assessment have been described.[13,14]

Level 1 screening is routinely done as part of recredentialing or revalidation. Level 2 assessment is used to screen for difficulties among those identified as at risk of poor performance because of risk factors. Level 3 assessment is a targeted intervention for those physicians whose performance has been identified as giving cause for concern.

Regulatory authorities and certifying bodies in many countries have struggled with the question of how to best assure the ongoing clinical competence of practicing medical practitioners. The American Board of Medical Specialties (ABMS) initiated Maintenance of Certification (MOC) in 2000 as a means to promote continuous professional development and lifelong learning in their diplomates.[15] MOC now requires diplomates to seek recertification on a periodic basis. Likewise, the Royal College of Physicians and Surgeons of Canada (RCPSC) Maintenance of Certification program and the General Medical Council (GMC) of the United Kingdom's revalidation process are designed to promote documentation of ongoing maintenance of competence. The Medical Board of Australia (MBA) recently commissioned the Collaboration for the Advancement of Medical Education Research and Assessment (CAMERA) at Plymouth University Peninsula Schools of Medicine and Dentistry (UK) to study international approaches to revalidation as a means to inform possible approaches for medical revalidation in Australia.[16]

Over the last 10 years, there have also been a number of changes to how hospital privileging decisions are made in the United States. In 2007, the Joint Commission introduced Ongoing Professional Practice Evaluation (OPPE) and Focused Professional Practice Evaluation (FPPE). OPPE is considered a screening tool (level 1) to identify those clinicians who might be delivering an unacceptable quality of care, while FPPE, the follow-up process, is designed to determine the validity of any positives found through OPPE.[17] Routine level 1 screening as part of the revalidation process has occurred in some provinces in Canada for a number of years.[14]

RISK FACTORS FOR UNDERPERFORMANCE

Potential risk factors for performance issues include length of time after graduation (greater time), practitioner age, male gender, doctors whose first medical qualification was gained outside the current practice country, and history of professionalism issues in training. There is also a literature that suggests that factors such as professional isolation, rural practice, and solo may be risk factors associated with underperformance.[18–30] External factors such as inadequate access to continuing education, poor initial training, solo practice, certification status, practice location, and organizational and systems factors all can contribute to errors in medical delivery and interact with individual factors in ways that may exacerbate or minimize deficiencies.[3]

Individual factors such as the effects of aging; health issues; psychiatric conditions such as depression, anxiety, and substance use issues; burnout; fatigue/sleep deprivation; personality characteristics; and external stressors all can negatively impact performance.[3,19,25,31–34] Lucey and Boote have referred to potential factors impacting performance as the seven D's. These include distraction (external stressors), deprivation (sleep), depression, drugs, disease, disability (learning), and disorder (personality).[35] Depression, drugs, drinking, and dementia are particularly associated with older practitioners.[36] A recent study found that cognitive impairment in physicians is responsible for 57% of adverse medical events, most of which were determined to be preventable.[30] The aging of the medical workforce has contributed to concerns about practitioner competency and patient safety. There is a robust literature that demonstrates that abilities such as novel or abstract problem-solving capability (fluid intelligence), processing speed, episodic memory, retrieval, sensory processing, and manual dexterity all decrease with age.[3,28,37,38]

DOMAINS OF UNDERPERFORMANCE

It is important to note that performance concerns are not unique to only cognitive and/or technical skills. Difficulties in any one of the American Board of Medical Specialty core competency areas or CanMEDS roles can contribute to patient safety issues. Cognitive skills such as knowledge, judgment, and clinical problem-solving; technical and psychomotor skills; and noncognitive skills including good interpersonal skills, positive attitudes, and professional behaviors are all critical to the provision of the highest level of patient care. While the importance of cognitive and technical skills in the provision of the highest level of patient care may seem more apparent, there is also a robust literature about the negative consequences associated with poor professionalism and interpersonal and communication skills.[2,39]

EVALUATION OF PERFORMANCE ISSUES

There are many manifestations of performance issues and multiple potential contributory factors to poor performance. Thus, comprehensive assessment is a key first step in the remediation process. Hauer and colleagues have presented a comprehensive approach to addressing strugglers across the continuum that includes assessment, diagnosis of problems, development of an individualized learning plan, provision of instruction, and reassessment and certification of competence.[5] The evaluation should determine the types and extent of performance issues and elucidate all potential causes of performances issues.

While many current approaches to addressing underperforming practitioners include an assessment component, the focus of the assessment is often directed at performance and educational issues without full consideration of the potential contribution of biological, psychological, and social processes. A recent review of 15 assessment and remediation programs in 5 countries indicated a wide variation in assessment approaches with the focus ranging from identifying and repairing specific knowledge and skills to wide interest in the biopsychosocial functioning of the physician with less attention on broader systems factors or contextual factors that might impact performance.[40,41] As it has become increasingly clear that doctors are often poor at taking care of their own health[42,43] and that mental and physical health issues are often present in practitioners identified as underperforming,[26,30,33,34,44] the importance of using a biopsychosocial approach as part of the evaluation process cannot be overstated.

The biopsychosocial approach systematically considers biological, psychological, and social factors pertinent to the individual and also should also consider the developmental stage of the individual, as each developmental stage is associated with unique health conditions, psychological factors, personal life, and organizational/systems stressors.[45] Assessment of biological factors includes consideration of whether factors such as age, genetics, infections, physical trauma, exposure to toxins, and poor nutrition could have contributed to medical and/or psychiatric conditions that may have negatively impacted practice performance or be an impediment to benefitting from remediation. Psychological factors include the thoughts, attitudes, beliefs, and perceptions of the individual and understanding how those cognitive patterns affect the individual's interpretation of events. Other important variables include perceived sense of control, sense of self-efficacy, level of motivation, perception of barriers, perceived sense of control over the environment, and insight. An assessment of social factors includes socioeconomical, socioenvironmental, and cultural factors pertinent to the individual. It is important to consider social factors pertaining to personal life as well as in the occupational environment. Personal stressors such as recent marriage, recent relocation, financial stressors, and birth of a child while occupational systems stresses such as extremely high workload, lack of appropriate equipment and/or staff, rotating day/night shifts, limited systems resources, and/or poor leadership can all negatively impact performance and thus need to be considered.

DEVELOPMENT OF A LEARNING PLAN

In developing a remedial learning plan, a thorough understanding of areas of knowledge and skill deficit is crucial. Gathering data informed by different frameworks is helpful. For example, a competency-based framework, considering which ABMS core competencies or CanMEDS roles are lacking, and a developmental framework, providing data on level of performance from knowledge, "knows" through performance in practice, "does", informs choice of assessment methods and remediation needs. Assessment methods can include multiple-choice tests for information at the lower levels of Miller's pyramid to chart reviews with chart-stimulated recall, sampling/review of clinical work, direct observation, simulation, and 360 surveys, which provide a sense of performance in practice. Optimally, these data combined with data gathered from the biopsychosocial evaluation inform recommendations for remediation and the development of an individualized learning plan. Consideration needs to be given to program format (lecture, small group discussion, workshop, rounds, focused reading, simulation, proctoring, etc.), setting, timing (frequency, duration of meeting, duration of training program), as well as content of the experience. It is possible that the participant will need more than one type of remedial program. See Table 20.1 for example of assessment and remediation strategies that incorporate these principles. In some cases, an integrated program similar to a mini-residency may be the best approach. Optimally, the training will help the participant effectively set learning goals, plan and use strategies to achieve those goals, manage their personal and professional resources, and reflect on their performance as they monitor and evaluate their progress at various stages of the learning process. This

TABLE 20.1
Example of assessment and remediation strategies that takes into account educational and biopsychosocial issues

Performance	Skill Domain	Professional Functioning		Biological		Psychological		Social	
		Assess	**Remediate**	**Assess**	**Remediate**	**Assess**	**Remediate**	**Assess**	**Remediate**
Does	Cognitive	360, Record review, quality data, observation, portfolio	Case-based learning, CSR	CSR, 360, observation	Small group	360, observation	Case-based learning	360, observation	Small group
	Non-cognitive	360, CSR, quality data, observation, portfolio	Case-based learning, CSR	360	Small group	360	Case-based learning	360	Small group
	Procedural/technical	Observation/proctor, quality data, portfolio, record review	Case-based learning, CSR	Proctor	Small group	360	Group/coach	360	Group/coach
Shows How	Cognitive	OSCE, SM, SP, CSR	Small group, CSR	CSR	Small group	CSR	Small group	CSR	Small group
	Non-cognitive	OSCE, SM, SP, CSR	Small group, CSR	SP	Role play	SP	Small group	SP	Role play
	Procedural/technical	Low fidelity SM, portfolio, case logs	Case-based learning, CSR, low fidelity SM	SM	Case-based learning	Portfolio	Case-based learning	SM	Case-based learning

Knows How	**Cognitive**	SOQ, low fidelity SM, vignette based MCQ	Role play	SM	Role play	SM	Role play	SM	Role play
	Non-cognitive	SOQ, low fidelity SM, vignette based MCQ	Role play	SM	Role play	SM	Role play	SM	Role play
	Procedural/ technical	SOQ, low fidelity SM, vignette based MCQ	SM	SM	Small group	SM	Small group	SM	Role play
Knows	**Cognitive**	MCQ	Focused reading	Physical[a]	TX	Multi-disciplinary assessment	Didactic CME	Multi-disciplinary assessment	Small group
	Non-cognitive	MCQ	Small group	Physical[a]	TX	Multi-disciplinary assessment	Didactic CME	Multi-disciplinary assessment	Small group
	Procedural/ technical	SOQ	Didactic CME	Physical[a]	TX	Multi-disciplinary assessment	Didactic CME	Multi-disciplinary assessment	Small group

It is common that a learner will require multiple remediation strategies.

[a]Can be part of the multi-disciplinary evaluation.

MCQ, written examination; SOQ, standardized oral examination; SM, simulation and models; SP, standardized patient; TX, treatment (if medical/psychiatric); CSR, chart stimulated recall; 360, multi-source feedback.

process of helping the learner to develop a schema in which to master processes that enhance learning is referred to as self-regulated learning (SRL). Reflection and reflective competency are important skills for the learner to develop as they promote competence and lifelong learning.[46,47] At the end of the remediation cycle, independent of type of remediation provided, it is important to do an assessment to determine that goals for remediation from both the biopsychosocial and educational perspective have been accomplished. Optimally, the assessment will be at the "does" level. It is also helpful to follow up to make sure that gains are maintained over time.

OUTCOMES OF REMEDIATION

Rosner and colleagues noted that performance outcome data following remedial CME were not available as most programs were in their infancy.[48] Unfortunately, more than 20 years later, there are still limited outcome data on remediation efforts in practicing physicians as few programs have published follow-up studies.[5,40,41] In addition, comparisons and generalization of results are difficult as remedial programs use different methods for assessment and remediation, exclusion criteria for entry into assessment and remediation programs, outcome measures (completion of training vs. implementation of learning), and length of follow-up when present varies. Also, sample sizes are often small. McAuley and colleagues reported that more than half of the 56 referred physicians who were reassessed during the study period satisfactorily addressed concerns while ~20% made some improvement and 27% failed or retired from practice.[29] Grant (1995) described the process and results of the Physician Prescribed Educational Program (PPEP).[49] While data were presented about phase I assessment results, little was written about phase II remediation results other than 45/47 participants were participating in or completed the program. Moran and colleagues (1996) reported significant improvement at 18 months in a small group of physicians that had participated in a focused CME activity designed to improve clinical practice.[50] In a remedial education program in Ontario based on 5 participants, only a small percentage of underperforming physicians (20%) improved postremedial efforts.[51] Goulet and colleagues have written extensively about remediation efforts provided through the College des Médicins du Quebec.[31,52–55] In their sample of 305 doctors, 70% of the retraining programs succeeded, 15% were partially successful, and 13% failed. In another report, they found statistically significant improvements in record keeping (20% before and 54% after remediation), clinical investigation plan (13% before and 59% after remediation), diagnostic accuracy (32% before and 61% after remediation), and patient treatment and follow-up (31% before and 67% after remediation). Recently, they reported follow-up data on 408 physicians participating in 465 remedial activities between 2003 and 2013. They report a 75% success rate in passing the remedial program. However, 36% of physicians (52 out of 143) who had a follow-up visit after a successful remediation were recommended for additional remediation. Lillis and colleagues reported that 75% of doctors who entered remedial education were considered to be practicing at an acceptable standard at the end of remediation.[56] A recent study by Guerrasio and colleagues describes remediation outcomes of medical students, residents, fellows, and attending physicians who attended a remediation program at one school of medicine's remediation program. Fourteen practicing physicians participated in the program. Two graduated, 7 were in good standing or unrestricted practice, 2 transferred, 2 remained on probation or restricted practice, and 1 withdrew.[57]

There are a few studies that describe outcomes following participation in remedial CME activities. Spickard and colleagues reported on 54 physicians participating in a remedial prescribing CME course between January 1997 and January 1999. All participants identified three to five changes they intended to make over the next 3 months. Participants were contacted 3 months after course completion, and 83% responded. Participants reported full implementation (90% to 100% of the time) of 40% of the commitments. The overall implementation rate was 73%. Reported barriers to implementation including competing priorities and lack of time were common barriers.

Samenow and colleagues described their experience with physicians who participated in a CME course targeting disruptive behavior. Behavioral change was monitored using a 360 survey delivered at course initiation and follow-up sessions (1, 3 and 6 months). Of the 20 physicians who consented to participate in the study precourse survey, data were obtained on 14 physicians, 3-month follow-up data on 13 physicians, and 6-month follow-up data on 5 physicians. Score patterns suggested improvement for 11 of the 13 physicians by others' report and 7 of the 13 physicians by self-report at 3-month follow-up. Six-month data were insufficient for statistical analysis. At the time of course completion, 93% of the participants reported that they had a better understanding of how their behavior affected patient care and that the course helped them change their attitudes and behaviors. Participants were also able to identify at least one specific change in their behavior both professionally and in their personal lives that they attributed to skills learned in the course.

Parran and colleagues reported on 358 learners who participated in a remedial CME course targeting professionalism between September 2005 and February 2012. Pre–post ethics questionnaire results were available for 118 participants as the pre–posttest was implemented in the 2010 academic cycle, while 269 physicians participated in the pre-/post-/follow-up reflective essay assignment, which was implemented in 2006. Participants had the opportunity to further reflect on their ethical challenge at the end of the course and at 12 weeks. They concluded that class participants recognized ethical principles and the importance of boundary maintenance in clinical practice but had an inability to apply those principles in the clinical practice setting.

FACTORS RELATED TO OUTCOME

There are a number of studies that describe factors related to successful remediation. Neuropsychological performance is a strong predictor of both level of performance on competency assessments and remediation outcome.[30,51,58–60] There is increasing evidence of the ecological validity of neuropsychological testing as well as the predictive validity of testing for a variety of behavioral and medical conditions.[61] Neuropsychological issues do not preclude successful remediation. However, it is optimal that the extent and causes of poor neuropsychological test performance are understood and diagnosed medical conditions are properly treated prior to the initiation of a remedial program. It is not surprising that neuropsychological testing has been demonstrated to be an important tool in both the assessment and evaluation process.

There is increasing evidence that poor health is a risk factor for underperformance and physicians are poor at addressing their own health.

Insight as well is an important variable for predicting successful remediation.[62] Those who perform poorly are less able to accurately judge their level of performance. This appears to be due to lack of the ability to produce correct responses and the expertise necessary to determine that they are not producing them.[63] One of the reported difficulties associated with remediating students with issues of professionalism is their lack of insight and difficulties in self-assessing their performance.[64] In our own data, we have found high levels of insight, and self-efficacy are strongly correlated with positive remedial outcome in a group of 54 physicians referred for remediation secondary to concerns surrounding a lack of professionalism.[65]

CHALLENGES

Underperforming physicians rarely self-identify. Given estimates of rates of underperformance and dyscompetence, it is clear that only a small percentage of those in need of remedial services are identified. There are a number of systems issues that contribute to difficulties in the proactive identification and successful remediation of underperforming physicians. Warning signs of difficulties may be ignored, clear policies for handling physicians with performance issues may be lacking, and discomforts in addressing the issues all contribute to the problem of underidentification[2] and diffusions of responsibility[66] all contribute to the problem of underidentification. Proactive processes such as OPPE and FPPE are relatively new processes. Identifying appropriate data points and data collection methods are challenging. This is particularly true if one is trying to assess noncognitive skills. Further, not all hospitals are Joint Commission approved and not all physicians are members of medical staff. Likewise, with the MOC process, not all physicians are board certified, and older physicians who are grandfathered appear to opt out of the MOC processes.[15] Thus, these processes cannot be applied to all practitioners and may miss those at highest risk for issues for dyscompetence. Additionally, the relationships among recertification, OPPE/FPPE, patient outcomes, and physician competence need more study. Another difficulty is that there can be confusion as to whether performance issues should be addressed as part of human resources (employment), well-being (impairment), or medical staff process. There are often concerns about potential litigation that could arise as part of the process. This can make colleagues uncomfortable to bring forth complaints and contribute to faculty and colleagues being hesitant to participate in assessment and/or remediation of an identified clinician. Often, systems, physicians, and staff are not aware of potential resources in their organization or, more broadly, that are available to deal with physicians who experience performance concerns.

Appropriate assessment and remediation are often lengthy and expensive processes. Most typically, the cost is borne by the referred physicians and includes cost for the program as well as lost revenue that results from time away from practice. Often, there is a lack of understanding on the part of the referred physician as well as the referring system of the possible personal, financial, and time demands associated with the process. Identifying proctors and mentors within the work setting can be difficult as they may be concerned about possible litigation or feel that the costs outweigh the benefits of participation. Systems issues can be a contributory factor to the problematic behavior, and these issues can often be difficult to address.

The importance of appropriate identification and remediation of underperforming and dyscompetent physicians is clear. The potential difficulties associated with physician underperformance and the challenges these types of cases present are highlighted in the case study described at the beginning of this chapter. These challenges include a lack of clarity as to what constitutes underperformance, difficulties in timely identification of underperforming physicians, the potential of patient harm prior to performance concerns surfacing, the heterogeneity of performances issues that can present, the multiple factors that can contribute to underperformance, and the lack of resources in addressing these issues. There is a need for a comprehensive assessment to ascertain the nature, extent, pattern of (acute onset vs. chronic pattern), and causes of performance issues. Optimally, the assessment will include evaluation of the physician's health and well-being, practice style and setting, knowledge, skills, attitudes, beliefs, behaviors, and ability to apply those appropriately in the practice setting. These data then inform the remediation plan. Factors that predict successful remediation include absence of neuropsychological deficits and by extension good physical and mental health and the presence of high levels of insight and self-efficacy. It is also important to be aware that systems issues can contribute to difficulties in both the identification and remediation of underperforming physicians. Being mindful of individual and systems factors, the complexity of these cases, and available resources provides the best opportunity for an optimal outcome.

FUTURE DIRECTIONS

There continues to be a lack of evidence to inform best practices in the identification, assessment, and remediation of underperforming and dyscompetent physicians. Lack of consistency in the use of terms, in methods of assessment and remediation, and in follow-up limit the interpretation and generalizability of results. Moving forward, it will be important to address these issues through theoretically grounded and appropriately structured research.

Proactive programs such as OPPE, FPPE, MOC, and physician review programs of the types currently done through Colleges in the Canadian provinces and being considered in other countries are important steps in identifying underperforming practitioners prior to their causing patient harm. While these are important steps forward, many obstacles remain. Our understanding of factors that contribute to underperformance and how underperformance manifests in practice is still developing. Thus, it remains difficult to gather data that inform such decisions. Also, when potential concerns about a practitioner's level of performance are surfaced at the work setting, appropriate action is not always taken in a timely fashion. This includes situations where there are concerns about knowledge and skills as well as behavioral problems such as professionalism issues, poor interpersonal and communication skills, and physical/mental health concerns. Colleagues, trainees, and even department chairs are often uncomfortable addressing performance issues in colleagues.[9,10,66,67] Faculty development programs that increase knowledge and skills and highlight the importance of early detection and the critical need to address performance issues in colleagues could potentially promote earlier and more consistent identification of practitioners with performance issues. Optimally, such programs would increase knowledge about indications/signs of performance issues, promote skills and ease in providing feedback about issues of concerns, and increase knowledge of resources available within one's institution and more broadly. Experiential exercises and opportunities to practice giving feedback would be important components of the professional development program.

Assessment of ongoing competence in airline pilots is more rigorous than that of practicing physicians.[68] Commercial airline pilots undergo regular medical certification, submit to random testing to detect possible substance abuse, and undergo assessment on a simulator at least once a year. They are subject to random performance checks, undergo specific training and testing routinely, and have age-related retirement. There has been discussion of mandatory retirement in physicians, and some health systems have begun mandatory age-related screening of physicians. While age is a demonstrated risk factor for dyscompetence, poor mental and physical health can also be associated with performance issues. Historically, the importance of self-care has not been stressed as part of the medical education curriculum, nor has it been emphasized for its importance through the developmental lifespan of the physician.[69] Moving forward, it will be important to place an increased emphasis on health and wellness as direct challenges to performance quality in the medical workforce and to help physicians view well-being as a core component of professionalism. CPD professionals could play a role in this through the design and provision of CPD programs highlighting the importance of well-being.

It will be important to continue to develop better measures for assessing the performance of practitioners in practice. Simulation technology holds great promise for both the assessment and remediation of health care providers across the educational continuum. There is a growing literature that demonstrates the value of simulation-based medical education (SBME) over more traditional clinical medical education in achieving specific clinical skill acquisition goals.[70,71] While specific studies on the application of simulation-based education to underperforming physicians are lacking, the potential value of SBME is apparent.

Physician performance issues are not unique. The rapid expansion of medical knowledge, increases in the complexity of health care delivery systems, the aging of the physician workforce, and challenges to physician health and well-being all suggest that physician performance difficulties will continue to be an issue moving forward. It will take a comprehensive and integrated approach before performance issues are proactively and consistently addressed and remediated. This will necessarily involve a systems component that provides education about the importance of and methods for promoting timely identification of performance issues, comfort in addressing them, and knowledge of and availability of appropriate resources. Physicians are in a unique position of trust. Their services are not optional or reviewable by those outside the profession. Responsibility for public trust is within the profession. Underperformance occurs at all stages, from medical school to practicing physicians. The search for excellence and the need for ongoing professional development should be the focus for every stage. The continuing drive for quality implies that the professional life of a physician is one of continuous quality improvement and an interconnected series of Shewhart cycles that involves ongoing assessment and improvement. This perspective must be instilled early in medical education and embraced whether the effort is focused on improving performance in an identified area of relative weakness or in striving for excellence where there is no deficit. This will involve faculty development for those involved in undergraduate and graduate training. Faculty and attendings need to recognize the importance of addressing performance issues in a timely fashion. They also need to gain comfort and skill in providing effective feedback. It is the hope and expectation that all physicians will come to embrace this characteristic of commitment to meeting the implicit public trust invested in them.

For the practitioners in difficulty, it will be important to help them understand the process as part of a quality cycle. The remediation program must include comprehensive assessment, development of an individualized remediation plan, provision of remediation, and assessment in practice post remediation. Best outcomes will occur if health and potential systems areas are addressed and if the learner is able to see the remediation process as the beginning of a series of ongoing quality and professional development cycles. For the field, research on methods of early identification, assessment, remediation strategies, and outcomes are needed to inform best practices moving forward.

REFERENCES

1. Federation of State Medical Boards. *Evaluation of Quality of Care and Maintenance of Competence. The Special Committee on Evaluation of Quality of Care and Maintenance of Competence* [Internet]. 1999.
2. Leape LL, Fromson JA. Problem doctors: is there a system-level solution? *Ann Intern Med.* 2006;144(2):107.
3. Williams BW. The prevalence and special educational requirements of dyscompetent physicians. *J Contin Educ Health Prof.* 2006;26(3):173–191.
4. Young A, Chaudhry HJ, Rhyne J, et al. A census of actively licensed physicians in the United States, 2010. *J Med Regulat.* 2013;99(2):11–24.
5. Hauer KE, Ciccone A, Henzel TR, et al. Remediation of the deficiencies of physicians across the continuum from medical school to practice: a thematic review of the literature. *Acad Med.* 2009;84(12):1822–1832.
6. Makary MA, Daniel M. Medical error—the third leading cause of death in the US. *BMJ.* 2016;353:i2139.
7. Rosenstein AH. Measuring and managing the economic impact of disruptive behaviors in the hospital. *J Healthc Risk Manag.* 2010;30(2):20–26.
8. Hickson GB, Entman SS. Physician practice behavior and litigation risk: evidence and opportunity. *Clin Obstet Gynecol.* 2008;51(4):688–699.
9. DesRoches CM, Rao SR, Fromson JA, et al. Physicians' perceptions, preparedness for reporting, and experiences related to impaired and incompetent colleagues. *JAMA.* 2010;304(2):187–193.
10. Campbell EG, Regan S, Gruen RL, et al. Professionalism in medicine: results of a national survey of physicians. *Ann Intern Med.* 2007;147(11):795–802.
11. St George I, Kaigas T, McAvoy P. Assessing the competence of practicing physicians in New Zealand, Canada, and the United Kingdom: progress and problems. *Fam Med.* 2004;36(3):172–177.
12. Evans R, Elwyn G, Edwards A. Review of instruments for peer assessment of physicians. *BMJ.* 2004;328(7450):1240.
13. Kaigas T. Monitoring and enhancement of physician performance (MEPP): a national initiative. *The College of Physicians and Surgeons of Ontario's (CPSO) Members' Dialog.* 1995.
14. Finucane P, Bourgeois-Law G, Ineson S, et al. A comparison of performance assessment programs for medical practitioners in Canada, Australia, New Zealand, and the United Kingdom. *Acad Med.* 2003;78(8):837–843.
15. Iglehart JK, Baron RB. Ensuring physicians' competence—is maintenance of certification the answer? *N Engl J Med.* 2012;367(26):2543–2549.
16. Archer J, Pitt R, Nunn S, et al. Revalidation: the evidence for revalidation and options for revalidation in the Australian context. *Medical Board of Australia,* 2015.
17. Wise RA. *Joint Commission Physician Blog [Internet]: The Joint Commission.* 2013. Available from https://www.jointcommission.org/jc_physician_blog/oppe_fppe_tools_privileging_decisions/. Accessed June 10, 2016.

18. Grace ES, Wenghofer EF, Korinek EJ. Predictors of physician performance on competence assessment: findings from CPEP, the Center for Personalized Education for Physicians. *Acad Med.* 2014;89(6):912–919.
19. Norton PG, Dunn EV, Soberman L. What factors affect quality of care? Using the Peer Assessment Program in Ontario family practices. *Can Fam Physician.* 1997;43:1739.
20. Norton P, Faulkner D. A longitudinal study of performance of physicians' office practices: data from the Peer Assessment Program in Ontario, Canada. *Jt Comm J Qual Improv.* 1999;25(5):252–258.
21. Morrison J, Morrison T. Psychiatrists disciplined by a state medical board. *Am J Psychiatry.* 2001;158(3):474–478.
22. Cardarelli R, Licciardone JC, Ramirez G. Predicting risk for disciplinary action by a state medical board. *Tex Med.* 2004;100(1):84–90.
23. Clay SW, Conatser RR. Characteristics of physicians disciplined by the State Medical Board of Ohio. *J Am Osteopath Assoc.* 2003;103(2):81–88.
24. Khaliq AA, Dimassi H, Huang C-Y, et al. Disciplinary action against physicians: who is likely to get disciplined? *Am J Med.* 2005;118(7):773–777.
25. Kohatsu ND, Gould D, Ross LK, et al. Characteristics associated with physician discipline: a case–control study. *Arch Intern Med.* 2004;164(6):653–658.
26. Donaldson LJ, Panesar SS, McAvoy PA, et al. Identification of poor performance in a national medical workforce over 11 years: an observational study. *BMJ Qual Saf.* 2014;23(2):147–152.
27. Papadakis MA, Hodgson CS, Teherani A, et al. Unprofessional behavior in medical school is associated with subsequent disciplinary action by a state medical board. *Acad Med.* 2004;79(3):244–249.
28. Williams BW, Flanders P. Physician health and wellbeing provide challenges to patient safety and outcome quality across the careerspan. *Australas Psychiatry.* 2016:1039856215626652.
29. McAuley RG, Paul WM, Morrison GH, et al. Five-year results of the peer assessment program of the College of Physicians and Surgeons of Ontario. *CMAJ.* 1990;143(11):1193.
30. Kataria N, Brown N, McAvoy P, et al. A retrospective study of cognitive function in doctors and dentists with suspected performance problems: an unsuspected but significant concern. *JRSM Open.* 2014;5(5):2042533313517687.
31. Goulet F, Hudon E, Gagnon R, et al. Effects of continuing professional development on clinical performance: results of a study involving family practitioners in Quebec. *Can Fam Physician.* 2013;59(5):518–525.
32. Pitkanen M, Hurn J, Kopelman MD. Doctors' health and fitness to practise: performance problems in doctors and cognitive impairments. *Occup Med (Lond).* 2008;58(5):328–333.
33. Harrison J. Doctors' health and fitness to practise: the need for a bespoke model of assessment. *Occup Med (Lond).* 2008;58(5):323–327.
34. Cohen D, Rhydderch M. Measuring a doctor's performance: personality, health and well-being. *Occup Med (Lond).* 2006;56(7):438–440.
35. Lucey C, Boote R. *Working With Problem Residents: A Systematic Approach Practical Guide to the Evaluation of Clinical Competence.* Elsevier Health Sciences; 2008:201–215.
36. Peisah C, Wilhelm K. Physician don't heal thyself: a descriptive study of impaired older doctors. *Int Psychogeriatr.* 2007;19(05):974–984.
37. Peisah C, Wilhelm K. The impaired ageing doctor. *Intern Med J.* 2002;32(9–10):457–459.
38. Eva KW. The aging physician: changes in cognitive processing and their impact on medical practice. *Acad Med.* 2002;77(10):S1–S6.
39. The Joint Commission. Behaviors that undermine a culture of safety. *Sentinel Event Alert.* 2008;(40):1–3.
40. Humphrey C. Assessment and remediation for physicians with suspected performance problems: an international survey. *J Contin Educ Health Prof.* 2010;30(1):26–36.
41. Humphrey C, Locke R. Provision of assessment and remediation for physicians about whom concerns have been expressed: an international survey. *National Clinical Assessment Service/King's College London International Survey.* 2007.
42. Gundersen L. Physician burnout. *Ann Intern Med.* 2001;135(2):145–148.
43. Peisah C, Wijeratne C, Waxman B, et al. Adaptive ageing surgeons. *ANZ J Surg.* 2014;84(5):311–315.
44. Williams B, Flanders P. An exploration of the potential relationship between health issues and problematic workplace behavior. *Federation of State Medical Boards 2016 Annual Meeting*; San Diego, CA: 2016.
45. Engel GL. The need for a new medical model: a challenge for biomedicine. *Holistic Med.* 1989; 4(1): 37–53.
46. Hargreaves K. Reflection in medical education. *J Univ Teach Learn Pract.* 2016;13(2).
47. Epstein RM, Hundert EM. Defining and assessing professional competence. *JAMA.* 2002; 287(2):226–235.
48. Rosner F, Balint JA, Stein RM. Remedial medical education. *Arch Intern Med.* 1994;154(3):274–279.

49. Grant WD. An individualized educational model for the remediation of physicians. *Arch Fam Med.* 1995;4(9):767–772.
50. Moran JA, Kirk P, Kopelow M. Measuring the effectiveness of a pilot continuing medical education program. *Can Fam Physician.* 1996;42:272.
51. Hanna E, Premi J, Turnbull J. Results of remedial continuing medical education in dyscompetent physicians. *Acad Med.* 2000;75(2):174–176.
52. Goulet F, Jacques A, Gagnon R. An innovative approach to remedial continuing medical education, 1992–2002. *Acad Med.* 2005;80(6):533–540.
53. Goulet F, Gagnon R, Gingras MÉ. Influence of remedial professional development programs for poorly performing physicians. *J Contin Educ Health Prof.* 2007;27(1):42–48.
54. Goulet F, Jacques A, Gagnon R, et al. Performance assessment. Family physicians in Montreal meet the Mark! *Can Fam Physician.* 2002;48:1337–1344.
55. Goulet F, ed. *Remediation of Practicing Physicians. Joint Conference of IPAC.* Wicklow, Ireland: Druids Glen Resort, Co; 2014.
56. Lillis S, Takai N, Francis S. Long-term outcomes of a remedial education program for doctors with clinical performance deficits. *J Contin Educ Health Prof.* 2014;34(2):96–101.
57. Guerrasio J, Garrity MJ, Aagaard EM. Learner deficits and academic outcomes of medical students, residents, fellows, and attending physicians referred to a remediation program, 2006–2012. *Acad Med.* 2014;89(2):352–358.
58. Korinek LL, Thompson LL, McRae C, et al. Do physicians referred for competency evaluations have underlying cognitive problems? *Acad Med.* 2009;84(8):1015–1021.
59. Perry W, Crean RD. A retrospective review of the neuropsychological test performance of physicians referred for medical infractions. *Arch Clin Neuropsychol.* 2005;20(2):161–170.
60. Turnbull J, Carbotte R, Hanna E, et al. Cognitive difficulty in physicians. *Acad Med.* 2000;75(2):177–181.
61. Lezak MD, Howieson DB, Bigler ED, et al. *Neuropsychological Assessment,* 5th ed. New York: Oxford University Press; 2012:1161.
62. Hays R, Jolly B, Caldon L, et al. Is insight important? measuring capacity to change performance. *Med Educ.* 2002;36(10):965–971.
63. Dunning D, Johnson K, Ehrlinger J, et al. Why people fail to recognize their own incompetence. *Curr Direct Psychol Sci.* 2003;12(3):83–87.
64. Sullivan C, Murano T, Comes J, et al. Emergency medicine directors' perceptions on professionalism: a Council of Emergency Medicine Residency Directors survey. *Acad Emerg Med.* 2011;18(s2):S97–S103.
65. Williams N, Welindt D, Williams BW, et al. *What's Insight got to do with it? The Role of Insight on Remediation Outcomes Federation of State Medical Boards 2016 Annual Conference; San Diego, CA*: 2016.
66. Sanfey H, Fromson JA, Mellinger J, et al. Surgeons in difficulty: an exploration of differences in assistance-seeking behaviors between male and female surgeons. *J Am Coll Surg.* 2015;221(2):621–627.
67. Sanfey H, Fromson J, Mellinger J, et al. Residents in distress: an exploration of assistance-seeking and reporting behaviors. *Am J Surg.* 2015;210(4):678–684.
68. Trunkey DD, Botney R. Assessing competency: a tale of two professions. *J Am Coll Surg.* 2001;192(3):385–395.
69. Beresin EV, Milligan TA, Balon R, et al. Physician Wellbeing: a critical deficiency in resilience education and training. *Acad Psychiatry.* 2016;40(1):9–12.
70. McGaghie WC, Issenberg SB, Cohen MER, et al. Does simulation-based medical education with deliberate practice yield better results than traditional clinical education? A meta-analytic comparative review of the evidence. *Acad Med.* 2011;86(6):706.
71. Scalese RJ, Obeso VT, Issenberg SB. Simulation technology for skills training and competency assessment in medical education. *J Gen Intern Med.* 2008;23(1):46–49.

PART V

IMPLEMENTING AND EVALUATING CHANGE IN PROFESSIONAL DEVELOPMENT

Enhancing Continuing Professional Development *with* Insights *from* Implementation Science

Gary A. Smith and Audriana M. Stark

Case

Attendance at CME and faculty development events at your institution is strong. However, when queried on the event-evaluation form to indicate how this information will be used in practice with patients or learners, most participants provide no response. Other evidence is likewise weak that participants are implementing the methods and processes with the necessary frequency and fidelity to generate the desired outcomes of continuing professional-development programs for patients and learners.

Questions

What might be the underlying causes of the implementation gap? How can the delivery of the programs potentially be more persuasive for adopting new practices to positive effect?

INTRODUCTION

In both continuing medical education (CME) and faculty development for teaching, program directors aim to change behavioral actions (delivery of care, teaching) of practitioners (physicians, faculty) with the intention to improve desirable outcomes (patient health, student learning). Nonetheless, there is a data-based perception[1-3] that the transfer of evidence-based interventions from workshops, trainings, and grand rounds to physician practice is low (risk-difference effect sizes <20%), and impact on patient outcomes is even lower (3% to 14%). Similarly, a recent review of higher-education faculty development[4] reveals no known study demonstrating a direct connection between faculty development programming and student learning, although that partly results from challenges with measuring such connections. Despite large investment of time and resources by professional-development offices and by program participants, the traditional, knowledge-delivery-focused programs appear to be inefficient for achieving stated goals.

This chapter draws upon knowledge from a broad base of professional-development and workplace-learning studies, to conceptualize the requirements for transfer of knowledge from research to practice that generates desirable outcomes. We synthesize a model for the design of professional learning to guide this transfer with an emphasis on the roles of CME and faculty development programs, hereafter collectively referred to as continuing professional development (CPD).

We draw from Rogers' Theory of Diffusion[5] and perspectives from implementation science.[6–8] Although "implementation science" commonly refers to transfer of research to practice in health care delivery,[6] the concept has been extended to other fields.[9,10] Implementation science has largely been engaged in North America and the United Kingdom and is closely equivalent to "knowledge translation" in the Canadian health-science and policy literature. The field is divided into dissemination and implementation sciences by some authors (e.g., Ref.[11]), and grew rapidly in little more than a decade to establish theoretical[12] and research-design foundations.[13,14] The potential application of implementation science to medical education for quality improvement has been outlined[15]; however, there is a general lack of operational models for applying implementation science to the design of CPD.

IMPROVEMENT PATHWAY FROM RESEARCH TO OUTCOMES

The process by which an innovation (also known as an evidence-based intervention[10]) is transformed from a knowledge source (e.g., research study or clinical trial) into changed behavior by people so as to produce an improved outcome has been extensively studied, and many frameworks exist. Critical to our purpose is recognition that professional-development programs employ interventions that generally focus on changing practitioner (physician or teacher) behavior, but that behavioral change, even if it occurs, may not lead to the desired end result (improved health care or student learning). The transfer of scientific knowledge to an effective practical result is much more difficult in human-service fields, such as the health and teaching professions, than for product manufacturing. With computers, pharmaceuticals, and other products, the research result is built into the product and the product *is* the innovation. With medicine and teaching, each practitioner must implement the innovation, which means that the outcome depends on the education of, and execution by, adopters who are affected by many individual and organizational variables.[9] Research into the necessary processes of evidence-based knowledge dissemination and implementation has arisen in order to improve rates of transfer in essential human services, such as health care and education.

A variety of largely linear models involving dissemination and implementation are described in the literature (e.g., Ref.[5,6,16]), while also acknowledging that nonlinearity is a common reality. Building from these models, we propose to CPD providers a pathway to improve outcomes (Fig. 21.1).

We adapt the term *implementation science* as the body of scientific research and methods to promote the systematic uptake of research findings and other evidence-based

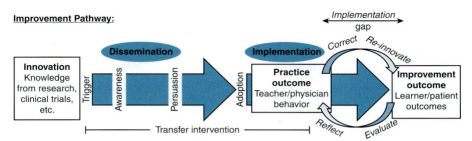

FIGURE 21.1. A schematic diagram of the pathway for disseminating and implementing an innovation (research) to generate practice and improvement outcomes. A trigger begins the transfer intervention. Potential adopters are made aware of the innovation and persuaded during the dissemination phase. The implementation phase begins if the decision is made to adopt the innovation. Implementation includes the practice outcome—changes in behavior resulting from the adopted practice, which concludes the transfer intervention. The change in behavior is intended to produce an improvement outcome—enhanced patient health or learner achievement. The improvement outcome is evaluated and reflected upon, leading to corrections for fidelity and potential reinnovation to address implementation gaps.

practices into routine practice in order to improve the quality and effectiveness of a delivered service,[7] such as patient care and teaching. The general improvement pathway (Fig. 21.1) contains two segments: (1) *dissemination* is the purposeful, strategic transfer of the innovation to potential adopters, while (2) *implementation* represents the process of putting the innovation to use and achieving desired results.

Consideration of what triggers the decision to transfer research to practice is generally not included in the implementation research. However, it is important to note that there is substantially more research pertinent to medical practice and teaching than is typically targeted for attention by practitioners; therefore, we consider this initiating professional-development step in our model (Fig. 21.1). Individual physicians or educators may encounter an innovation through reading journals or attending conferences and then begin their own pathway toward a change in practice. More often, we suggest, purposeful selection of dissemination and implementation initiatives originates within formal programs. CPD is typically based on needs assessments that reveal individuals' motivations for increased competency or as priorities that the offices recognize as emerging within the profession. Serving individuals' needs for maintenance of certification also triggers CME providers to disseminate updates on evidence-based medical practice. In other cases, institutional priorities established outside of the CPD programs may select innovations to be disseminated and implemented. Examples include quality-improvement initiatives, changing delivery-of-care policies, or curriculum revisions. Although these latter triggers originate outside of the professional-development offices, CPD providers commonly provide programming to disseminate the selected innovations.

Dissemination of a selected innovation, or related innovations, involves two fundamental functions (Fig. 21.1). The first is making physicians and educators *aware* of innovations from relevant clinical trials or education research, which is the familiar function of workshops, grand rounds, conferences, distributed information briefs, and peer-reviewed publications. The second is to present and demonstrate the innovations in a fashion that *persuades* practitioners to invest effort to implement them.

An innovation may diffuse through an organization in an unplanned, untargeted, and uncontrolled fashion. The distinction of dissemination as an active process and diffusion as a passive process is foundational in implementation-science studies[8,10] and traces to Lomas.[17] Given the close linkages between Rogers' Theory of Diffusion and the later dissemination and implementation research, we find it important to note that Rogers included active, strategic practices within his definition of diffusion,[5] leading to regrettable confusion about contexts for the application of Rogers' work. We will return to the importance of Rogers' framework for what is now referred to by many implementation-science authors as dissemination rather than diffusion.

Building off of Fixsen and colleagues[6] we recognize two distinct outcomes (Fig. 21.1). *Practice outcome* refers to the adoption of the innovation resulting from a successful transfer intervention beyond the dissemination process—going from research to practice. Stated practice outcomes, for example, relate to physicians following the expected protocol or evidence-based practice and educators using a new research-based pedagogy or curriculum. Although this behavior change is a necessary step, the ultimate goal is the improvement of patients' health and learners' achievement, which are examples of the *improvement outcome*.

The *adoption* decision, whether by individuals or an organizational unit, marks the end of dissemination and the beginning of implementation (Fig. 21.1). However, simply using the innovation—the practice outcome—does not assure an optimal, intended result for patients or learners—the improvement outcome. A remaining gap (Fig. 21.1) may result from lack of fidelity in implementing the clinical or teaching protocol or from incongruence between the innovation, researched and/or trialed in one context, and the context of the implementation setting. Minding the implementation gap requires an iterative process, shown by the curved arrows in Figure 21.1 that further link the two outcomes. This process includes evaluating results, reflecting on what is affecting positive or negative implementation outcomes, correcting misapplication of the intended protocol, or potentially changing the protocol (reinnovate[6]) in order to reach the improvement outcome.

It is particularly important for CPD providers to note the critical transitions that exist (1) between dissemination and implementation (adoption) and (2) between initial implementation that meets the practice outcome and the improvement outcome (Fig. 21.1). CPD directors typically focus on the dissemination stage with goals directed toward the practice outcome, but implementation-science research provides a framework, explored in the next section, for including these administrators in a process that concludes with the improvement outcome.

IMPROVEMENT DRIVERS FROM RESEARCH TO OUTCOMES

While the dissemination and implementation pathway may appear simple, the factors that drive improvement are complex and multidimensional. It has long been recognized as naïve to assume that educating individuals about an innovation—the hallmark of professional-development programs—will automatically generate practice and improvement outcomes. We adapt the implementation drivers concept[18,19] as improvement

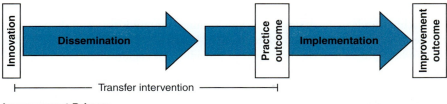

Improvement Drivers:

FIGURE 21.2.   The improvement drivers include the organizational context, workplace learning, and continuing-professional-development programs. Professional learning occurs through both the CPD program (longitudinal programs, training and workshops, and consultations) and workplace learning (coaching, reflective practice, communities of practice) within the encompassing organizational context (cultures of learning and improvement, supportive leadership, decision-data support system). The influence of professional-development programs typically fades near the completion of the transfer.

drivers (Fig. 21.2) that describe the position of CPD programs within dissemination and implementation efforts. CPD is only one part of professional learning,[20] which includes a broad base of workplace-learning experiences within authentic environments rather than in educational contexts. Notably, the impact of CPD programs commonly fades after the adoption stage (Fig. 21.2), placing increased importance on workplace learning for accomplishing practice and improvement outcomes. However, regardless of individuals' professional-learning achievements, the enclosing context of organizational characteristics, mostly unrelated to learning interventions, has an important influence on the outcomes.

Continuing Professional Development Programs

CPD programs represent the formal professional-learning elements that disseminate innovations and, to varying degrees of success, promote adoption that leads to practice outcomes, as shown by the overlap in Figure 21.2, between the dissemination pathway and professional-development programs as a driver. CPD offices provide enrolled learning events in the form of workshops, training sessions, conferences, and grand rounds. These traditional program offerings, as noted in the introduction, are not perceived to be highly effective in reaching practice or improvement outcomes.

Greater success is associated with longitudinal programs, such as teaching fellow and teaching academy programs,[21,22] faculty learning communities,[23] workshop or conference series,[24] and simulation-based mastery learning[25–27] relative to single events. Longitudinal programs have the benefit of providing for cognitively beneficial spaced learning,[28] practice and feedback with introduced protocols and pedagogies, and the greater likelihood of individual scholarship. These programs are resource intensive for CPD offices and require extended, recurring time commitment for participants. As a result, longitudinal programs have potentially high-impact outcomes but directly affect a small percentage of physicians and educators.

Consultation at the request of teachers is a common component of faculty-development programs but is atypical of CME offices. Offering consultation services permits for just-in-time assistance that is customized to educators' needs. Assistance from faculty developers generally comes in the form of expertise in learning theories, education research, and teaching methods independent of subject-matter expertise, which resides with the teacher. With health care innovations, methodological and content expertise are inseparable, so it is unrealistic for CME providers to offer comparable consultant services. In both programs, there may be limited benefits from offered events that feature external experts who are unavailable at later times to answer participants' questions about adoption or to provide feedback on participants' implementation efforts.

Workplace Learning

Learning during work, across all employment sectors, is responsible for perhaps as much as 70% of professional learning with formal workshops and training accounting for only 10%.[29] Likewise, faculty mostly learn about teaching directly from teaching experiences and from colleagues rather than faculty developers.[30–32] A review of several studies in physician training[6] corroborates the conclusion that formal workshops and training are only successful at achieving practice and improvement outcomes when combined with effective workplace learning practices. Greenhalgh and others[33] conclude that the adoption of innovations by individuals is powerfully influenced by the structure and quality of their workplace social networks.

Workplace learning (Fig. 21.2) includes all elements of learning for work, learning at work, and learning from work[34] and involves experiences with peers, mentors, coaches, patients, and students. These experiences range from casual conversations, observations of peers at work, brief academic detailing sessions, paper or e-mail information briefs, informal or scheduled group meetings, and deliberate coaching.[35] Therefore, CPD programs are only one part of the necessary professional learning, and CPD providers should promote a permeable boundary between the functions of their offices and the overall hospital, clinic, and classroom environments where physicians, residents, and educators implement the innovations[36] (Fig. 21.2).

Coaching that provides ongoing expert guidance and feedback is essential to mastery learning and effective implementation. It is important to practice in a real setting (not just role-plays or mock-ups at the workshop, or a simulation) and to get feedback on that practice. Practitioners must know what actions constitute the best practices, have the knowledge tools to perform those actions, and possess the ability and efficacy to perform those actions. Implementation researchers emphasize, therefore, that training and coaching should become one continuous action.[6] A classic example from teacher training showed that even when practice opportunities were included in workshops, there was only a 5% transfer to classroom practice, whereas transfer increased to 95% when on-the-job coaching was added to workshops as part of the transfer intervention.[37] Given evidence for the efficacy of coaching in combination with training, professional-development directors should identify where these coaches exist and collaborate on the training-coaching continuum. Expert coaches may emerge from longitudinal programs or may be recruited for intensive mastery training ahead of broader dissemination and implementation efforts (e.g., Ref.[27])

Workplace learning may occur by leveraging dispersed expertise through peer relationships in communities of practice (CoPs). Participants in a CoP have a common motivated interest in a particular issue and compose a social structure focused on sharing, creating, and curating knowledge and skills pertinent to that issue. CoPs focused on health care or education interventions may emerge naturally among motivated, curious practitioners or be fostered from longitudinal programs.[6,36,38–40] When seeded or nurtured by CPD providers, CoPs extend professional learning beyond formal programming without expending office resources and can serve as a permeable interface between the formal programs and the workplace.[40]

Physician and educator reflection in practice and reflection on practice are also important elements of workplace learning.[36] Although reflection is a personal process, it occurs within an overall social context with inputs from peers, coaches, supervisors, mentors, patients, and learners. Audits and feedback regarding patient-care metrics, teaching evaluations from learners, and peer observations of teaching are all sources of information that can be combined with personal experience for reflective learning.

Organizational Context

Improvement outcomes not only require changes in the knowledge and skills of the individuals who implement innovations but are dependent upon, and sometimes require changes in, organizational structure and culture—values, philosophies, norms, symbols, ethics, policies, procedures, decision-making, leadership, personnel interactions—that routinely bring about and support changes by individuals.[6,10] Organizational goals, resource availability, and managerial support are powerful predictors of an employee's transfer of learned skills.[35] Likewise, these organizational components are critical to achieving practice and improvement outcomes in both health care[13,41,42] and teaching[36] and envelop professional learning (Fig. 21.2).

Leaders establish value systems and rewards that motivate employees to adopt innovations and recognize the inherent risks of implementing complex innovations. Leaders protect physician and educator time and allow on-the-job autonomy and flexibility to implement and practice innovations.[42] While high-level administrators may support or even initiate an innovation intervention, it is important that department chairs and program directors support these efforts because they directly evaluate employees, approve workload distribution, allocate resources, and play an important role to establish workplace morale.

The organization also needs decision-support data systems that provide information for assessing implementation gaps and achievements. Feedback for improvement during implementation requires access to data that mark milestones and inform decisions.[18]

Diffusing an innovation among individuals requires an organizational culture, influenced by both leadership and the interpersonal relationships among employees, that favors continuous improvement through ongoing learning. The *culture of learning and improvement* (Fig. 21.2) is strongly linked to social capital and absorptive capacity.[13] Social capital describes the network of relationships that increase knowledge and resources through cooperative learning and bonding between individuals. Social capital can be built through communities of practice.[40] Absorptive capacity is the set of attributes that permit the organization to acquire, assimilate, and transform knowledge for beneficial use.[43] High absorptive capacity requires an organization that supports innovations by individuals and changes to accommodate innovations that can succeed only by involving the whole organization. The knowledge necessary for adoption and implementation of a complex innovation within an organization is socially constructed and commonly contested, which entails ongoing negotiation among implementers and leaders.

Therefore, it is important for CPD providers to be well connected with leadership at multiple levels and to have a sense of the culture that exists among departments. Professional developers need to know opinion leaders[44] who will advocate innovations and who can support potential implementers through coaching or networking when they leave the workshop or training and return to their work environment. Without buy-in for innovation, transfer interventions that are triggered within the CPD are likely to fail.[36]

STIMULATING IMPLEMENTATION THROUGH CONTINUING PROFESSIONAL-DEVELOPMENT TRANSFER INTERVENTIONS

Although CPD programs should not expect to achieve practice outcomes or improvement outcomes without compatible workplace learning and organizational contexts (Fig. 21.2), it is important for directors to consider best practices for their program. The transfer of research evidence into health care or teaching practice includes interventions by CPD providers that we suggest should be linked to implementation-science research. In particular, we build upon Rogers'[5] attributes of adopted innovations and commitment-to-change research that underlies the common activity, included in the case that opened this chapter, of surveying participant intention to implement an advocated practice.

Rogers' identified five attributes of an innovation that explain about half of the variance in the adoption rate: relative advantage, compatibility, trialability, observability, and complexity.[5] These attributes were extended into implementation-science research (e.g., Ref.[12,13,33,44]). Importantly, we assert that these attributes are not only a function of the innovation but are also explicitly connected to the transfer intervention—how information about the innovation is disseminated and the guidance provided during initial implementation. Dearing[44] notes that the attributes should be used in the design of communication messages and images about interventions. Closely related is the adaptability of an innovation, which has been viewed as a positive attribute[5] or a negative attribute.[6] While other authors[33,45] provide longer lists of characteristics that promote or hinder implementation, we focus on these six because of their high correspondence to effective implementation[5,6] and close relationship to CPD program planning.

We propose these attributes as a first step to developing evidence-based practices for the design and delivery of CPD programs. We operationalize each attribute as a series of questions that CPD providers can ask as they design and develop programs for maximizing adoption. We also provide examples of what each attribute could look like in practice.

Relative Advantage

Relative advantage is the degree to which an innovation is superior to the potential adopter's existing practice.[5] If the benefits outweigh the cost of adoption, then a relative advantage exists and the innovation is more likely to be adopted. The autonomous worker will decide whether to use lessons from programs depending on his or her experience, goals, and motivations.[46] The innovation has to be something that practitioners are interested in or believe in or that resonates with their future directions.[38] Tapping into and framing the transfer intervention within these desires can create a perceived relative advantage for potential adopters.

CPD programs must make the case for why the new innovation is more advantageous to the individual than the practice that she or he is currently using. While showing data to illustrate a relative advantage is alluring (e.g., Ref.[47]), presenting research evidence alone is not enough to persuade someone to adopt an innovation.[5,6,48] People prefer personal evidence over empirical evidence[32] and place more trust in the advantages that are pointed out by colleagues and opinion leaders than those presented in the research literature.

We operationalize relative advantage using a series of questions that investigate whether or not CPD directors are making the case for the innovation's advantages:

- Are we credibly demonstrating how learning, learner affect, or patient outcome can be expected to improve?
- Are we reducing uncertainty about implementing the changes?
- Is the advantage relevant and valued by the individual?

Through CPD events and consultations, directors and facilitators can address these questions by providing opportunities for participants to reflect upon and explain the perceived goals, advantages, and disadvantages of their current practice. To the extent possible, the transfer intervention can be explained in terms of outcomes that are individualized to participant needs. Clear, evidence-based arguments for a change in practice should draw upon robust, published data but also be combined with the experiences and knowledge of the facilitators and peers in the institution.

Compatibility

Compatibility is the degree to which an innovation is consistent with the existing values, past experiences, and needs of the potential adopter.[5] Compatibility is the second most influential attribute when considering a timely rate of adoption. Innovations that are incompatible with beliefs, values, and practices are more difficult, if not impossible, for people to adopt without experiencing an associated transformative change in values and beliefs. When innovations are relevant and perceived to improve task performance, they are more easily adopted.[33]

Professional developers should resist the urge to treat potential adopters as "empty vessels" but rather activate existing notions and ideas in ways that link the innovation with program participants' prior knowledge and can, therefore, be a worthwhile modification to their practice. Below are the questions that professional-development directors can ask of themselves and those who will facilitate activities through their offices to determine whether the innovation is compatible with the potential adopter's values and beliefs:

- Is the advocated innovation aligned with what participants are already doing or an idea with which they are already familiar?
- Are we knowledgeable of how the advocated innovation aligns with the existing values and beliefs of the potential adopters?
- Are we relating the changes in practice to accomplish the innovation to what the potential adopters identify as *their* needs?

Program activities and individual consultations must respect the beliefs and values of the participants and the priorities that they have for their work. Participants should be provided the opportunity to reflect upon and explain what aspects of the innovation are compatible with these personal attributes as a foundation for contemplating adoption. Furthermore, participants can be prompted to relate the innovation to something familiar that they already do or use.

Observability

Observability is the degree to which the benefits of the innovation are visible.[5] Rates of adoption are higher when potential adopters see the benefits from the innovation through the work of a trusted advisor, opinion leader, or colleague. Adoption also is more likely when an individual experiments with the innovation on his or her own and witnesses the benefits. Exemplary demonstrations increase the likelihood of adoption partly by making a costly, worrisome, and complex intervention more understandable through visibility of its processes and the observation of its positive outcomes.[42] Observation is also critical for practices that require a high degree of tacit knowledge, which is not easily communicated explicitly and can be difficult to replicate when adopters are experimenting with the innovation.[49]

The following questions are posed to investigate whether ample opportunity to observe practices and outcomes are being provided in order to persuade potential adopters to invest in the innovation:

- Are we modeling what we advocate for others to adopt through our own practices in the CPD program?
- Are we providing opportunities for adopters to observe the innovation and its benefits in the program? In the workplace?

- Are we facilitating networks of opinion leaders and early adopters to be observed and to share their expertise?
- Do we, when possible, translate tacit knowledge into explicit knowledge?

Observation opportunities should, ideally, be included within formal programs and fostered in the workplace. Teaching strategies and methods, for example, can be modeled by workshop design; role-playing can be used during training to illustrate both teaching and clinical-communication methods; simulation can be used for observing procedures. However, it is likely that many observations that are essential to adoption take place in the work environment among colleagues. Observing peers who use the advocated practices may be more persuasive than formal demonstrations, but need not be left to chance. CPD providers should recommend observation of early adopters working in authentic contexts and facilitate networking and communities of practice that lead to productive workplace observations and discussions.

Complexity

Complexity is the perceived degree of difficulty in understanding or using the innovation[5] and is *negatively* correlated with the rate of adoption. Therefore, CPD providers must strive to reduce the perceived complexity, and hence the uncertainty, of the innovation. One of the most common reasons for failed change is that adopters find the change too difficult.[50]

People may differ in their perceptions of how complex an innovation would be for them in their context. The gap between current practice and desired practice will vary with each physician or teacher. People with background knowledge that can be leveraged may perceive the innovation as less complex than may someone without such existing knowledge. Each incremental adoption can lower the threshold for subsequent related innovation adoption. However, if an innovation appears too complex from the start, potential adopters may lack the efficacy needed to implement it if the gap between current and desired practice are too large. Therefore, it is important for CPD providers to guide each participant forward within his or her own zone of feasible innovation.[51] We recommend answering these questions to measure the degree of difficulty that is perceived by the potential adopters:

- Will the perceived complexity of the innovation impede adoption?
- Are we maintaining low cognitive load in our explanations of potentially novel ideas or methods?
- Are we providing simple, step-by-step processes?
- Are we seeking whether adopters view innovations as too complex?

In order to reduce complexity, it is important that workshops, trainings, and presentations be thoughtfully designed. Complex processes and procedures should be reduced to easily understood steps. Event participants can be queried to make sure that the pace and complexity of the presentation are within grasp, including anonymous questioning with audience-response systems to identify and clarify misunderstandings.

Another strategy is to ask participants to write down what they find most confusing (the "muddiest point"[52]) and then respond to these concerns to decrease uncertainty. Even designing presentation slides to reduce cognitive load is shown to enhance learning of complex topics.[53,54] Providing augmentation or follow-up support reduces the perceived complexity with some innovations and points to the importance of longitudinal programs or consultations following one-time workshops and trainings.

Trialability

Trialability is the degree to which the innovation can be experimented with on a limited basis.[5] When a potential adopter is provided opportunities to experiment with the innovation in increments or doses, they are more likely to try the innovation. Thus, trialability has a positive relation with the rate of adoption of an innovation.

Implementation-science researchers agree that small changes are more likely to occur than large ones[16] and trialability paves paths for adoption. In one study,[55] teachers did not change their beliefs or attitudes about an innovation until it had been tested and the outcomes were confirmed. Achieving desired outcomes during a trial laid the foundation for full adoption of the innovation. Moore and others[56] identified "trying out what was learned" as a crucial stage prior to physicians "incorporating what was learned" during training into practice. People undertake an important meaning-making process through trialing the innovation. Creating opportunities to practice a skill, especially in the context where the skill will be put to use can contribute significantly to the adoption of the innovation and the transfer of program learning into the workplace.

The following questions stimulate thinking about how facilitators provide opportunities for trial and incremental adoption:

- Are we providing opportunities for participants to experiment with the innovation as a part of the continuing professional-development program? In the workplace?
- Are we providing incremental pathways within the zone of feasible innovation to adoption of innovative/unfamiliar approaches?
- Are we following up with participants after their trial to see what challenges or strengths they experienced when using the innovation?

When possible, CPD events should be designed to provide opportunities for participants to practice the innovation with feedback provided by the expert facilitators and peer discussion. Longitudinal simulation-based mastery learning, for example, has shown both high practice and improvement outcomes.[25,26]

Participants can also be encouraged to try out parts of a complex innovation and then add additional steps as self-efficacy and comfort grow. An example would be faculty developer advocacy for shifting to learner-centered instruction by incrementally adding innovations in preclass learning-progress assessment, in-class active learning, use of audience-response systems, and postclass learning assessment. All of these strategies go together well in a flipped-learning model, but ultimate instructor success in flipping their course may be enhanced by adding the components over time rather than replacing didactics all at once.

Adaptability

A contested attribute of implementation is the concept of adaptability—the degree of change or modification of an innovation by an adopter to suit the needs of the setting or to shape it for the local context. Rogers[5] refers to adaptability as "reinvention" and views it as a positive spin-off of an original innovation that enables incremental adoption rather than no adoption. Reinvention of an innovation to suit needs may ease people into adopting an innovation that they otherwise may have rejected. Rogers advocates this adapt-to-adopt model.

Later work in implementation research views adaptability as a potential threat to the innovation and the associated outcomes of the innovation. Fidelity, or the degree to which an intervention is implemented as it was prescribed in the original protocol,[57] can be compromised when people modify the model from the original intention. Nearly all of the data included in one review[6] indicate that high-fidelity implementation of evidence-based programs produce better outcomes for consumers. Thus, adaptability is scrutinized by research in implementation science rather than promoted, as done by Rogers.[5]

A useful example is studies that show mixed results for the impact of using audience-response technology in medical professional development.[58–60] However, none of these implementations followed the evidence-based practice of peer instruction. Even among physics faculty, where peer instruction originated, there is significant awareness of the method but low rates of implementation with fidelity.[61] Adaptations, or reinvention, of the practice compromise the core features of the innovation and render ambiguous research results.

Therefore, implementation science places a strong focus on implementing with fidelity and only adapting—reinnovating (Fig. 21.1)—if necessary and appropriate.[6] This approach is important from a research perspective because it prevents an innovation from being discounted as a failure if loss of fidelity is the underlying cause of defect rather than the innovation itself. If, however, the innovation was implemented with fidelity and the improvement outcome was not achieved, then the context for that failure can be investigated and an alternative intervention plan may arise.

We recommend a blended approach for adapting innovation. CPD providers can help navigate the reinvention process to ensure minimal loss of fidelity by being aware of what features are critical to the innovation and guiding people through adaptations so as to not lose the core components. Interventions can be designed to invite productive process adaptations so that fidelity of outcomes is heightened, not lessened.[44] Careful supervision, coaching, and continual evaluations of processes and outcomes should take place to minimize a loss of fidelity through a process known as "guided adaptability."[44] Below are questions to reduce the risk of losing fidelity when facilitating adaptations to innovations:

- Are we persuasive against overadoption of practices that we feel are less impactful or counterproductive?
- Are we providing alternative pathways to adoption of innovative/unfamiliar approaches that preserve the core components of the innovation?
- Are we following the implementation process to monitor fidelity and advise accordingly?

Workshops, trainings, presentations, and consultations should always provide research evidence for *why* the innovation works.[44,49] If adopters understand the mechanisms and causes for the improvement outcomes, they will better understand what core components cannot be altered if they are to expect success. CPD providers and facilitators must remain available during implementation to guide adaptations that preserve the core components in order to generate the benefits of increased compatibility and decreased complexity without jeopardizing improvement outcomes that negate the relative advantage of implementing the innovation.

Commitment to Change

End-of-event surveys commonly ask participants to select one or more elements from the presented information that they will incorporate into their practice, such as the case that opens this chapter. Research about the commitment to change is made ambiguous by the varied ways in which the commitment question is posed, the period within which implementation is expected, and the reliance on participants' self-report of their implemented changes.[50,62,63] Nonetheless, where randomized control trials are used,[63] it appears that participants who state commitment at the time of an event are much more likely to make a change in practice than those who do not. This correlation explains the popularity of the survey item for program evaluation.

However, the opening case reveals two problems. First is the concern when a significant proportion of program participants do not make a commitment. Aside from disliking surveys, the lack of responses suggests that either the event was unpersuasive or it affirmed existing practice rather than encouraging adoption of a new practice. Examining program design within the context of the six attributes discussed above, along with other survey questions, is helpful for evaluating why participants may not feel able to commit to a change. Assessing participant needs and existing practice in advance of developing programs helps to assure that the innovation requires formal program support. Second is that while research indicates that high percentages (generally >52%) report making commitment to changes,[62,63] the previously summarized data[1-3] show a limited impact of CME events on improvement outcomes. This inconsistency implies that either the self-reported changes are inaccurate or that the achieved practice outcomes are being implemented with insufficient fidelity. Therefore, while we feel that obtaining commitment to change at the time of CPD events is important, it is also essential for CPD providers and facilitators to follow up with participants through the implementation stage. Otherwise, if the CPD program focuses only on dissemination (Fig. 21.2), then implementation gaps may remain with insufficient workplace learning and organizational climate to support changes that achieve the improvement goals.

FUTURE DIRECTIONS

Implementation science informs at least two avenues for defining the missions and planning the activities of CME and faculty-development programs. First, we expect that CPD programs will increasingly become connected to the organizational drivers that are essential to achieving improvement outcomes. Second, we anticipate increasing study of the design and implementation of transfer interventions that assure that CPD providers are applying evidence-based practices in their endeavors to promote the successful implementation of evidence-based innovations.

Learning is an ongoing process that includes social processes with peers and experts and is framed by both opportunities and barriers within the organization. CPD programs tend to focus on events, whether single or in series, that disseminate information with an anticipation of observing practice outcomes and a hope that those practices will generate improvement outcomes. CPD initiatives must move into the workplace to coach, consult, support opinion leaders, and cultivate champions, especially among department and program leaders that strongly influence the organizational culture. CPD providers can seed or nurture emerging and existing communities of practice that foster workplace learning.[40] Directors and facilitators of formal programming need to be visible on the wards, in the classroom, in the conference room, and in individuals' offices rather than only at workshops, trainings, and grand rounds.

CPD offices must reach beyond their focus on learning to form partnerships with leaders and units elsewhere in the organization in order to achieve improvement outcomes. The growing shift from individual development to organization performance improvement argues for CPD programs to be full partners alongside the other drivers of improvement or be "doomed to play only small roles in organizations with minimal impact and great risk of downsizing and outsourcing."[64]

Anticipating that formal CPD programs will continue to be drivers of dissemination and implementation, it is essential that there be a strong, scholarly framework for designing those programs. Professional-learning design should draw on theoretical foundations in humanist, constructivist, and social-cognitivist learning theories, core concepts of adult learning, instructional design, and psychology and management of change processes. The six operationalized attributes of innovations and transfer interventions, presented here, can form the basis of initial research questions.

We suggest that design-based research, which emerged as the foundational methodology of learning scientists in school and college settings, is appropriate for simultaneously designing and studying transfer interventions. Design-based research integrates the design of forms of learning with the systematic study of those forms of learning within the context of instruction in order to generate humble theory specific to the domain of the study that goes beyond identifying what works to elucidating why it works.[65] Even broader research perspectives would include design-based-implementation research[66] that seeks to not only understand how to better build the skills of implementers but also how to build the capacity of the organization to implement and sustain innovations within a domain of learning, such as academic medical centers.

REFERENCES

1. Forsetlund L, Bjørndal A, Rashidian A, et al. Continuing education meetings and workshops: effects on professional practice and health care outcomes (review). *Cochrane Database Syst Rev.* 2009;(2):CD003030.
2. Cervero RM, Gaines JK. *Effectiveness of Continuing Medical Education: Updated Synthesis of Systematic Reviews.* Chicago, IL: Accreditation Council for Continuing Medical Education; 2014.
3. Lau R, Stevenson F, Ong BN, et al. Achieving change in primary care—causes of the evidence to practice gap: systematic reviews of reviews. *BMJ Open.* 2015;5:e009993.

4. Saroyan A, Trigwell K. Higher education teachers' professional learning: process and outcome. *Stud Educ Eval.* 2015;46:92–101.

5. Rogers EM. *Diffusion of Innovations,* 5th ed. New York: Free Press; 2003.

6. Fixsen DL, Naoom SF, Blase KA, et al. *Implementation Research: A Synthesis of the Literature.* Tampa, FL: University of South Florida, Louis de la Parte Florida Mental Health Institute, The National Implementation Research Network (FMHI Publication #231); 2005.

7. Eccles MP, Mittman BS. Welcome to Implementation Science. *Implement Sci.* 2006;1:1.

8. Dearing JW, Kee KF. Historical roots of dissemination and implementation science. In: Brownson RC, Colditz GA, Proctor EK, eds. *Dissemination and Improvement Research in Health: Translating Science to Practice.* New York: Oxford; 2012:55–71.

9. Fixsen DL, Blase KA, Naoom SF, et al. Core implementation components. *Res Soc Work Pract.* 2009;19(5):531–540.

10. Rabin BA, Brownson RC. Developing the terminology for dissemination and implementation research. In: Brownson RC, Colditz GA, Proctor EK, eds. *Dissemination and Improvement Research in Health: Translating Science to Practice.* New York: Oxford; 2012:23–51.

11. Brownson RC, Colditz GA, Proctor EK, eds. *Dissemination and Improvement Research in Health: Translating Science to Practice.* New York: Oxford; 2012.

12. Nilsen P. Making sense of implementation theories, models and frameworks. *Implement Sci.* 2015;10:53.

13. Damschroeder LJ, Aron DC, Keith RE, et al. Fostering implementation of health services research findings into practice: a consolidated framework for advancing implementation science. *Implement Sci.* 2009;4:50.

14. Michie S, van Stralen MM, West R. The behaviour change wheel: a new method for characterising and designing behaviour change interventions. *Implement Sci.* 2011;6:42.

15. Price DW, Wagner DP, Krane NK, et al. What are the implications of implementation science for medical education? *Med Educ Online.* 2015;20:11.

16. Grol RPTM, Bosch MC, Hulscher MEJL, et al. Planning and studying improvement in patient care: the use of theoretical perspectives. *Milbank Q.* 2007;85(1):93–138.

17. Lomas J. Diffusion, dissemination, and implementation: Who should do what? *Ann N Y Acad Sci* 1993;703:226–237.

18. Blase KA, Van Dyke M, Fixsen DL, et al. Implementation science: key concepts, themes, and evidence for practitioners in educational psychology. In: Kelly B, Perkins DF, eds. *Handbook of Implementation Science for Psychology in Education.* New York: Cambridge University Press; 2012:13–34.

19. Fixsen D, Blase K, Naoom S, et al. *Implementation Drivers: Assessing Best Practices.* Chapel Hill, NC: University of North Carolina; 2015. http://nirn.fpg.unc.edu. Accessed May 14, 2016.

20. Webster-Wright A. Reframing professional development through understanding authentic professional learning. *Rev Educ Res.* 2009;79(2):702–739.

21. Yelon SL, Ford JK, Anderson WA. Twelve tips for increasing transfer of training from faculty development programs. *Med Teach.* 2014;36(11):945–950.

22. Onyura B, Ng SL, Baker LR, et al. A mandala of faculty development: using theory-based evaluation to explore contexts, mechanisms and outcomes. *Adv Heal Sci Educ.* 2016. [In Press].

23. Cox MD, Richlin L, eds. Building faculty learning communities. *New Direct Teach Learn.* 2004;(97):1–157.

24. Knight AM, Carrese JA, Wright SM. Qualitative assessment of the long-term impact of a faculty development programme in teaching skills. *Med Educ.* 2007;41(6):592–600.

25. Cook DA, Brydges R, Zendejas B, et al. Mastery learning for health professionals using technology-enhanced simulation. *Acad Med.* 2013;88(08):1.

26. McGaghie WC, Issenberg SB, Barsuk JH, et al. A critical review of simulation-based mastery learning with translational outcomes. *Med Educ.* 2014;48(4):375–385.

27. McGaghie WC, Barusk JH, Cohen ER, et al. Dissemination of an innovative mastery learning curriculum grounded in implementation science principles: a case study. *Acad Med.* 2015;90(11):1–8.

28. Moulton CA, Dubrowski A, Macrae H, et al. Teaching surgical skills: what kind of practice makes perfect?: a randomized, controlled trial. *Ann Surg.* 2006;244(3):400–409.

29. Jennings C, Wargnier J. *Effective Learning with 70:20:10.; CrossKnowledge.* 2011. http://www.crossknowledge.net/crossknowledge/whitepapers/effective-learning-with-70_20_10-whitepaper.pdf. Accessed December 9, 2015.

30. Knight P, Tait J, Yorke M. The professional learning of teachers in higher education. *Stud High Educ.* 2006;31(3):319–339.

31. Oleson A, Hora MT. Teaching the way they were taught? Revisiting the sources of teaching knowledge and the role of prior experience in shaping faculty teaching practices. *High Educ.* 2013;68(1):29–45.

32. Andrews TC, Lemons PP. It's personal: biology instructors prioritize personal evidence over empirical evidence in teaching decisions. *CBE Life Sci Educ.* 2015;14:1–18.
33. Greenhalgh T, Robert G, MacFarlane F, et al. Diffusion of innovations in service organizations: systematic review and recommendations. *Milbank Q.* 2004;82(4):581–629.
34. Swanwick T. See one, do one, then what? Faculty development in postgraduate medical education. *Postgrad Med J.* 2008;84(993):702–739.
35. Salas E, Cannon-Bowers JA. The science of training: a decade of progress. *Annu Rev Psychol.* 2001;52:471–499.
36. O'Sullivan PS, Irby DM. Reframing research on faculty development. *Acad Med.* 2011;86(4):421–428.
37. Joyce B, Showers B. *Student Achievement Through Staff Development*, 3rd ed. Alexandria, VA: Association for Supervision and Curriculum Development; 2002.
38. Smith K. Lessons learnt from literature on the diffusion of innovative learning and teaching practices in higher education. *Innov Educ Teach Int.* 2012;49(2):173–182.
39. Steinert Y. Learning from experience: from workplace learning to communities of practice. In: Steinert Y, ed. *Faculty Development in the Health Professions.* Dordrecht, The Netherlands: Springer; 2014:141–158.
40. Stark AM, Smith GA. Communities of practice as agents of future faculty development. *J Fac Dev.* 2016;30(2):59–67.
41. Chaudoir SR, Dugan AG, Barr CH. Measuring factors affecting implementation of health innovations: a systematic review of structural, organizational, provider, patient, and innovation level measures. *Implement Sci.* 2013;8:22.
42. Rousseau DM, Gunia BC. Evidence-based practice: the psychology of EBP implementation. *Annu Rev Psychol.* 2015;55(4):1013–1016.
43. Zahra SA, George G. Absorptive capacity—a review, reconceptualization, and extension. *Acad Manag Rev.* 2002;27(2):185–203.
44. Dearing JW. Applying diffusion of innovation theory to intervention development. *Res Soc Work Pract.* 2009;19(5):503–518.
45. Grol R, Wensing, M. Characteristics of successful innovations. In: Grol R, Wensing M, Eccles M, eds. *Improving Patient Care; the Implementation of Change in Clinical Practice.* Oxford, UK: Elsevier; 2005:60–70.
46. Yelon SL, Sheppard L, Sleight D, et al. Intention to transfer: how do autonomous professionals become motivated to use new ideas. *Perform Improv Q.* 2004;17(2):82–103.
47. Freeman S, Eddy SL, McDonough M, et al. Active learning increases student performance in science, engineering, and mathematics. *Proc Natl Acad Sci.* 2014;111(23):8410–8415.
48. Kezar A, Gehrke S, Elrod S. Implicit theories of change as a barrier to change on college campuses: an examination of STEM reform. *Rev High Educ.* 2015;38(4):479–506.
49. Smith GA. Why college faculty need to know the research about learning. *InSight.* 2015;10:9–18.
50. Wakefield JG. Commitment to change: exploring its role in changing physician behavior through continuing education. *J Contin Educ Health Prof.* 2004;24(4):197–204.
51. Rogan JM, Anderson TR. Bridging the educational research-teaching practice gap: curriculum development, part 2: becoming an agent of change. *Biochem Mol Biol Educ.* 2011;39(3):233–241.
52. Angelo TA, Cross KP. *Classroom Assessment Techniques: A Handbook for College Teachers,* 2nd ed. San Francisco, CA: Jossey Bass; 1993.
53. Mayer RE. Applying the science of learning to medical education. *Med Educ.* 2010;44(6):543–549.
54. Issa N, Mayer RE, Schuller M, et al. Teaching for understanding in medical classrooms using multimedia design principles. *Med Educ.* 2013;47:388–396.
55. Guskey TR. Staff development and the process of teacher change. *Educ Res.* 1986;15(5):5–12.
56. Moore DE Jr, Green JS, Gallis HA. Achieving desired results and improved outcomes: integrating planning and assessment throughout learning activities. *J Contin Educ Health Prof.* 2009;29(1):1–15.
57. Slaughter SE, Hill JN, Snelgrove-Clarke E. What is the extent and quality of documentation and reporting of fidelity to implementation strategies: a scoping review. *Implement Sci.* 2015;10:129.
58. Grzeskowiak LE, Thomas AE, To J, et al. Enhancing continuing education activities using audience response systems: a single-blind controlled trial. *J Contin Educ Health Prof.* 2015;35(1):38–45.
59. Hettinger A, Spurgeon J, El-Mallakh R, et al. Using audience response system technology and PRITE questions to improve psychiatric residents' medical knowledge. *Acad Psychiatry.* 2014;38(2):205–208.
60. Miller RG, Ashar BH, Getz KJ. Evaluation of an audience response system for the continuing education of health professionals. *J Contin Educ Health Prof.* 2003;23(2):109–115.
61. Dancy M, Henderson C, Turpen C. How faculty learn about and implement research-based instructional strategies: the case of peer instruction. *Phys Rev Phys Educ Res.* 2016;12(010110):1–27.
62. Shershneva MB, Wang MF, Lindeman GC, et al. Commitment to practice change: an evaluator's perspective. *Eval Health Prof.* 2010;33(3):256–275.

63. Domino FJ, Chopra S, Seligman M, et al. The impact on medical practice of commitments to change following CME lectures: a randomized controlled trial. *Med Teach.* 2011;33(9):e495–e500.

64. Holton EF III. Theoretical assumptions underlying the performance paradigm of human resource development. *Hum Resour Dev Int.* 2002;5(2):199–215.

65. Cobb P, Confrey J, Lehrer R, et al. Design experiments in educational research. *Educ Res.* 2003;32(1):9–13.

66. Fishman BJ, Penuel WR, Allen A-R, et al. Design-based implementation research: an emerging model for transforming the relationship of research and practice. In: Fishman BJ, Penuel WR, eds. *National Society for the Study of Education Yearbook: Vol 112 Design Based Implementation Research.* New York: National Society for the Study of Education; 2013:136–156.

Chapter 22

UNDERSTANDING *and* EFFECTING HEALTH CARE ORGANIZATIONAL CHANGE

Morris J. Blachman

Case

It is apparent that health systems around the globe are changing, the result of demands for more efficient, cost-effective, and evidence-based care; patient satisfaction; and wishes of government, insurers, and the health care industry. Your CME/CPD unit is caught in this transformation, being called upon to educate about the changes and to aid in integrating and aligning its functions with the needs of the health system. To a large extent, you feel that this will take time and have a potentially major effect, both positively and potentially negatively, on your organization.

Questions

What organizational and management principles could be effective here? How can you apply them to your situation and your role as a thought leader in CME/CPD? What are some keys to success?

INTRODUCTION

Organizational Change: The future has arrived! In July 2016, Alvin Toffler passed away. He was the author of many works, but was best known for his 1970 book, *Future Shock*. Toffler made the point then that we had entered a time when we were experiencing change at such a rapid pace that it was becoming increasingly difficult to keep up. He also observed this was likely to continue to accelerate.[1] Many might long for what may now seem like simpler times. The 21st century has brought not only rapid change in the health care landscape but continuous change as well. In some sense, that might not be as novel a concept as it might seem. After all, Heraclitus told us that "There is nothing permanent except change" some 25 centuries ago.

What are the changes that will likely embroil health care, medical schools, health systems and academic medical centers, and specialty societies in the next 5 to 10 years? As other chapters in this volume attest, these institutions and the practitioners, teachers, and leaders associated with them will be grappling with a dizzying array of changes. There will be a new paradigm of practice with activities and terms such as value-based payment (rather than fee for service); patient-centric; learner-centric; cost-effective, team-based care; population health and community-based health care delivery; high reliability performance; performance improvement culture; personal (individual) and precision medicine; process engineering; and ongoing quality improvement.

Health care institutions and the physicians practicing within and outside of them will be facing a steep learning curve. The nearly ubiquitous call for "Lifelong Learning" is one indication of the recognition that the only reasonable way health care practitioners can keep up is to pursue learning in an ongoing manner. Equally important, the institutions must find ways to learn and to adapt to these rapidly changing conditions.

Both the institutions and individuals will have to become far more agile in embracing and responding to the transformation. The institutions are likely to adopt new organizational structures moving away from the more traditional hierarchical styles. J.P. Kotter, one of the world's leading experts on institutional change, comments that the old institutions are no longer capable of meeting the needs of the 21st century environment. He warns that to be successful means recognizing how the context is changing and implementing what changes organizations need to make to meet those new challenges.[2]

This requirement to adjust and improve in the face of change[3] will likely lead health care institutions to seek to become learning organizations.[4-6] The changing context impacting these health care institutions will, in turn, generate changes to which the clinicians who populate these institutions will also need to adapt. Early stages of the ways in which this process can affect the institutions are already being observed. For example, in the United States any ACGME-accredited institution needs to implement the Clinical Learning Environment Review (CLER) requirements. Likewise, efforts are under way around the globe to make sure new physicians are appropriately educated in evidence-based cost-effective medicine and well versed in quality improvement and patient safety. This will necessitate considerable adjustment on the part of faculty in both modeling the new behaviors as well as teaching residents in this new context. As one observer noted, "This will require a new species of faculty."[7,8]

Why does this matter in the CPD world? It matters because it poses a set of challenges and a set of opportunities.

CPD CHALLENGES

CPD offices will be challenged to step up and not only meet current professional development needs but also keep pace with the changes in those needs as they unfold in the future.[6] This shift could be substantial. The American Hospital Association Physician Leadership Forum's 2014 publication, Continuing Medical Education as a Strategic Resource made the point that CME has an important role to play to "enhance and strengthen" the partnership between physicians and hospitals as they work to "transform the delivery model."[9]

CPD offices will be challenged to do a better job utilizing evidence-based and evidence-informed educational design taking into account the latest research on learning.

This requires developing a scholarly underpinning for the offices so that they can not only consume new learning but contribute to it as well. As implementation science grows, the practices of the CPD office will need to keep pace, ensuring that the learner is given the best opportunity to meet their professional needs across all the domains of competence.

Lastly, CPD offices also need to be attentive to the likely changes in institutional demands on them. The new models of health care delivery and reimbursement will push institutions to squeeze out costs and demonstrate quality outcomes. Those pressures will likely trickle down to demands on the CPD office. It will also be critical to demonstrate CPD's strategic value contribution to the realization of the institution's goals.

Managing a CPD office in the 21st century requires an entirely different array of skills, and, as the future unfolds, those skill sets will continue to change as well. CPD offices will be challenged to meet these unfolding needs. Kotter's admonition is not only applicable to institutions but is also appropriate to apply to the entire CPD enterprise. As the CPD world ponders these challenges, it also needs to consider a quote often attributed to W. Edwards Deming "You do not have to change. You do not have to survive either." The CPD enterprise does have a choice in how it confronts these challenges; we have the opportunity not only to survive but to flourish.

CPD OPPORTUNITIES

Albert Einstein once said, "In the middle of difficulty lies opportunity." CPD has opportunities as a strategic asset and as a change agent and enabler of change.

CPD as a Strategic Asset

CPD is uniquely positioned to address all the roles the physician might play in the Academic Health Center (as a clinician, as a faculty person, as a researcher, and as a leader), and it can attend to the professional development needs of community faculty and physicians. CPD can assist all of them to become effective "Learners in Practice."

The CPD office is the locus of expertise in planning, delivering, evaluating, and sustaining physician professional development. It can also be a source of expertise in learning, an office designed to absorb and utilize new knowledge/scholarship. In essence, it needs to be a mini learning organization. As a matter of best practice, the CPD office should deliver evidence-based and evidence-informed services. In addition, as a mini learning organization, it can be a model to other offices and the overarching institution demonstrating the utility and value of being organized that way.

In response to the quality and financial challenges faced by health care institutions, CPD can be one of the drivers of cultural and organizational change—helping define learning opportunities that provide strategic support for the organization's direction and priorities. CPD offices have the opportunity to become an exemplar in the midst of their health care institution. To do so means creating the functions, knowledge base, and skill sets necessary to function effectively that way.

CPD as a Change Agent and an Enabler of Change

The AHA study spoke to the strategic potential of CPD in their recommendations to the Hospital and Health System Field: "Use CME to advance the strategic aims of the organization… engage physicians as partners in strengthening organizational competencies…[and] communicate the value of strategically oriented CME to the physician community to engage them as partners in improvement efforts."[9] The study also referenced a wide array of areas (such as strategic planning, clinical integration, community health management, and quality improvement) where CME/CPD could be strategically of value to hospitals and health care institutions.[9]

In his seminal article, What Do I Need to Learn Today?—The Evolution of CME, Graham Mc Mahon, MD, pointed out that CME professionals and offices are beginning to play important and strategic roles in their health systems. And, he argued that CPD can make far more valuable contributions than it does now. However, that will require "*the engagement of health care leaders, educators, and learners – and won't succeed until health care systems, and institutions recognize education's strategic value in driving change.*"[10] Others have made similar observations. Ron Cervero and Julie Gaines, in their 2014 systematic review of the literature on CME effectiveness, noted that CME was ensnared "amidst the struggle between the educational agendas and political-economic agendas…"[11]

CPD offices have two noteworthy opportunities that arise from these challenges. The first is to become a mini learning organization and develop the capacity to meet physician and other health professional changing professional development needs, both within institution and in the community, well into the future. The second is help the institutional decision-makers recognize and embrace the *strategic value* CPD can bring in driving change in full alignment with the *strategic direction* of the institution in which it is embedded.

STRATEGIC MANAGEMENT

Consider the challenge set out in the beginning of this chapter. To be successful, CME/CPD professionals need to engage in change management within their office. They need to be agile not only in assisting others to adapt to change but to meet the change challenges. The change to adopt is directional, is transformational, and needs to be in alignment with the purpose of both the CPD office and the institution(s) within which it is embedded or associated.

How does one go about these two tasks of internally transforming as well as becoming an integral part of the broader institution's strategic operations? One promising avenue is to engage in strategic management. Strategic management is an intentional and logical process that sets direction, establishes actions, evaluates results, and redirects resources as needed to stay on course. Strategic management is not simply an event; it is a way of conducting business. It incorporates strategic planning and sets the context in which operational management occurs.[12] One might think about this as similar to having a blueprint to guide in construction of a building or a home or even a large development complex. It also can be a constructive way to exercise power in a responsible

Strategic Management Process

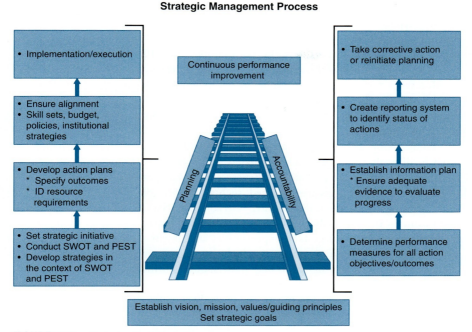

FIGURE 22.1.   Strategic management process.

manner. A strategic management logic model shares many features with the logic model of good CME activity planning and design. A visual representation of the process is shown in Figure 22.1.

Back to the case laid out at the beginning of the chapter. What are the steps the CPD leadership might take to accomplish the establishment of a meaningful strategic action plan?

Good strategic management begins with a very thoughtful discussion that establishes with clarity a Vision statement, a Mission statement, and a set of Values and/or Guiding Principles. The Vision and Mission state who you aspire to be and what you do. The values/guiding principles state ***how*** you do what you do. The Vision is always aspirational; it is something which you continuously strive to achieve. For example, "to be internationally recognized for…" Such a vision implies not only reaching that goal, but sustaining it and that requires continuous striving. The Mission is a statement of what you actually do to move toward that vision. For example, "to develop, implement, manage, evaluate and improve high quality educational experiences that enhance physicians' core competencies and promote the values of medicine's humane tradition."

Lessons from the management literature suggest that how one behaves can be as critical to success as what one does. Values and Guiding Principles are usually chosen to emphasize the particular standards by which the organization or unit wants to behave and to be known. Examples of Values include terms such as "Integrity," "Honesty," "Empathy," etc. Examples of Guiding Principles are "We will be learner-centric"; "We will hold ourselves accountable for all our actions"; etc.

The next step is to consider what are the outcomes or goals for which the office is already accountable (accreditation, mandates, regulations, etc.) and then what are the outcomes or goals the office wants to achieve in order to pursue the aspirations of the vision and to accomplish the mission. For example, the CPD office in the case mentioned at the beginning of this article may determine it needs to become a learning organization (within its own office) or to be invited to be a regular participant for all system educational planning meetings or to be a regular member of the groups put together to design institutional quality improvement efforts, for the purpose of providing expert advice on learning, etc.

Undertaking such a large change initiative can be a daunting task as change can often be difficult and might generate anxiety and opposition. Leadership will want to have a good sense of the probability of success and what can be done to enhance that probability. Once the goals are identified, such as, for example, to turn the CPD office into a learning organization, the next step is to conduct a SWOT (strengths, weaknesses, opportunities, threats) analysis. The SWOT addresses internal factors in strengths and weaknesses and external factors in opportunities and threats. This analysis gives a good sense of the environment or context in which the office is trying to create and manage change. The SWOT is designed to help understand both the challenges and opportunities for achieving the desired goals. The articulation of these items is to inform the actions that will be designed to pursue the goals. Eventually, the questions will be how these strengths that have been identified can be leveraged; what can be done to mitigate the weaknesses; how the office can take advantage of existing opportunities to help the office move more rapidly or forcefully toward the goal; and finally, how the threats can be avoided, effectively countered, or lessened.

The next step is to determine the strategic initiatives that if properly followed are likely to lead to achieving the goals. For example, if the office does not currently engage actively in learning from, and employing the results of, the published literature, one strategic initiative might be to create a scholarly underpinning for the office. It might be operationalized in action plans by setting a 3-year formalized internal staff professional development program. The strategic initiative would include developing the behaviors, skills, and processes that would result in personnel who have developed the new competencies and an office actively engaged in the scholarly practice of learning from the professional literature.

As the strategic initiatives are considered and the action plans that flow from them are developed, it will be important to determine the resource requirements (personnel, skill sets, funds, culture, etc.) necessary to success. A meaningful strategic plan has to be appropriately resourced for success. Leadership is responsible to make sure the office has the capacity to carry out the strategies and that the office is in a state of readiness to implement the plan. Once the planning has proceeded to this point, the next step is implementation or execution.

Parallel to the planning track is the establishment of an accountability track. Figuring out what one wants to do and developing the plan to do it are two necessary steps to planned success, but they are not sufficient. Two additional steps are required: first, the plan must be implemented; and second, the success of the plan must be evaluated so that any necessary midcourse corrections can be made to assure the plan is bringing about the results desired. The accountability track is developed in tandem with the planning track. Performance measures are developed for all action plan objectives or outcomes. The question to be answered here is: What do we need to know to assess progress toward the objectives/outcomes stipulated? This means determining the kind of evidence/information that is necessary to collect to evaluate the progress. This can be thought of as an information plan because it requires thinking through what of that evidence or information is already available or which might be accessible from elsewhere or might have to be created.

Next, establish a reporting system that is transparent and communicates progress toward the outcomes/goals. This can be a relatively simple system that tracks the progress for each objective and color codes the results on a spread sheet with the outcome displayed in Green (if progress is on track), in Yellow (if progress is slower than expected or is slightly veering off track), or in Red (if progress is stopped or going in the wrong direction).

Establish a mechanism or process for ensuring that corrective action is taken to redirect when appropriate. The redirection could be to follow the same basic path, with minor corrections, or it could be to go back to the planning track and rethink the action plan. In the case we discussed, suppose a journal club had been the vehicle for the professional development and very little change was taking place. Members of the office were not reading or using the literature to inform their work. One might rethink the action plans and turn to individual development plans as a means to develop the scholarly interest and capability.

This iterative process sets the overall context for the direction of the office and ensures that the goals are always in sight and that movement in the right direction takes place through continuous performance improvement.

Keys to Success in Strategic Management

Bringing about significant change is difficult and requires both patience and perseverance. The process, as iterated above, is labor and time intensive. Learning and change take time. The two most important factors in successful transformation are the active engagement of the leadership (in this case, within the office) and the development of a culture (shared understanding) that supports the process. To ensure a shared understanding, the Vision, Mission, and Values/Guiding Principles need to be clear and consistently pursued. All those engaged in bringing about the change need to communicate. That communication must be clear and multidirectional and flow freely.

Leadership must assure that there is sufficient capacity to carry out the strategies and action plans. In addition, every aspect of the office or organization should be in alignment with the strategic direction including the budget, array of personnel and skill sets, programmatic decisions, etc. Staff need to be included as active participants.

Leadership also needs to know through the accountability track: what is working, what is not working, and what needs to be modified so it will work. Finally, leadership must hold themselves as well as staff accountable. Walk the Talk. As Ralph Waldo Emerson put it, "Put your creed into deed."

While strategic planning and management give us clarity in overall direction and address big issues, many of the changes that need to be made are often very specific and more limited. They fall more under operational management. Change still needs to be managed at that level.

POWER MAPPING

How are these very specific changes to be addressed? One tool to use is: "Power Mapping." This tool helps determine how and where to exercise the power necessary to deal effectively with the issue. But, it requires that there is clarity as to what outcome or outcomes need to be accomplished.

Power Mapping is a tool designed to aid in decision-making and the development of action plans to achieve these very specific results. It is outcome driven, embedded in strategic thinking, assessment based, culturally sensitive, and pathway organized. As shown in Table 22.1, the process is carefully ordered and begins by identifying the specific action

TABLE 22.1
Power Mapping

Elements	Factors
What needs to change	• Know what needs to change
	• Set realistic goals
	• Set specific outcomes
Location of decisions	• Administrative unit
	• Corporate management
	• Board
Identify people or organizational level responsible for permitting or prohibiting an action	• Supporters
	• Uncommitted
	• Opponents
Key individuals	• Level of competence
	• Level of energy
	• Level of trust
	• Motivation
	• Degree of empathy
	• Personal characteristics
	• Flexibility
	• Accommodating
	• Dedication/commitment
	• Mobility interes
	• External power linkages
	• Colleagues
	• Family
	• Friends
	• Networks
	• Personal and professional goals

| **TABLE 22.1** |
| **Power Mapping (*Continued*)** |

Elements	Factors
Decision-making process	• Merit of the case • Institutional position • Ideology • Tradition • Experience • GURU/Gray eminence • Power bloc • Majority • Consensus • Exchange/Barter • Referent group
Negotiation style	• Compromise • Rigid • Market • On the job training/learning • Outcome oriented
Scenario management	• Know the limits of the possible • Develop 2–3 causal pathways • Consider probability of success for each pathway • Consider how to increase the probability for each pathway • Avoid organizing to fail

Resource consideration	• What is readily available, could be reallocated, or needs to be developed
	  • Personnel
	  • Money
	  • Organizational
	  • Political capital

Evaluation	• Assess progress • Correct or rethink as indicated by findings

or actions desired in clear and concrete terms. In essence, it requires knowing WHAT needs to change. That, in turn, will lead to figuring out the particular decisions that need to be made to achieve the outcome. Set realistic goals concerning the change(s) you wish to make.

Next, identify the locus where the decision will be made (C-Suite; Administrative Unit or Office (Dean, Department Chair, etc.) and identify the specific people or organizational unit responsible for permitting or prohibiting whatever action you want to have taken. Once the key people have been identified, determine their formal positions in the organizational structure (wiring diagram) as well as their informal power position(s). Assess, as best as possible, where they stand (or are likely to stand) in relation to issue or outcome desired. Are they supporters (high or low), uncommitted (neutral), or opponents (high or low)? In addition, for each key individual under consideration, assess their personal characteristics specifically in relation to the decision(s) being sought. This will include such items as their motivation, level of energy, level of trust, empathy, competence, flexibility, degree of dedication, past experience in handling similar issues, etc.

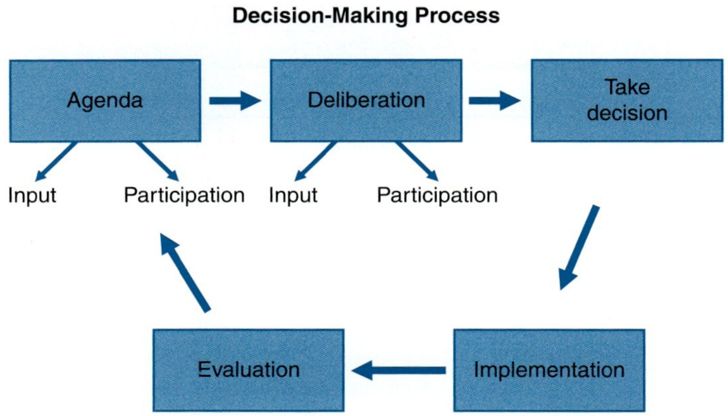

Decision-Making Process

FIGURE 22.2.　Decision-making process.

Get to know how the decision-making process works for that unit or system. Every decision-making process is a cycle with five components: (1) agenda setting, (2) deliberation, (3) taking the decision, (4) implementation, and (5) evaluation (see Fig. 22.2). Although every decision is composed of these five components, they are often not broken out so neatly. The first three components often are run together. It is important to recognize the differences in each of those components so that the intervention can be most effective.

The degree to which decision-makers are open to have others engaged in any given segment of the process can be different and needs to be assessed so you can figure out where you can have an impact. For example, suppose the action being sought is to have someone from the CPD office to be made a part of a committee that addresses the professional development needs of physician leadership throughout the system. The decision-maker may simply make that decision on her or his own without consulting anyone else. Or, she or he may simply ask for input from others, looking to see if anyone else might be invested in the decision. This latter form of participation allows those asked to provide the input to give it to the decision-maker who then exercises power by deciding to use the input or not.

Alternatively, the decision-maker may decide to open up the process of setting the agenda and ask for active participation involving some format permitting exchange of ideas among the participants. Setting the agenda is always a political process in which power is exercised. Knowing how that decision-maker will react allows the office strategic manager to plan how to be most effective. Likewise, it matters who is able to participate in the deliberation/discussion of the issue. Again, this may be done through input or by participation.

Another step will be the actual taking of the decision. How is that accomplished? There are a number of ways committees take decisions. It is important to know what moves the committee or most influences it. Learning what style is used is empowering as it makes it easier to figure out how best to influence the process. For example, are decisions in that committee usually made based on the "merits of the case"? Is there some set of principles that determine the decision (only physicians can be on this committee or only people with a certain level of authority can be on this committee)? Is there a "Guru or Gray Eminence" to whom most generally turn to guide them in their decisions?

The answers to these questions should guide where and how the CPD office might influence the decision-making process and outcome.

Other broad questions that are worthy of consideration relate to the actual process of decision-making, the culture of the group and process, and negotiating style as described below:

What is the actual process by which decisions are taken? There are a number of questions that might guide the exploration:

- Is it strictly a quantitative, majority vote?
- Is it done by consensus or unanimity?
- Do they rely on how some other groups have made similar decisions?
- Is it based on some quid pro quo?

What is the culture of the decision-making group and process?

- Do they operate more in secrecy or openness?
- Is there trust or mistrust?
- Do they rely more on principles or people/feelings?
- Are they direct or indirect in discussion?
- Do they come to decision closure rapidly or do they seem to be open ended?

If the culture or issue is one that is likely to be addressed through some form of negotiation, what is the negotiating style?

- Is it one of seeking compromise?
- Is it a rigid "take it or leave it"?
- Is it like a market where the expectation is a lot of haggling?
- Is it outcome oriented, open on process and methods, but strong on adhering to the outcome?[13]

Finally, after developing all the information needed for the Power Mapping, engage in scenario assessment. Consider at least two or three options that might be alternative ways of thinking about how to go about pursuing the desired outcome(s). Keep in mind how the CPD action aligns with the action being sought. As was the case with strategic planning, pursuit of any objective will require resources. Consider what resources each of the options that are derived from the scenarios will require: personnel, funds, time, and political capital. Also, consider how opposition to the goal might affect the amount of resource needed.

Estimate the probability of success and in running through the scenarios consider how you can design not only to achieve your goal but also to avoid failing. Think through the unintended, but knowable consequences of each scenario. Develop milestones or markers to evaluate how well (or not) you are progressing. Be willing to make midcourse corrections (replay the scenarios and make adjustments).

FUTURE DIRECTIONS

The year 2022 will not look like 2017, but it will likely resemble 2017 more than 1970. The past several decades have brought enormous changes in medical knowledge, medical practice, medical treatments, medical technology, in cultural expectations, and in understanding the dynamics of learning and education. There is no reason to believe that what Alvin Toffler brought into public consciousness in 1970 will be reversed.[1] Quite the contrary, change is most likely to accelerate.[3]

For the CPD world, Toffler's Future Shock has moved from a prescient title to a reflection of history. Across the globe, the demands on CPD to keep up with the changes will grow, but there is ample opportunity to meet those challenges now, if the CPD community chooses to do so. The key is not just what will be done by CPD offices in the future; it is what will be done today and tomorrow. "Strategic planning does not deal with future decisions. It deals with the futurity of present decisions."[14] As Graham McMahon put it, "I envision a future in which educational expectations and professional competency obligations are aligned and integrated and in which all physicians have an educational 'home' that helps them navigate their continuing growth—so that education is intertwined with practice throughout their careers."[10]

REFERENCES

1. Toffler A. *Future Shock*. New York: Random House; 1970.
2. Kotter JP. Accelerate. *Harvard Business Review*. 2012. 4. Reprint R1211B.
3. Kotter JP. *Accelerate: Building Strategic Agility for a Faster-Moving World*. Boston, MA: Harvard Business Review Press; 2014.
4. Senge PM. *The Fifth Discipline. The Art and Practice of the Learning Organization*. London, UK: Random House; 1990.
5. Garvin DA, Edmondson AC, Gino F. Is yours a learning organization? *Harvard Business Review*. 2008. Reprint R0803H.
6. Crites GE, McNamara MC, Akl EA, et al. Evidence in the learning organization. *Health Research Policy and Systems*; March 2009. http://www.health-policy-systems.com/content/7/1/4. Accessed July 31, 2016.
7. Raymond JI. Palmetto Health Columbia, South Carolina, Graduate Medical Education (GME) Strategic Planning Session, September 2013.
8. Baxley EG, Lawson, L, Garrison HG, et al. The teachers of quality academy: a learning community approach for preparing faculty to teach health system science. *Acad Med*. 2016;91(12):1655–1660.
9. Combes JR, Arespacochaga E. *Continuing Medical Education as a Strategic Resource*. Chicago, IL: American Hospital Association's Physician Leadership Forum; 2014.
10. McMahon GT. What do I need to learn today?—the evolution of CME. *N Engl J Med*. 2016;374(15): 1403–1406.
11. Cervero RM, Gaines JK. *Effectiveness of Continuing Medical Education: Updated Synthesis of Systematic Reviews*. Chicago, IL: ACCME; 2014.
12. Steiner GA. *Strategic Planning: What Every Manager Must Know*. New York: Free Press; 1997.
13. Fisher R, Ury W, Patton B. *Getting to Yes: Negotiating Agreement without Giving in*, 3rd ed. New York: Penguin Books; 2011
14. Drucker PF. *Management: Tasks, Responsibilities, Practices*. New York: Harper & Row Publishers, Inc.; 1993.

Chapter 23

LEARNING *to* LEAD *in an* ACADEMIC HEALTH SYSTEM

Mary G. Turco, Allison T. McHugh, and Richard I. Rothstein

Case

Following your institution's receipt of a large philanthropic gift, you have been charged with the design and implementation of new leadership development programs for your academic health system. You have many ideas for programs and opportunities at varying levels of leadership, which include interprofessional team learning and alignment with the needs and mission of your organizations—the medical school and nursing school, the hospital and medical center, the clinical practices, and the integrated, affiliated regional health system. You have read some of the literature on leadership and canvassed programs at other institutions but remain uncertain about your final plans.

Questions

Why must you develop leaders for the currently evolving health system? How do you equip leaders to lead themselves, others, the system, and interprofessional teams to effect change successfully? What programs and opportunities facilitate learning to lead? How might you successfully design and implement a new leadership development program?

INTRODUCTION

Developing confident, effective leaders for evolving 21st century health systems around the world is an enormously important educational challenge. In their prescient 2010 study *Health Professionals for a new century: transforming education to strengthen health systems in an interdependent world*, Julio Frenk and coauthors, all international thought leaders in health professionals' education, named multiple systemic reasons why the education of health professionals has not kept pace with the world's health challenges including a myriad of new "infections, environmental, and behavioral risks" that "threaten [the] health security of all."[1] Among the reasons were a mismatch of competencies to patient and population needs, poor teamwork, persistent gender stratification of professional status, predominant hospital orientation at the expense of primary care, and *weak leadership* to improve health system performance.[1] The authors called for a redesign of professional health education across the continuum, including continuing professional development (CPD), to match the work of Flexner (Medicine)[2] Welch-Rose (Public Health)[3] and Goldmark (Nursing) in the early 20th century.[4] They demanded "a new century of transformative professional education" so as to create a more "equitable and better performing health systems…with consequent benefits for patients and populations everywhere in our interdependent world."[1]

The focus of this chapter is helping health professionals learn to lead so as to eliminate the problem of weak leadership in our health systems. In doing so, it can be argued that dilemmas with competencies, teamwork, gender stratification, and primary care may also be addressed. First, however, the quality of leadership must improve. Frenk and colleagues asked for a redesign of professional health education across the continuum of *all* health professions. These redesigns must include adding or strengthening leadership training. Those charged with equipping individuals to effect change in complex health care organizations must see to it that leadership training across the continuum teaches individuals to lead themselves, others, the system, and interprofessional teams, including its *interprofessional leadership teams.*

This change in the culture of health professions leadership education requires a new mental model that values interdisciplinary and interprofessional leadership. Professionals who possess the new mental model can effectively lead their clinic, center, system, or nation in delivering better education and health care. In some cases, they can learn to lead the world. Collectively they can save many lives and solve global health threats. Twenty-first century leaders who learn a new mental model are like educators in the early 20th century who embraced Flexner's, Welch-Rose's, and Goldmark's vision for a new education system to meet a new health delivery era. The adoption of 20th century education reforms contributed to the doubling of life span during that century.[1] Interestingly, the 20th century health professions educators who adopted the new mental models of that age *privileged* undergraduate and graduate *medical* education over *continuing* medical education and *all other categories of health professions' undergraduate, graduate, and continuing education.* Today, that privileging is unacceptable. The education and leadership development of all professions in relationship to each other is key to "tackling" our 21st century challenges. Our planet now has 7-plus billion people, some of whom "are trapped in health conditions of a century earlier."[1] All health professions must generate leaders to meet this challenge.

The following sections of this chapter focus on how to equip individuals as they move across the educational continuum to lead themselves, others, the system, and teams; programs that facilitate leadership education; guidance from the literature for designing and implementing a new leadership development program; and thoughts on future directions for leadership education to meet the 21st century's pressing health challenges and threats.

EQUIPPING LEADERS TO LEAD SELF, OTHERS, THE SYSTEM, AND INTERPROFESSIONAL TEAMS

There are no simple, generalizable methods to teach leadership for all of the challenges health professionals face. There are, however, better ways to think about leadership education so as develop interventions that fit the particular contexts in which leadership problems exist. Regher has advised educators to reflect on their own context and incorporate their own interpretations to develop meaningful educational interventions.[5] The following sections offer leadership theory and informed ways to think about leadership so as to equip individuals to lead.

Learning to Lead the Self

In his popular, practical, and internationally recognized book on leadership, Northouse[6] reflects on the multitude of ways to define or conceptualize leadership, identifying four components as central. Leadership (a) is a process, (b) involves influence, (c) occurs in groups, and (d) involves common goals. He defines leadership as "a process whereby an individual influences a group of individuals to achieve a common goal." Northouse elaborates that defining leadership as a process "means that it is not a trait or characteristic that resides in the leader, but rather a transactional event that occurs between the leader and the followers...an interactive event." Successful leadership requires the leader to influence followers, with bases of power that are divided between those coming from *position* power (legitimate, reward, coercive, and information) and those from *personal* power (referent and expert).[7,8] Types of positional and personal power appear in Table 23.1.

These bases of power enable a leader to influence others. This traditional thinking puts the leader "out there, wielding power, providing answers, and standing apart."[10] Common wisdom suggests that the more a leader knows about standard leadership skills (such as establishing vision, mission and goals, strategic planning, change management),

TABLE 23.1
Position and Personal Power Types[a]

POSITION POWER TYPES

Legitimate/Positional:
"Power exerted by an individual in a formal, designated position of leadership or authority"
Reward:
Power that "may provide either material or psychological reward."
Coercive:
Power "that results actual of imagined negative consequences that accrue to an individual who does not complete a task successfully."
Information:
"Power of information to aid decision making in a particular situation."

PERSONAL POWER TYPES

Referent:
Power that "results from the sometimes intangible personal characteristics and inter-professional skills of the influencing agent."
Expert:
Power "held by those having particular (perhaps unique) knowledge" that can influence "other's beliefs and actions."

[a]French[7] and Raven[8] six bases of power as described by Gabel.[9]

the better her or his effectiveness. However, Souba calls for new thinking on leadership. He argues that leadership training must first transform people by changing their "mental maps and thought patterns." Behaviors then change, and organizational transformation follows. He states that "this new way of understanding leadership requires that leaders spend much more time learning about and leading themselves."[11] Leaders play a critical role to help others (and themselves) revise their outmoded ways of thinking. Souba elaborates that leadership and other roles are "social constructions" and that people "let the roles we understand ourselves to play in life define our identity." He suggests that leaders consider that one's "roles are not really who you are." Rather, each person is the "most genuine and earnest commitments that you make in life." A leader gives her or his word to these commitments and brings them to life through the word in action. "Real commitments are those that help others, improve the human condition, and move the world forward." Souba calls these powerful commitments that each individual makes in life her or his "stand."[12] One's stand comes from within and is an expression of one's convictions. To take a stand requires a promise to be responsible for the commitment.

The leading of oneself requires energetic self-reflection and attention to personal leadership principles, which "distinguish *being* a leader as the ontological basis for what leaders know."[12] These include *awareness* (reflecting on how effective you are being, what's happening around you, and noticing if you are not achieving your vision), *commitment* (being committed to and standing for something bigger than yourself creates a context to overcome barriers along the way and the commitment becomes who we are), *integrity* (honoring the commitments you make to yourself and others, keeping your word), and *authenticity* (being clear about who you are, what you believe in, what your core values are, and then living according to that vision of yourself). These personal leadership principles offer an alternative to what Souba[11] calls the 6 Achilles' Heels. The 6 Achilles' Heels are commonly considered indicators of success that make a person feel worthy and valuable: *achievement* (the pressure to excel, accomplish, and perform), *authority* (the need to control, dominate, and have clout), *admiration* (the fixation with being liked, popular, accepted, and approved of), *affluence* (the obsession with wealth and material possessions), *appearance* (the addiction to bodily features and "looks"), and *attention* (the need to be noticed and in the spotlight). A desire for approval can lead to conventionality and inauthenticity, rather than adherence to authentic commitment. Souba goes on to suggest that most of a human being's life is "an experienced/constructed reality that is significantly affected by conversational language." This human design process is determined by the unique **Me** (my genetic profile, experiences, memories, assumptions, beliefs, personality, feelings) constructing **My mental maps** (how I make sense of my life and my world; my thinking; my reality) leading to **My choices and behaviors** (what I do; my deeds; my conduct; the actions I take) and resulting in **My performance and results** (my effectiveness at work and at home; the quality of my life).[12]

In *The Science of Leading Yourself: A Missing Piece in the Health Care Transformation Puzzle*, Souba suggests that the science of leading oneself is dependent on anchoring effective leadership in the leader's way of being—a "first-person, as-lived experience."[13] This is an ontological phenomenological perspective in which "(1) our actions as leaders are correlated with the way in which the leadership situation we are dealing with occurs for us, and (2) this 'occurring' is shaped by the context we bring to that situation."[12]

Warren Bennis wrote that "becoming a leader is synonymous with becoming yourself. It's precisely that simple, and it's also that difficult."[14] Knowing oneself means acting, speaking, listening, and effectively using language to distinguish and shape reality. While conventional leadership activities (strategy, vision, communication, management) results are needed for determining performance and its measurement, the being and action of individual leadership are transforming. Awareness, commitment, integrity, and authenticity constitute a framework to address successfully the changing landscape of health care delivery and its effects on professionalism.

The question has been posed: "What can you say about the future you're committed to such that it will grant you the being and acting required to take on your leadership challenge and the obstacles you will encounter along the way?"[13] Knowing yourself and how you are as a leader, your being and acting, will equip you for the leadership challenges and opportunities in the process of leading others on the team, in the academic health system (AHS), and in the greater communities. To enable individuals to learn to lead themselves, opportunities must exist—throughout one's education—for guided self-reflection. Educators across the continuum and professions can create these opportunities in courses, electives, special interest groups, and mentoring relationships. CPD leaders familiar with the leadership literature and with institutional and community content experts can work with faculty, program directors, and human resource instructors to design and deliver such important activities.

Learning to Lead Others

The ability to know yourself is a key component of what has been referred to as emotional intelligence (EI), which has been demonstrated to be extremely important for leadership success in all venues, mattering even more than intelligence quotient (IQ).[15] The original framework for emotional intelligence was framed as "a set of skills hypothesized to contribute to the accurate appraisal and expression of emotion in oneself and in others, the effective regulation of emotion in self and others, and the use of feelings to motivate, plan, and achieve in one's life."[16] There is an emerging attention to the application of emotional intelligence in the health care leadership world, following much consideration and understanding of its role in the traditional business world. To foster a culture of collaboration needed for the evolving health care systems, emotional intelligence has been suggested as a critical health care leadership competency.[17] In a systematic review of the current literature, three themes concerning physician leadership and emotional intelligence were identified: "(1) emotional intelligence is broadly endorsed as a leadership development strategy across providers and settings, (2) models of emotional intelligence and leadership practices vary widely, and (3) emotional intelligence is considered relevant throughout medical education and practice."[18]

There is a striking need to emphasize the awareness and development of emotional intelligence across the continuum of learning and the disciplines. Using focus groups of medical professionals at an academic medical center to elicit participants' perceptions of qualities necessary for effective *physician* leadership, investigators found that four themes emerged: management of the team, establishing a vision, communication, and personal attributes.[19] For *nursing* leaders, who are critical members of the health care team and partners in the transformation of health care, multiple investigators determined qualities and competencies necessary for effectiveness and success: emotional intelligence, self-awareness, mindfulness, a passion for developing and inspiring others (mentorship), an ability to communicate effectively, authenticity, accountability, vision, attitude, and an ability to influence others through relationships, integrity, and trust.[20–22] Nursing leaders must also remain committed to excellence, reward and recognize others, build a culture around service, and align behaviors with goals and values.[23] Comack describes the use of the acronym LEADS—**L**eading self, **E**ngaging others, **A**chieving results, **D**eveloping coalitions, and **S**ystem transformation—as an evidenced-based framework for establishing qualities and competencies for physicians, nurses, and other health care leaders.[24]

In all health care leaders, it is the personal attributes related to knowing and leading oneself and emotional intelligence that have primal importance, since these are carefully observed, known, discussed, and valued by the followers. This is *leadership capital* that can be well spent to engender loyalty, establish culture, facilitate change, and create powerful alliances and collaborations that are needed for the transitions underway in health systems and clinical practice. To enable individuals to learn to lead with emotional intelligence, a variety of opportunities can be offered in live, online, or hybrid activities across the continuum. Emotional intelligence instruction can be done well in triads and teams, inside or outside the school or workplace, in one-time or ongoing activities, to create a culture of collaboration.

Learning to Lead the System and Interprofessional Health Care Teams

The evolution of expanded health systems, moving beyond the academic medical center to networks of affiliated and aggregated practices and institutions, has placed additional importance on the leadership skills of their physician, nurse, and other health care team leaders. Traditionally, most clinician leaders have spent countless hours honing their clinical and academic skills, but not all have put the same effort toward the development and improvement of their leadership capabilities. In a recent reflection about academic leadership, Naylor stated that "top-performing leaders seem to be self-effacing team builders who eschew rapid-cycle strategic planning and management trends, focusing instead on strategic and incremental changes that will gradually transform their organizations."[25] Naylor added that "Academic physicians and search committees often concentrate on personal achievement and intellectual or technical mastery in research and clinical care" and noted that "In contrast, the literature on leadership suggests 'other-directed' skills matter more, e.g. mentorship, learning and teaching competencies, and so-called emotional intelligence."[25]

Bachrach has written that physicians are taking on a "greater role in business decision making and are found at the negotiating table with leaders from business, insurance, and other integrated health care delivery systems." Physicians who lead "strategic business units" within the academic medical center "are expected to acquire and demonstrate enhanced business acumen."[26] The same is true for nurse leaders, many of whom now have oversight of one or several business units within health care organizations and the responsibility to communicate organizational mission and vision within these units. Huston describes the many skills needed for the "nurse leader of 2020."[27] Not only do they need business acumen and an ability to create organizational culture that promotes quality and safety, but they also need a global perspective of health care and professional issues, technology skills, decision-making skills rooted in empirical science, political and team-building skills, and the ability to establish expectations and manage in a complex rapidly changing health care environment.[27] The introduction and refining of these necessary business-oriented skills and a focus on other leadership traits are necessary components for sustainable health system success.

In the United States and elsewhere, health system redesign is moving from the traditional unidirectional core academic medical center with surrounding referral network to an integrated, affiliated collective developing a shared set of goals and utilizing bidirectional cohesive assimilation of information, finance, governance, patient care, research, and teaching activities. The "top-down," traditional, and "vertical" decision-making authority/process that was generally hierarchical, gendered, and based on position and profession in the organization is being replaced by horizontal decision-making authority/process by interdisciplinary and interprofessional teams that are less hierarchical and gendered in makeup.[28] Interdependent triads of physician, nursing, and administrative leaders affect local affairs and influence autonomy. Increasingly, clinician leaders are empowered with authority and responsibility for team-based leadership for patient care and scholarship while fostering a culture that follows that of the parent organizations but allows for attendance to local needs. Frontline clinicians leading local systems and teams have four key tasks: (1) establishing the group's purpose by emphasizing that the goals are shared and the needed actions are collective, (2) ensuring that clinical microsystems can execute to achieve these goals, (3) monitoring system performance, and (4) improving performance.[25] Bohmer notes that this "model of clinical leadership runs counter to much current practice. A focus on promoting collective action, ceding control to the inter-professional team, and showing the way by asking others how to get there are contrary to mainstream medical training and culture and the current tort environment."[28] Leaders must engage collaboratively in leadership education activities to learn to lead change together in the clinical training and cultural and legal environment.

PROGRAMS AND OPPORTUNITIES TO FACILITATE LEARNING TO LEAD CHANGE

In calling for a redesign of professional health education with attention to leadership across the continuum and professions in 2010, Frenk and coauthors echoed or predicted numerous reports and articles demanding curriculum change in undergraduate and/ or graduate education as well as continuing education.[1] In the United States, since the start of the 21st century, there have been numerous calls for leadership education, in some cases with defined competencies, including those from the Institute of Medicine,[29] Nursing Educators,[30] Carnegie Foundation,[31] Association of American Medical Colleges (AAMC),[32] American Association of Colleges of Nursing (AACN),[33] practice programs,[34] and individual States.[35] As an example, the AACN recommended that nursing baccalaureate programs teach "knowledge of the care delivery system, how to work in teams, how to collaborate effectively within and across disciplines, the basic tenets of ethical care, how to be an effective patient advocate, theories of innovation, and the foundations for quality and safety improvement."[36]

Health professions schools are responding with leadership electives, courses, interest groups, mentoring programs and awards, and dual-degree programs. The University of California at Los Angeles (UCLA) School of Medicine has, as an example, developed the PRIME Program, which addresses issues of self-care, burnout, and relationship management, while preparing students for future challenges working with underserved communities.[37] Graduate medical education (GME) programs in the United Kingdom[38] and United States have responded by offering their trainees resident-as-leader training, chief resident professional development, targeted graduate-level leadership programs, and online and library resources about leadership. Dartmouth developed a Leadership Preventive Medicine Residency Program and a Chief Residents Leadership Forum. Duke University created a Management and Leadership Pathway for Residents.[39] Some of the literature suggests, however, that many programs to date do not have evidence of change[40] or are not planned as well as they could be.[41] Nevertheless, the variety of graduate-level programs is evolving quickly. In the future, it will not be enough for a health professional to earn an undergraduate degree and complete a preceptorship or residency and/or fellowship with "some" leadership education and experience. Tomorrow's health system leaders will be expected/required to earn advanced degrees and certificates and/or participate in executive education and CPD programs to lead change.

There is no general repository of advanced leadership education and/or CPD opportunities for health care professionals beyond their preceptorship, residency, and fellowship. However, hundreds of programs and organizations exist worldwide. An overview of some of the degree and certificate programs, executive education/ CPD activities, and professional organizations that academic health system leaders can access for strategic professional development follows. Individuals, including CPD leaders charged to build a new leadership program, should have a working knowledge of these options and be sure sufficient resources exist or are created institutionally (e.g., scholarship, professional development benefits, etc.) to enable attendance or participation.

Health Professions Education

In 2012, Tekain and Harris developed a list of the then 76 masters-level programs in Health Professions Education (HPE) in the world. They provided a table and noted that the programs were maldistributed across Europe, North America, Asia, Latin America, the Middle East, Australia, and Africa.[42] By 2014, however, Tekian and colleagues Roberts, Batty, Cook, and Norcini noted the "proliferation" of Masters degree programs in HPE (MHPE) to 121.[43] These programs teach competencies that prepare graduates to be education leaders, scholars, and innovators "who have the potential to positively transform the education of health professionals, and in turn the future of health care." The authors called the Masters programs the "most visible markers of faculty development" and noted that they are needed to address the "increased globalization of medicine and science." Graduates strengthen academic missions because they "lead education institutions, develop curricular and assessment, and improve instruction and perform research."[43]

Doctoral programs have seen similar growth. In 1998, there were five HPE doctoral programs across the world.[44] As of 2014, there were 24 doctoral programs worldwide that offer a doctor of philosophy (PhD) in HPE, a PhD in Education or Health Sciences, or a doctor of education (EdD) with a concentration in HPE.[45] Some academic institutions train fellows for doctoral degrees in HPE, and some medicine and dentistry degrees focus on education. There is no current, comprehensive table of programs available worldwide, but a table developed in 2014 provides a list with application requirements and 2014 costs.[35] At the time the table was developed, the programs were located in Europe, North America, Africa, Australia, or New Zealand. Applicants from Latin America, the Middle East, and Russian Republics, to date, were required to pursue degrees in these locations.

Business Administration (MBA), Health Administration (MHA), and Health Management

Approximately half of the 145 accredited MD-granting medical schools in the United States offer a combined MD/MBA curriculum.[46] Several of Canada's 17 medical universities (including MD-granting schools plus dentistry, pharmacy, nursing) offer the MD/MBA as well including McGill and Calgary. [http://www.canadian-universities.net/MBA/Health_and_Medical_MBA.html] Ottawa offers an MD/MHA (Masters in Health Administration) and Calgary offers an MBA/MSW (Masters in Social Work). Canadian health professions schools offer a variety of health management degrees including MBAs, MHAs, Masters in Public Health (MPH), and Masters in Public Administration (MPA). [http://www.canadian-universities.net/MBA/Health_and_Medical_MBA.html]   Many young professionals are completing dual-degree programs not available to earlier generations. Some observers argue, however, that taking business or administration courses in medical or other health professions schools, before having professional experience or standing, may not be as useful as earning the degree later.[46]

Weil notes that, based on a 2012 study, the Association of the University Programs in Health Administration (AUPHA) identified 300 Masters-level programs in health science administration in the United States and that these programs graduate over 3,000 students annually in a mix of Masters in Business Administration (MBA), Masters in Public Health (MPA), and Masters in Health Administration (MHA).[46]

Nursing Advanced Degree Options

Nurses with a BSN can, like physicians and others, pursue a Masters degree outside Nursing including the MBA, MPH, and Masters in Health Care Delivery Sciences (MHCDS). They can also earn a Masters in Nursing in a variety of areas of expertise including Leadership, Education, Health Policy, Business, and Advanced Practice. Significant numbers of American nurses now also earn doctoral degrees (PhDs) in Nursing Practice or Executive Leadership among many other fields. These programs are offered with live, hybrid (live and online), or fully online courses.

External Executive Management and Leadership Programs

A popular option for experienced, ascending healthcare professionals is executive MBA programs. Among the institutions in the United States that offer this option live are Harvard, Michigan and Yale, while many universities offer an executive MBA option online.[38] The American College of Physician Executives (ACPE), in conjunction with Carnegie Mellon University, Thomas Jefferson University, University of Massachusetts, and University of Southern California, offers a Masters of Medical Management (MMM) for doctors of medicine and osteopathy only. Dartmouth offers an executive Masters in Public Health online from The Dartmouth Center for Health Policy and Clinical Practice (TDI) for all health professions and a hybrid (live and online) executive Masters in Health Care Delivery Science for midcareer health professionals of all disciplines. In 2017, the University of Pennsylvania plans to launch an online Masters in Health Care Innovation.

Professional associations have executive certificate programs. In the United States, the AAMC offers an executive development seminar in Organizational Leadership in Academic Medicine for Associate Deans and Department Chairs new in their roles, as well as a "Successful Medical School Department Chair" online series. The AAMC also offers the Leadership Education and Development Certificate Program (LEAD). The Executive Leadership in American Medicine (ELAM) program for women in medicine is located at Drexel University. Many medical societies offer fellowships in Leadership, for example the Society of Teachers of Family Medicine's Emerging Leaders and Leading Change Fellowships, and the American College of Physicians' Leadership Academy. Nurses can gain executive skills in programs offered by the American Organization of Nurse Executives (AONE).[33] AONE focuses on a range of competencies from leading oneself, others and the health care environment to leading strategy, human resources, and finance, and understanding health policy, payment reform, value based care, and the regulatory and legal aspects of health care.[22]

Other organizations that guide nurse executives' practice in the United States are the American Nurses Credentialing Center (AANC) which certifies nurses within specialties including the board certified nurse executive, and the Organization for Nurse Leaders (ONL).[33] ONL is aligned with AONE and the Robert Wood Johnson-Institute for Medicine "Campaign for Action" in which states organize specific Action Coalitions to lead nursing and health care initiatives.[33] Many medical and nursing leaders are also members of the Academy of Health Care Executives (ACHE) which provides knowledge of the health care environment critical for roles in the executive suite.

Sigma Theta Tau International (STTI), the international Honor Society of Nursing, is a key promoter of nurse leaders. Founded in 1922 by Indiana University School of Nursing, its mission is to advance world health and celebrate nursing excellence in scholarship, leadership, and service. Members include 135,000 active nurses from across 85 countries, 39% of who have Masters or Doctoral Degrees. There are 500 Sigma Theta Chapters at 695 organizations across the globe. STTI promotes a culture of lifelong learning and inquiry and supports nurses as scholars by offering research programs and supporting the *Journal of Nursing Scholarship* which is a peer reviewed professional journal distributed to over 125,000 nurses globally.[47] In addition to STTI, the International Council of Nurses (ICN) and its Burdett Global Nursing Leadership Institute (GNLI), established 2009, provide leadership development for nurses in senior executive positions who have a "passion for caring for the world's populations" [http://leadership.icn.ch/gnli/]. To lead globally, they are taught policy development and political skills, influence and negotiation, in addition to strategic thinking and an ability to create and maintain alliances, relationships and coalitions.[46,48]

The most up-to-date information about degree and certificate programs, executive education/CPD leadership programs, and professional organizations' offerings worldwide can be found via searches on the Internet.

DESIGNING AND IMPLEMENTING A NEW LEADERSHIP DEVELOPMENT PROGRAM

While a variety of degree, certificate or executive programs and professional organization options are helpful to individual leaders, many academic health systems also desire a customized, internal management and leadership program. Such programs can now be found throughout the world. In the United States and Canada examples exist at Mayo Clinic, Brigham and Women's Hospital, M.D. Anderson Center, Cleveland Clinic Foundation, McGill University, Johns Hopkins, Harvard-Macy Institute, Emory University, University of Washington, Duke University, University of Michigan, Stanford University, University of California Davis, and University of California San Diego.[44] Information about these and other programs can be found at the AAMC's "Medical School Based Career and Leadership Development Programs" List.[32] Dartmouth created an internal program that educates—together—the triads of physician, nursing and administrative leaders empowered with authority and responsibility for team-based leadership of patient care and scholarship. The academic health system leader in the chapter case, charged to "design and implement new leadership development programs" for the academic health system, must first consider her or his unique institutional context, review exemplary programs already in existence, and complete a careful reading of the literature—before building an internal program.

Guidance from the Literature

In 2015, Frich, Brewster, Cherlin, and Bradley completed an extensive systematic review of medical literature published between 1950 and 2013 on physician leadership development programs that included an assessment. The goal was to "characterize the setting, educational content, teaching methods, and learning outcomes achieved."[49] Of the 600 studies the investigators discovered, 45 met their criteria and 35 were studied closely.[50] Most programs used didactics (lecture) with interactive seminars and groups. Very few covered self-reflection, emotional intelligence or collaboration. Reviewers found "that physician leadership development programs are associated with increased self-assessed knowledge and expertise but few studies examined outcomes at a system level." They also found "important educational gaps" including a lack of programs that "integrate non-physician and physician professionals, limited use of more interactive learning and feedback to develop greater self-awareness, and an overly narrow focus on individual-level rather than system-level outcomes."[49]

The reviewers noted that building leadership capacity in groups and organizations includes "promoting a culture of accountability and alignment."[40,51,52] Their review also pointed out that local leadership programs have wide variation of approaches to leadership development among health care organizations.[53] The educational content spanned common topics, including leadership, teamwork, financial management, conflict management, quality improvement, communication, and health policy/strategy. Not unexpectedly, most studies reported basic learning outcomes (reaction to the program or self-reported knowledge). The highest educational outcome, system results/performance, was reported in six studies and included increased quality of care (objective or self-reported), patient satisfaction, advancing to higher leadership roles, or implementation of business plans. In comments on the importance of this review and analysis, Steinhilber and Estrada stated that "the study by Frich et al. supports the belief that physician leadership programs are important for quality of care, professional advancement, and patient satisfaction. It also sheds light on the need for more programs and improved ways to measure outcomes of such programs."[50]

The work of Frich and colleagues was preceded by reviews conducted by Straus, Soobiah, and Levinson in 2013,[54] and by Steinert, Naismith and Mann in 2012.[55] The title of the Straus, Soobiah, and Levinson project was *The impact of leadership training programs on physicians in academic medical centers: a systematic review.* Its purpose was "to identify the impact of leadership training programs at academic medical centers (AMCs) on physicians' knowledge, skills, attitudes, behaviors, and outcomes." In 2011, the authors reviewed studies in MEDLINE, EMBASE, CINAHL, Cochrane Central Register "reporting on the implementation and evaluation of a leadership program for physicians in AMCs." They also consulted experts.[54] From over 2,000 citations they discovered 11 articles about 10 studies that "showed that leadership training programs affected participants' advancement in academic rank (48% vs. 21%, p = 0.005) and hospital leadership position (30% vs. 9%, p = 0.008) and that participants were more successful in publishing papers (3.5 per year vs. 2.1 per year, p < 0.001) compared with nonparticipants."[54] It is important to note that Straus' and colleagues' analysis led to the conclusion "that leadership programs have modest effects on outcomes important to AMCs [academic medical centers]. Given AMCs' substantial investment in these programs, rigorous evaluation of their impact is essential. High-quality studies, including qualitative research, will allow the community to identify which programs are most effective."[54]

Steinert, Naismith, and Mann's study was titled a *Systematic review of Faculty Development initiatives designed to improve leadership abilities.* They synthesized the existing evidence that addressed the question "what are the effects of faculty development interventions designed to improve leadership abilities on the knowledge, attitudes, and skills of faculty members in medicine and on the institutions in which they work?" Their Medline, EMBASE, CINAHL, Web of Science, ERIC, and ABI/Inform search covered the period 1980–2009.[47] From 687 unique records they identified 48 articles that met their criteria and described 41 studies of 35 separate interventions (workshops, short courses, fellowships, and long term programs). Most research methods were quantitative; 12 used mixed methods.[56]

The reviewers' conclusions were that the outcomes of the interventions were that participants found programs to be useful and of both personal and professional benefit; reported positive changes in attitudes toward their own organizations as well as their leadership capabilities; increased knowledge of leadership concepts, principles, and strategies with gains in specific leadership skills (e.g., personal effectiveness and conflict resolution), and increased awareness of leadership roles in academic settings; made self-perceived changes in leadership behavior including changes in leadership styles, and application of new skills to the workplace (e.g., departmental reorganization and team building), adopted new leadership roles and responsibilities, and created new collaborations and networks. Steinert et al. found that key features that led to positive outcomes were "multiple instructional methods within single interventions; experiential learning and reflective practice; individual and group projects; peer support and the development of communities of practice; mentorship; and institutional support."[47] Programs should be grounded in a "theoretical framework; articulate a definition of leadership; consider the role of context; explore the value of extended programs and follow-up sessions; and promote the use of alternative practices including narrative approaches, peer coaching, and team development."[47]

Steinhilber and Estrada summarized the guidance in the two systematic reviews for designing and evaluating leadership development programs. Programs must (1) have a strong study design; (2) define the competencies necessary to succeed as a leader; (3) include other health professionals; and, (4) aim for system and organizational effectiveness outcomes.[50] According to Straus et al., programs should also (1) clearly define the target population and intervention; (2) assess outcomes blindly; (3) and include validated instruments.[41,54] In addition, programs should include qualitative methods for evaluation (case study method or realist evaluation), and mitigate the risk of bias. Reviewers caution implementers not to attribute causality to specific leadership development programs without supporting evidence, which is difficult to obtain.[41,45] Steinhilber and Estrada offer five recommendations for becoming a more effective leader gleaned from the systematic reviews. (1) Learn from peers at regional and national conferences "to gain advice from others on similar paths." (2) Use respected leaders at your institution as role models. (3) Read the work of leadership experts in other disciplines to create a "portfolio of leadership tactics." Consider organizing a Chair's leadership book club and invite junior faculty. Also consider using Steven Sample's *Contrarian's Guide to Leadership*, Jim Collins' *Good to Great*, and Daniel Pink's *Drive*.[57–59] (4) Welcome regular evaluation and make change if necessary. (5) And, most importantly, practice leadership "deliberately."[50]

There are many ways to use a philanthropic gift to design and implement strategic leadership development programs for an academic health system. Before beginning, one must understand *why* strong leaders are needed in the context in which the system is evolving. One must adopt a theory of leadership to guide *how* leaders will be equipped to lead. Health professions' leadership is uniquely challenging. That theory must address leading oneself and others as well as the system within a culture of shared authority—a new mental model that values interdisciplinary and interprofessional leadership teams. One must be familiar with the leadership activities offered at the undergraduate and graduate levels in their organizations and work to complement them. One must be knowledgeable about external and internal degree, certificate and CPD programs, as well

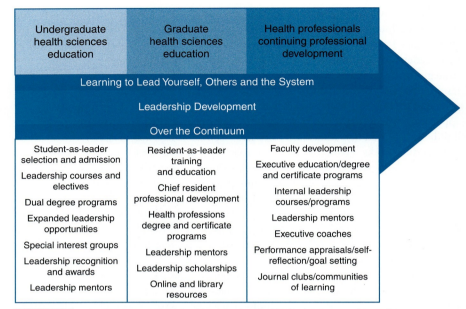

FIGURE 23.1. Leading in an academic health system: Leadership development over the continuum.

as professional organizations, and create or grow resources to underwrite attendance for leaders everywhere in the system—the schools, hospital/medical center, clinical practices, and integrated/affiliated regional health system sites. If a customized, local program is required, assessing exemplars and reviewing the most recent and comprehensive literature can assure success. The 21st century leadership program involves a comprehensive, integrated, robust strategy built across curricula and disciplines. The concept is illustrated in Figure 23.1.

In an era of unprecedented health challenges and threats across the world, such a strategy can meet the challenge to eliminate weak leadership and provide strategic, innovative, and sustainable leadership development education across the academic health system to transform health care.

FUTURE DIRECTIONS

Three issues that will be important in leadership education in academic health systems in the future are committing to interdisciplinary centers of inquiry, matching prowess in translational and implementation science with that in discovery, and endorsing a health system leader–innovator promotion track.

Committing to Interdisciplinary Centers of Inquiry

In the future, academic health systems must commit to inter-disciplinary centers of inquiry that offer mentorship and sponsorship (for scholarships and professional organizational membership) for key clinical team leaders. In many AHSs, extensive support exists for physicians' culture of inquiry and professional development needs. This is not the case with other health professionals' research and practice. Ives Erickson argues that for nurses to join the culture of inquiry fully "it is important to define a strategy that embeds nursing knowledge into clinical practice."[60] She proposes a framework that aligns stakeholders across inter-professional teams to guide professional practice, and an infrastructure "to explore, develop, learn and articulate" the contributions to patient care, the institution, and the profession made by all disciplines.[57]

Nonphysician professionals in specialty areas attend journal clubs, precept students and trainees, attend CPD programs, become specialty certified, and review the literature. As these health professionals do continuous self-improvement, institutions must build a formal infrastructure to grow and develop partnerships for professional development, research, education, and leadership. Partnerships with trained nurse-scientists and pharmacist-scientists, for example, can assist faculty with a research agenda, program of research, or funding for research. Mentorship programs can grow research, contribution to the literature, evidence-based practice, participation in professional organizations, certifications, and leadership work.

Matching Prowess in Translational and Implementation Science with That in Discovery

Engaged leaders are developing the "rapid-learning health systems" of the future "which leverage recent developments in health information technology and a growing health data infrastructure to access and apply evidence in real time, while simultaneously drawing knowledge from real-world care-delivery processes to promote innovation and health system change on the basis of rigorous research."[61] In an extension of the conceptualization of rapid learning, current challenges to be addressed include "implementing a new clinical research system with several hundred million patients, modernizing clinical trials and registries, devising and funding research on national priorities, and analyzing genetic and other factors that influence diseases and response to treatment."[60]

Next steps should also aim to improve comparative effectiveness research; build on investments in health information technology to standardize handling of genetic information and support information exchange through apps and software modules; and develop new tools, data, and information for clinical decision support. Further advances will require "commitment, leadership, and public-private and global collaboration."[62] Our academic health systems must develop leaders who contribute to the discovery and translation of new knowledge from real-world data for the improved benefit of the populations they serve. The Institute of Medicine defines a Learning Health System as "one in which knowledge generation is so embedded into the core of the practice of medicine that it is a natural outgrowth and product of the healthcare delivery process and leads to continual improvement in care."[63] "Academic health centers must match their prowess in the science of discovery with an equally earnest effort in translational and implementation science focused on health system improvement."[64]

Endorsing a Health Systems Leader–Innovator Promotion Track

One issue that has prevented some clinicians from taking on leadership roles has been the lack of perceived value that these activities have toward academic promotion when compared with traditional measurements of scholarship like publications, funded research, and teaching. "Academic health centers have traditionally used their promotions criteria to signal their values; creating a health systems innovator promotion track could be a critical step towards creating opportunities for innovators in academic medicine."[65] Adding the attribution and measurement of innovation in leadership to the standard promotions criteria will encourage more activity by clinicians in expanding system-wide administrative roles. Most progressive academic health systems have created innovation or value institutes with rapid deployment teams for implementing processes of change. Leaders have challenges to engage their staff and colleagues in improvement efforts directed by analytics and measurement, and spread the innovations across the network region. The "creation of a work environment that builds on mutually respectful relationships and valued interdependencies" has supporting evidence for effect, and a conceptual framework to enhance provider engagement employing *practice talk* has been recently proposed.[66]

Leaders will also need to address how value-based care may impact the education of medical and other health profession students, and the training of residents and fellows and other learners, "in environments where there may be less autonomy and more standardization."[67] That there will be many opportunities to demonstrate leadership innovation in academic health systems should not be in doubt. Disruptive innovation will be needed to balance the tensions of preparing for accountability and value-driven payment models while continuing the tertiary care academic referral business model.[68] The effect of health reform on academic health centers was summarized recently into six formidable challenges: finding the best mission balance; preparing for the era of no open ended funding; developing an integrated, inter-professional vision; broadening the institutional perspective; addressing health beyond clinical care; and, finding the right leadership for the times."[69] The authors posit that "search committees used to seek out the most distinguished researchers to head their institutions; current realities require search committees to prioritize considerations like management skills, relationship building, and emotional intelligence." Once the right leaders are hired and developed, they must be promoted.

R E F E R E N C E S

1. Frenk J, Chen L, Bhutta ZA, et al. Health professionals for a new century: transforming education to strengthen health systems in an interdependent world. *Lancet.* 2010;376(9756):1923–1958.
2. Flexner A, Pritchet H, Henry S. *Medical Education in the United States and Canada Bulletin Number Four (the Flexner Report).* New York: The Carnegie Foundation for the Advancement of Teaching; 1910.
3. Welch WH, Rose W. *Institute of Hygiene: A Report to the General Education Board of Rockefeller Foundation.* New York: The Rockefeller Foundation; 1915.
4. Committee for the Study of Nursing Education, Goldmark JC. *Nursing and Nursing Education in the United States: Report of the Committee for the Study of Nursing Education, and Report of a Survey by Josephine Goldmark, Secretary.* New York: MacMillan Company; 1923.
5. Regehr G. It's NOT rocket science: rethinking our metaphors for research in health professions education. *Med Educ.* 2010;44(1):31–39.
6. Northouse PG. *Leadership: Theory and Practice.* Thousand Oaks, CA: Sage Publications; 2015.
7. French JR, Raven B. The bases of social power. *Classics of Organization Theory.* In: Cartwright D, ed. Ann Arbor, MI: Institute of Social Research; 1959:311–320.

8. Raven BH. The bases of power: origins and recent developments. *J Soc Iss.* 1993;49(4):227–251.
9. Gabel S. Perspective: physician leaders and their bases of power: common and disparate elements. *Acad Med.* 2012;87(2):221–225.
10. Souba WW. The leadership dilemma. *J Surg Res.* 2007;138(1):1–9.
11. Souba C. Leading again for the first time. *J Surg Res.* 2009;157(2):139–153.
12. Souba WW. The being of leadership. *Philos Ethics Humanit Med.* 2011;6:5.
13. Souba WW. The science of leading yourself: a missing piece in the health care transformation puzzle. *Open J Leader.* 2013;2(3):45.
14. Bennis WG. *On Becoming a Leader.* New York: Addison-Wesley Publishing Co.; 1994.
15. Goleman D. *What Makes a Leader: Why Emotional Intelligence Matters,* 1st ed. Florence, MA: More Than Sound; 2014.
16. Salovey P, Mayer J. Emotional intelligence. *Imagin Cogn Pers.* 1989;9:185–211.
17. Lobas JG. Leadership in academic medicine: capabilities and conditions for organizational success. *Am J Med.* 2006;119(7):617–621.
18. Mintz LJ, Stoller JK. A systematic review of physician leadership and emotional intelligence. *J Grad Med Educ.* 2014;6(1):21–31.
19. Dine CJ, Kahn JM, Abella BS, et al. Key elements of clinical physician leadership at an academic medical center. *J Grad Med Educ.* 2011;3(1):31–36.
20. Frankel A. What leadership styles should senior nurses develop. *Nurs Times.* 2011;104(35):23–24.
21. Frandsen B. *Nursing Leadership: Management and Leadership Styles.* AANAC; 2014:1–11.
22. Sherman R, Pross E. Growing future nurse leaders to build and sustain healthy work environments at the unit level. *Online J Issues Nurs.* 2010;15(1).
23. Guyton N. Revitalized practice? Take nine. *Nurs Manag (Springhouse).* 2007;38(4):67–69. http://ovidsp.ovid.com/ovidweb.cgi?T=JS&NEWS=n&CSC=Y&PAGE=fulltext&D=ovft&AN=00006247-200704000-00015. doi:10.1097/01.NUMA.0000266725.17137.f3.
24. Comack MT. A journey of leadership: from bedside nurse to chief executive officer. *Nurs Adm Q.* 2012;36(1):29–34.
25. Naylor CD. Leadership in academic medicine: reflections from administrative exile. *Clin Med.* 2006;6(5):488–492.
26. Bachrach DJ. Developing physician leaders in academic medical centers. Part 1: their changing role. *Med Group Manage J.* 1995;43(6):8, 40, 44.
27. Huston C. Preparing nurse leaders for 2020. *J Nurs Manag.* 2008;16(8):905–911.
28. Institute of Medicine. Transforming leadership. In: *The Future of Nursing: Leading Change, Advancing Health.* Washington, DC: National Academies Press; 2011:221–251.
29. Bohmer RM. Leading clinicians and clinicians leading. *N Engl J Med.* 2013;368(16):1468–1470.
30. Institute of Medicine. *Crossing the Quality Chasm: A New Health System for the 21st Century,* 1st ed. Washington, DC: National Academy Press; 2001:1–8.
31. Fitzpatrick JJ. The future of nursing: leading change, advancing health. *Nurs Educ Perspect.* 2010;31(6):347–348.
32. Cooke M, Irby DM, O'Brien BC. *Educating Physicians: A Call for Reform of Medical School and Residency,* Vol. 16. John Wiley & Sons; 2010.
33. *Medical School Based Career and Leadership Development Programs.* Washington, DC: Association of American Medical Colleges; 2011:1–54.
34. American Organization of Nurse Executives. *Nurse Manager Skills Inventory.* Washington, DC: Nurse Manager Leadership Partnership; 2006.
35. O'Connell MT, Pascoe JM. Undergraduate medical education for the 21st century: leadership and teamwork. *Fam Med.* 2004;36(suppl):51.
36. *Creativity and Connections: Building the Framework for the Future of Nursing Education and Practice.* Massachusetts Organization of Nurse Executives; 2010:1–51.
37. Warde CM, Vermillion M, Uijtdehaage S. A medical student leadership course led to teamwork, advocacy, and mindfulness. *Fam Med.* 2014;46(6):459–462.
38. Bekas S. Leadership development in UK medical training: pedagogical theory and practice. *Teach Learn Med.* 2015;27(1):4–11.
39. Ackerly DC, Sangvai DG, Udayakumar K, et al. Training the next generation of physician-executives: an innovative residency pathway in management and leadership. *Acad Med.* 2011;86(5):575–579.
40. Malling B, Mortensen L, Bonderup T, et al. Combining a leadership course and multi-source feedback has no effect on leadership skills of leaders in postgraduate medical education. An intervention study with a control group. *BMC Med Educ.* 2009;9(1):1.
41. Fraser TN, Blumenthal DM, Bernard K, et al. Assessment of leadership training needs of internal medicine residents at the Massachusetts general hospital. *Proc (Bayl Univ Med Cent).* 2015;28(3):317–320.

42. Tekian A, Harris I. Preparing health professions education leaders worldwide: a description of masters-level programs. *Med Teach.* 2012;34(1):52–58.

43. Tekian A, Roberts T, Batty HP, et al. Preparing leaders in health professions education. *Med Teach.* 2014;36(3):269–271.

44. Cusimano MD, David MA. A compendium of higher education opportunities in health professions education. *Acad Med.* 1998;73(12):1255–1259.

45. Tekian A. Doctoral programs in health professions education. *Med Teach.* 2014;36(1):73–81.

46. Weil TP. Leadership in academic health centers in the US: a review of the role and some recommendations. *Health Serv Manage Res.* 2014;27(1–2):22–32.

47. Sigma theta tau/NLN grant. (resource center)(sigma theta tau international foundation for nursing/national league for nursing). *Nurs Educ Perspect.* 2007;28(2):103.

48. Ferguson SL. The ICN-burdett global nursing leadership institute creates outstanding world class nurse executives. *Nurse Leader.* 2015;13(5):49–51.

49. Frich JC, Brewster AL, Cherlin EJ, et al. Leadership development programs for physicians: a systematic review. *J Gen Intern Med.* 2015;30(5):656–674.

50. Steinhilber S, Estrada CA. To lead or not to lead? Structure and content of leadership development programs. *J Gen Intern Med.* 2015;30(5):543–545.

51. Conger JA, Benjamin B. *Building Leaders: How Successful Companies Develop the Next Generation.* 1999.

52. Gronn P. Distributed leadership as a unit of analysis. *Leadership Quart.* 2002;13(4):423–451.

53. Anderson MM, Garman AN. *Leadership Development in Healthcare Systems: Toward an Evidence-Based Approach.* National Center for Healthcare Leadership; 2014:1–18.

54. Straus SE, Soobiah C, Levinson W. The impact of leadership training programs on physicians in academic medical centers: a systematic review. *Acad Med.* 2013;88(5):710–723.

55. Steinert Y, Naismith L, Mann K. Faculty development initiatives designed to promote leadership in medical education. A BEME systematic review: BEME guide no. 19. *Med Teach.* 2012;34(6):483–503.

56. Steinert Y, Mann K, Centeno A, et al. A systematic review of faculty development initiatives designed to improve teaching effectiveness in medical education: BEME guide no. 8. *Med Teach.* 2006;28(6):497–526.

57. Sample S. *Contrain's Guide to Leadership,* 1st ed. Jossey-Bass; 2002.

58. Collins JC. *Good to Great,* 1st ed. New York: HarperBusiness; 2001.

59. Pink DH. *Drive.* Edinburgh [u.a.]: Canongate Books; 2010.

60. Erickson JI. Reflections on leadership talent: a void or an opportunity? *Nursing Adm Q.* 2013;37(1):44. http://www.ncbi.nlm.nih.gov/pubmed/23222753

61. Greene SM, Reid RJ, Larson EB. Implementing the learning health system: from concept to action. *Ann Intern Med.* 2012;157(3):207–210.

62. Etheredge LM. Rapid learning: a breakthrough agenda. *Health Aff (Millwood).* 2014;33(7):1155–1162.

63. *The Learning Healthcare System: Workshop Summary.* Institute of Medicine; 2007.

64. Grumbach K, Lucey CR, Johnston SC. Transforming from centers of learning to learning health systems: the challenge for academic health centers. *JAMA.* 2014;311(11):1109–1110.

65. Ellner AL, Stout S, Sullivan EE, et al. Health systems innovation at academic health centers: leading in a new era of health care delivery. *Acad Med.* 2015;90(7):872–880.

66. Hess DW, Reed VA, Turco MG, et al. Enhancing provider engagement in practice improvement: a conceptual framework. *J Contin Educ Health Prof.* 2015;35(1):71–79.

67. Pines JM, Farmer SA, Akman JS. "Innovation" institutes in academic health centers: enhancing value through leadership, education, engagement, and scholarship. *Acad Med.* 2014;89(9):1204–1206.

68. Stein D, Chen C, Ackerly DC. Disruptive innovation in academic medical centers: balancing accountable and academic care. *Acad Med.* 2015;90(5):594–598.

69. Wartman SA, Zhou Y, Knettel AJ. Health reform and academic health centers: commentary on an evolving paradigm. *Acad Med.* 2015;90(12):1587–1590.

Chapter 24

ARTICULATING *the* VALUE *of* CONTINUING MEDICAL EDUCATION

Todd Dorman

Case

As chair of the CME/CPD committee, you have invited your organization's CEO to attend one of your monthly meetings. The goal is to demonstrate to him the following CME values: accomplishments of your program over a set period of time; what its potential is in both the short and long term; and what are its needs to be successful—financial, logistical, human, and cultural. You are apprehensive, since funding for other programs is being either cut or taken away altogether.

Questions

How would you organize the presentation to be an effective, coordinated statement of the value of CME/CPD? What are the elements you need to consider for a continued dialog to achieve your goal? Who are the key stakeholders who need to hear this message after you gain the CEO's interest?

INTRODUCTION

We all want value for our effort whether that effort is based on energy, time, or money. This is true in our personal and professional lives. Consequently, the same is true for administrators and our health system. Value from the effort to improve is critical. Without such value, it can be hard to justify ongoing contributions of energy, time, and money. In addition to what we on the health system side value, the patient and family expect certain values as well. For these latter stakeholders, value is so important that loss of value translates into loss of trust. Consequently, we need to understand the value of CME/CPD from each stakeholder's perspective (Fig. 24.1). This chapter will address what we understand about value in the CME/CPD field. By the end of this chapter, you should be able to describe the value of CME/CPD, its effectiveness, and its ability to be a strategic lever for improvement and a strategic imperative for

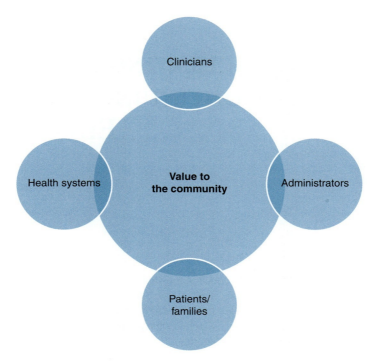

FIGURE 24.1. Value perspectives.

protecting the public trust. Since the value proposition is dependent on local context, the principles described herein are applicable nationally and internationally. In addition, you should have a better understanding of how to present this material to your organizational leadership.

WHAT DO WE MEAN BY VALUE?

Although value is most commonly defined from an economic perspective as a ratio of quality to cost (Value = Quality/Cost), it actually has many dimensions and such a narrow perspective, as defined economically, simply does not do it justice. As implied above, at the opposite end of the spectrum from such a purely economic perspective is the fact that value is in the eye of the beholder and thus is associated with an emotive response like trust (Fig. 24.2).

The major definitions for value, from a business perspective, fall into the following categories[1]:

- **General**: Price × Quantity = Value
- **Accounting**: Monetary worth of an asset, business entity, or service.
- **Economics**: Worth of all the benefits and rights arising from ownership. Refers to intrinsic value.

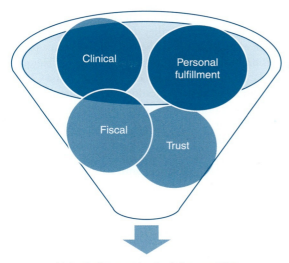

Value is the promise to deliver and the
belief by the recipient that it will indeed
be experienced

FIGURE 24.2.   The value proposition.

- **Marketing**: Extent to which a good or service is perceived by its customer to meet his or her needs or wants, measured by customer's willingness to pay for it. It commonly depends more on the customer's perception of the worth of the product than on its intrinsic value.
- **Mathematics**: Magnitude or quantity as in a numbers.

Obviously, each of these definitions comes into play in different circumstances and possibly by different stakeholders. Given the complexity of the health environment and the need for a balanced perspective across stakeholders, the most important definition is actually an integration across these categories. This integrated definition is important because it encompasses the monetary considerations important to the payers for CME/CPD, the benefits to the provider and patient, and the intrinsic value that is connected to public trust. Such an integrated definition also allows for a full appreciation of the value of CME/CPD.

It is important to recognize that the concept of value can also be viewed from a business model perspective. In such an analysis, one considers the drivers of revenue and expense and then can categorize different models or centers. The most common types of centers are

- Profit center
- Cost center
- Investment center
- Revenue center

Historically, the most common type that was applied to CME/CPD was a profit center.[2] There are numerous problems with this historic approach. A profit center controls all aspects of revenue and expense, and thus all aspects of margin or profitability are controlled. In many circumstance in CME/CPD, this is simply not true. An activity director may have a significant say over the cost of an activity as they determine the registration fee based upon their perception of the market. In addition, they may insist upon a paper syllabus as compared to an online version or may insist upon a certain level of banquet services, all of which drive cost and make it out of the independent control of the CME/CPD unit. Alternatively, like in a for-profit Medical Education and Communication company, it is very appropriate to function as a profit center for obvious reasons.

It is important to note that being a profit center typically includes establishing a targeted margin. Such approaches can potentially put the very nature of the required independence from industry at question. The pressure to make a certain margin places a pressure on decision-making that subconsciously can impact contracting on the revenue or expense side, and such pressure should be minimized or avoided. Finally, it should be noted that from a pure terminology perspective, one cannot be a profit center in a not-for-profit environment.

The model most suited, especially in academic health systems and professional societies, for CME/CPD is as a value center. A value center is a subtype of a cost center. A cost center does not have to finish the fiscal year with expense in excess of revenue, but can in fact generate a positive margin. That may seem counterintuitive, but the concept of a cost center is that they can't and don't control all the sources of revenue and expense and thus are at risk of having a balanced or negative margin. Thus, being a cost center does carry some risk. When finances get tight, money management principles dictate that one try to find expenses to eliminate as one can usually enact cuts immediately, whereas revenue enhancement takes time. That being said, being a cost center that indeed breaks even or has a positive margin offers some protection. Importantly, being a cost center that can demonstrate value is critical to long-term survival. This is where the integrated definition comes into play. In many circumstances, the value may occur in a different budget merely from bookkeeping practice or the value may be secondary to cost avoidance.

For example, meeting attendance might be booked under meeting budgets or in a marketing budget or possibly even under a membership budget as can be seen in professional societies. Thus, the value realized can appear in someone else's budget. There are bookkeeping methods to address this through allocation of revenue or cost models, but in the end, the activity was bringing value that may not have been recognized. An example of intrinsic value is when we educate, develop, and improve the performance of our own health system. Thus, for many stakeholders, the value from CME/CPD can be seen in enhanced effectiveness and efficiency. These also might accrue benefit to a different budget, possibly even a budget of a different but related corporation, such as when a health system benefits based upon work the school has performed.

VALUE AS DEFINED BY EFFECTIVENESS

There are many who would argue that measuring effectiveness is the first step to determining if CME/CPD has value. Despite what some continue to insinuate, evidence of the impact and effectiveness of CME/CPD already exists and in some domains is quite strong.

Approximately one decade ago, a monograph on the effectiveness of CME/CPD was published. The monograph was the end product of work done through an evidence-based practice center and as such was funded through the AHRQ.[3] The results were clear. Despite the fact that CME/CPD historically utilized few adult education principles, the literature supported the fact that CME/CPD was indeed effective. The level of effectiveness was different depending on whether one evaluated knowledge exchange and retention or practice change and patient outcome. These results have been supported by a number of other publications and a Cochrane review.[4]

CME/CPD is effective, but there is a still a large opportunity to improve. CME was designed originally to be focused solely on physician education and not interprofessional education. CME/CPD was designed to focus on knowledge improvement and not on performance improvement.[5] This is not because CME/CPD in its earlier years ignored or missed the value of showing the linkage between education and outcomes, but because few in health care education were focused on outcomes and most did not even believe that outcome metrics could be crafted and implemented.

CME/CPD is well suited to provide high-quality education utilizing active teaching and learning methodologies and a broad array of instructional designs. It can provide awareness of problems and new information. CME/CPD can utilize simulation for interprofessional training and task training. It can facilitate ethics education and has been shown to enhance openness to change and self-transcendence.[6]

VALUE TO CLINICIANS

Clinicians value CME/CPD from a more personal perspective. The vast majority of health care providers are dedicated to improvement, and education plays a central role in their ability to improve. Education helps them understand their present performance and the gap to the ideal, and then education can help move them to close that gap.

This dedication to improvement is an internal motivator. Importantly, clinicians have a strong desire for their patients to improve, and thus CME/CPD has value to physicians based upon the connection between lifelong learning and improvement. Additionally, most physicians value knowledge even for knowledge sake. In other words, they love to learn.

Physicians also believe that CME/CPD helps demonstrate their commitment to themselves and thus their patients. Consequently, CME/CPD is also valued as a support mechanism for reputation of the individual and the profession. Wenghofer and colleagues have shown that physicians who participate in CME/CPD are less likely to receive quality of care complaints (OR 0.604; $p = 0.028$).[7]

Academic physicians also value activities that are supportive of their development and the development of others. Thus, CME/CPD becomes a tool they utilize to educate the team and others. It is a tool to share experiences and help focus on case-based and problem-based patient care solutions. Through teaching in CME/CPD activities, academic physicians can add to their ability to be promoted, especially if such educational opportunities happen on a national and international basis.

Finally, physicians have to meet ever-increasing regulatory burdens. CME/CPD is valued for its ability to help physicians meet such burdens while staying focused at improvements in performance and outcome. These burdens come from The Joint Commission in the form of ongoing professional practice evaluations, state licensure requirements from state boards, hospital credentialing requirements, and Maintenance of Certification (MOC) requirements for ongoing board certification.

VALUE TO ADMINISTRATORS

Historically, many administrators merely saw CME/CPD as a profit center. I have addressed why this is not correct and why it might create a subconscious ethical dilemma. Administrators, though, are indeed stakeholders in this domain, and they need and should expect certain returns, especially if they are investing in the cost of CME/CPD. From a pure staff development issue, they will easily understand the need to invest in the ongoing professional development of all team members. It was once famously stated that we need to invest in our staff even though they then decide to leave for a job elsewhere, because we should never forget what would happen if we don't invest in them and they then choose to stay. What does need to change, though, is that they need to not only invest in staff but invest in the team and thus the need for more interprofessional education. The translation to effectiveness and efficiency will be easily addressed under such an approach.

Business office leadership frequently determines value by calculating a return on investment, and when considering the outcomes of education, this approach may not be practical. Investing in the team has some inherent costs. What is important is that a return on education should be considered. That return might include revenue in other domains like quality indicator reimbursement, which we will discuss in a subsequent section. Importantly, cost avoidance can mitigate some of the expenses and is frequently not appreciated. For example, if all physicians in a health organization had to go off-site and possibly even out of state to garner enough credits at high-quality CME/CPD with objectives that match those of the individual and their organization, then those costs might be avoided by offering CME/CPD locally. Furthermore, time away from practice can impact practice revenue. Avoidance of that loss of revenue is just the type of hidden cost that can be easily missed when considering a return on investment/education.

Finally, health organizations are a business in the community. Administrators should also consider value to the community. One such value is indeed a fiscal value. Visitors coming to attend CME/CPD activities typically spend money in the community. Contacting the local or state travel and tourism board to learn how much on average an in-state and out-of-state visitor brings as a margin the community can be eye opening. Even if the calculation is small, the fact remains that the CME/CPD enterprise is indeed contributing, on behalf of the parent organization, to the community in real and tangible ways. In fact, often local and state government officials will ask organizations like health systems how they contribute, and this fiscal contribution is often overlooked. It should be noted that utilization of community resources supports employment in the community and can also contribute to the reputation of the community as a destination.

VALUE TO HEALTH SYSTEMS

Not only can the reputation of the community be enhanced, but the reputation of the health system is increased as providers not affiliated with the health system have chosen to seek education from them. This is true whether the individuals have traveled to attend live conferences, workshops, or simulations or whether that interaction was supported through other media such as on-demand material available on the Web.

Internally, the health system can and will benefit from the opportunity to train teams in interprofessional activities. As care is delivered by a team, training staff to interact professionally, to communicate effectively, and to function in an interdisciplinary manner is associated with enhanced patient outcomes. Such an approach might also contribute to employee engagement and satisfaction and contribute to reductions in turnover. Such reductions can be associated with reduced quality/safety events and reductions in the inherent cost of staff replacement.

Educational approaches that bring providers together enhance communication and support longitudinal care models. Familiarity with the needs and abilities of other providers allows providers to better prepare patients and families for ongoing supportive care across the continuum.

However, education should never be done to garner referrals as this is not acceptable by ethical or regulatory standards. High-quality education might naturally impact referrals. For example, if providers learn how to improve their care at an educational activity and see the educator/speaker/facilitator as approachable, they may choose of their own volition to refer a patient with a medical problem appropriate for that provider or specialist. Additional referrals occur only if certain conditions are met. The referred patient should be helped by the referral, the patient should be satisfied with the care provided, and the patient should be returned to the primary provider. In addition, the referring physician should receive a written communication regarding what care transpired and ongoing recommendations regarding care. As stated, although referrals should not be an aim of education, education about when to and when not to refer patients is acceptable as such knowledge should enhance care.

CME/CPD can and does help retrain and remediate providers who have left the field for a variety of reasons and are now ready to return. Such approaches can help health systems through the return of highly experienced individuals, in supporting diversity efforts, and can be especially useful in specialties in which shortages already exist. In addition, CME/CPD can help support education that allows individuals to assume new roles within the health system, thus translating experience and dedication into development growth. Finally, education can be a strategic tool to accomplish high-value care.

VALUE TO PATIENTS/FAMILIES

Patients and their families value CME for the trust it engenders as clinicians demonstrate their dedication to personal growth and improvement. The knowledge that their physicians are working hard to stay abreast of new innovations in health and wellness allows for confidence in their health care team. It supports their need for ensuring they receive the best treatments in a timely fashion.

There are those that argue that the public expects physicians to be at the top of their game through ongoing education efforts and so that they really do not value it. This seems to be an oversimplification. Patients would be disappointed to learn that their physician is not engaging in such ongoing iterative development. Patients expect their physicians to be so engaged and the knowledge of that engagement can indeed be reassuring.

VALUE TO COMMUNITIES

As previously mentioned, there is economic value to the local and state economy. That value can be calculated in the manner described. When marketing the educational activity, one simultaneously is marketing the location. This can enhance the image of the locale as well. Additionally, there are other benefits to the community that would be valued, including enhanced relationships. General education activities might enhance the relationship and provide additional value. For example, a number of CME/CPD providers run mini–medical school courses for the community to improve medical understanding especially for the media.

IN SUMMARY

CME/CPD has been shown to be effective. In health systems, communities of practice, and other health care settings, CME/CPD is the only viable means of education and communication. While other methods can be brought into play (the weekly newsletter from the CEO), nothing can match the performance-enhancing role of thoughtful, accredited CME/CPD. It brings value to the physicians, the health system, the community, and most importantly the patients and their families.

PRESENTING YOUR CASE

The type of presentation and content of the presentation are dependent upon the audience. Clinicians tend to principally want to see clinical data but are accepting of satisfaction data, whereas fiscally oriented individuals want to see new revenue, avoided expense, or risk mitigation. Most leaders like short presentations. Frequently, a successful strategy is to have a handout that has more material than is being presented. The additional material should include background data and more in-depth data. The in-depth data should be included in anticipation of additional questions. All data should be benchmarked if possible. Stressing how performance and outcomes align with organizational strategic priorities is usually quite fruitful.

FUTURE DIRECTIONS

Predicting the future of value assessment in CME/CPD is easy. There are a few areas that it seems obvious what will happen. These include additional studies evaluating effectiveness of models of education with the goal being finding the most efficacious strategies in order to maximize value, no matter the definition. Such studies are needed by educational providers, by administrators, and by health systems. Even patients and families would want such information to know that their physicians are utilizing the best approaches to provide them with the best treatment. There also will be a growth of on-demand education and a drop in multiday live meetings. The on-demand material will be supportive off-line and at the point of care. There will be links built into EMR to facilitate access in situ and just in time.

The costs associated with live meetings can be significant, and the time away from practice can be difficult. Utilizing mixed instructional methodologies with mixed media will be the approach in the future. For example, a 4-day live course would be converted to a half-day live activity that is more workshop, hands on, and small group exercises sandwiched between print material in advance of these workshops and then case vignettes several months later to evaluate for retention and to reinforce knowledge and the ability to apply what was learned.

Given the need to provide care across the longitudinal axis, there will be a growth in education designed to integrate thoughts, experience, and knowledge base across providers from different time frames of care. For instance, the work being done in post–intensive care syndrome will lead to a better understanding of these patients and lead to strategies to mitigate long-term events through such strategies deployed during critical illness. This will require these providers to work together and thus to educate together.[8,9]

Associated with such a need will be a growth in interprofessional education. The team performance will be critical in the care of patients, and leveraging the right team member at the right time will be vitally important. Each team member will need to be able to function at the upper end of his or her field, but not in isolation. Thus, they will not simply need to be educated together but to practice problem solving together in a true interprofessional manner.

Financial models of education started shifting almost a decade ago, and based upon data from the ACCME, it appears that they continue to shift. There is less funding from industry and a concomitant growth in funding from physicians or their employers. As this shift occurs, each of these groups will want to get the maximum amount of value for what they spend, and so the value of CME/CPD will grow in importance as these funding models shift.

Finally, there will be a growth in improvement-focused CME. In part, this will be connected to MOC for some boards and consequently will facilitate physician regulatory burden. In addition, such an approach will help get every member of the team focused at improvement and knowledgeable in improvement sciences. Significant benefits to patient care should ensue. Improvement in domains measured by payment-associated quality indicators will provide a feedback to the new funders that will be greatly appreciated.

REFERENCES

1. http://www.businessdictionary.com/definition/value.html. Accessed June 30, 2016.
2. http://www.dummies.com/how-to/content/managerial-accounting-types-of-responsibility-cent.html. Accessed June 30, 2016.
3. Marinopolous SS, Dorman T, Ratanawongsa N, et al. The Effectiveness of CME. *AHRQ Evidence Reports and Technology Assessments No. 149*. 2007. http://archive.ahrq.gov/downloads/pub/evidence/pdf/cme/cme.pdf
4. Forsetlund L, Bjørndal A, Rashidian A, et al. Continuing education meetings and workshops for health professionals. *Cochrane Database Syst Rev.* 2009;(2):CD003030.

5. Legare F, Freitas A, Thompson-Leduc P, et al. The majority of accredited continuing professional development activities do not target clinical behavior change. *Acad Med.* 2015;90:197–202.

6. Altamirano-Bustamante MM, Altamirano-Bustamante NF, Lifshitz A, et al. Promoting networks between evidence-based medicine and values-based medicine in continuing medical education. *BMC Med.* 2013;11:39.

7. Wenghofer EF, Campbell C, Marlow B, et al. The effect of continuing professional development on public complaints: a case–control study. *Med Educ.* 2015;49:264–275.

8. Jensen JF, Thomsen T, Overgaard D, et al. Impact of follow up consultations for IC survivors on post-ICU syndrome. A systematic review and meta-analysis. *Intensive Care Med.* 2015;41(5):763–775.

9. Elliott D, Davidson JE, Harvey MA, et al. Exploring the scope of post-intensive care syndrome therapy and care: engagement of non-critical care providers and survivors in a second stakeholder meeting. *Crit Care Med.* 2014;41(12):2518–2526.

Chapter 25

PRINCIPLES *of* EFFECTIVE RESEARCH *in* CONTINUING PROFESSIONAL DEVELOPMENT *in* *the* HEALTH PROFESSIONS

Curtis A. Olson and Betsy White Williams

Case

As you review the annual report of your unit—outlining the year's achievements relative to the number of programs, their attendees, the scope and breadth of topics covered, summaries of the countless evaluations, results of accreditation processes—several thoughts occur to you. What was the impact of your program overall? How might you evaluate its effect on each attendee? These questions, and many others, lead naturally to a discussion of research, something not in your comfort zone. In these changing times, evidence of the presence or effect of lifelong learning is critical/important.

Questions

What are the core principles of effective educational research? How can those principles be used to guide learners who attend your programs? Are needs being met at the patient, provider, and system levels?

INTRODUCTION

This case scenario speaks to the relevance of research to educational practice. A primary focus of research efforts in the field of continuing professional development (CPD) is producing knowledge, theories, and heuristics that increase our understanding of learning, teaching, and education and give guidance to our efforts to help others learn. Many research skills and methods can be used to enhance educational program evaluation as well. We begin this chapter by exploring the linkages between research and evaluation in some depth.

It has been said that developing an effective educational program is often less like engineering a superhighway than finding one's way through a swamp, a step at a time.[1] Oxman et al.'s[2] review of 102 studies on the effectiveness of various types of educational interventions led them to conclude there is no *magic bullet*—no single intervention or combination of interventions that will be effective in all situations. Subsequent reviews of the literature (e.g., Cervero and Gaines' 2014 review of literature reviews of CPD effectiveness[3]) have supported this conclusion.

Thought leaders in medical education research have attributed this inability to identify proven, reproducible educational interventions that succeed independent of context to variability—differences in how a given intervention is implemented across sites, differences in learners, and the inherent complexity of the social context.[4] There are many variables associated with an educational intervention and the environment in which it is implemented, and interaction of these variables can produce different effects.[5] Traynor and Eva put it this way:

> The fact that my workshop yielded beneficial learning outcomes cannot be expected to have a great impact on other educators, as it will be virtually impossible for me to explain and explore every specific aspect of the educational experience. Relevant variables include the content covered, the way it was delivered, my enthusiasm as the instructor, the motivation and emotions of the students, the link between each of those factors and the students' previous experiences with me and with other educational activities.[6] (p. 213)

This is especially true in situations characterized by high complexity,[7] such as an effort to directly improve clinical practice using an interprofessional education intervention. When the subject matter is straightforward, the intended educational outcome is modest (e.g., knowledge gain), and we have a high degree of control over the key factors in the learning environment (as would be the case for a computer-based educational program designed to teach individuals basic concepts of quality improvement), the level of complexity is relatively low. Under these circumstances, the research evidence (see, for example, Means et al.[8]) and resources such as instructional design models[9] provide us with useful guidance. However, as the complexity of the educational problem increases (e.g., as the emphasis shifts to how to get clinicians to complete our computer-based educational program or to how to empower clinical teams to change their practice), the evidence base is less helpful.[9]

As educators, in complex situations we can draw on the available research evidence and integrate that information with best practice, model programs, theory, expert advice, and our own experience to develop an intervention. However, in the end, we must be empiricists who are able to integrate research and evaluation, to combine *evidence-based practice* and *practice-based evidence*. That is, we must use the best available evidence to design the intervention, put it to the test, examine the results, learn what we can, and make adjustments to the intervention and the mental schema that guide our practice. However, our capacity to obtain and use evaluation data to determine if an intervention is working the way it is supposed to—a critical component in an empirical approach to designing effective programs—is underdeveloped. It is difficult to learn from experience and make progress if we lack information telling us if we have fallen face-first into the swamp or are standing on solid ground. As models such Shewhart's Plan–Do–Check–Act cycle[10] or Kolb's experiential learning cycle[11] demonstrate, evaluation plays critical role in the process of monitoring the outcomes and impact of interventions and learning how to make educational interventions more effective.

The implication is that to optimize the value of CPD as a means of improving clinical practice and patient outcomes, there is a pressing need to expand our capacity to conduct targeted and useful evaluations of educational interventions. As a field, we need a cadre of experienced, skilled people who, working as part of a team, can develop evaluations tailored to the specific context. They must be able to define evaluation questions, collect and analyze data, interpret and report the results, and consider the implications for future practice. *The critical point is that there is substantial overlap in the knowledge and skills needed for evaluation and those required for doing research.*

This analysis has two major implications. First, the overlap between evaluation and research shows that developing research capacity and improving educational practice are deeply intertwined. We would argue that improving one's research skills and using them to conduct better evaluations of educational interventions is a uniquely valuable form of professional development for researchers and practitioners alike. The program planning cycle—developing an intervention, implementing it, evaluating progress, and making course corrections—is at its heart a learning cycle, and the better the evaluation, the better the data on the program's effectiveness, and the greater the potential for learning. Second, it means doing research need not be something done apart from practice; it can be an integral part of practice. A single investigation can meet the information needs of evaluation stakeholders, and at the same time contribute to the field's knowledge base, thereby greatly increasing the potential impact of our work. To accomplish this, we need more "scholarly practitioners."[12]

This chapter on principles for effective research is intended, therefore, as much for practitioners in continuing education of health professionals as for those who consider themselves researchers. Indeed, it seeks to blur the traditional distinction between the producers of knowledge (researchers) and the users of knowledge (practitioners). Our ultimate goal is to encourage CPD professionals to be practitioner–researchers who can contribute to research and other forms of scholarship while fulfilling their other responsibilities. We would like to see members of the CPD field acquire an enhanced capacity to apply concepts and methods from the domain of educational research, whether for evaluating an educational program, advancing the field, or both. We also hope to persuade department heads, CEOs, administrators, and managers that developing increased research capacity—whether through hiring, collaboration, or professional development of members of existing CPD staff—is fundamental to changing clinical practice.

In this chapter, we draw on our experience as researchers, authors, reviewers, and editors to offer 10 guiding principles for effective research in the field of continuing professional development for health professionals, which for our purposes includes medicine, nursing, allied health, dentistry, and pharmacy.[13] Several of the principles are corrective, reflecting common problem areas in CPD research. Others suggest future directions, pointing toward knowledge gaps and methods of inquiry we believe deserve greater attention.

BASIC ASSUMPTIONS

As authors, we come to this task with a particular interest, a point of view that stems from our beliefs about the goals of CPD research. As scholars working in the field, we are part of a diverse scientific community, an eclectic group that has differing views on what counts as real research.[14] It can be difficult at times to find common ground on fundamental assumptions and goals, much less reach consensus. Therefore, we want to make our basic assumptions clear. Our views on how to conduct effective educational research and even our conception of what it means for research to be effective are intimately linked to these foundational beliefs.

We begin this discussion by focusing on two dualisms: *research and evaluation*, and *applied and basic research*. In the process, we raise issues such as what should be considered research in the CPD field and what criteria should be used to assess effectiveness of that research. We then use a framework developed by Albert[15] to describe a continuum of perspectives held by medical education researchers on these issues[16] and identify where we stand in relation to that spectrum. This discussion provides an essential prelude to our discussion of the 10 principles. We believe lack of understanding or disagreement about the relationship of research to evaluation and basic to applied research is at the root of many common problems in the design, conduct, and reporting of research and evaluation studies.

How Does Research Differ from Evaluation?

As implied above, this question has no definitive answer. One difficulty in marking the differences between research and evaluation is the significant overlap between them. Distinguishing between them based on methodology is difficult. Both make extensive use of social science methods and many evaluation studies are done to research standards. In our view, the two most important differences are (1) the primary *source of the problems and questions* addressed and (2) and the standards used to determine the *quality and value of the evidence* produced.

1. Source of problems and questions. The National Academy of Science definition states that the object of research is to "extend human knowledge of the physical, biological, or social world beyond what is already known."[17] In other words, research addresses gaps or problems in our knowledge. Designing a study requires an understanding of what is known and not known. Gaps in knowledge and theory, as recorded in the scholarly literature, are the primary source of research problems and questions. The importance of grounding research in the scholarly literature is evidenced in the introduction to many research reports, which includes a review of the relevant literature providing an argument that a gap exists and defining its contours. The results of research may provide useful guidance to educational practice, but that is a secondary concern.

Evaluation, on the other hand, gives priority to the needs of the evaluation stakeholders. For example, stakeholders may face important decisions about an educational program or want information about how to improve a program. An evaluation is done to get the answers they need for their intended purpose. An evaluation may just happen to speak to a gap in our knowledge base or it may focus on an area that has already been heavily researched, but these are secondary considerations when focusing and designing the evaluation. Not surprisingly, this is a major reason why many program evaluations submitted to education journals as original research go unpublished.

Evaluations can in many cases be designed to serve both purposes; however, this seldom happens without careful advance planning. To paraphrase Norman,[18] the statement "This was a great project. We should write this up and publish it" often leads to an exercise in futility.

2. Quality and value. Research and evaluation are governed by different quality standards. Michael Quinn Patton (cited in Mathison[19]) argued that differences in quality standards for research and evaluation derive from their different purposes and whose interests are served by the standards. In Patton's view, a primary purpose of research is to enhance understanding. Research standards are set by peer reviewers, granting agencies, authoritative methodological sources, editors, and so on. Quantitative research is judged on criteria such as validity, reliability, attention to causality, and generalizability. Similar criteria such as credibility, verifiability, and reflexivity (attention to researcher bias) apply to qualitative research.[20] The value of research rests not only on its quality but also the importance of the contribution it makes to knowledge and theory.

On the other hand, argued Patton, the primary purpose of evaluation is usually defined by the how the stakeholders intend to use the results. This focus on stakeholder needs is nearly universal and is widely considered a distinguishing feature of evaluation.[19] Like research, evaluation standards are set by peer reviewers, granting agencies, authoritative methodological sources, editors, and so on. And, according to Patton, the quality of an evaluation is judged on many of the same criteria as research. The Program Evaluation Standards,[21] for example, address five key attributes of evaluation quality (Table 25.1). The attribute *Accuracy* includes standards for validity, reliability, and reduction of error and bias. However, as this table shows, evaluation quality is also assessed by examining other attributes: *Utility, Feasibility, Propriety, and Accountability.* Each of these four attributes is closely tied to the evaluator's responsibility to be responsive to stakeholder needs and the larger evaluation context. The overall quality of an evaluation is heavily influenced by its practical value.

TABLE 25.1
Overview of the *Program Evaluation Standards*

Attribute	Description
Accuracy	The accuracy standards are intended to increase the dependability and truthfulness of evaluation representations, propositions, and findings, especially those that support interpretations and judgments about quality.
Utility	The utility standards address the extent to which program stakeholders find evaluation processes and products valuable in meeting their needs.
Feasibility	The feasibility standards are intended to increase evaluation effectiveness and efficiency.
Propriety	The propriety standards support what is proper, fair, legal, right, and just in evaluations.
Accountability	The evaluation accountability standards encourage adequate documentation of evaluations and a metaevaluative perspective focused on improvement and accountability for evaluation processes and products.

Yarbrough D, Shulha L, Hopson R, et al. *The Program Evaluation Standards: A Guide for Evaluators and Evaluation Users*, 3rd ed. Thousand Oaks, CA: Sage Publications; 2011, used with permission.

Basic versus Applied Research

Some, including the authors, would argue against Patton's view that research is aimed primarily at understanding and enlightenment and instead make a distinction between basic and applied research.[22] In this view, the role of basic research is increasing our understanding of the world. It is considered highly autonomous in the sense that research problems are determined internally by the investigators. Conversely, the goal of *applied research* is to solve practical problems. Like evaluation, its role is instrumental. The investigators may be accomplished scientists but the state of scientific knowledge does not determine the choice of questions or problems. In Roll-Hansen's words,

> It is an instrument in the service of its patron. Applied research helps interpret and refine the patron's problems to make them researchable, and then investigates possible solutions. The practical problems of the patron set the frame for the activity. Applied research is in this sense subordinate to social, economic and political aims.[22] (p. 5)

Although applied research shares evaluation's focus on the needs of stakeholders, applied research is not, however, synonymous with what Patton means by "evaluation." Not all evaluation is done, or needs to be done, to research standards.

WHERE WE STAND

Our discussion of research versus evaluation and basic versus applied research frames the issue of where we stand on the nature and purpose of CPD research, the appropriate balance between science and service to stakeholders, and how our views compare with other researchers in the field. We explain and situate our views using a conceptual framework developed by Albert.[15] Albert developed a continuum representing the range of opinions in medical education research on the types of research that bring the most value to the field (Fig. 25.1). One end of the continuum is the

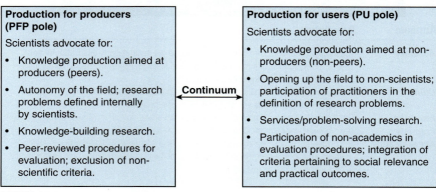

FIGURE 25.1.   Two poles of research in the field of medical education. (From Albert M, Hodges B, Regehr G. Research in medical education: balancing service and science. *Adv Health Sci Educ.* 2006;12:103–115, with permission of Springer.)

pole of *production for producers*. Researchers at this end argue that research should, above all else, advance knowledge and be governed by strict scientific criteria of excellence. They assert that researchers should be allowed a high degree of autonomy in the face of external demands. The right to participate in the field rests exclusively on scientific competence. Excluded are those who want to influence research to serve other ends, such as educational practice. The drive to understand medical education, rather than solve practical education problems, is the primary and proximal motivational force.

At the other end are researchers who support *production for users*, giving greater weight to relevance and utility. Their goal is the production of knowledge that responds to the problems and needs of the users. They argue that criteria for judging excellence of research should include "the utility of the research, its capacity to identify solutions to a real world problem, and its potential conversion into an innovation..."[16] (p. 106)

We understand CPD as an applied field and strongly believe that CPD research should be tied to problems of educational practice. But ours is a soft rather than a hard view of what "tied to problems of practice" means. This perspective allows for a short-term focus on building knowledge (production for producers), provided there are good reasons to expect an effect on practice in the longer term. Consider the example of the seminal study by Fox et al. of learning and change among physicians.[23] As described by the authors, the goal of this study was to build a richer, empirically grounded foundation for the field and provide a theoretical framework that could guide subsequent studies to determine why some educational interventions are more successful in changing clinical practice than others. It was not, in other words, designed to directly solve a specific practical problem.

> It was agreed that rather than looking toward education as a cause, and change as an effect, an alternative approach was necessary. [Our] research efforts should focus on how and why different changes occurred. This would enable an identification of relationships that could explain change in terms of its causes, and describe the role of learning in the change process.[24]

The authors offered no detailed account of how the study would enhance educational practice. However, understanding the phenomenology of learning has long been accepted as fundamental to improving educational practice. Accordingly, this study would meet our criterion of "tied to problems of educational practice."

In effect, our perspective encompasses the entire continuum in Figure 25.1; we believe that, in practice, even basic science *cannot be completely autonomous*. Although scientists leaning toward production for producers seek autonomy for the field, social needs and the public good must inevitably enter into the choice of research questions lest the field undermine its claim for public support. Furthermore, we believe that the goals of basic and applied research are not mutually exclusive but can be combined in a single study. As Stokes observed, the annals of science are

> ...rich with cases of research that [are] guided both by understanding and by use, confounding the view of basic and applied science as inherently separate realms.[24]
> (p. 25)

In short, our foundational assumptions are that evaluation and research serve different, but not incommensurable purposes; that there is substantial overlap between the knowledge and skills required for research and evaluation; that both effective research and evaluation are cornerstones for progress in CPD practice; and that the value of educational research, whether basic or applied, ultimately rests on its contribution to educational practice. With that as background, we now turn to the 10 principles.

TEN PRINCIPLES FOR EFFECTIVE CPD RESEARCH IN THE HEALTH PROFESSIONS

A list of the 10 principles can be found in Table 25.2. These principles can be used to improve the quality and usefulness of CPD research. Although they are numbered, the reader should not infer that their ordering implies that some are inherently more important than others. Space constraints do not allow us to discuss the principles in depth, much less describe in detail how to implement them. Accordingly, this list is best used as a stimulus to reflection and further learning; several resources for that purpose have been compiled in Appendix C. Finally, use of the principles requires flexibility, adaptation, and interpretation. Discussing them with peers and mentors and exploring how they apply in specific contexts will greatly enhance their value.

TABLE 25.2
Ten Principles for Effective Research in Continuing Professional Development in the Health Professions

Gaining Entry/Moving Forward
1. Learning to conduct effective research in CPD should be seen as a purposeful, ongoing process of professional development.
2. Education researchers should endeavor to develop a program of research.

Research Design
3. Educational research should address an important gap in the field's knowledge base or develop new knowledge.
4. Educational research should contribute to understanding and solving important problems of educational practice.
5. Educational research should be informed by theory or a clearly articulated conceptual framework.
6. Educational research should employ recognized methodologies and meet the quality standards associated with those methodologies.

Dissemination
7. Reports of intervention studies should clearly and accurately describe the constituent elements of the educational intervention, the rationale for key program design decisions, and the salient aspects of the context of the intervention.
8. Researchers should be responsible stewards of research resources.

Looking Forward
9. Future research should give greater attention to understanding and facilitating team learning and change.
10. Future research on the effectiveness of educational interventions should give less attention to "does it work?" and more to "when does it work and how?"

Gaining Entry/Moving Forward

1. Learning to conduct effective research in CPD should be seen as a purposeful, ongoing process of professional development. One's professional development in research is a lifelong project. Research is a broad and rich domain that is continually evolving; new problems, new ways of conceptualizing old problems, and methodological advances all contribute to change. Doing research and staying abreast of ongoing changes make it a field with special appeal to people who are avid lifelong learners and enjoy investigating challenging problems.

A good starting point for novices and seasoned investigators alike is to take stock of their current research knowledge, skills, and experience and build on that foundation. We have included a self-efficacy tool for assessing one's research skills (Table 25.3). This tool, adapted from a validated instrument for clinical research developed by Bakken and colleagues[25] at the University of Wisconsin–Madison, lists key competencies involved in both quantitative and qualitative research.

Taking stock serves several purposes; among them are identifying existing areas of relevant experience and training, prioritizing goals for personal professional development, and even identifying the skills needed to ensure a well-rounded research team.

TABLE 25.3
Assessment of Self-Efficacy in Education Research

Education Research Self-Efficacy Assessment

INSTRUCTIONS: The following items are tasks related to performing education research. Please rate your ability to successfully perform each task by selecting a single number from 0 to 10 that best describes your **level of confidence**. Please indicate how confident you are in successfully performing each task *today*. Rate your degree of confidence by recording a number from 0 to 10 where 0 = "I cannot do this task at all" and 10 = "I am highly confident I can do this task."

Current Confidence
Level (0–10)

1. Content Knowledge: Reading the Research Literature
   a. Read the research literature critically.
   b. Identify an area of interest within a given body of literature.
   c. Understand theory and findings in your area of interest.
   d. Explain in a general way the importance of theory to research.
   e. Recognize the classic studies, traditional designs, common forms of measurement, common variables, and common methodological problems related to one's own research area.
   f. Critically synthesize the literature relevant to your research question.
2. Methodological Skills: Research Purpose, Hypotheses, Variables, and Operational Definitions
   a. Identify and describe a clear focus, problem, or general question to investigate.
   b. Refine the problem so it can be investigated.
   c. Establish a clear purpose for the research.
   d. For quantitative studies, translate the general question in specific hypotheses, operationalize variables and terms, determine how each variable will be measured, and evaluate the validity and reliability of a given measurement.

(Continued)

TABLE 25.3
Assessment of Self-Efficacy in Education Research (*Continued*)

Education Research Self-Efficacy Assessment

3. Methodological Skills: Research Design and Procedures (Descriptive, Explanatory, or Exploratory studies)
   a. Identify appropriate theories, conceptual frameworks, and/or inquiry paradigms to guide the inquiry.
   b. Categorize research designs (e.g., prospective vs. retrospective).
   c. State the purpose, strengths, and limitations of different research paradigms and designs.
   d. Compare major types of studies such as case reports, case controls, cross-sectional, longitudinal, and epidemiological studies, survey studies, field research, and evaluation studies.
   e. Explain important threats to validity and reliability or trustworthiness for various designs.
   f. State the relationship between the chosen research design, the type of data collected, and the data analysis approach.
   g. Prepare for and use consultation from design specialists.
   h. Thoroughly analyze the dominant research designs used in your area of study.
   i. Recognize sources of error and bias in one's study and approaches to minimize error.

4. Methodological Skills: Data Collection and Analysis (Quantitative)
   a. Distinguish inferential from descriptive statistics.
   b. Determine the universe, population, appropriate sample, sample size, and sampling technique for a study.
   c. Understand basic statistical concepts (e.g., statistical significance, P-values).
   d. Understand commonly used statistical tests (e.g., t-tests, Chi square).
   e. Construct a plan for managing data files and for analyzing those data.
   f. Interpret printouts on common analyses from statistical packages for one's research area.
   g. Develop graphs, diagrams, and other graphics to summarize and communicate data.
   h. Report results correctly and be able to cite strengths and limitations of the study.
   i. Prepare for and use consultation from computer analysts and statisticians.
   j. Understand more advanced statistical tests used in one's research area (e.g., discriminant analysis).

5. Methodological Skills: Data Collection and Analysis (Qualitative)
   a. Determine from where and whom data will be collected.
   b. Determine key phases of the inquiry.
   c. Select/develop appropriate instrumentation (e.g., inquiry team composition, training).
   d. Plan data collection and recording modes.
   e. Plan data analysis procedures.
   f. Plan logistical procedures for project, field excursions, and postexcursion activities
   g. Plan to enhance trustworthiness of inquiry (credibility, transferability, dependability, confirmability).
   h. Conduct interviews, observation, and documentary review as appropriate to area of inquiry.

TABLE 25.3
Assessment of Self-Efficacy in Education Research (*Continued*)

Education Research Self-Efficacy Assessment

6. Methodological Skills: Data Evaluation and Discussion
   a. Explain the outcome of an analysis.
   b. Conduct additional literature review as needed to elaborate upon findings and their implications for a given body of research.
   c. Integrate findings into existing literature.
   d. Express appropriate cautions about interpreting results.
   e. Place one's study in the context of existing research and justify how it contributes to important questions in the area.
7. Leadership/Project Management Skills:
   a. Develop plans for implementing a study, including timeline, budget, requirements for personnel, facilities, and supplies.
   b. Identify collaborators within and outside of the discipline who can offer guidance to the project.
   c. Hire, manage, and evaluate personnel involved with a study.
   d. Prepare and submit required reports, budget requests, and other administrative documents.
   e. Implement and direct a research project.
8. Ethics/Human Subjects Protection
   a. Secure permission from human subjects, research, and other institutional review committees and boards.
   b. Understand and apply the process of obtaining informed consent.
   c. Identify issues relating to research integrity.
   d. Know institutional and governmental policies concerning the ethical conduct of research.
   e. Seek and utilize institutional sources of support when faced with an ethical dilemma.
   f. Write a consent form for human subjects research.
9. Reporting on Research
   a. Prepare and deliver poster or oral presentations for professional audiences.
   b. Deliver a focused and well-organized lecture.
   c. Write journal articles, research proposals, and grant applications according to general and specific format guidelines.
   d. Employ appropriate English usage, style, grammar, and composition in professional writing.
10. Grant Writing
    a. Identify appropriate funding sources.
    b. Prepare a research proposal suitable for submission in your research area.
11. Technology Tools: Using Appropriate Hardware and Software
    a. Use computer technology for presentations (e.g., PowerPoint, LCD projector, PDA).
    b. Use technological tools for data collection (e.g., smartphones, audio recording equipment, Web-based surveys) as appropriate for area of inquiry.
    c. Use data analysis software (e.g., SPSS, Minitab, NVIVO, Atlas.ti).
    d. Use reference management tools (e.g., EndNote) to manage bibliographies.
    e. Use word processing software to produce grants, journal publications, and other scientific documents.
    f. Use survey design software (e.g., SurveyPro, Qualtrics).
    g. Conduct searches of the literature using common interfaces (e.g., PubMed, ERIC).

Adapted from Mullikin EA, Bakken LL, Betz NE. Assessing research self-efficacy in physician scientists: the clinical research appraisal inventory. *J Career Assess.* 2007;15(3):367–387.

Combined with the information in this chapter, the results of this assessment can be used to develop a personal professional development plan that includes a rationale that links growth in specific research skills to organizational or departmental priorities (e.g., demonstrating to internal organizational stakeholders that your programming is effective and worth supporting). Having a formalized plan can aid in enlisting the support of managers, directors, or chairs.

Identifying areas for further development provides direction to a search for learning opportunities. Several universities offer degree or certificate programs that address educational research, many of which are specific to one or more health professions (e.g., see Tekian's 2014 article on doctoral programs in health professions education[26]). Professional societies and major conferences focusing on education of health professionals often offer educational opportunities that include workshops, mentoring, and fellowships. We refer you again to Appendix C for specific resources.

The local environment or community often provides many options. Those who work in an academic environment, especially research institutions with well-developed research infrastructures, typically have access to training in topics such as recruitment of subjects, navigating the human subjects review process, procedures for protecting human subjects, grant writing, and specific research methodologies. Research interest groups are also common. Because many of these topics are relevant across multiple discipline and institutions, they are often available online, as is access to interest groups.

Many research competencies, such as learning how to conduct a semistructured interview or to "think like a researcher" are best learned in a staged process of observation and supervised practice. One especially valuable professional development activity is working on a more senior investigator's study, provided it is understood that the primary goal is to learn. This allows a more junior researcher to be a "legitimate peripheral participant," doing work on the project that someone needs to do and yet offers the opportunity for learning.[27] A useful concept is "zone of proximal development." To paraphrase Vygotsky, the ZPD is the distance between what a learner can do without assistance and what he or she can do with assistance.[28] Learning from the experience will be much diminished if the learners are assigned tasks they already know how to do or are too far over their head.

Even novices will likely discover they have relevant knowledge and skills, some of which might be at the level of a more experienced researcher. For example, several years of experience recruiting community-based job placement sites for dental hygienists could be of high value in recruiting clinical practices to take part in a CPD effectiveness study. The self-assessment tool in the appendix mentioned earlier can help identify these areas.

Apprenticeship modes of learning must, however, be supplemented by other activities that promote a deeper understanding of the purpose of study such as reading and discussing articles and other resources relevant to the task. Educational research requires flexibility and adaptation. If one can perform a research task sufficiently well for the present study but does not know why the task is structured as it is, what alternative approaches exist, and what criteria for research quality apply, it becomes much more difficult to transfer what is learned into a different context.

The lack of a clinical background or training in educational research need not be barrier. In fact, a background in communications, psychology, public health, or engineering is considered an asset by many. Norman[29] argued that a noteworthy strength of medical education research is that it brings together various disciplinary perspectives. Only in recent years have research training program graduates prepared to work in health professions education begun entering the field. Historically, nearly all came from other disciplines. That experience demonstrated the relevance and value of perspectives and procedures from many different fields of study to medical education research.

2. Education researchers should strive to develop a program of research. At some point in their careers, many researchers will want to develop a program of research rather than do an aggregation of studies on largely unrelated topics. This is a lesser concern for people who are just beginning their research careers and are actively working on developing a solid base of knowledge and skills, but it is worth exploring options even early on. Holzemer defines a program of research as

> ... a coherent expression of a researcher's area of interest that has public health significance, builds from the published research literature in the field, has relevance for clinical ... practice, and captures the passion and commitment of the researcher.[30] (p. 1)

It is typically organized around a central theme (the researcher's area of interest) and shows a logical progression of inquiry. Defining a program of research gives investigators the opportunity to consider what they want to be known for and find an area about which they are curious, intrigued, or passionate and, in so doing, create a niche that allows them to become a recognized expert. It also affords them the efficiencies that come from building on one's own work and opportunity to develop a high degree of proficiency using the research methodologies best suited for the questions being investigated. The research published by Joan Sargeant at Dalhousie University in Halifax provides an example (Table 25.4).

Research Design

3. Educational research should address an important gap in the field's knowledge base or develop new knowledge. The decision to undertake a study and the choice of a research

TABLE 25.4
Example of Publications Constituting a Program of Research

- Sargeant J, et al. (2005). Exploring family physicians' reactions to **multisource feedback:** perceptions of credibility and usefulness. *Medical Education*
- Sargeant J, et al. (2007). Challenges in **multisource feedback**: intended and unintended outcomes. *Medical Education*
- Sargeant J. (2008). "To call or not to call": making informed **self-assessment**. *Medical Education*
- Sargeant J, et al. (2011). How do **physicians assess their family physician colleagues' performance**? Creating a rubric to inform assessment and feedback. *J Contin Educ Health Prof*
- Sargeant J. (2012). How external performance standards inform **self-assessment**. *Medical Teacher*

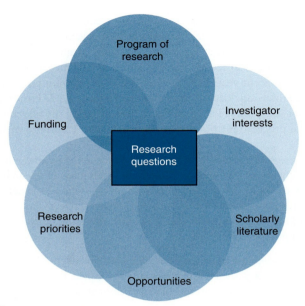

FIGURE 25.2. Selected factors influencing the choice of research question.

question to guide that study are influenced by several factors (Fig. 25.2). However, careful consideration should be given to how a study builds upon and adds to knowledge and theory. The idea for a research project might originate from somewhere other than the literature. The process can be thought of as a dialogue between research interests and capabilities, one's professional development goals, the opportunities that exist in the environment, gaps in the literature, and funding priorities. The ideal is to find the area where these factors overlap.

Wherever the process begins, engaging the literature early on is essential. Research needs and priorities are often identified in systematic reviews, editorials, society publications, and conference proceedings. A review of existing research around a topic of interest provides valuable information not only about what is already known but also about the methodologies used, how research questions have been framed, and tools such as tests and surveys that are available. Articles also help to identify potential collaborators and other information that can aid in your investigation.

It is also important to consider early on which journals might publish one's work. A review of the literature can help identify journals with an interest in the topic and define the target audience. An excellent resource is the regularly updated and comprehensive list published by the American Association of Medical Colleges of journals that publish scholarly works in education.[31]

4. Educational research should also contribute to understanding and solving important problems of educational practice. As indicated above, we strongly believe that whether research is considered basic or applied, the justification for the research and argument for its significance ultimately requires a plausible connection to problems of educational practice. Problems can arise from many sources including one's own experience, but the argument for the existence and importance of the problem must draw on the scholarly literature.

Another and often taken for granted aspect of this principle concerns the nature of educational problems. Deciding what is an educational problem as opposed to a clinical, organizational, or personnel management problem is something some investigators find difficult or give too little attention. For example, a study examining the impact of an innovative shift scheduling approach on the quality of care provided by the emergency department or an examination of the impact of patient education on shared decision-making in the primary care setting does not speak directly to problems of CPD practice. Additional guidance on this topic can be found in a 2016 *JCEHP* editorial.[32]

It is also important to establish that the educational problem is an *important* one. Reviews of the literature typically yield studies, analyses, and opinion pieces describing the problem of interest and its consequences and calling for further study.

5. Educational research should be informed by theory or a clearly articulated conceptual framework. Studies in the CPD field are generally undertheorized, making little or no mention of theory. Among those that do mention a theory, many give it only lip service.[33] The authors describe a theory and then neglect to explain how it guided construction of the research questions, development of the intervention, analysis of the results, and so on.

"Theory" need not necessarily be a formal theory such as the theory of planned behavior or social cognitive theory. It can also take the form of logic model or program theory clarifying linkages between components of the educational intervention and the intended outcomes. A good basic resource is the guide developed by the Kellogg foundation.[34] A more advanced treatment may be found in Huey Chen's work on theory-driven evaluation.[35,36]

Also common is the lack of clarity about the meaning of key concepts and supposed relationships between them because the study lacks a clearly defined conceptual framework. For example, some research reports use education and learning interchangeably as if there was no important distinction to be made between them, leading to laments such as the following:

> I fear that this may get worse; what I call here non-theoretical grabbing at data. Conceptual confusion drives me crazy: distributed learning, flexible learning, open learning, e-learning.... Have you ever been to a conference on learning and then half the people were talking about teaching?[37]

Another common example is authors who describe their educational intervention as "interprofessional" without clarifying how they are using the term and providing evidence that the intervention meets the criteria their definition entails.

We agree with Georges Bordage who has argued that, whether the investigators are aware or not, every study has a conceptual framework or theory behind it.[38] What varies is how explicitly that framework is described and how well grounded it is in theory, established models, or evidence-based practices. We further agree with Bordage's assertion that

> We all have assumptions, explicit or implicit, about the way things are and how they work. It is the researchers' and authors' responsibility to make those assumptions explicit to the readers and to connect their work to the literature in the field.[38] (p. 313)

Bordage's essay provides an excellent explanation of conceptual frameworks and how they relate to theory; he also provides three case examples, including one drawn from CPD, showing how conceptual frameworks can be used to frame, understand, and create solutions for educational problems.

6. Educational research should employ recognized methodologies and meet the quality standards associated with those methodologies. This principle address several common problems associated with the research methods used in CPD research and how their use is justified. Too often, we see studies that make little or no effort to justify the methodology used, describe the steps taken to enhance the credibility and trustworthiness of the results, or acknowledge important major limitations of the methodology employed (e.g., self-reported changes in practice, pretest–posttest design). Another problem is researchers who report using a methodology (e.g., Delphi), an analytical procedure (e.g., constant comparison), or an outcome measure (e.g., multiple choice test of knowledge) and neglect to demonstrate that their approach meets the quality standards for these methods. Another problem is failure to recognize that some research methods come in variations. In grounded theory, for example, there are the classic, Straussian, and constructivist approaches, each built on different assumptions about the nature of theory and role of the investigator.[39] The procedures for each vary in significant ways and they employ different strategies for ensuring quality. Specifying the type of grounded theory employed in a study is essential if reviewers and editors are to know how to properly evaluate the study.

7. Reports of intervention studies should clearly and accurately describe the constituent elements of the educational intervention, the rationale for key program design decisions, and the salient aspects of the context of the intervention. A frequent observation made by authors of published systematic reviews of the CPD effectiveness literature is that the components of educational interventions are often poorly described and the terminology used to identify those components (e.g., audit and feedback, peer detailing) is not clearly defined making it difficult to draw conclusions about the relationship between the educational methods used and observed outcomes.

Another issue is weak or missing descriptions of the *context* of the educational intervention. As Pawson and Tilley noted,

> Programs are always introduced into pre-existing social contexts and ... these prevailing social conditions are of crucial importance when it comes to explaining the successes and failures of social programs.[40]

However, deciding which aspects of the context are relevant is a challenging task, even for seasoned investigators. There is a lack of consensus around what context is and how it should be described. A theory or conceptual framework may identify relevant aspects of the environment. There is also an emerging literature focused squarely on this topic that can provide guidance.[41,42] For example, the problem of describing the context of interventions is not unique to education; it is also an issue for the quality improvement field. The SQUIRE guideline (Standards for QUality Improvement Reporting Excellence), developed for reporting quality improvement projects, can be useful in deciding what to include and where in a research report the issue of context might be addressed.[43] Although developed primarily for studies of clinical interventions, the TIDieR guideline (Template for Intervention Description and Replication)[44] provides a useful guide that calls attention to key elements constituting a detailed and balanced description of an educational intervention.

Looking Forward

To this point, the seven principles we have described are largely corrective in their intent. They address common gaps and shortcomings in the design and reporting of education research in the CPD field. Researchers who follow these principles can not only greatly enhance the value of research to the CPD field but will also distinguish their research from much of the work currently being done. We now turn to three principles that chart future directions for the CPD research enterprise.

8. Researchers should be responsible stewards of research resources. This principle allows us to emphasize three specific ethical obligations of researchers that deserve special attention as CPD moves forward. The first concerns responsible use of a finite resource: survey populations. A JCEHP editorial[45] argued that the populations we survey in our studies should be considered a commons—that is, a resource shared within a community—with a finite capacity for carrying a survey burden (defined here simply as the number of surveys received by an individual). As a shared resource, we need to consider the impact of our research practices on not just our own self-interests but those of the research community at large. The survey burden for virtually all populations has increased dramatically, driven by factors such as widespread access to online survey tools. Some factors are more specific to the education domain, such as accrediting bodies that regard routine surveys as a prima facie indicator of continuous quality improvement and responsiveness to learner needs. We can abuse this shared resource in many ways including doing a census survey when sampling could be used and conducting unnecessary surveys (the data are already available or the data collected serve no valuable purpose). We believe that all researchers have an obligation to survey populations and the research community to

> ... preserve and protect the resource that is arguably the most important component of successful educational research and evaluation surveys—the goodwill and cooperation of the people comprising the populations we seek to understand.[45] (p. 94)

Another important obligation is to our human subjects. Most if not all journals in the health professions education field require either human subjects review and approval by a recognized body or a formal exemption from human subjects review issued by a recognized body (i.e., authors are not permitted to decide for themselves that their study is exempt). It should be standard research practice to get either an approval or exemption from the appropriate authority. However, even when a study qualifies for an exemption (e.g., involves interviewing participants in a CPD activity as part of a program evaluation), we are obliged to consider potential harms to our informants and take appropriate steps to minimize the risks. All research has the potential to harm subjects. Even a seemingly benign investigation can result in a someone being ostracized, ridiculed, or even dismissed from their position. We can inadvertently coerce subjects into participating. We can fail to respect their autonomy and volition by not providing them with the information needed to give their informed consent.

The third obligation is to disseminate research, making it accessible to other investigators and practitioners in the field. Doing effective research is resource intensive. We should not only be judicious about how those resources are deployed but also act to increase the potential for return on investment by presenting at conferences, preparing and submitting a manuscript for publication, self-archiving a report of the research online, and so on. Although we consider dissemination an important obligation, it is also important to attend to copyright issues. Authors' rights to distribute their published works vary by publisher. Some publishers allow authors to put the accepted version of the manuscript (after it has been reviewed, edited, and accepted but before the publisher has formatted, copyedited, and typeset the manuscript for distribution) on a personal Web site or their organization's intranet. Detailed copyright information for specific journals can be obtained from RoMEO, which is a "searchable database of publisher's policies regarding the self-archiving of journal articles on the web and in Open Access repositories" (http://www.sherpa.ac.uk/romeo/index.php).

9. Future research should give greater attention to understanding and facilitating team learning and change. The shift toward interdisciplinary clinical practice and team-based care creates new needs and opportunities for researchers in the CPD field. Among other things, it can require a shift in the unit of analysis from an individual to a group or a practice. As we become more aware of constructs such as collective competence[46] and transactive memory,[47] it becomes clearer that we need a deeper understanding of team learning and change. If our aim is to facilitate group learning, we clearly need a much richer understanding of what it is and how it occurs by conducting studies at the group level.

10. Research on the effectiveness of educational interventions should give less attention to "does it work?" and more to "when does it work and how?" Several thought leaders in medical education research have argued it is time to shift our emphasis away from effectiveness and outcomes studies and give more attention to questions about how and why educational interventions work.[3–6,13] One approach to studying the "black box" between the intervention and the observed outcomes is to include a component that looks at the mechanisms by which the intervention led to the observed outcomes and the contextual factors that influenced the process. At present, the CPD research field lacks widely used and tested methodologies for achieving this goal. Pawson and Tilley's realistic evaluation approach[40] is one candidate. Although no known studies have applied this approach in the CPD context, we can benefit from the examples provided by research on undergraduate and graduate health professions education. These early experiences have stimulated an active discourse about how it can be adapted and used, from which we can also benefit.

Another approach is Success Case Method (SCM).[48] For example, Olson and colleagues[49] used SCM to study how and why several practice-based educational interventions yielded significant changes in tobacco cessation counseling in primary care settings. Although developed as an evaluation method to assess the impact of training in organizations, it can be viewed as a form of qualitative research and conducted to research standards by, for example, treating each instance of success as a case study and using cross-case analytical methods to strengthen the trustworthiness of the findings.

A third approach is theory-based evaluation or one of its variants such as logic model-based evaluation.[34–36] Put simply, this approach is based on a theory or model of how the intervention is expected to produce the intended results. This program-specific theory guides an evaluation to determine if and how the intervention contributed to any observed results.

Regehr's analysis of the state of medical education research[5] led him to a different perspective on getting beyond the "did it work" question. He suggests we shift the main emphasis of education research to basic research and away from the applied model of solving problems of educational practice. His analysis touches on several concerns but of particular relevance is the problem of context specificity of educational interventions: that is, a study that shows a workshop was effective in one setting is often of little import for those working in other settings. The problem is the relentless complexity and dynamism of the environments in which educational interventions (and research on those interventions) are conducted. As a result, cross-context predictions become meaningless. His analysis led to a thought-provoking conclusion, which is worth quoting at length:

> I would like to suggest that the science of education is not about creating and sharing better *generalisable solutions* to common problems, but about creating and sharing *better ways of thinking* about the problems we face.... Thus, the value of our scientific discourse (our talks and papers) will arise not from our ability to create a general solution that will apply to everyone's problems or even our ability to solve each other's problems, but rather from our ability to help each other think better about our own versions of the problems. Likewise, the value of reading the literature will not depend on our finding a solution that we can blindly adopt, but, rather, on reflecting on how to incorporate others' interpretations of a problem into our own context, on what needs to be adapted to make those interpretations relevant to our context, and on why that adaptation is necessary.[5] (p. 37)

There are many ways to "use the research,"[50] and in this passage, Regehr emphasizes but one: its instrumental use. He also does not address the varying levels of complexity and reproducibility associated with different educational interventions and the contexts in which they are deployed. However, we believe his provocative suggestion deserves further discussion among the CPD research community.

FUTURE DIRECTIONS

We have described 10 principles we consider most important given the current state of the CPD field and the problems and opportunities that lie ahead. Going forward, we need to continuously strive to improve research in the field, recognize progress, and identify areas for improvement. If we have been successful in writing this chapter, the principles we have described will aid in that effort.

At the same time, we recognize this list is by no means complete and reflects our assumptions, experience, and judgments. We have undoubtedly omitted principles that others would consider essential. If this chapter prompts self-reflection and a rigorous and critical debate over the contents of the list or the contribution research makes to educational practice, we will consider that a success as well.

Nevertheless, we strongly believe the impact of implementing these principles on CPD research and practice can be positive and substantial. They point the way toward deeper understanding and increased effectiveness in the continuing professional development of health professionals. As Donald Schon famously wrote:

> In the varied topography of professional practice, there is a high, hard ground where practitioners can make effective use of research-based theory and technique, and there is a swampy lowland where situations are confusing "messes" incapable of technical solution. The difficulty is that the problems of the high ground, however great their technical interest, are often relatively unimportant to clients or to the larger society, while in the swamp are the problems of the greatest human concern.[51] (p. 42)

In other words, the greatest progress in CPD requires not only building superhighways but also finding our way across uncertain ground, taking a step at a time, using research and evaluation to both guide and monitor our progress. We hope these 10 principles will aid in that endeavor.

R E F E R E N C E S

1. Erickson F, Gutierrez K. Culture, rigor, and science in educational research. *Educ Res.* 2002;31(8):21–24.
2. Oxman AD, Thomson MA, Davis DA. No magic bullets: a systematic review of 102 trials of interventions to improve professional practice. *CMAJ.* 1995;153(10):1423–1431.
3. Cervero RM, Gaines JK. The impact of CME on physician performance and patient health outcomes: an updated synthesis of systematic reviews. *J Contin Educ Health Prof.* 2015;35(2):131–138.
4. Cervero RM. Place matters in physician practice and learning. *J Contin Educ Health Prof.* 2003;23:S10–S18.
5. Regehr G. It's NOT rocket science: rethinking our metaphors for research in health professions education. *Med Educ.* 2010;44(1):31–39.
6. Traynor R, Eva KW. The evolving field of medical education research. *Biochem Mol Biol Educ.* 2010;38(4):211–215.
7. Mennin S. Complexity and health professions education. *J Eval Clin Pract.* 2010;16(4):835–837.
8. Means B, Toyama Y, Murphy R. *Evaluation of Evidence-Based Practices in Online Learning: A Meta-Analysis and Review of Online Learning Studies.* Washington, DC: U.S. Department of Education, Office of Planning, Evaluation, and Policy Development; 2010.
9. Branch RM, Kopcha TJ. Instructional design models. In: Spector JM, Merrill M, Elen J, et al., eds. *Handbook of Research on Educational Communications and Technology,* 4th ed. New York: Springer; 2014:77–87.
10. Moen R, Norman C. *Evolution of the PDCA Cycle.* 2006. http://pkpinc.com/files/NA01MoenNormanFullpaper.pdf. Accessed August 17, 2016.
11. Kolb DA. The process of experiential learning (Chap. 2). *Experiential Learning: Experience as the Source of Learning and Development.* Englewood Cliffs, NJ: Prentice-Hall; 1984:21–38.

12. Olson CA. On the need for scholarly practitioners in CPD. *J Contin Educ Health Prof.* 2011;31(3): 137–139.
13. Cook DA, Levinson AJ, Garside S, et al. Internet-based learning in the health professions: a meta-analysis. *JAMA.* 2008;300(10):1181–1196.
14. Shavelson RJ, Towne L, eds. *Scientific Research in Education.* Washington, DC: National Academy Press; 2002.
15. Albert M. Understanding the debate on medical education research: a sociological perspective. *Acad Med.* 2004;79(10):948–954.
16. Albert M, Hodges B, Regehr G. Research in medical education: balancing service and science. *Adv Health Sci Educ.* 2007;12:103–115.
17. National Academy of Science, National Academy of Engineering, Institute of Medicine of the National Academies. *On Being a Scientist : A Guide to Responsible Conduct in Research,* 3rd ed. Washington, DC: National Academies Press; 2009.
18. Norman G. Data dredging, salami-slicing, and other successful strategies to ensure rejection: twelve tips on how to not get your paper published. *Adv Health Sci Educ.* 2014;19(1):1–5.
19. Mathison S. What is the difference between evaluation and research—and why do we care? In: Smith NL, Brandon PR, eds. *Fundamental Issues in Evaluation.* New York: Guilford Press; 2008:183–196.
20. Cohen DJ, Crabtree BF. Evaluative criteria for qualitative research in health care: controversies and recommendations. *Ann Fam Med.* 2008;6(4):331–339.
21. Yarbrough D, Shulha L, Hopson R, et al. *The Program Evaluation Standards: A Guide for Evaluators and Evaluation Users,* 3rd ed. Thousand Oaks, CA: Sage Publications; 2011.
22. Roll-Hansen N. *Why the Distinction Between Basic (Theoretical) and Applied (Practical) Research Is Important in the Politics of Science.* 2009. http://www.lse.ac.uk/cpnss/research/concludedresearchprojects/contingencydissentinscience/dp/dproll-hansenonline0409.pdf. Accessed July 24, 2016.
23. Fox RD, Mazmanian PE, Putnam RW, eds. *Changing and Learning in the Lives of Physicians.* New York: Praeger; 1989.
24. Stokes DE. *Pasteur's Quadrant: Basic Science and Technological Innovation.* Washington, DC: Brookings Institution Press; 1997.
25. Mullikin EA, Bakken LL, Betz NE. Assessing research self-efficacy in physician scientists: the clinical research appraisal inventory. *J Career Assess.* 2007;15(3):367–387.
26. Tekian A. Doctoral programs in health professions education. *Med Teach.* 2014;36(1):73–81.
27. Lave J, Wenger E. *Situated Learning: Legitimate Peripheral Participation.* New York: Cambridge University Press; 1991.
28. Vygotsky L. Interaction between learning and development. *Mind and Society.* Cambridge, MA: Harvard University Press; 1978:79–91.
29. Norman G. Fifty years of medical education research: waves of migration. *Med Educ.* 2011;45(8):785–791.
30. Holzemer WL. Building a program of research. *Jpn J Nurs Sci.* 2009;6(1):1–5.
31. Blanco M, Love N. *Annotated Bibliography of Journals for Educational Scholarship (Revised).* 2016. https://www.aamc.org/download/456646/data/annotated-bibliography-of-journals-march-2016.pdf. Accessed July 24, 2016.
32. Olson CA. What is an educational problem? Guidance for authors submitting to JCEHP. *J Contin Educ Health Prof.* 2016;36(1):1–3.
33. Klette K. *The Role of Theory in Educational Research.* Lysaker, Norway: The Research Council of Norway; 2012.
34. W.K. Kellogg Foundation. *Logic Model Development Guide: Using Logic Models to Bring Together Planning, Evaluation, and Action.* Battle Creek, MI: W.K. Kellogg Foundation; 2004.
35. Chen HT. *Practical Program Evaluation: Assessing and Improving Planning, Implementation, and Effectiveness.* Thousand Oaks, CA: Sage; 2005.
36. Chen HT. *Theory-Driven Evaluations.* Newbury Park, CA: Sage Publications; 1990.
37. Bernath U, Vidal M. The theories and the theorists: why theory is important for research. *Distances et Savoirs.* 2007;5:427–458.
38. Bordage G. Conceptual frameworks to illuminate and magnify. *Med Educ.* 2009;43(4):312–319.
39. Kenny M, Fourie R. Tracing the history of grounded theory methodology: from formation to fragmentation. *Qual Rep.* 2014;19(103):1–7.
40. Pawson R, Tilley N. *Realistic Evaluation.* London, UK: Sage Publications; 1997.
41. Grant RE, Sajdlowska J, Van Hoof TJ, et al. Conceptualization and reporting of context in the North American continuing medical education literature: a scoping review protocol. *J Contin Educ Health Prof.* 2015;35(suppl 2):S70–S74.
42. Bates J, Ellaway RH. Mapping the dark matter of context: a conceptual scoping review. *Med Educ.* 2016;50(8):807–816.

43. Ogrinc G, Mooney SE, Estrada C, et al. The SQUIRE (Standards for QUality Improvement Reporting Excellence) guidelines for quality improvement reporting: explanation and elaboration. *Qual Saf Health Care*. 2008;17:i13–i32.

44. Hoffmann TC, Glasziou PP, Boutron I, et al. Better reporting of interventions: template for intervention description and replication (TIDieR) checklist and guide. *BMJ*. 2014;348:g1687.

45. Olson CA. Survey burden, response rates, and the tragedy of the commons. *J Contin Educ Health Prof*. 2014;34(2):93–95.

46. Lingard L. Paradoxical truths & persistent myths: reframing the team competence conversation. *J Contin Educ Health Prof*. 2016;36(suppl 1):S19–S21.

47. Wegner DM. Transactive memory: a contemporary analysis of the group mind. In: Mullen B, Goethals GR, eds. *Theories of Group Behavior*. New York: Springer-Verlag; 1986:185–208.

48. Brinkerhoff RO. *The Success Case Method: Find Out Quickly What's Working and What's Not*. San Francisco, CA: Berrett-Koehler; 2003.

49. Olson CA, Shershneva MB, Brownstein MH. Peering inside the clock: using success case method to determine how and why practice-based educational interventions succeed. *J Contin Educ Health Prof*. 2011;31(suppl 1):S50–S59.

50. Olson CA. Is the research on continuing education of health professionals underutilized? *J Contin Educ Health Prof*. 2011;31(2):77–78.

51. Schon D. *The reflective practitioner: how professionals think in action*. San Francisco, CA: Jossey-Bass; 1984.

Chapter 26

PROJECTING *the* FUTURE *of* CONTINUING PROFESSIONAL DEVELOPMENT

Paul E. Mazmanian and David A. Davis

Case

Like others, your CME/CPD program has traditionally been evaluated using a logic model and assessments of learners using competency-based methods (e.g., OSCEs). You wonder about how these apply in the "real world," especially as health care evolves. You recognize that clinical and system performance will be tracked closely by information technology, patient-based scoring, and system report cards. It is also a world in which individual practitioners' competencies will be assessed in interprofessional collaboration, communication, and professionalism, for example.

Questions

How can we prepare ourselves now for this future? What elements are relevant for CME/CPD? What other directions are important to consider in projecting professional development in the future?

INTRODUCTION

Global forces drive change in health, continuing medical education (CME)/continuing professional development (CPD), and the assessment of health care systems, including health care providers. This chapter explores a number of these forces, focusing on the roles of CPD and health system leaders in projecting a vision of the future of CPD. Assessment provides a lens for sharpening our analysis for improved CPD; without measurement, there can be no certainty for improvement. Further, the chapter uses an organizational structure similar to that found in the Introduction to this book to frame several forces of change. They may be grouped as macro (created by and affecting large, national or transnational issues and players), meso (affecting local health systems or teams), or micro (affecting the individual clinician). Each set of forces plays a role in promulgating change and thus the future. Taken in context, these forces not only constitute the subject matter of this chapter but also challenge persons responsible for facilitating the CPD of others to take stock of their own professional values, ethics, and skill sets, in negotiating the demands of better assessment and creating more innovative approaches for translating knowledge into improved patient care and community health.

MACRO FORCES: WORKFORCE SHORTAGES, INEQUITY, AND CREDENTIALING IN HEALTH CARE

In health care settings worldwide, it is almost impossible to avoid discussions of major forces for change—value and cost, patient centeredness, quality improvement, patient safety, and their influence on assessment. This chapter accepts their influence and recognizes the effect of workforce imbalances, health care resources, and credentialing on the organization of care.

Global Shortages and Disparities

In a world economy marked by disparities in resources, one striking feature is evident: there is a global shortage of health professionals, most severe in low- and middle-income countries. The World Health Organization (WHO) reports 230 medical doctors per 100,000 people in the United States but only 1.1 per 100,000 in Malawi. Overall, the total professional health workforce of sub-Saharan Africa approximates 1 per 1000 people—the lowest ratio of any region in the world; yet, the burden of disease in the region is among the highest. In many countries, shortages are made more acute by the uneven distribution of professional health workers practicing in urban versus rural and underserved areas. In South Africa, for example, 46% of the population lives in rural areas, but only 12% of doctors and 19% of nurses are deployed in nonurban settings. Poor working conditions and low pay make it difficult to retain qualified health professionals in hard-to-reach populations. In contrast, some countries are unable to use all the providers they have educated, limited by budgetary restraints.[1]

Even in well-resourced countries a host of workforce problems can undermine the ability of health systems to respond effectively to the challenges they face. Those problems can include low workforce motivation, looming shortages of certain types of health care workers, accelerating labor migration, and distributional imbalances based on geography, gender, occupation, or institutional type. Qualitative imbalances may include underqualification or misqualification of health care workers.[1] Regardless of their geographic location, however, health systems ordinarily involve three major interests: (1) the individual as a health care worker and learner, (2) the health care organization (private or public) as an employer, and (3) the patient as a recipient and payer.[2] Occasionally, these interests not only overlap but conflict with one another, based at least in part on who pays for education or health care services.

A major outcome of workforce imbalances is inequity: it is evident throughout health care. While exacerbated in low-resource countries, contemporary health systems face a serious paradox. In some countries, decades-long investments in health care coupled with major developments in biomedical research have resulted in remarkable expansions of knowledge, skills, and resources to address many high-priority health problems. On the other hand, attempts to reform health care have had limited success in developing more effective, efficient, safe, and equitable delivery systems to achieve the fundamental goal of improving patient care for all, including community health outcomes.[2] This trend is worsened in low-resourced settings.

Credentialing of Organizations

Among the forces operating at the macro level, accreditation is an important and potentially powerful player. *Accreditation* is a voluntary process by which a nongovernmental agency grants a time-limited recognition to an institution, organization, business, or other entity after verifying that it has met predetermined and standardized criteria.[3–5] Educational programs or health care institutions seek accreditation as a signal to the public and other stakeholders that the institution has met previously determined standards. There may be formal linkages across the individual and organizational credentialing interests, whereby award of the organizational credential depends, in part, on the credentialing status of individuals within that organization.[3,4] For example, the Magnet Recognition Program of the American Nurses Credentialing Center encourages a program to attract and retain top talent; improve patient care, safety, and satisfaction; foster a collaborative culture; advance nursing standards and practice; and grow business and financial success.[6]

In the United States, the Joint Commission (an independent, not-for-profit organization that accredits and certifies several thousand health care organizations and programs in the United States) provides a useful example of the role and future-shaping potential of organizational accreditation. The mission statement of the Joint Commission is to continuously improve health care for the public, in collaboration with other stakeholders, by evaluating health care organizations and inspiring them to excel in providing safe and effective care of the highest quality and value.[7] The United States generally accepts that attaining education is evidence of acquired skill, and the credentialing process facilitates skill acquisition through additional training and assessment.[4] The Joint Commission requires documentation of licensed medical staff to meet accreditation requirements for health care organizations, including hospitals, doctors' offices, nursing homes, office-based surgery centers, behavioral health treatment facilities, and providers of home care services.[7]

Those responsible for assisting physicians with their CPD will recognize the complexity of regulations governing incentives for individual physicians, health care organizations, and the public. They will also see the potential for competing interests of stakeholders to conflict. In order for a health care organization to participate in and receive payment from the Medicare or Medicaid programs of the U.S. Centers for Medicare and Medicaid Services (CMS), it must meet the eligibility requirements for program participation, including a certification of compliance with the Conditions of Participation (CoPs) or Conditions for Coverage (CfCs). Certification is based on a survey conducted by a state agency on behalf of the federal government, CMS, or a national accrediting organization approved by CMS as having standards and a survey process that meets or exceeds Medicare's requirements. Health care organizations that achieve such accreditation are determined to meet or exceed Medicare and Medicaid requirements.[8]

Worldwide, there is remarkable variation in approaches to organizational accreditation. For example, the Council of Health Service Accreditation of Southern Africa approves programs for quality and safety of health care services in South Africa. It is the only internationally accredited quality improvement and accreditation body for health care facilities based in Africa.[9] In Europe, no single EU body oversees the accreditation of health care organizations.[10] In North America, Accreditation Canada and the Joint Commission approve programs in Canada[11] and the United States, respectively.[7] In Australia, accreditation of health care organizations is administered by the Australian Commission on Safety and Quality in Health Care.[12] In New Zealand, HealthCERT, a program of the Ministry of Health, is responsible for accreditation of health care organizations.[13] Joint Commission International (JCI) offers education, publications, advisory services, and international accreditation and certification. JCI accredits programs in Brazil, China, and the Russian Federation.[14] For the organization, accreditation indicates attainment of specified organizational benchmarks and carries the potential of leading to organizational change. To the extent qualified care givers are credentialed and required for accreditation, the person and the organization are fundamentally linked (and hopefully improved) by the credentialing processes.[4]

The "Good Doctor": Quality and Safety

While the focus of all health care is on the patient, the individual clinician is situated at the center of the team providing that care. With no codified ideal or genetic tests to identify what it means to be a "good doctor," measuring physician (and ultimately all health professional) performance becomes complex, requiring continuous rethinking and reframing of strategies by which to judge competence. For example, regardless of medicine's long-term devotion to the values of lifelong learning and self-assessment, the current body of literature does not conclusively identify the most effective continuing education methods, their correct mixture, or the total "dose" of continuing education needed to maintain clinical competence or to improve clinical outcomes.[15] Further, unguided self-assessment continues to produce notoriously flawed results.[16–19] Accordingly, the tradition of physician self-regulation is threatened by the patients, public, and private payers, who demand increased safety and accountability from the individuals and systems providing care.[20]

In response to this picture, the past two decades have seen remarkable growth in effort, innovative change, and documented progress in research on credentialing of health care providers.[5,21,22] These changes have roots inside and outside of medicine, with no stronger internal influences than the widespread recognition of the ineffectiveness of classroom lectures[23], the limited ability of physicians to accurately self-assess,[16] and the reality of quality of care disasters like the Bristol Royal Infirmary in the United Kingdom,[22,24] the failed communication of blood type for transplant surgery at a major research university in the United States, and similar events elsewhere.[22,24,25] Regardless of context—rural, urban, public, private, or highly technical academic medical center—the individual health care provider, practicing alone or in teams, bears major responsibility for assuring competent performance, patient safety, and improved quality.[4,5,22–24]

Credentialing of Health Care Providers

For those in health care education, training, workforce development, or employment, the term *credential* is synonymous with verification of qualification or competence, an indication that an individual, group, or organization has been evaluated by a qualified and objective third-party credentialing body and has met standards that are defined, published, psychometrically sound, and legally defensible.[3,26,27] There are three major types of credentials for health care providers. *Licensure* is the mandatory process by which a governmental agency grants time-limited permission to an individual to engage in a given occupation, after verifying that he or she has met predetermined and standardized criteria. Licensure offers title protection for those who meet the criteria. *Certification* is the voluntary process by which a nongovernmental entity grants a time-limited recognition and use of a credential to an individual, after verifying that he or she has met predetermined and standardized criteria. It is the vehicle that a profession or occupation uses to differentiate among its members, using standards, sometimes developed through a consensus-driven process, based on existing legal and psychometric requirements. *Registration* has several definitions, often associated with nursing, especially in North America: two are offered here. First, similar to licensure, it is the process by which a governmental agency grants a time-limited status on a registry, determined by specified knowledge-based requirements (e.g., experience, education, examinations), thereby authorizing those individuals to practice. A second meaning of registration is a listing of practitioners maintained by a governmental entity, without educational, experiential, or competency-based requirements.[3–5]

For the individual physician and other health professionals, licensure and certification are intended to recognize achievement, and competence, the latter now subcategorized by professional bodies. In the United States, these descriptive competencies include medical knowledge and clinical practice, practice-based learning and systems-based practice, professionalism, and interprofessional collaboration.[28] Generally speaking, licensure indicates attainment of a minimal threshold of competence while specialty certification generally includes requirements for advanced training and additional assessment. For example, in the US medical system, licensure and initial certification by the American Board of Medical Specialties include requirements for completion of an accredited training program.[29] Once initially certified, in the United States, physicians may maintain their credential by participating in a robust continuous professional development program termed Maintenance of Certification, which includes a structured approach for enhancing patient care and improving patient outcomes, through focused assessment and improvement activities.[30] Similar systems exist in Canada[31] and in the United Kingdom.[32] Figure 26.1 provides a visual representation of the physician journey from admission to the profession through undergraduate training and practice life. It portrays

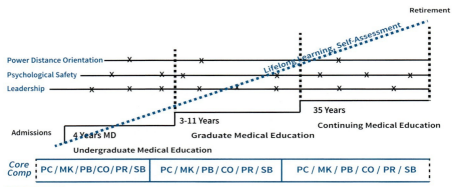

FIGURE 26.1. Lifelong learning, self-assessment, and the core competencies. The following numbers and definitions of competencies align with the numbers for UME, GME, and continuing medical education. (1) Patient Care, PC: The learner must be able to provide patient care that is compassionate, appropriate, and effective for the treatment of health problems and the promotion of health. (2) Medical Knowledge, MK: The learner must be able to demonstrate knowledge about established and evolving biomedical, clinical, and cognate (e.g., epidemiological and social behavioral) sciences and the application of this knowledge to patient care. (3) Practice-Based Learning and Improvement, PB: The learner must be able to investigate and evaluate his or her patient care practices, appraise and assimilate scientific evidence, and improve his or her patient care practices. (4) Interpersonal and Communication Skills, CO: The learner must be able to demonstrate interpersonal and communication skills that result in effective information exchange and teaming with patients, patients' families, and professional associates. (5) Professionalism, PR: The learner must be able to demonstrate a commitment to carrying out professional responsibilities, adherence to ethical principles, and sensitivity to a diverse patient population. (6) Systems-Based Practice, SB: The learner must be able to demonstrate an awareness of and responsiveness to the larger context and system of health care and the ability to effectively call on system resources to provide care that is of optimal value. http://www.acgme.org/Portals/0/PDFs/ACGMEMilestones-CCC-AssesmentWebinar.pdf

the profession's commitment to the policies and values of life-long learning and self-assessment. It also recognizes six core competencies developed by the ACGME and the ABMS. During the last two decades, with content and process derived in part from work of competency-based movements in Canada, the United Kingdom, and elsewhere.[30–32] Finally, it presents examples of psychological constructs of value in questions of health care provider and organizational fit.[33]

A scan of at eight major economies selected from five continents indicates a wide variety of physician credentialing practices and a lack of standardized language for describing and discussing validation systems. For example, initial licensing in Canada and the United States generally requires a combination of 4 years of medical school after undergraduate education and high-stakes testing during postgraduate training. In contrast, South Africa permits admission to medical training from high school; initial licensure requires 6 years of study, 2 years of internship, and 1 year of community service. Specialization occurs during postgraduate education of 4 years or more.[9] Terms such as revalidation, recertification, maintenance of competence, and maintenance of licensure carry different connotations in different regions.[21]

Education and licensure requirements for physicians practicing in the European Union (EU)[10] vary by member states, but the privilege to practice in one state must be recognized by all. The recognition of professional traineeship completed in one member state must be based on a clear written description of learning objectives and assigned tasks determined by the trainee's supervisor in the host state. The Royal Australasian College of Physicians[34] oversees 4 to 6 years of training, plus 1 year of internships and multiyear residencies with two high-stakes assessments. Further, in China, the education program leading to a medical license takes 5 years followed by 3 to 5 years of residency and required passage of the National Medical Licensing Examination.[35]

MICRO- AND MESO-FORCES: FEEDBACK, PROFESSIONALISM, AND EMERGING DESIGNS

Assessment of Feedback

Although present for decades, a cluster of newer and emerging forces occupies an expanding role in the delivery of safe care to patients and therefore to CPD's future directions. These forces include but are not limited to: (1) the assessment of feedback, (2) the assessment of professionalism (explored from micro and macro perspectives, as well as meso or midlevel); (3) interprofessional education and collaborative care; (4) the Learning Health Care System and its possible unintended consequence, clinician burnout; and (5) three major concepts offering opportunity for improvement—metacognition and deliberate practice, health information technology, and research involving less studied assessment tools: neuroimaging, social network analysis, and portfolio learning for improved performance.

A seminal study from 1985 found that only 30% of the information needs of physicians were met during a patient visit, and usually, they were met through consultation with another physician or health professional. Print sources were not used due to age of textbooks in the office, poor organization of journal articles, inadequate indexing of books and drug information sources, lack of knowledge of appropriate source, and the time required to find the desired information.[36]

Learning in the workplace continues to be a central component of lifelong learning in medicine. A long history of research on the topic suggests that learning in the medical workplace is triggered regularly by the need to solve a problem,[37,38] with colleagues, books, and electronic resources,[38–40] the ongoing methods for answering questions that arise during practice. Most importantly, feedback has been recognized as an important learning tool for informing a physician's clinical performance.[38,41]

Despite its acknowledged value in learning, delivery of feedback based on observation of performance occurs infrequently.[41,42] Further, self-assessment without observation and feedback is ineffective.[16,43] Recent feasibility testing of an evidence-based model for facilitating performance feedback to enhance acceptance and utilization suggests four phases of importance to the learner and to the CPD provider: (1) build relationships to supersede recipients' sensitivity to receiving performance reports, (2) explore recipients' general reactions to their feedback report including specific items to determine whether the recipient's self-assessment was confirmed, (3) assure a clear understanding of the report's context and the opportunities it affords for change and learning, and (4) coach for performance change, with a plan and focus on realistic goals.[44] In short, there are formidable gaps between capabilities and performance. The design of feedback will likely play an important role in the future success of CPD planning and assessment.

NEWER AND EMERGING FORCES

The Assessment of Professionalism

In 1980, Richards and Cohen reviewed the literature to learn why physicians attend traditional CME programs.[45] They found the reasons for participation included (1) an integral part of professionalism, (2) an interest in topical subjects, (3) a means of validating or modifying prior learning or behavior, (4) a means of attaining an identified learning objective, and (5) a change of pace from practice routine and an opportunity for social contact with other physicians. Richards and Cohen concluded that: (1) a commitment to the ongoing improvement of craftsmanship through the continuous learning of facts, concepts, and skills is basic to the very notion of a professional, (2) society, too, maintains that belief, and (3) the proliferation of laws and regulations governing physician participation in CME is essential to the satisfactory practice of medicine.[45]

While the fundamental concepts, proposed centrality and operationalization of professionalism are not new, its measurement and complexity continue to puzzle and provoke educators, policy makers, and researchers in the health professions.[46] Major challenges arise from the notion that professionalism occupies a continuum stretching from the individual (attributes, capacities, behaviors) through the interpersonal domain (interactions with other individuals and with contexts) to the macrosocietal level where phenomena such as social responsibility, morality, political agendas, and economic imperatives reside. A reciprocity exists here: an individual's professional behavior may be influenced by context; similarly, individuals within an institution may influence its collective professional values.

Hodges and Ginsburg[46] suggest that professionalism is a complex and multidimensional construct, its assessment requiring consideration of individual, interpersonal, and societal dimensions. For consistency in our discussion, their general recommendations are broken out below in each dimension at an individual (micro level).

- *Quantitative or qualitative instruments* should be employed in behavioral assessments, having demonstrable reliability and defensibility.
- *Triangulation* may be ensured by the use of multiple kinds of measures, by multiple observers, synthesized over time with data gathered in multiple complex and challenging contexts.
- *Identification and documentation of negative behaviors* requires thoughtful instrument design and validity research. This process is distinct from one which recognizes, documents, and reinforces positive professional behaviors.
- *An overall assessment program* is more important than its individual tools. It should employ a variety of tools in a safe climate and provide rich feedback, anonymously when appropriate, and follow-up of behavior change over time. Effective assessment and feedback programs incorporate faculty/monitor training.

The Hodges and Ginsburg[46] recommendations for assessment of professionalism as an interpersonal phenomenon align loosely with what Nelson, Batalden, and Godfrey[47] describe as mesosystem actions taken by midlevel managers responsible for large clinical programs, clinical support services, and administrative services. The recommendations include:

- *Comprehensiveness.* Because professionalism implies a set of behaviors and responses to situational and contextual phenomena, assessment should include the decisions, responses, and behaviors of all actors in the learning or practice setting (perhaps using multisource feedback), gathering longitudinal data from both teachers and learners as well as from other key players such as health care professionals, administrators, and patients.
- *Assessment of the learning/practice environment* is important, including feedback to improve performance of teams and to improve structural elements such as policies. Monitoring the learning environment for interpersonal phenomena is also critical.
- *Benchmarking.* While consensus on what are appropriate professional responses to complex problems and situations may not always be achieved, assessment and feedback should request a collective perspective when possible.

For the assessment of professionalism as an institutional/societal phenomenon (macro level), the Hodges and Ginsburg[46] recommendations include the following:

- *Professionalism* can be understood in the context of the goals, aspirations, and collective behaviors of health care and educational institutions and of the profession itself.
- *Assessment* involves characterizing social expectations, through dialogue and meaningful input from public state holders, and measuring the degree to which the profession (as a whole or in subsets) meets them. Accreditation requirements at every level require teaching and evaluating professionalism. Effectiveness should be measured in terms of clear institutional and social outcomes.
- *Critiquing* the dominance of certain ways that expectations and practices are framed or enforced (e.g., cultures, generational, gendered, hierarchical) should lead to improved institutions and organizational climate and practice.
- *Professional lapses* may arise from particular kinds of problematic social interactions.
- The *hidden curriculum* and tacit problematic organizational or institutional norms are important in assessing and contextualizing professional or unprofessional behaviors of learners, teachers, or institutions, including health care systems.[46]

Irby and Hamstra[48] suggest three frameworks may be especially useful when considering the assessment of physicians for professionalism. The oldest is virtue based, focusing on the inner habits of the heart, the development of moral character and reasoning, plus humanistic qualities of caring and compassion: the "good physician" is a person of character. Another of the frameworks involves identity formation, with a focus on identity development, including socialization into the community of practice. Here, the "good physician" integrates into his or her identity a set of values and dispositions consonant with the physician community. He or she aspires to a professional identity reflected in the very best physicians.

The behavior-based framework dominates professionalism today. It emphasizes milestones, competencies, and measurable behaviors. The "good physician" is a person who consistently demonstrates competence in performing patient care tasks. While virtue-based professionalism involves internalization and commitment to a core set of values and actions guided by moral reasoning, professional identity formation requires positive role models to sensitize learners in advance to situations where negative role models might be encountered. Finally, behavior-based professionalism requires clear expectations and teaching to behaviors, including feedback to reinforce correct or desirable behavior and to sanction unprofessional behavior.[48]

Interprofessional Education and Collaboration

Explicit feedback, strengthened evidence, population-based outcomes, and novel longitudinal study design are themes extending throughout recent investigations involving interprofessional education (IPE), collaborative care, and quality. In 2015, the Institute of Medicine (IOM) studied how to measure the impact of interprofessional education on collaborative practice and patient outcomes.[49] IOM recognized that it is possible to link the learning process with downstream person-, population-, or system-directed outcomes, provided that well-designed studies are intentionally targeted to answering such questions.[49] IOM also recognized numerous gaps in the evidence linking IPE to patient, population, and system outcomes.

Without a purposeful, collaborative, and comprehensive system of engagement between the education and health care delivery systems, evaluating the impact of IPE interventions on health and system outcomes will be difficult. The (IOM) report recommended that interprofessional stakeholders, funders, and policy makers commit resources to a coordinated series of well-designed studies of the association between interprofessional education and collaborative behavior, including teamwork and performance in practice. These studies should investigate the measurement of interprofessional collaboration (including intermediate learning outcomes) effectively across a range of learning environments, patient populations, and practice settings. Further, longitudinal studies—those that are necessarily more complex, spanning the education continuum, following trainees over time, and encompassing classrooms, simulation laboratories, and practice settings—are generally lacking.[49]

The Learning Health Care System

In studying opportunities to manage the complexity of biomedical and clinical knowledge while providing more efficient, lower-cost health care, the IOM focuses advancement on the ideal of a continuously learning health care system. It is one in which science, informatics, incentives, and culture align for continuous improvement and innovation; best practices are seamlessly embedded in the care process; patients and families are active participants in all elements; and new knowledge is captured as an integral by-product of the care experience.[50]

The Committee on the Learning Health Care System (CLHCS) in America recognized that individual physicians, nurses, technicians, pharmacists, and others involved in patient care work diligently to provide high-quality compassionate care to their patients, but the system does not always support them in their work.[50] It lags in new discoveries—in disseminating data in real time, organizing, and coordinating the enormous volume of research and recommendations—and in providing incentives for choosing the smartest route to health, not just the easiest. The IOM suggests these broad issues prevent clinicians from providing the best care to their patients and limit their abilities to continuously learn and improve.

Offsetting these issues, four trends present opportunities for health system and CPD leaders. *Vast computational power* makes it possible to harvest useful longer-term information from actual patient care, as opposed to time-limited studies. *Connectivity* allows that information be accessed in real time virtually anywhere, by professionals and patients, permitting unprecedented diffusion of information less expensively, quickly, and on demand. *Progress in human and organizational capabilities and management science* can improve the reliability and efficiency of care, permitting more scientific deployment of human and technical resources to match the complexity of systems and institutions. *Increasing empowerment of patients* unleashes the potential for the participants, in concert with clinicians, in the prevention and treatment of disease—tasks that increasingly depend on personal behavior change.[50]

Use of health information technology assumes importance that is of particular interest to health systems and CPD providers. Issues requiring further study are numerous in this area: building relationships with end users, assessing their reactions to the process and content; and coaching for performance,[44] while planning for longer-term studies to eliminate dependence on coaches, and increasing access to innovations that reduce pain, suffering, and expense associated with the long lag time from discovery to application in practice.[50]

The IOM Committee on the Learning Health Care System[50] recommends that research funding agencies promote research designs and methods that draw naturally on existing care processes and that also support ongoing quality improvement efforts. Clinicians and health care organizations should adopt tools that deliver timely and reliable, clinical knowledge to the point of care. Organizations should implement incentives that encourage the use of those tools and improve coordination and communication within and across organizations. Health care delivery organizations and clinicians, partnering with patients, families, and community organizations, should develop coordination and transition processes, data-sharing capabilities, and communication tools to ensure safe, seamless care.

While each recommendation regarding the learning health care system appears valuable to achieving better care at lower costs, assessment of communication and other behaviors requires rigorous design and implementation across all levels: micro, meso, and macro. Because physicians perform differently under controlled conditions, two designs appear attractive. A longitudinal study of communication using questionnaires administered periodically and correlated with practice behaviors would enable the assessment of gaps between specific communication skills and actual performance. On the other hand, a social network analysis utilizing the electronically communicated records of physicians and others in the health care system and community could enable an assessment of current and desired communication patterns.[51] In either case, a carefully designed mechanism to feedback results should lead to specific improvements.

Clinician Burnout

A focus on health reform generally and the learning health care system specifically may miss a critical element—the well-being of the professionals who work within the system.[52-54] As noted earlier in the current chapter, studies of feedback reveal conflicts between personal and professional values of health care professionals and the larger health care–related organizations and commercial entities with which they are associated. These conflicts can place the well-being of health professionals at risk for demoralization and burnout.[53] The risk of burnout can be assessed throughout the career of the health care provider, using brief validated scales to track the learner and to correlate scores with select performance measures in health care settings. Although not a comprehensive workup of mental state, such a strategy may serve as an early warning system to prevent more difficult or complex emotional challenges later in practice. The relationship between an individual's sense of self-efficacy, motivation to change, and implementation of activities to improve suggests methods of addressing physicians' sense of self-efficacy has the potential to improve the efficacy of their continuing education.[55]

Deliberate Practice: Purposeful, Informed, Based on Feedback

The complexity of the clinical setting exerts competing demands on the health care provider and it tests the capacity of persons to self-regulate their learning.[56] Emerging metacognitive models may help health care learners and CPD leaders alike to gain perspective on the prodigious growth of new medical knowledge and the complexity and uncertainty that strain the emotions of caregivers during daily practice.[57-59] As individual health care providers exert metacognitive processes to analyze and thus discipline the way they think, feel, and act, learning health care organizations must accept responsibility for helping health care providers maintain their professionalism. Professionalism and metacognitive growth may be served for development by deliberative practice, a stepwise approach to building or modifying previously acquired skills by focusing on particular aspects of those skills and working specifically to improve them. Over time this step-by-step improvement leads to expert performance. Because of the way new skills are built atop existing skills, it is important for faculty or teachers to provide beginners with the correct fundamental skills, in order to minimize the chances that learners will need to relearn those fundamental skills later, at a more advanced level.

Ericsson and Pool[60] describe deliberate practice as possessing seven characteristics. *First*, deliberate practice develops skills that others already have mastered and for which effective training techniques have been established. Training should be overseen by a coach or teacher who is familiar with the abilities of expert performers and with ways those abilities can best be developed. *Second*, deliberate practice takes place outside one's comfort zone and requires a learner to try things just beyond his or her current abilities. Thus, it demands near-maximal effort, which is generally not enjoyable. *Third*, deliberate practice includes well-defined, specific goals to improve an aspect of target performance, not a vague, overall improvement. Once an overall goal has been set, a teacher or coach develops a plan for making a series of small changes that will add up to the desired larger or more complex changes. Improving some aspect of the targeted performance allows a learner to see that his or her performances have been improved by the training. *Fourth*, deliberate practice is *deliberate*, requiring full attention and conscious actions. *Fifth*, deliberate practice involves feedback and modification of efforts in response to that feedback. Early in the training process, much of the feedback comes from the coach, while with time and experience, learners begin to monitor themselves. *Sixth*, deliberate practice both produces and depends on effective mental representations. Improving performance goes hand in hand with improving mental representations; as one's performance improves, the representations become more detailed and effective, making it possible to improve even more. They show the right way to do something and allow one to notice when doing something wrong to correct it. *Seventh* and finally, deliberate practice nearly always involves building or modifying previously acquired skills by focusing on particular aspects of those skills.[60]

In short, deliberate practice differs from other sorts of purposeful exercise in two important ways. It requires a field that is already reasonably well developed, one in which the best performers have attained a level of performance, clearly setting them apart from novices. Further, it requires a coach or instructor to provide practice activities designed to help a learner improve his or her performance. With this definition, there is a distinction between purposeful practice (in which an individual tries very hard to push himself or herself to improve) and practice that is both purposeful and informed. In particular, deliberate practice is informed and guided by the best performers' accomplishment and by an understanding of what the expert performers do to excel. Deliberate practice is purposeful practice that articulates where it is going and how to get there.[60]

Imaging the Neurophysiology of Decision-Making

CPD providers, leaders, and health systems must share a common conviction that clinical decision-making should be an integral part of medical education at the undergraduate and postgraduate levels and throughout CPD. How doctors think and how they make decisions have major implications for patient safety.[58,61] While most studies in the area have been behavioral or observational, recent imaging studies suggest a strong neurophysiological basis, requiring attention and further study.

The imaging studies suggest the following impressions: (1) decision-making and conflict in decision-making can be modeled[62]; (2) voluntary and involuntary risk taking may be identified and imaged in the human brain[63]; (3) human choices have been successfully attributed to the dopaminoceptive system; humans can structure their search for and use of relevant information adaptively selecting between decision strategies[64]; (4) compared with recall questions, problem-solving questions induce medical students to use higher cognitive functions and lower emotions stress[65]; and (5) there appears to be a neurophysiological mechanism fundamental to value-based decisions, wherein the brain weighs costs and benefits by combining neural benefit and cost signals into a single, difference-based neural representation of net value, which is accumulated over time until the individual decides to accept or reject an option.[66] The CPD provider might imagine coaching a learner toward alignment with an image of experts' decision-making, scanned and aggregated for training toward best clinical decision-making and administered as much for learning as for simultaneous assessment of action. This is not to overstate or overpromise the immediate application of such an approach but to suggest its potential for longer-term applied research, improving human potential, especially as imaging opportunities and electronically supported clinical decisions move closer in proximity to the bedside in learning health care systems.

FUTURE DIRECTIONS

Future directions must draw on the past and be informed by the forces for change articulated in this chapter. Writing in 1987, Manning and Petit advised: "Changes in continuing medical education (CME) during the past three decades have been controversial and complex.[67] A 1950s style, small-scale, voluntary activity has evolved into broad-scale programs with accredited sponsors and with ties to relicensure. Within the next three decades, CME will be directed by methods chosen by specialty boards for recertification and by exploitation of computer and telecommunication technology. Written recertification examinations can waste physicians' time studying material that will not improve care of their patients. We hope improved methods of analysis of individual practices, on-the-spot access to pertinent medical information, and better communication among physicians can be incorporated into recertification procedures."[67]

Not to embellish the past but to contextualize our present knowledge and focus on future directions, a select study of learning and change merits more detailed analysis.[37] Several references in the current review derive from the project, published in 1989 and supported by the Society of Medical College Directors of Continuing Medical Education (SMCDCME), the predecessor organization to the Society for Academic Continuing Medical Education (SACME). Often described as the Change Study, it involved 24 member institutions whose society representatives conducted more than 340 individual interviews with practicing physicians.[37] Seven hundred seventy-five unique changes were analyzed. Seventeen research team members wrote for the published Change Study.[37] Several of those writers are contributors to the current volume; they and many of their SMCDCME colleagues continued to lead research, planning, and policy making in international circles, while training others to continue the growth of scholarship in CPD. Such collaborative work and professional development, sponsored by SACME or a similar organization, appears centrally important to the continued future success of CPD, its study, and improvement.

Each element in the current brief overview—at macro, meso, and micro levels—speaks to the need for understanding and engagement by the CPD professional, the clinician–learner, and the health system in which he or she functions. Future considerations are clustered by the main actors—the clinician–learner, the evaluator or assessor, and the system or CPD leader. It is important to respect the linkages between, and mutual dependence of, each of these three agents: the success of the CPD leader is tied to the success of the learner, the assessor, and the CPD planner, each functioning in a complex system of care and public health. Derived from assessment and uses of health information technology (HIT), including registries and claims data, those linkages provide opportunities for a future converging of learner assessment, performance improvement, and credentialing, essential catalysts for patient safety, the bedrock for health care quality improvement.

The Clinician–Learner

Perhaps the most important lesson from the literature and this review of forces for change is this: physicians and other health professionals must strive *throughout their practice lives* to ensure their practices are, at all times, current, collaborative, caring, and competent. This involves sustained curiosity and a commitment to professionalism,[40,68] to the professional identity of what it means to be a good doctor, and to lifelong learning that takes advantage of ongoing opportunities to improve self-assessment, identifying gaps in competencies and addressing them. To accomplish the alliterative "4c" goal, clinicians must recognize that they alone cannot determine their own learning needs[16,17] requiring objective data and even external observer–coaches to achieve it while surfacing their own critical thinking in the context of their adult professional development,[69,70] including age and stage of career—breaking in to the profession, fitting in with colleagues, or getting out of health care, for retirement or other reasons.[71]

Thus, clinicians of the future are advised to explicitly (1) set learning goals based on *objective* performance data and select activities that enable the identification of gaps in practice; (2) select educational activities that meet clinical performance needs individually and in teams, seeking interactions with others who build on the learners' knowledge and skills and enable not only the observation but also testing of new skills in the practice setting; (3) participate in learning activities with clearly stated, *specific* objectives that enable measured progress over a predetermined period of time; and (4) match the education or training environment to the practice contexts where performance will be demonstrated. Future clinicians will also become familiar with the concept of mastery learning and adaptation for portfolios in which cumulative longitudinal data regarding performance (360 degree assessments, patient feedback, utilization data, and others) and educational achievements are collected for scrutiny by others.[72]

Not to be taken lightly in the quest for optimal patient care, clinicians and their educator/leaders will need to normalize, articulate, address, and monitor their well-being.[52–55] Recognizing, accepting, and addressing the early signs of stress and burnout is important to clinician, family, and (ultimately) patient health.[73,74]

Evaluators and Assessors

Among the future trends apparent in this review is the growing need for and importance of assessment and evaluation and those with skills, competence, and dedication to these tasks. Such individuals are encouraged to (1) develop consensus about an evaluation design that links evaluation to instructional objectives and includes an assessed need or gap in performance, a carefully delineated instructional strategy, evaluation tools, and costs; (2) select or develop observational tools to reliably evaluate knowledge, competence, and performance; (3) assess satisfaction and perceived value for each component of multifaceted interventions, including the overall impact of instruction on performance and patient health; (4) evaluate demonstration of knowledge, skills, and attitudes (KSAs) in variable contexts, including transfer of KSAs to practice; and (5) ensure that high-stakes testing takes place in the workplace or in similar simulated and standardized settings. Further, assessors must cast a critical eye on the competency-based assessment movement to assure that, among its useful and clinically driven goals, individual clinician values, experience, moral character, and professional identity are not ignored.[47,48,72,75]

While these skills can apply at the micro level, they can also be projected onto the macro or national level. Here, the future holds the promise of large data repositories, with "Big Data" analytics enabling researchers to focus on what happens in entire populations, describing it, analyzing patterns, and generalizing new hypotheses regarding learning, care, and those who deliver services.[76–78] It also points toward closer alignments or even mergers of organizations invested in the assessment and certification of individual clinical competence, the evaluation and accreditation of education and health care systems, and the certainty of accountable, safe, health care, all the while staying mindful that learned professions must comply with requirements of access and free trade.[79,80] Here, at the macro level, assessors will become increasingly skilled in determining inequities in workforce training and deployment, in resource allocation, and in other values to drive the curriculum of CPD.

CPD Planners

Highly important to the future of CPD is that of the professional CPD planner, developer, and manager. While the role is addressed elsewhere in this text (see Chapter 4), specific suggestions flowing from this chapter's context follow. Planners are advised to undertake the following efforts: (1) provide reliable data for learners to reflect upon present levels of performance compared with desired levels of performance; (2) offer consultation to help learners specify achievable and measurable goals while enabling comfortable communication and practice of what is learned among individuals or teams; (3) design activities with the goal of helping individuals or teams of learners adopt change incrementally, assuring compatibility with present systems and advantage over present behaviors and measuring results including clinical progress and costs; and (4) design education and training activities that provide more immersive and realistic contexts to practice or learn the intended knowledge, skills, or attitudes.[72]

Finally, planners must become aware of the need to address new content areas (critical decision-making, evidence-based medicine, cost/value, quality improvement, and patient safety, among many others), "new" or better defined competencies (such as professionalism), a much-broadened array of educational methods and designs (e.g., using information technology, performance feedback, or coaching), and a widely varying audience, including health professionals of many kinds. In this last context, attending to the needs of low-resourced settings might mean the training of nontraditional health care providers to deliver care.[1] In contrast, in regions where health professionals are underemployed, or returning to work after extended absences, retraining programs may need to be developed and assessed.[55,81]

Considerations for the CPD and System Leader

Including health systems themselves, all the forces for change articulated throughout this chapter, lead to the speculation that true leadership in CPD (and leadership in health care in general) means an understanding of the needs of health systems and populations as a whole. Thus, this section targets both system and CPD leadership, assuming that wise and seamless systems will recognize and support the overlap. Several key ingredients form these considerations: outcomes orientation; assessment, evaluation, and scholarship in the field; the role of stakeholders in the system; and the development of a meaningful, patient- and system-focused curriculum.

Outcomes orientation. From the particular perspective of the CPD leader, specific lessons or preparations for the future will need to—at all times—consider the outcome. This close approximation of CPD and the assessment of its effect is both the major thesis of this chapter and a key driving element in the future success of CPD. While including the highest level outcomes as objectives in plans for change, outcomes can also include process measures, patient outcomes, and community health data as targets and planning tools. Credentialing may be considered a concurrent reminder/guide reflecting mean or minimum standards.[72]

Assessment, evaluation, and the scholarship of improved professional development. Social science alone does not promise better policy or health care. It is simply a guide to understanding problems, the conditions that give rise to them, and the outcomes likely to occur when policy addresses them. In this very specific sense, social and natural sciences present a more reliable guide than what is otherwise available to leaders in health care and education.[82] It is insufficient to plan and implement educational or other evidence-based interventions: they must also be evaluated and shared, not only to improve locally facilitated activities but also to enable transfer and replicability into other contexts. Further, longitudinal studies of performance must be completed, using both information ordinarily available on physician performance and methods to understand correlational behaviors and attitudes of individuals performing in organizations and systems of care. Properly designed and rigorously executed, these studies should help individual performers and systems to adapt and to make better decisions.

Two particular areas of study appear attractive to the futurist. At the micro level, neural imaging to understand the pathophysiology of learning and decision-making offers a relatively new tool for the CPD scholar. Further, at the meso level, social network analysis affords the promise of understanding knowledge transfer, collegial interaction, and the culture of physician and other health professional interaction. For example, investigating the use of smartphones in health care, including applications and outcomes, should enable higher reliability and real-time studies of higher-quality evidence, interprofessional communication, and processes of care, in learning.[83,84]

Such studies will build on the evidence in continuing education and training, which currently holds (1) effects are inconsistent across practitioners, settings, and behaviors, and gaps in performance present opportunities for improvement; (2) interactive learning and opportunities to practice skills can affect change; (3) sequenced and multifaceted activities can effect change in practice and patient outcomes; and (4) educational content similar to the practice environment is more likely to affect change than dissimilar training content. However, providing varied cases and contexts is effective for transfer of training to multiple contexts.[72] Especially for workplace-based assessment, these data may be entered into learning portfolios that document work experience, observed clinical encounters, discussions of individual cases, and feedback on routine performance.[38]

Stakeholders in the health care system. Many components make up the systems in which doctors and other health professionals function—patients, health care providers, insurers and other payers, and the health care system itself. The CPD leader must look internally to reconcile allegiances to the practicing physician, the health system, the patient, and community. Conflicts of interest between personal and professional values of health professionals and larger health care organizations and commercial entities with which they are associated may contribute not only to unrest in the health care workforce but also to demoralization, burnout, and poor patient care.[53,85]

Toward a curriculum for CPD leadership. The curriculum for CPD leaders is full and expanding at a rapid pace. First, it includes an increased understanding of the health system, incorporating items such as health information technology, utilization of tests and other resources, measures, and incentives. Leaders in CPD will require fundamental understandings of causation, for example, what constitutes causal explanation and what warrants causal inference as opposed to descriptive regularity.[86] They will need to learn how to assess needs and negotiate interventions within the context of care, selecting content and designing learning activities for individuals and for teams of health care providers serving patients enrolled in diverse models of care. They will also need to augment performance improvement interventions that may suffer from rushed implementation or otherwise poor consideration of innovations in the science of learning or the complexities of care.

Second, as a result of the first, CPD leaders will require sensitivity to quality issues. They will need to understand and use (1) training for reflection on the part of the health care learner whose actions constitute an emerging system of education and care, (2) incentives for providers to use established guidelines for better outcomes or for increased efficiency, (3) health care product assessment for safety and quality, and (4) patient engagement.

Third, in order to be effective, the CPD leader must ensure a visible commitment to a string of values: (1) a "relentless operational ethos" of continuous improvement and assessment yielding better value for patients and systems; (2) the merit of automated, reliable information to and from the point of care to assess needs and outcomes; (3) evidence-based protocols for effective, efficient, and consistent care; (4) optimized resource utilization, including personnel, physical space, and other considerations; (5) integrated care, that is, the right care in the right setting with the right providers and team; (6) tailored community and clinic support for resource-intensive patients; (7) embedded safeguards, for example, supports and prompts to reduce injury and infection; and finally, (8) transparency—visible progress in performance, outcomes, and costs.[50]

Well-being. Finally, the CPD leader is challenged to consider the well-being of the individual learner as well as that learner's performance. Historically, the emphasis has been on the actions and outcomes of the clinician as a learner, but the stress on delivery systems has not gone without affecting the well-being of health care providers whose actions help to define the effectiveness of the systems themselves. Of late, more attention has been drawn to the well-being of the learner him/herself as a performer within the system of care.[54] Psychological studies have surfaced a wealth of elements affecting health professional well-being: individual differences regarding affiliation, dominance, and team performance; attitudes toward patient safety; error reporting confidence; feelings toward a hierarchy of authority involving rank, rewards, and distribution of power; psychological safety, including the management of mistakes; and feelings about competence or achievement of work.[33,87]

In analyzing the fit and function of caregivers in their clinical environments, it is ironic that the healthy intellect of those who maintain responsibility for the health of others has been discounted so completely for so long. A gentler, more comprehensive and learner-oriented approach to CPD might help to reconcile the stressors between the demands for competency and accountability and performance as well as the compassion for learner well-being. Such an approach would embrace lifelong learning as "…a process whereby physicians or health care providers who no longer attend school on a regular full-time basis…undertake sequential and organized activities with the conscious intention of bringing about changes in information, knowledge, understanding, or skill, appreciation and attitudes; or for the purpose of identifying or solving personal, professional, or community problems."[88,89]

REFERENCES

1. WHO. *Transformative Scale up of Health Professional Education.* World Health Organization; 2011. http://apps.who.int/iris/bitstream/10665/70573/1/WHO_HSS_HRH_HEP2011.01_eng.pdf. Accessed July 25, 2016.
2. Horsley T, Grimshaw J, Campbell C. *Policy Brief 14: How to Create Conditions for Adapting Physicians' Skills to New Needs and Lifelong Learning.* World Health Organization; 2010. http://www.euro.who.int/__data/assets/pdf_file/0020/124418/e94294.pdf. Accessed June 27, 2016.
3. Durley CC. *The NOCA Guide to Understanding Credentialing Concepts.* National Organization for Competency Assurance; 2005. www.cvacert.org/documents/credentialingconceptsNOCA.pdg. Accessed August 22, 2016.
4. McHugh MD, Hawkins RE, Mazmanian PE, et al. *Challenges and Opportunities in Nurse Credentialing Research Design.* Discussion Paper. Washington, DC: Institute of Medicine; 2014. http://name.edu/wp-content/uploads/2015/credentialingresearchdesign. Accessed August 22, 2016.
5. Institute of Medicine (IOM). *Future Directions of Credentialing Research in Nursing: Workshop Summary.* Washington, DC: The National Academies Press; 2015.
6. Nurse Credentialing.org Magnet. http://www.nursecredentialing.org/Magnet/ProgramOverview. Accessed August 23, 2016.
7. The Joint Commission. https://www.jointcommission.org/about_us/about_the_joint_commission_main.aspx. Accessed August 26, 2016.
8. The Joint Commission. *Facts about Federal Deemed Status and State Recognition.* The Joint Commission. Published on November 15, 2015. https://www.jointcommission.org/facts_about_federal_deemed_status_and_state_recognition/. Accessed August 26, 2016.
9. The Council for Health Service Accreditation in Southern Africa (COHSASA). http://www.cohsasa.co.za/. Accessed August 26, 2016.
10. Sole M, Pantelli D, Risso-Gill I, et al. How do medical doctors in the European Union demonstrate that they continue to meet criteria for registration and licencing? *Clin Med.* 2014;14(6):633–639. http://www.clinmed.rcpjournal.org/content/14/6/633.full.pdf+html. Accessed August 26, 2016.
11. Accreditation Canada. https://accreditation.ca/. Accessed August 26, 2016.
12. Australian Commission on Safety and Quality in Health Care. http://www.safetyandquality.gov.au/. Accessed August 26, 2016.
13. Ministry of Health. http://www.health.govt.nz/. Accessed August 26, 2016.
14. Joint Commission International. *JCI-Accredited Organizations.* http://www.jointcommissioninternational.org/about-jci/jci-accredited-organizations/. Accessed July 19, 2016.
15. Institute of Medicine (IOM). *Redesigning Continuing Education in the Health Professions.* Washington, DC: National Academies Press; 2010.
16. Davis DA, Mazmanian PE, Fordis M, et al. Accuracy of physician self assessment compared with observed measures of competence: a systematic review. *JAMA.* 2006;296(9):1094–1102. doi:10.1001/jama.296.9.1094.
17. Davis DA. How to help professionals maintain and improve their knowledge and skills: triangulating best practices in medicine. In: Anders Ericsson K, ed. *Development of Professional Expertise: Toward Measurement of Expert Performance and Design of Optimal Learning Environments.* Cambridge, UK: Cambridge University Press; 2009:180–202.
18. Miller SH. American Board of Medical Specialties and repositioning for excellence in lifelong learning: maintenance of certification. *J Contin Educ Health Prof.* 2005;25(3):151–156.

19. American Board of Medical Specialties. 2016. http://www.abms.org/media/84748/abms_memberboard-srequirementsproject_moc_artii.pdf. Accessed June 27, 2016.

20. Hawkins RE, Irons MB, Welcher CM, et al. The ABMS MOC part III examination: value, concerns, and alternative formats. *Acad Med.* 2016;91(11):1509–1515. doi: 10.1097/ACM.0000000000001291.

21. Horsley T, Lockyer J, Cogo E, et al. National programmes for validating physician competence and fitness for practice: a scoping review. *BMJ Open.* 2016;6(4):e010368. doi:10.1136/bmjopen-2015-010368.

22. Dauphinee WD. An international review of the recertification and revalidation of physicians: progress toward achieving best practices. In: McGaghie WC, ed. *International Best Practices for Evaluation in the Health Professions.* London, UK: Radcliffe Publishing; 2013:281–310.

23. Davis DA, Thomson MA, Oxman AD, et al. Changing physicians performance. A systematic review of the effect of continuing medical education strategies. *JAMA.* 1995;274(9):700–705. http://www.ncbi.nlm.nih.gov/pubmed/7650822. Accessed August 26, 2016.

24. Alaszewski A. The impact of the Bristol Royal Infirmary disaster and inquiry on public services in the UK. *J Interprof Care.* 2002;16(4):371–378. doi: 10.1080/1356182021000008319.

25. Tanne JH. When Jesica died. *BMJ.* 2003;326(7391):717. http://www.ncbi.nlm.nih.gov/pmc/articles/PMC1125622/. Accessed August 26, 2016.

26. Hickey JV, Unruh LR, Newhouse RP, et al. Credentialing: the need for a national research agenda. *Nurs Outlook.* 2014;62(2):119–127.

27. U.S. Department of Labor, Employment and Training Administration. 2014. http://wdr.doleta.gov/directives/attach/TEGL15-10a2.pdf. Accessed July 22, 2016.

28. American Board of Medical Specialties (ABMS). *Based on Core Competencies.* American Board of Medical Specialties. http://www.abms.org/board-certification/a-trustedcredential/based-on-core-competencies/. Accessed August 26, 2016.

29. United States Medical Licensing Examination (USMLE). http://www.usmle.org/. Accessed July 22, 2016.

30. American Board of Medical Specialties Maintenance of Certification (ABMS MOC). *Certification Matters.* ABMS MOC. http://www.certificationmatters.org/about-boardcertified-doctors/about-the-abms-moc-program.aspx. Accessed August 26, 2016.

31. Royal College of Physicians and Surgeons of Canada. *The Maintenance of Certification Program.* The Royal College of Physicians and Surgeons of Canada. http://www.royalcollege.ca/rcsite/cpd/mainte-nance-of-certification-program-e. Accessed August 12, 2016.

32. Care Quality Commission. *Guidance for Providers on Meeting the Regulations.* Care Quality Commission; 2015. http://www.cqc.org.uk/sites/default/files/20150324_guidance_providers_meeting_regulations_0pdf. Accessed August 26, 2016.

33. Appelbaum NP, Dow A, Mazmanian PE, et al. The effects of power, leadership and psychological safety on resident event reporting. *Med Educ.* 2016;50(3):343–350.

34. The Royal Australasian College of Physicians. https://www.racp.edu.au/. Accessed August 26, 2016.

35. National Medical Examination Center (NMEC). http://www.nmec.org.cn/EnglishEdition.html. Accessed August 26, 2016.

36. Covell DG, Uman GC, Manning PR. Information needs in office practice: are they being met? *Ann Intern Med.* 1985;103(4):4596–599. doi:10.7326/0003-4819-103-4-596.

37. Fox RD, Mazmanian PE, Putnam RW. The theory of learning and change. In: Fox RD, Mazmanian PE, Putnam RW, eds. *Changing and Learning in the Lives of Physicians.* New York: Praeger Publishers; 1989:161–175.

38. Singh T, Norcini JJ. Workplace-based assessment. In: McGaghie WC, ed. *International Best Practices for Evaluation in the Health Professions.* Chapter 12. London, UK: Radcliffe Publishing; 2013:257–279.

39. Davis D. The clinical environment. In: Fox RD, Mazmanian PE, Putnam RW, eds. *Changing and Learning in the Lives of Physicians.* New York: Praeger Publishers; 1989:99–109.

40. Putnam RW, Campbell MD. Competence. In: Fox RD, Mazmanian PE, Putnam RW, eds. *Changing and Learning in the Lives of Physicians.* New York: Praeger Publishers; 1989:79–87.

41. Veloski J, Boex JR, Grasberger MJ, et al. Systematic review of the literature on assessment, feedback, and physicians' clinical performance. BEME Guide No. 7. *Med Teach.* 2006;28(2):117–128.

42. Ivers N, Jamtvedt G, Flottorp S, et al. Audit and feedback: effects on professional practice and healthcare outcomes. *Cochrane Database Syst Rev.* 2012;6(6):CD000259.

43. Eva KW, Regehr G. Self-assessment in the health professions: a reformulation and research agenda. *Acad Med.* 2005;80(10 suppl):546–554.

44. Sargeant J, Lockyer J, Mann K, et al. Facilitated reflective performance feedback: developing an evidence- and theory-based model that builds relationship, explores reactions and content, and coaches for performance change (R2C2). *Acad Med.* 2015;90(12):1698–1706.

45. Richards RK, Cohen RM. Why physicians attend traditional CME programs. *J Med Educ.* 1980;55(6):479–485. http://www.ncbi.nlm.nih.gov/pubmed/7381898. Accessed August 29, 2016.

46. Hodges BD, Ginsburg S. Assessment of professionalism. In: McGaphie WC, ed. *International on Practices for Evaluation in the Health Professions.* London, UK: Radcliffe Publishing Ltd.; 2013:139–167.
47. Nelson EC, Batalden PB, Godfrey MM. *Quality by Design: A Clinical Microsystems Approach.* San Francisco, CA: Jossey-Bass; 2007.
48. Irby DM, Hamstra SJ. Parting the clouds: three professionalism frameworks in medical education. *Acad Med.* 2016. [Epub ahead of print]. doi: 10.1097/ACM.0000000000001190.
49. Institute of Medicine (IOM). *Measuring the Impact of Interprofessional Education on Collaborative Practice and Patient Outcomes.* Washington, DC: National Academies Press; 2015.
50. Institute of Medicine (IOM). *Best Care at Lower Cost: The Path to Continuously Learning Health Care in America.* Washington, DC: The National Academies Press; 2013.
51. Lurie SJ, Fogg TT, Dozier AM. Social network analysis as a method of assessing institutional culture: three case studies. *Acad Med.* 2009;84(8):1029–1035.
52. Shanafelt TD, Boone S, Tan L, et al. Burnout and satisfaction with work-life balance among US physicians relative to the general US population. *Arch Intern Med.* 2012;172(18):1377–1385. doi:10.1001/archinternmed.2012.3199.
53. Gabel S. Demoralization in health professional practice: development, amelioration, and implications for continuing education. *J Contin Educ Health Prof.* 2013;33(2):118–126.
54. Shanafelt TD, Hasan O, Dyrbye LN, et al. Changes in burnout and satisfaction with work-life balance in physicians and the general US working population between 2011 and 2014. *Mayo Clin Proc.* 2015;90(12):1600–1613.
55. Williams BW, Kessler HA, Williams MV. Relationship among practice change, motivation, and self-efficacy. *J Contin Educ Health Prof.* 2014;34(1):5–10.
56. Sandars J, Patel R. Self-regulated learning: the challenge of learning in clinical settings. *Med Educ.* 2015;49:548–555.
57. Croskerry P. The importance of cognitive errors in diagnosis and strategies to minimize them. *Acad Med.* 2003;78(8):775–780.
58. Cutrer WB, Miller B, Pusic MV, et al. Fostering the development of master adaptive learners: a conceptual model to guide skill acquisition in medical education. *Acad Med.* 2017;92(1):70–75. doi:10.1097/ACM.0000000000001323.
59. Eichbaum QG. Thinking about thinking and emotion: the metacognition approach to the medical humanities that integrates the humanities with the basic and clinical sciences. *Perm J.* 2014;18(4):64–75.
60. Ericsson A, Pool R. *Peak: Secrets from the New Science of Expertise.* New York: Houghton Mifflin Harcourt; 2016.
61. Croskerry P, Petrie DA, Reilly JB, et al. Deciding on fast and slow decisions. *Acad Med.* 2014;89(2):197–200.
62. Pochon JB, Riis J, Sanfey AG, et al. Functional imaging of decision conflict. *J Neurosci.* 2008;28(13):3468–3473.
63. Rao H, Korczykowski M, Pluta J, et al. Neural correlates of voluntary and involuntary risk taking in the human brain: an fMRI Study of the Balloon Analog Risk Task (BART). *Neuroimage.* 2008;42:902–910.
64. Gluth S, Rieskamp J, Buchel C. Neural evidence for adaptive strategy selection in value-based decision-making. *Cereb Cortex.* 2014;24:2009–2021.
65. Chang HJ, Kang J, Ham BJ. A functional neuroimaging study of the clinical reasoning of medical students. *Adv Health Sci Educ Theory Pract.* 2016;21(5):969–982. doi: 10.1007/s10459-016-9685-6.
66. Basten U, Biele G, Heekeren HR, et al. How the brain integrates costs and benefits during decision making. *Proc Natl Acad Sci U S A.* 2010;107(50):21767–21772.
67. Manning PR, Petit DW. The past, present, and future of continuing medical education: achievements and opportunities, computers, and recertification. *JAMA.* 1987;258(24):3542–3546.
68. Lanzilotti SS. Curiosity. In: Fox RD, Mazmanian PE, Putnam RW, eds. *Changing and Learning in the Lives of Physicians.* New York: Praeger Publishers; 1989:30–43.
69. Lockyer JM, Parboosingh J. Relationships with medical institutions. In Fox RD, Mazmanian PE, Putnam RW, eds. *Changing and Learning in the Lives of Physicians.* New York: Praeger Publishers; 1989:111–122.
70. Paul HA, Osborne CE. Relating to others in the profession. In: Fox RD, Mazmanian PE, Putnam RW, eds. *Changing and Learning in the Lives of Physicians.* New York: Praeger Publishers; 1989:123–133.
71. Bennett NL, Hotvedt MO. Stage of career. In: Fox RD, Mazmanian PE, Putnam RW, eds. *Changing and Learning in the Lives of Physicians.* New York: Praeger Publishers; 1989:65–77.
72. Mazmanian PE, Feldman M, Berens TE, et al. Evaluating outcomes in continuing education and training. In: McGaghie WC, ed. *International Best Practices for Evaluation in the Health Professions.* London, UK: Radcliffe Publishing Ltd.; 2013:199–227.
73. Caplan R, Gallis H. Financial well-being. In: Fox RD, Mazmanian PE, Putnam RW, eds. *Changing and Learning in the Lives of Physicians.* New York: Praeger Publishers; 1989:55–64.

74. Parochka J, Fox RD. Family and community. In: Fox RD, Mazmanian PE, Putnam RW, eds. *Changing and Learning in the Lives of Physicians*. New York: Praeger Publishers; 1989:152–159.

75. Berwick DM. Era 3 for medicine and health care. *JAMA*. 2016;315(13):1329–1330. doi:10.1001/jama.2016.1509. Accessed July 18, 2016.

76. Monsen K. Knowledge discovery data analytics methods: 4 challenges and opportunities in credentialing research methodologies. In: Institute of Medicine (IOM). *Future Directions of Credentialing Research in Nursing: Workshops Summary*. Washington, DC: The National Academies Press; 2015. doi:10.17226/18999.

77. Tsugawa Y, Jena AB, Figueroa JF, et al. Comparison of hospital mortality and readmission rates for medicare patients treated by male vs female physicians. *JAMA Intern Med*. 2017;177(2):206–213. doi: 10.1001/jamainternmed.2016.7875.

78. Cook DA, Andriole DA, Durning SJ, et al. Longitudinal research databases in medical education: facilitating the study of educational outcomes over time and across institutions. *Acad Med*. 2010;85(8):1340–1346. doi: 10.1097/ACM.0b013e3181e5c050.

79. Ameringer CF. Introduction. *The Health Care Revolution*. Berkeley and Los Angeles, CA: University of California Press; 2008:10.

80. Mazmanian PE, Fried PO. Regulations. In Fox RD, Mazmanian PE, Putnam RW, eds. *Changing and Learning in the Lives of Physicians*. New York: Praeger Publishers; 1989:135–150.

81. Varjavand N, Novack H, Schindler BA. Returning physicians to the workforce: history, progress, and challenges. *J Contin Educ Health Prof*. 2012;32(2):142–147.

82. Prewitt K, Schwandt TA, Straf ML, eds.; Committee on the Use of Social Science Knowledge in Public Policy; Division of Behavioral and Social Sciences and Education; National Research Council. *Using Science as Evidence in Public Policy*. Washington, DC: The National Academies Press; 2012.

83. Ozdalga E, Ozdalga A, Ahuja N. The smartphone in medicine: a review of current and potential use among physicians and students. *J Med Internet Res*. 2012;14(5):e128.

84. Ventola CL. Mobile devices and apps for health care professionals: uses and benefits. *P T*. 2014;39(5):356–364. http://www.ncbi.nlm.nih.gov/pmc/articles/PMC4029126/. Accessed August 29, 2016.

85. Goddard AF. Lessons to be learned from the UK junior doctors' strike. *JAMA*. 2016;316(14):1445–1446. doi:10.1001/jama.2016.12029.

86. Freese J, Kevern JA. Types of causes. In: Morgan SL, ed. *Handbook of Causal Analysis for Social Research*. Dordrecht: Springer Science and Business Media; 2013:27–41.

87. Dow AW, DiazGranados D, Mazmanian PE, et al. Applying organizational science to health care: a framework for collaborative practice. *Acad Med*. 2013;88(7):952–957.

88. Mazmanian P, Duff W. Beyond accreditation and the enterprise of CME: an alternative model linking independent learning centers and health services research. In: Davis DA, Fox RD, eds. *The Physician as Learner*. Chicago, IL: American Medical Association; 1994.

89. Liveright AA, Haygood N, eds. *The Exeter Papers: Report of the First International Conference on the Comparative Study of Adult Education*. Boston, MA: Center for the Study of Liberal Education for Adults of Boston University; 1968:8.

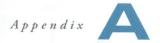
Elements *of the* Educational Activity Planning Process: Historical *versus* Contemporary Views

Ginny Jacobs-Halsey and David A. Davis

The field of CME/CPD has undergone significant changes over the past several years, and it continues to rapidly evolve. These developments are in response to health care's growing need for a more focused, strategically aligned, and impactful approach to professional and organizational development. Most notably, there are heightened expectations of faculty to move from a teacher-centered to a creative, learner-centered approach. Also, there is an increased emphasis on learner engagement and a drive to improve one's ability to assess educational outcomes. In keeping with the Plan-Do-Study-Act template utilized throughout Chapter 4, the following table addresses each of the key elements in planning an educational activity by reflecting on that was then (historical view) and then capturing that which provides future directions (contemporary view).

Element(s)	Historical View (that was then)	Contemporary View (future directions)
Plan		
Assess needs	Conducted by content experts (often single activity director with input from others) No patient involvement	Planning teams comprised of health system leaders, interprofessional team members, and patients actively engaged in collaborative process by identifying and responding to needs Routine input from (and involvement by) patients and patient advocate groups
Ensure alignment	Narrow in scope, aligned with departmental or teacher or personal agenda	Expanded to encompass broader systems view, coordination of care; movement from educational to performance objectives Increased number of performance improvement activities being made available (PI-CME, MOC) in tandem with certified education
Do		
Develop content	Therapeutics	Prevention, screening, management, best evidence; application of knowledge (see flipped classroom on next page)

(*Continued*)

Element(s)	Historical View (that was then)	Contemporary View (future directions)
Address competencies	Medical knowledge or patient care (most common) Tendency to delivery best care as seen through the lens of the provider Tendency to focus on competency needs for one profession and not deliberately address the special needs of the team	Expanded content to address additional competencies (e.g., system-based practice, professionalism, and interpersonal communication skills) Cultural competence seen as foundational pillar for reducing disparities through culturally sensitive and unbiased quality care Increased emphasis on interprofessional collaborative practice competency domains (values/ethics, roles/responsibilities, communication, teamwork) Special emphasis on learners' ability to self-assess and provide constructive feedback
Select appropriate and effective format	Didactic (lecture-based) courses Online tools applied, but typically with static delivery	Point-of-care learning Multiple formats Interactive design Flipped classroom (i.e., materials shared prior to live activity to facilitate advanced review and/or discussion) Online tools utilize smart technology, tailored curriculum
	Providers	*Health care professional teams*
Assess and address learner motivation	Credit hours, opportunity to complete educational requirements at vacation destination	Demonstrated competence, improved performance, application of QI principles, completion of maintenance of certification (MOC) requirements
Develop faculty skills	Teacher-centered approach **(expertise)** Emphasis on presenter's ability to convey their vast knowledge and expertise on a topic	Learner-centered approach **(facilitation)** Seek to meet the learners "where they are." Increased value on facilitation skills
Select Delivery Methods		
Methods	Single mode of delivery (typically live or online)	Multiple modes of delivery; blended learning
Level of interactivity/ learner engagement	Anonymous learners were allowed.	Engaged participants expected
Sequencing	Annual course offerings viewed as one and done; events do not necessarily connect. Just-in-case education Grand rounds, M&M conferences offered as independent sessions held at regularly scheduled day/time	Series of educational activities linked to one another—goals established for overarching educational initiatives Just-in-time education Regularly scheduled series (RSS) enhanced to address overarching objectives and have curriculum build over the series. morbidity, mortality, and improvement (MM&I)—introduce focus on improvement

Element(s)	Historical View (that was then)	Contemporary View (future directions)
Use of technology	Minimal use of technology	Increased use of technical tools to engage learners (e.g., point-of-care clinical decision support software, simulations, audience response systems, survey/polling software, etc.)
Materials (type and timing)	Heavy reliance on PowerPoint slides. Slides occasionally made available at time of presentation to follow along	Reduced reliance on text-heavy slides. Tendency to provide selected slides with opportunity for note-taking. Shift to flipped classroom concept where materials are shared in advance. Steps taken to drive more reflection and discussion
Physical space	Primary educational setting—ballroom space with goal of achieving maximum capacity. Focus is on information disseminated by the 'sage on the stage'	Attempts being made to create learning communities. Round-table setup becoming more popular to allow for small group work and peer-to-peer discussions
Study		
Measure effectiveness and impact	Happiness indexes. Simple evaluation administered immediately post session. Focused on "intent to change"	Evaluate change in behavior and performance improvements. Assess quality of patient care. Evaluation contains question related to planned changes. Follow-up data and/or surveys conducted to assess actual change in practice
	CME units operate as silos. Educational portfolio lacks deliberate strategic connection to institution's overarching goals	Education aligned (ultimately integrated) with institution's mission and strategic priorities
Act		
Review outcomes	One and done. Variable amount of time devoted to postcourse review	Ongoing. Formal debriefs routinely conducted with specific action plans implemented
Debrief/make plans for improvement	Episodic approach to future planning. Success metrics focused on number of participants and financial results	Continuous Quality Improvement (CQI) principles applied. Deliberately build on lessons learned

Point-of-Care Information Resources: A Selected List *of* Apps, Databases, *and* Web Sites

Sarah Knox Morley

This appendix is a supplement to *Chapter 9: Accessing Online Information Resources for Point of Care (POC) Learning*. The proliferation of electronic resources makes it nearly impossible to create a comprehensive listing. Publishers develop new products or purchase competitors at an astonishing rate. Free Web sites come and go or lose market share when their content loses currency.

This appendix provides a selected list of generally accepted sources available at the time of publication and is a resource familiar to the author. The list includes both no-cost and fee-based online information resources for answering clinical questions. A description and Web site (or hypertext transfer protocol; http) are provided for each resource. This list represents general medicine, nursing, and pharmacy materials that are not specialty-specific resources. Likewise, many of these resources are available to those outside the United States; however, the list itself does contain only US resources.

Readers of this text most likely have their own list of cherished resources. When using a resource (new or old), always evaluate the content for accuracy, bias, currency, and relevance. The list will be updated periodically for SACME members.

AccessMedicine: http://mhmedical.com/
One of several online resources from McGraw Hill publishing containing full text textbooks; Diagnosaurus 2.0 (Differential Diagnosis by symptoms, diseases, organ systems); Diagnostic Tests; Images; Video and Audio.

AccessPharmacy: http://mhmedical.com/
Full text books, multimedia, and case files.

AHRQ ePSS: http://epss.ahrq.gov/PDA/index.jsp
U.S. Preventive Services Task Force (USPSTF) recommendations.

BMJ Best Practice: http://bestpractice.bmj.com/best-practice/welcome.html
Research evidence, clinical guidelines, online medical formularies, CME/CPD, and patient education leaflets.

BMJ Clinical Evidence: http://clinicalevidence.bmj.com/x/index.html
Systematic reviews of research evidence based on key clinical questions.

BioMed Central: https://www.biomedcentral.com/
Freely accessible articles from 290 peer-reviewed journals in the fields of biology, clinical medicine, and health.

CINAHL Complete: https://www.ebscohost.com/nursing/products/cinahl-databases/cinahl-complete
An EBSCO*Host* database covering nursing, allied health, and consumer health literature. Includes *Evidence-Based Care Sheets*, concise two-page summary on key topics, including diagnosis, treatment, and disease transmission.

Clinical Key: https://www.clinicalkey.com/#!/
A resource containing online reference books, journal articles, practice guidelines, drug information, and images.

Cochrane Library: http://www.cochranelibrary.com/
A collection of evidence-based medicine databases with full text and abstracts; includes the Cochrane Database of Systematic Reviews.

Drug Information Portal: http://druginfo.nlm.nih.gov/drugportal/drugportal.jsp
A compilation of free drug resources from the National Library of Medicine (NLM) (e.g., AidsInfo, DailyMed, LactMed, ToxNet)

DynaMed Plus: http://www.dynamed.com/
Clinical topic summaries, current evidence-based point-of-care reference with links to full text articles and guidelines, medical images and graphics, and Micromedex content; incorporates *ACP Smart Medicine* for ACP members.

EPocrates Plus: https://www.epocrates.com/products/goPremium
A point-of-care drug information app with additional resources for locating guidelines, general disease monographs, and alternative medications.

Essential Evidence Plus: http://www.essentialevidenceplus.com/
Topic reviews, Cochrane abstracts, calculators, and guidelines.

Guideline Central: https://www.guidelinecentral.com/
Free guideline summaries from over 35 medical societies and government agencies.

Lexicomp Online: http://www.wolterskluwercdi.com/lexicomp-online/
Drug information, including drug monographs, interactions, calculations, IV compatibility, toxicology, and patient education.

MedCalc 3000: http://medcalc3000.com/
Pertinent medical formulae, clinical criteria sets, and decision tree analysis tools.

Medscape: http://www.medscape.com/
Medical news, point-of-care drug and disease information, professional education, and CME.

Micromedex Clinical Knowledge: http://micromedex.com/clinical-knowledge
Drug, toxicology, acute care, patient education, and alternative medicine database.

National Guideline Clearinghouse: https://www.guideline.gov/
Publicly available site for evidence-based clinical practice guidelines.

Natural Medicines: https://naturalmedicines.therapeuticresearch.com/
An evidence-based resource for complementary and alternative therapies including evidence tables.

New England Journal of Medicine **Clinical Videos:** http://www.nejm.org/multimedia/medical-videos

An online resource containing peer-reviewed procedural techniques.

NEJM Journal Watch: http://www.jwatch.org/

A current awareness service for practicing clinicians, nurses, and students; clinical summaries and expert opinion covering 12 specialties.

Nursing Reference Center: https://www.ebscohost.com/nursing/products/nursing-reference-center

A compilation of evidence-based resources, patient education handouts, point-of-care drug information, and CEU.

Psychiatry Online: http://psychiatryonline.org/

A Web-based portal featuring the Diagnostic and Statistical Manual of Mental Disorders (DSM) and other books and journals from American Psychiatric Publishing, Inc.

PsycINFO: http://www.apa.org/pubs/databases/psycinfo/

A mental and behavioral health database with links to full text articles.

PLOS Public Library of Science: https://www.plos.org/

An open access peer-reviewed scientific journal.

PubMed (MEDLINE): http://www.ncbi.nlm.nih.gov/pubmed

The NLM freely available biomedical database containing over 23 million citations with links to many free full text articles.

PubMed Health: http://www.ncbi.nlm.nih.gov/pubmedhealth/

Another NLM database specializing in reviews of clinical effectiveness research; contains summaries and full text of selected systematic reviews of clinical trials.

Stat!Ref: http://www.statref.com/

A collection of electronic books and tools in a variety of medical specialties, pharmacology, and nursing; includes Essential Evidence Plus and MedCalc 3000.

TRIP and TRIP PRO: https://www.tripdatabase.com/

A clinical search engine with filters to search for evidence-based content.

UpToDate: http://www.uptodate.com/home

An online resource with over 10,000 topic reviews in 22 medical specialties, includes calculators and patient education materials.

VisualDX: https://www.visualdx.com/

A visual clinical decision support system for dermatologic, infectious, and drug-induced diseases.

Educational Research: Relevant Databases, Web Sites, Organizations, Funding Sources, Certificate Programs, Books, *and* Articles

Betsy White Williams, Dillon Welindt, and Curtis A. Olson

This appendix serves as a complement to Chapter 25 *Identifying Principles of Effective Educational Research*. Resources include links to relevant databases, Web sites, organizations, funding sources, certificate programs, books, guides, and journal articles. These can assist the reader in conducting and becoming more proficient in medical education research and program evaluation. The articles are grouped into sections based on content. A link to journals that publish medical education research is also provided.

Readers should be aware of resources pertaining to scholarship and medical education research that are available at their own institution. The specific links for all of these programs are not provided in this appendix. Many academic medical centers and medical schools have certificate programs, workshops, and other resources that promote scholarship and research. We would recommend that you check your institution for these resources. Finally, while an extensive search was undertaken, the authors do not represent this to be an exhaustive list. Moving forward, the list will be updated and available to SACME members.

DATABASES

Name: CINAHL Complete (EBSCO)
Link: https://health.ebsco.com/products/cinahl-complete
Description: The Cumulative Index to Nursing and Allied Health Literature provides access to journals about nursing, allied health, biomedicine, and health care.

Name: Education Resource Information Center (ERIC)
Link: https://eric.ed.gov/
Description: ERIC is an Internet-based digital library of education research and information sponsored by the Institute of Education Sciences (IES) of the U.S. Department of Education. ERIC provides access to bibliographic records of journal and nonjournal literature from 1966 to the present.

Name: EMBASE
Link: https://www.embase.com/login
Description: EMBASE provides relevant, up-to-date biomedical information to the global biomedical research community.

Name: Google Scholar
Link: https://scholar.google.com/
Description: Google Scholar is a Web search engine that indexes the full text or metadata of scholarly literature across an array of publishing formats and disciplines. It includes most peer-reviewed online academic journals and books, conference papers, theses and dissertations, preprints, abstracts, technical reports, and other scholarly literature, including court opinions and patents.

Name: Health and Psychosocial Instruments (HaPI)
Link: http://www.ovid.com/site/catalog/DataBase/866.jsp
Description: Health and Psychosocial Instruments (HaPI) is a database that provides access to information on approximately 15,000 measurement instruments (i.e., questionnaires, interview schedules, checklists, coding schemes, rating scales, etc.) in the fields of health and psychosocial sciences.

Name: ProQuest Education Journals
Link: http://www.proquest.com/products-services/pq_ed_journals.html
Description: This Education Database includes over 1,000 full-text journals and 18,000 dissertations, supporting research on the theory and practice of education. Education Database covers not only the literature on primary, secondary, and higher education but also special education, home schooling, adult education, and hundreds of related topics.

Name: PsycINFO
Link: http://www.apa.org/pubs/databases/psycinfo/
Description: This database contains more than 4 million bibliographic records centered on psychology and the behavioral and social sciences.

Name: Public Library of Science (PLOS)
Link: https://www.plos.org
Description: PLOS is an Open Access publisher with a mission to accelerate progress in science and medicine by leading a transformation in research communication.

Name: PubMed
Link: http://www.ncbi.nlm.nih.gov/pubmed
Description: PubMed consists of more than 26 million citations for biomedical literature from MEDLINE, life science journals, and online books. Citations may include links to full-text content from PubMed Central and publisher Web sites.

Name: RoMEO
Link: http://www.sherpa.ac.uk/romeo/index.php
Description: A searchable database of publisher's policies regarding the self-archiving of journal articles on the Web and in Open Access repositories.

Name: The Web of Science
Link: http://wokinfo.com/training_support/training/web-of-knowledge/
Description: *The Web of Science* (formerly Web of Knowledge) provides information in the sciences, social sciences, arts, and humanities.

WEB SITES

Name: CAFM Research Alliance (CERA)
Link: http://www.stfm.org/Research/CERA
Description: CERA is a resource available through the Society of Teachers of Family Medicine (STFM). CERA attempts to increase the quality and frequency of research and scholarly activity among members of Council of Academic Family Medicine organizations.

Name: DR MERL
Link: https://drmerl.wordpress.com/
Description: Dependable Reviews of Medical Education Research Literature (DR MERL) is a collection of reviews of the latest research in medical education. The reviews are on topics in undergraduate and graduate medical education.

Name: Educational Scholarship Resources in Medical Education
Link: https://www.aamc.org/members/gea/gea_sections/mesre/
Description: The mission of the Section for Medical Education Scholarship Research and Evaluation (MESRE) of the AAMC is to enhance the quality of research in medical education and to promote its application to educational practice. Included on their site is an annotated bibliography of journals for educational scholarship. The link is: https://www.aamc.org/download/456646/data/annotated-bibliography-of-journals-march-2016.pdf

Name: George T. Harrell Health Science Library—Medical Education Research
Link: http://harrell.library.psu.edu/mededresearch
Description: This Web site provides guidance for individuals who are new to medical education research. Information includes resources on processes, methodologies, and search methodologies.

Name: Health Education Assets Library (HEAL)
Link: http://content.lib.utah.edu/cdm/search/collection/uu-heal
Description: The HEAL is a collection of over 22,000 freely available digital materials for health sciences education. The collection is housed at the University of Utah J. Willard Marriott Digital Library.

Name: MedEdPORTAL
Link: https://www.mededportal.org
Description: MedEdPORTAL is a site for peer-reviewed educational scholarship, innovations to improve patient care, and continuing education activities to support lifelong learning.

Name: MedEdWorld

Link: http://www.mededworld.org/Home.aspx

Description: MedEdWorld, launched by the Association of Medical Education in Europe, is an international health professions community of individuals and educational organizations. Topics are appropriate and relevant for those involved in health professions education—including teachers and trainers, educationists, researchers, and administrators.

Name: MESRE Annotated Bibliography

Link: https://www.aamc.org/download/456646/data/annotated-bibliography-of-journals-march-2016.pdf

Description: This is an annotated bibliography of educational scholarship journals. The Medical Education Scholarship, Research, and Evaluation Committee (MESRE) of the AAMC compiled the bibliography.

ORGANIZATIONS

Organization: Agency for Healthcare Research and Quality

Link: http://www.ahrq.gov/

Description: The Agency for Healthcare Research and Quality's (AHRQ) mission is to produce evidence to make health care safer, higher quality, more accessible, equitable, and affordable and to work within the U.S. Department of Health and Human Services and with other partners to make sure that the evidence is understood and used.

Organization: American Board of Medical Specialties

Link: http://www.abms.org/about-abms/research-and-education-foundation/

Description: The American Board of Medical Specialties (ABMS) is the oversight board that works in collaboration with its 24 specialty Member Boards that maintain the standards for physician certification. Numerous resources can be found on the ABMS including a link for the ABMS Research and Education Foundation (REF). The REF is a not-for-profit organization that supports the ABMS in its mission of improving health care quality and the continuous professional development of physician specialists through a variety of research and education initiatives.

Organization: Academic Health Sciences Network

Link: http://ahsn.ca

Description: The Academic Health Science Network is a part of the Association of Faculties of Medicine of Canada (AFMC). The AHSN Symposium is an opportunity to discuss the future of academic health sciences in Canada, exchange information, build community, and generate actions for the year ahead.

Organization: Academy of Medical Educators

Link: http://www.medicaleducators.org/

Description: The Academy of Medical Educators (AoME) is a multiprofessional organization for those involved in medical education. The mission of AoME is to provide leadership, promote standards, and support all those involved in the academic discipline and practice of medical education.

Organization: Accreditation Council for Graduate Medical Education (ACGME)
Link: https://www.acgme.org/acgmeweb/
Description: The ACGME sets standards for US graduate medical education (residency and fellowship) programs, the institutions that sponsor them, and renders accreditation decisions based on compliance with those standards. They have a number of resources including webinars and meetings.

Organization: Alliance for Continuing Education in the Health Professions (ACEHP)
Link: http://www.acehp.org/
Description: The Alliance is an organization that supports professional health care educators across health care professions who seek to develop, deliver, and manage relevant, health care continuing education. They have an annual meeting, webinars, a number of publications, and other resources that are helpful to those involved in CME/CPD. ACEHP is a partner with AHME and SACME in publishing the peer-reviewed Journal for Continuing Education in the Health Professions (JCEHP). The Alliance also cosponsors the quadrennial CME Congress with AHME, SACME, and the Canadian Association for Continuing Health Education.

Organization: American Educational Research Association (AERA)
Link: http://www.aera.net/
Description: AERA is an organization concerned with improving the educational process by encouraging scholarly inquiry related to education and evaluation and by promoting the dissemination and practical application of research results. They have events, meetings, and publications that are helpful to those involved in educational research.

Organization: American Evaluation Association
Link: http://www.eval.org/
Description: The American Evaluation Association attempts to improve evaluation practices and methods, increase evaluation use, promote evaluation as a profession, and support the contribution of evaluation to the generation of theory and knowledge. The organization has numerous resources including live conferences, interest groups, and webinars (live and archived). The organization publishes the quarterly New Directions for Evaluation as well as the American Journal for Evaluation. They also publish Guiding Principles for Evaluators, which is a free pamphlet available to members as well as nonmembers.

Organization: Association of American Medical Colleges (AAMC)
Link: http://www.aamc.org/start.htm
Description: The AAMC serves the academic medicine community to improve the health of all. They have a number of resources for medical students, residents, and professionals in academic medicine. Resources include an annual meeting, the

Research in Medical Education meeting as well as MedEdPORTAL, and the MERC certificate program. AAMC has a number of written resources and reports and also publishes the peer-reviewed journal Academic Medicine.

Organization: Association for the Behavioral Sciences and Medical Education (ABSAME)
Link: http://www.absame.org/
Description: ABSAME is an interdisciplinary professional society dedicated to strengthening behavioral science teaching in medical schools, in residency programs, and in continuing medical education.

Organization: Association of Faculties of Medicine of Canada (AFMC)
Link: https://www.afmc.ca
Description: AFMC has represented Canada's 17 faculties of medicine since 1943. AFMC works to represent and support the mandates of research, medical education, and clinical care with social accountability. The Health Research division of AFMC is primarily responsible for the development and implementation of the Association of Faculties of Medicine of Canada (AFMC) Research Mandate.

Organization: Association for Hospital Medical Education (AHME)
Link: www.ahme.org
Description: AHME's members include several hundred teaching hospitals, academic medical centers, and consortia who provide medical education across the continuum. AHME aims to promote improvement in medical education to meet health care needs. The organization also serves as a forum and resource for medical education information. AHME has a number of conferences and educational offerings and is a partner with ACEHP and SACME in publishing the peer-reviewed Journal for Continuing Education in the Health Professions (JCEHP). The Association also cosponsors the quadrennial CME Congress with ACEHP, SACME, and the Canadian Association for Continuing Health Education.

Organization: Association for Medical Education in Europe (AMEE)
Link: http://www.amee.org/home
Description: AMEE is an organization that promotes international excellence in education in the health care professions across the continuum of undergraduate, postgraduate, and continuing education. AMEE sponsors a number of conferences, certificate programs, webinars, and launched MedEdWorld. The organization also publishes the peer-reviewed journal Medical Teacher, as well as AMEE guides and Best Evidence in Medical Education systematic reviews.

Organization: Association for the Study of Medical Education (ASME)
Link: http://www.asme.org.uk/
Description: ASME is a membership society whose mission is to meet the needs of teachers, trainers, and learners in medical education by supporting research-informed, best practice across the continuum of medical education. ASME produces the journals

Medical Education and the Clinical Teacher. It also sponsors a number of conferences and workshops including researching medical education.

Organization: Australian and New Zealand Association for Medical Education (ANZAME)
Link: http://www/anzame.org
Description: The organization was formed in 1972 to help develop medical education as a scientific discipline. The organization holds an annual conference and publishes the peer-reviewed journal Focus on Health Professional Education.

Organization: Best Evidence Medical Education (BEME)
Link: http://bemecollaboration.org/
Description: The BEME Collaboration (Harden et al., 1999) is an international group of individuals, universities, and professional organizations committed to the development of evidence-informed education in the medical and health professions. Included on their Web site are research methodology guides and articles in aide of research. The link for those resources is: http://bemecollaboration.org/Publications+Research+Methodology/development

Organization: International Association of Medical Science Educators (IAMSE)
Link: http://www.iamse.org/
Description: IAMSE is a professional development society organized and directed by health professions educators whose goals include promoting excellence and innovation in teaching, student assessment, program evaluation, instructional technology, human simulation, and learner-centered education. It sponsors the peer-reviewed journal Medical Science Educator as well as several manuals. The organization offers webinars as well as meetings.

Organizations: Medical Education Scholarship Research and Evaluation (MESRE) Section of AAMC (MESRE)
Link: https://www.aamc.org/members/gea/gea_sections/mesre/
Description: The mission of the Section for Medical Education Scholarship Research and Evaluation (MESRE) is to enhance the quality of research in medical education and to promote its application to educational practice.

Organization: Society for Academic Continuing Medical Education (SACME)
Link: http://www.sacme.org
Description: SACME's mission is to promote the highest value in patient care and health of the public through the scholarship of continuing medical and interprofessional education. SACME has an annual meeting and offers other educational offerings including the Virtual Journal Club and a mentorship program. They also have grant funding available through the Manning Award. With its partner organizations ACEHP and AHME, SACME publishes the peer-reviewed Journal for Continuing Education in the Health Professions (JCEHP). SACME also cosponsors the quadrennial CME Congress with ACEHP, AHME, and the Canadian Association for Continuing Health Education.

Organization: Society of Directors of Research in Medical Education (SDRME)
Link: http://www.sdrme.org/
Description: The **Society of Directors of Research in Medical Education** (SDRME) is an organization dedicated to enhancing the quality of education in medical schools. Its slogan is "Advancing Medical Education Through Quality Research." The site contains a number of written resources and helpful links.

Organization: Society of Teachers of Family Medicine (STFM)
Link: http://www.stfm.org
Description: The Society of Teachers of Family Medicine (STFM) is an association that includes medical school professors, preceptors, residency program faculty, residency program directors, and others involved in family medicine education. Resources include the Council of Academic Family Medicine Educational Research Alliance (CERA). The link is: http://www.stfm.org/Research/CERA

POSSIBLE FUNDING SOURCES

Name: Carolinas HealthCare System
Link: https://www.carolinashealthcare.org/documents/carolinashcsystem/cfe/stefanidis-edu-research-funding.pdf
Description: This list provides funding sources in the United States for educational research, as well as search engines for research funding.

Name: The Association for Surgical Education
Link: http://surgicaleducation.com/wp-content/uploads/2015/12/Sources-of-Funding-for-Medical-Educational-Research-Grants.docx
Description: This site includes a list of potential sources for medical education research funding.

Name: University of Kansas Medical Center
Link: http://www.kumc.edu/school-of-medicine/ame/resources/funding-sources-for-medical-education-research.html
Description: This site includes a list of sources for medical education research funding.

Organization: Association for Surgical Education
Link: https://surgicaleducation.com
Description: The Association for Surgical Education's primary goal is to promote the art and science of education in surgery. They offer a number of resources including workshops, courses, and links to education scholar programs. These resources can be found at https://surgicaleducation.com/getting-started-2. They also have a link to sources of funding for medical education research.

Organization: Department of Innovation in Medical Education (DIME-University of Ottawa)
Link: http://www.med.uottawa.ca/aime/eng/funding.html
Description: The goal of this research grant is to support projects that involve scholarship in health professions education within the Faculty of Medicine at the University of Ottawa. The project may involve any aspect relevant to health professions education including, but not limited to, undergraduate, postgraduate, assessment, and faculty development.

Organization: Aetna Foundation
Link: http://www.aetna.com/foundation/
Description: Aetna Foundation funding is provided only to nonprofit organizations with 501(c)(3) or similar tax-exempt status and educational institutions.

Organization: Agency for Healthcare Research and Quality Grants On-Line Database
Link: http://www.gold.ahrq.gov/
Description: The Agency for Healthcare Research and Quality's mission is to improve the quality, safety, efficiency, and effectiveness of health care for all Americans. Information from AHRQ's research helps people make more informed decisions and improve the quality of health care services.

Organization: The American Association of Medical Colleges
Link: https://www.aamc.org/initiatives/awards/
Description: Each year at [their] annual meeting, the AAMC presents its major awards honoring individuals and programs making significant contributions to our community in the fields of medical education, research, and community service.

Organization: American Educational Research Association
Link: http://www.aera.net/grantsprogram/
Description: With funding from the National Science Foundation (NSF), the American Educational Research Association (AERA) offers the AERA Grants Program, which provides small grants and training for researchers who conduct studies of education policy and practice using quantitative methods and including the analysis of data from the large-scale data sets sponsored by National Center for Education Statistics (NCES) and NSF.

Organization: Association for the Study of Medical Education
Link: http://www.asme.org.uk/grants-awards/current-grants-awards/
Description: ASME's mission: "To meet the needs of teachers, trainers and learners in medical education by supporting research-informed, best practice across the continuum of medical education." The link provides information on all grants and awards offered by ASME.

Organization: The Canadian Institute of Health Research
Link: http://www.cihr-irsc.gc.ca/
Description: As the Government of Canada's health research investment agency, the Canadian Institutes of Health Research (CIHR) supports health research in biomedical, clinical, health systems services, and population health.

Organization: The Arnold P. Gold Foundation: Picker Gold Challenge Grants
Link: http://www.gold-foundation.org/programs/picker-gold-challenge-grants-for-residency-training/
Description: Since 2008, the Arnold P. Gold Foundation and The Picker Institute have partnered on the Picker Gold Graduate Medical Education Challenge Grant Program, which supports the research and development of successful patient-centered care initiatives and best practices in the education of our country's future practicing physicians.

Organization: The Max Bell Foundation
Link: http://www.maxbell.org/
Description: Max Bell Foundation is a Canadian independent grantmaking foundation that pursues its mission and strategic priority by supporting Canadian-registered charities with Project Grants, Internship Grants, and Senior Fellow Grants.

Organization: Medical Council of Canada
Link: http://mcc.ca/about/research-and-development/grants/
Description: To support medical assessment research, the Medical Council of Canada (MCC) offers research grants to interested faculty members, staff members, or graduate students of Canadian medical faculties. Grants are intended to support and provide a principal investigator with the financial resources required to further complete his or her research while promoting the Council's vision of striving for the highest standard of medical care for Canadians.

Organization: Ontario Ministry of Health and Long-Term Care
Link: http://www.health.gov.on.ca/en/pro/ministry/research/
Description: The Ministry of Health and Long-Term Care's vision for research is to improve the health care and outcomes of Ontarians by investing strategically in policy-relevant and applied health system research. The Ministry of Health and Long-Term Care funds health system and population health research largely through the Health System Research Fund. Other health research investments are made through the Ministry of Research and Innovation.

Organization: Ministry of Research, Innovation, and Science
Link: https://www.ontario.ca/page/ministry-research-innovation-and-science
Description: Ministry of Research, Innovation, and Science supports research, commercialization, and innovation taking place across Ontario through a range of programs and services like the Ontario Research Fund, Innovation Demonstration Fund, and Ontario Venture Capital Fund.

Organization: National Institutes of Health Office of Extramural Research
Link: http://grants.nih.gov/grants/oer.htm
Description: The NIH provides financial support in the form of grants, cooperative agreements, and contracts to support the advancement of the NIH mission to enhance health and extend healthy lives.

Organization: National Board of Medical Examiners
Link: http://www.nbme.org/research/stemmler.html
Description: According to the NBME site, the goal of the Stemmler Fund is to provide support for research or development of innovative assessment approaches that will enhance the evaluation of those preparing to, or continuing to, practice medicine. Expected outcomes include advances in the theory, knowledge, or practice of assessment at any point along the continuum of medical education, from undergraduate and graduate education and training, through practice. Pilot and more comprehensive projects are both of interest. Collaborative investigations within or among institutions are eligible, particularly as they strengthen the likelihood of the project's contribution and success.

Organization: PSI Foundation
Link: http://www.psifoundation.org/
Description: The Foundation was established with the mission of improving the "health of Ontarians." The Foundation's granting interests are in two areas: education of practicing physicians and health research with an emphasis on research relevant to patient care.

Organization: Robert Wood Johnson Foundation
Link: http://www.rwjf.org/en.html
Description: The Robert Wood Johnson Foundation funds program and policy initiatives in four areas, which are each critical to health equity: Health Systems; Healthy Kids, Healthy Weight; Healthy Communities; Health Leadership.

Organization: Society for Academic Continuing Medical Education
Link: http://sacme.org/SACME_Grants
Description: Funding is available through the Manning Award. Also available are mentorship and fellowship opportunities.

Organization: The Spencer Foundation
Link: http://www.spencer.org/mission
Description: The Foundation is intended to investigate ways in which education, broadly conceived, can be improved around the world. The Foundation is committed to supporting investigation of education through its research programs and to strengthening and renewing the educational research community through its fellowship and training programs and related activities.

Organization: Social Sciences and Humanities Research Council
Link: http://www.sshrc-crsh.gc.ca/home-accueil-eng.aspx
Description: The Talent program promotes the acquisition of research skills and assists in the training of highly qualified personnel in the social sciences and humanities.

Organization: The College of Family Physicians Canada
Link: http://cfpc.ca/Research/
Description: The CFPC's Research Department is part of the College's Academic Family Medicine Division. The Research Department supports the Section of Researchers,

provides research advice to the CFPC, organizes the Family Medicine Innovations in Research and Education Day activities and the FMF research stream, and oversees a number of research programs.

CERTIFICATE AND DEGREE PROGRAMS

Program: The Council of Emergency Medicine Residency Directors (CORD) Medical Education Research Certificate Program

Link: http://www.cordem.org/i4a/pages/index.cfm?pageID=3344

Description: The Council of Emergency Medicine Residency Directors (CORD) recently partnered with the AAMC to create a research training opportunity faculty within emergency medicine. This program adds a mentored education research project to the traditional independent learner model of the MERC workshops.

Program: Essential Skills in Continuing Education and Professional Development (ESCEPD) Course

Link: https://www.amee.org/conferences/amee-2016/programme/courses/essential-skills-in-continuing-education-and-profe

Description: The ESME courses, offered and accredited by AMEE, are aimed at practicing teachers in medicine and the health care professions, both basic scientists and clinicians.

Program: The Harvard Macy Institute

Link: http://www.harvardmacy.org/index.php/hmi-courses

Description: The Harvard Macy Institute offers a number of course for those involved in health education including A Systems Approach to Assessment in Health Professions Education.

Program: Medical Education Research Certificate Program

Link: https://www.aamc.org/members/gea/merc/

Description: The Medical Education Research Certificate (MERC) program provides knowledge to promote the understanding of the purposes and processes of medical education research. The program also is designed to help participants become informed consumers of medical education research literature, and to be effective collaborators in medical education research. The courses are targeted for clinicians and other educators who desire to learn research skills that will enable collaborative participation in medical education research projects.

Program: Doctoral Programs in Health Professions Education List

Citation: Supplemental digital content AM Last Page: overview of doctoral programs in health professions education. *Acad Med.* 2014;89(9).

Description: This supplemental content provides a list of international doctoral programs for health professions education.

BOOKS

Citation: Norman GR, van der Vleuten CP, et al. *International Handbook of Research in Medical Education*. Vol. 7. Springer Science & Business Media; 2002.
Link: http://www.springer.com/us/book/9781402004667
Abstract: This edited book provides a review of current research findings and contemporary issues in health sciences education. The orientation is toward research evidence as a basis for informing policy and practice in education. The handbook includes 33 chapters organized into six sections: Research Traditions, Learning, The Educational Continuum, Instructional Strategies, Assessment, and Implementing the Curriculum.

Citation: Cleland J, Durning SJ. *Researching Medical Education*. John Wiley & Sons; 2015.
Link: http://www.wiley.com/WileyCDA/WileyTitle/productCd-111883920X,subjectCd-ED04.html
Abstract: The book includes contributions from a team of international clinicians and nonclinical researchers in health education, representing a range of disciplines and backgrounds. This book introduces readers to the basic building blocks of research and a range of theories and how to use them. It also illustrates a diversity of methods and their use and gives guidance on practical researcher development. The book links theory, design, and methods across the health profession education.

Citation: Cargill M, O'Connor P. *Writing Scientific Research Articles: Strategy and Steps*, 2nd ed. John Wiley & Sons; 2013.
Link: http://www.wiley.com/WileyCDA/WileyTitle/productCd-1118570707.html
Abstract: The book provides clear processes for writing each section of a manuscript. Each learning step uses practical exercises to develop writing and data presentation skills.

Citation: Dornan T, Mann KV, Scherpbier AJ, et al. *Medical Education: Theory and Practice*, 1st ed. Elsevier Health Sciences; 2010.
Link: http://store.elsevier.com/Medical-Education-Theory-and-Practice/isbn-9780702035227/
Abstract: This book interweaves practice, theory, innovation, and research. It provides a contemporary overview of the field followed by a discussion of the theoretical foundations of medical education. The remainder of the book reviews a wide range of educational contexts, processes, and outcomes.

Citation: Gunderman RB. *Achieving Excellence in Medical Education*, 2nd ed. London, UK: Springer Verlag; 2011.
Link: http://www.springer.com/us/book/9780857293060
Abstract: This book explores two essential questions facing medical educators and learners: (1) "What is the vision of educational excellence?" and (2) "How can performance be enhanced?" The book includes information on resources for promoting excellence in medical education, discussions of new educational technologies, and medical education's role in preparing future leaders.

Citation: Swanwick T. *Understanding Medical Education: Evidence, Theory and Practice*, 2nd ed. John Wiley & Sons; 2013.

Link: http://www.wiley.com/WileyCDA/WileyTitle/productCd-1118472403.html

Abstract: This book provides a comprehensive resource of the theoretical and academic bases to modern medical education practice.

Citation: Heiman G. *Basic Statistics for the Behavioral Sciences*, 7th ed. Cengage Learning; 2013.

Link: http://www.cengage.com/search/productOverview.do?N=16&Ntk=P_EPI&Ntt =2748415891642071544966635647212282521 2&Ntx=mode%2Bmatchallpartial

Abstract: This book provides an overview of basic statistics. Selection of topics in the book was guided by three considerations: (1) "What are the most useful statistical methods?"; (2) "Which statistical methods are the most widely used in journals in the behavioral and social sciences?"; and (3) "Which statistical methods are fundamental to further study?"

Citation: Miller DM, Linn RL, Gronlund NE. *Measurement and Assessment in Teaching*, 11th ed. Pearson Higher Ed., 2013.

Link: https://www.pearsonhighered.com/product/Miller-Measurement-and-Assessment-in-Teaching-11th-Edition/9780132689663.html

Abstract: This book emphasizes the construction and use of tests and assessments that are valid and reliable. Examples illustrating sound assessment construction principles, comprehensive coverage of approaches to testing and assessment, and up-to-date concepts of validity in context of standards-based education are included. This is a basic book in tests and measurement. It is not however specific to medical education.

Citation: Mertens DM. *Transformative Research and Evaluation*. Guilford Press; 2008.

Link: http://www.guilford.com/books/Transformative-Research-and-Evaluation/Donna-Mertens/9781593853020

Abstract: This book provides a framework for making methodological decisions and conducting research. Mertens discusses how to formulate research questions based on community needs, develop researcher–community partnerships grounded in trust and respect, and skillfully apply quantitative, qualitative, and mixed-methods data collection strategies. Practical aspects of analyzing and reporting results are addressed, and numerous sample studies are presented. This book is not specific to medical education.

Citation: Walsh K. *The Oxford Text of Medical Education*. Oxford University Press; 2013.

Link: http://oxfordmedicine.com/view/10.1093/med/9780199652679.001.0001/med-9780199652679

Abstract: This book covers topics including curriculum, identities in medicine and social context, delivery, supervision, the stages of medical education, selection and dropout, assessment, quality issues, scholarship and research, medical education in emerging and developing markets, and the future of medical education.

Citation: Rao PS, Richard J. *Introduction to Biostatistics and Research Methods.* PHI Learning Pvt. Ltd.; 2012.
Link: https://phindia.com/bookdetails/introduction-to-biostatistics-and-research-methods-rao-p-s-s-sundar-richard-j–isbn-OTc4LTgxLTIwMy00NTIwLTE
Abstract: The book acquaints readers with various topics pertaining to research methods.

Citation: Abdulrahman KAB, Mennin S, Harden R, et al. *Routledge International Handbook of Medical Education.* Routledge; 2015.
Link: https://www.routledge.com/
Abstract: Among the offerings in this book are chapters on how to implement a meaningful assessment program; how teaching expertise and scholarship can be developed, recognized, and rewarded; and methods for ensuring the quality of educational program.

Citation: Allen AK. *Research Skills for Medical Students.* Sage; 2012.
Link: https://us.sagepub.com/en-us/nam/research-skills-for-medical-students/book238668
Abstract: This book is targeted to novice investigators. It provides information to aid novice investigators utilize study designs and data collection tools and analyze effectively.

Citation: Van den Akker J, Gravemeijer K, McKenney S, et al. *Educational Design Research*, 1st ed. Routledge; 2006.
Link: https://www.routledge.com/
Abstract: The content for this book stems from an educational design research seminar organized by the Netherlands Organization for Scientific Research, in particular, its Program Council for Educational Research (NWO/PROO).

Citation: Wager E. *Getting Research Published: An A to Z of Publication Strategy*, 3rd ed. CRC Press.
Link: https://www.crcpress.com/Getting-Research-Published-An-A-Z-of-Publication-Strategy-Third-Edition/Wager/p/book/9781785231384
Abstract: This book covers the ethics and conventions involved in research. It provides suggestions for publishing in peer-reviewed journals and at conferences. The book includes suggestions on how to choose the right journal and many other problems that can be associated with getting a manuscript published.

Citation: Straus S, Tetroe J, Graham ID. *Knowledge Translation in Health Care: Moving from Evidence to Practice*, 2nd ed. John Wiley & Sons; 2013.
Link: http://www.wiley.com/WileyCDA/WileyTitle/productCd-1118413547.html
Abstract: This book provides a practical introduction to knowledge translation for those working within health policy and funding agencies and as researchers, clinicians, and trainees. Using practical examples, it explains how to use research findings to improve health care in real life.

Citation: Institute of Medicine. Committee on Planning a Continuing Health Care Professional Education Institute. *Redesigning Continuing Education in the Health Professions.* National Academies Press; 2010.
Link: http://www.nap.edu/catalog/12704/redesigning-continuing-education-in-the-health-professions
Abstract: Redesigning Continuing Education in the Health Professions illustrates a vision for a better system through a comprehensive approach of continuing professional development and posits a framework upon which to develop a new, more effective system. The book also offers principles to guide the creation of a national continuing education institute.

Citation: Davis DA, Fox RD. *The Continuing Professional Development of Physicians: From Research to Practice.* American Medical Association Press; 2003.
Link: https://commerce.ama-assn.org/store/catalog/productDetail.jsp?skuId=sku1240032&productId=prod1240023
Abstract: The Continuing Professional Development (CPD) of Physicians takes the concept of CPD and explores it from theory into practice as an agent for positive physician performance change.

Citation: Johnson B, Christensen L. *Educational Research: Quantitative, Qualitative, and Mixed Approaches.* Sage; 2014.
Link: https://us.sagepub.com/en-us/nam/educational-research/book237507
Abstract: This introductory research methods textbook provides readers an understanding of the multiple research methods and strategies—including qualitative, quantitative, and action research, as well as mixed methods inquiry—used in education and related fields. Included in the book are chapters that provide information on how to read and critically evaluate published research; write a proposal, construct a questionnaire, and conduct an empirical research study on their own; and ultimately write up results in a research report using APA style.

Citation: Wallen NE, Fraenkel JR. *Educational Research: A Guide to the Process.* Lawrence Erlbaum Associates, Inc.; 2001.
Link: https://www.routledge.com/
Abstract: This book emphasizes the process of research through examples with chapters on research methodology. Part I covers the basic research process including an example of a student research proposal. Part II provided more detail about research methodology.

Citation: Cohen L, Manion L, Morrison K. *Research Methods in Education,* 7th ed. Routledge; 2013.
Link: https://www.routledge.com/
Abstract: This is the 7th edition of this book. In the current edition, the authors include more information on current developments in research practice, action research, questionnaire design, ethnographic research, conducting needs analysis, constructing and using tests, observational methods, reliability and validity, ethical issues, and curriculum research.

Citation: Green JL, Camilli G, Elmore PB. *Handbook of Complementary Methods in Education Research*, 3rd ed. Routledge; 2016.
Link: http://www.aera.net/Publications/Books/Handbook-of-Complementary-Methods
Abstract: The *Handbook of Complementary Methods in Education Research* is a successor volume to AERA's earlier editions of *Complementary Methods for Research in Education*. The new volume presents a range of research methods used to study education. Methods are described in detail, including its history, its research design, the questions that it addresses, ways of using the method, and ways of analyzing and reporting outcomes.

Citation: Creswell JW. *Educational Research: Planning, Conducting, and Evaluating Quantitative*, 5th ed. New Jersey: Upper Saddle River; 2015.
Link: https://www.pearsonhighered.com/program/Creswell-Educational-Research-Planning-Conducting-and-Evaluating-Quantitative-and-Qualitative-Research-Enhanced-Pearson-e-Text-with-Loose-Leaf-Version-Access-Card-Package-5th-Edition/PGM19679.html
Abstract: This book is an introductory educational research text. It includes integrated treatment of quantitative and qualitative methods. It is written in clear and practical language.

Citation: Lo B, Field MJ. *Conflict of Interest in Medical Research, Education, and Practice*. National Academies Press; 2009.
Link: http://www.nap.edu/catalog/12598/conflict-of-interest-in-medical-research-education-and-practice
Abstract: This Institute of Medicine report examines conflicts of interest in medical research, education, and practice. Included are discussions of the development of clinical practice guidelines. It focuses on conflicts of interest across the spectrum of medicine and its identification of overarching principles for assessing both conflicts of interest and conflict of interest policies.

Citation: Alliance for Continuing Education in the Health Professions. *The Insiders Guide to Medical Education Grants*. Alliance for Continuing Education in the Health Professions; 2016.
Link: http://www.acehp.org/p/pr/vi/prodid=36
Abstract: Included in this book are discussions of grant development, financial reconciliation, and educational outcomes. The format makes use of cases, samples, strategies, and helpful tips.

Citation: Pawson R, Tilley N. *Realistic Evaluation*. Sage; 1997.
Link: https://us.sagepub.com/en-us/nam/realistic-evaluation/book205276
Abstract: This book discusses program evaluation needs and methods to improve the process of program evaluation. The book presents an overview of "realistic evaluation" as a paradigm, which is founded in scientific realist philosophy. The approach is based on the notion that programs deal with real problems rather than mere social constructions and that the primary intention of evaluation is to inform realistic development.

Citation: Chen H-T. *Practical Program Evaluation: Assessing and Improving Planning, Implementation, and Effectiveness.* Sage; 2005.
Link: https://us.sagepub.com/en-us/nam/practical-program-evaluation/book235546
Abstract: This book is intended to clarify evaluation concepts for practical use. This is described through three essential steps: identification of stakeholder needs, optimal evaluation approach suited to those needs, and implementing that approach. This book emphasizes a theory-driven approach toward evaluating programs.

ARTICLES

Writing Tips

1. Blanco M, Lee M, McMahon K, et al. RIME grantsmanship: how to write promising grant proposals. *MedEdPORTAL*. 2012.
2. Blanco MA, Lee MY. Twelve tips for writing educational research grant proposals. *Med Teach*. 2012;34(6):450–453.
3. Cook DA. Twelve tips for getting your manuscript published. *Med Teach*. 2016;38(1):41–50.
4. Cook DA, Bordage G. Twelve tips on writing abstracts and titles: how to get people to use and cite your work. *Med Teach*. 2016;38(11):1100–1104.
5. Coverdale JH, Roberts LW, Balon R, et al. Writing for academia: getting your research into print: AMEE Guide No. 74. *Med Teach*. 2013;35(2):e926–e934.
6. Dereski M, Engwall K. Tips for effectively presenting your research via slide presentation. *MedEdPORTAL*. 2016;12:10355.
7. Rabin E. How to write an abstract of a research project. *MedEdPORTAL*. 2012;8:9245.
8. Swanberg S, Dereski M. Structured abstracts: best practices in writing and reviewing abstracts for publication and presentation. *MedEdPORTAL*. 2014;10:9908.

Articles on Methods

1. Artino AR Jr, Durning SJ, Creel AH. AM last page: reliability and validity in educational measurement. *Acad Med*. 2010;85(9):1545.
2. Artino AR Jr, Gehlbach H, Durning SJ. AM last page: avoiding five common pitfalls of survey design. *Acad Med*. 2011;86(10):1327.
3. Blanchard R, Scott J. Connecting mixed methods as an education research strategy. *MedEdPORTAL*. 2014;10.
4. Boet S, Sharma S, Goldman J, et al. Review article: medical education research: an overview of methods. *Can J Anaesth*. 2012;59(2):159–170.
5. Bunniss S, Kelly DR. Research paradigms in medical education research. *Med Educ*. 2010;44(4):358–366.
6. Carey T, Sanders G, Viswanathan M, et al. Framework for considering study designs for future research needs. *Methods Future Research Needs Reports No. 8*. AHRQ, 2007:12.
7. Cook DA. Randomized controlled trials and meta-analysis in medical education: what role do they play? *Med Teach*. 2012;34(6):468–473.
8. Cook DA. Much ado about differences: why expert-novice comparisons add little to the validity argument. *Adv Health Sci Educ Theory Pract*. 2015;20(3):829–834.
9. Cook DA. Tips for a great review article: crossing methodological boundaries. *Med Educ*. 2016;50(4):384–387.
10. Cook DA, Beckman TJ. Reflections on experimental research in medical education. *Adv Health Sci Educ*. 2010;15(3):455–464.
11. Cook DA, Bordage G, Schmidt HG. Description, justification and clarification: a framework for classifying the purposes of research in medical education. *Med Educ*. 2008;42(2):128–133.
12. Cook DA, Bowen JL, Gerrity MS, et al. Proposed standards for medical education submissions to the Journal of General Internal Medicine. *J Gen Intern Med*. 2008;23(7):908–913.
13. Cook DA, Brydges R, Ginsburg S, et al. A contemporary approach to validity arguments: a practical guide to Kane's framework. *Med Educ*. 2015;49(6):560–575.
14. Cook DA, Hatala R. Got power? A systematic review of sample size adequacy in health professions education research. *Adv Health Sci Educ*. 2015;20(1):73–83.

15. Cook DA, Kuper A, Hatala R, et al. When assessment data are words: validity evidence for qualitative educational assessments. *Acad Med.* 2016;91(10):1359–1369.
16. Cook DA, Levinson AJ, Garside S. Method and reporting quality in health professions education research: a systematic review. *Med Educ.* 2011;45(3):227–238.
17. Cook DA, Levinson AJ, Garside S. Method and reporting quality in health professions education research: a systematic review. *Med Educ.* 2011;45(3):227–238.
18. Cook DA, Lineberry M. Consequences validity evidence: evaluating the impact of educational assessments. *Acad Med.* 2016;91(6):785–795.
19. Cook DA, Reed DA. Appraising the quality of medical education research methods: the medical education research study quality instrument and the Newcastle–Ottawa scale-education. *Acad Med.* 2015;90(8):1067–1076.
20. Cook DA, West CP. Conducting systematic reviews in medical education: a stepwise approach. *Med Educ.* 2012;46(10):943–952.
21. Egan-Lee E, Freitag S, Leblanc V, et al. Twelve tips for ethical approval for research in health professions education. *Med Teach.* 2011;33(4):268–272.
22. Frambach JM, van der Vleuten CP, Durning SJ. AM last page: quality criteria in qualitative and quantitative research. *Acad Med.* 2013;88(4):552.
23. Grant RE, Sajdlowska J, Van Hoof TJ, et al. Conceptualization and reporting of context in the North American continuing medical education literature: a scoping review protocol. *J Contin Educ Health Prof.* 2015;35:S70–S74.
24. Hanson JL, Balmer DF, Giardino AP. Qualitative research methods for medical educators. *Acad Pediatr.* 2011;11(5):375–386.
25. Hoffmann TC, Glasziou PP, Boutron I, et al. Better reporting of interventions: template for intervention description and replication (TIDieR) checklist and guide. *BMJ.* 2014;348:g1687.
26. Huggett KN, Gusic ME, Greenberg R, et al. Twelve tips for conducting collaborative research in medical education. *Med Teach.* 2011;33(9):713–718.
27. Hutchinson L. Evaluating and researching the effectiveness of educational interventions. *BMJ.* 1999;318(7193):1267.
28. Schifferdecker K. When quantitative or qualitative data are not enough: application of mixed methods research in medical education. *MedEdPORTAL.* 2008;4:1146.
29. Keune JD, Brunsvold ME, Hohmann E, et al. The ethics of conducting graduate medical education research on residents. *Acad Med.* 2013;88(4):449–453.
30. Kuper A, Reeves S, Levinson W. An introduction to reading and appraising qualitative research. *BMJ.* 2008;337:a288.
31. Lichtenstein AH, Yetley EA, Lau J. Application of systematic review methodology to the field of nutrition. *J Nutr.* 2008;138(12):2297–2306.
32. Lingard L, Albert M, Levinson W. Grounded theory, mixed methods, and action research. *BMJ.* 2008;337:a567.
33. Maudsley G. Mixing it but not mixed-up: mixed methods research in medical education (a critical narrative review). *Med Teach.* 2011;33(2):e92–e104.
34. Myers E, Sanders G, Ravi D, et al. Evaluating the potential use of modeling and value-of-information analysis for future research prioritization within the Evidence-based Practice Center Program. *Methods Future Research Needs Reports No. 5.* AHRQ, 2007:11.
35. Norman G, Eva KW. Chapter 21. Quantitative research methods in medical education. In: Swanwick T, ed. *Understanding Medical Education: Evidence, Theory and Practice.* Wiley-Blackwell; 2010: 315–337.
36. Olson CA. Reflections on using theory in research on continuing education in the health professions. *J Contin Educ Health Prof.* 2013;33(3):151–152.
37. Prideaux D, Bligh J. Research in medical education: asking the right questions. *Med Educ.* 2002;36(12): 1114–1115.
38. Ramani S, Mann K. Introducing medical educators to qualitative study design: twelve tips from inception to completion. *Med Teach.* 2016;38(5):456–463.
39. Reeves S, Albert M, Kuper A, et al. Why use theories in qualitative research? *BMJ.* 2008;337:a949.
40. Reeves S, Kuper A, Hodges BD. Qualitative research methodologies: ethnography. *BMJ.* 2008;337: a1020.
41. Robinson KA, Saldanha I, Mckoy NA. Frameworks for determining research gaps during systematic reviews. *Methods Future Research Needs Report No. 2.* AHRQ, 2007:11.
42. Robinson KA, Whitlock E, O'Neil ME, et al. *Integration of Existing Systematic Reviews*; 2012:14.
43. Schneider B, Carnoy M, Kilpatrick J, et al. *Estimating Causal Effects using Experimental and Observational Designs.* Washington, DC: American Educational Research Association; 2007.

44. Tabrizi J. Qualitative research in medical education. *Res Med Educ.* 2011;3(1):54–59.
45. Thompson M, Tiwari A, Fu R, et al. *A Framework to Facilitate the Use of Systematic Reviews and Meta-analyses in the Design of Primary Research Studies.* AHRQ; 2007:12.
46. Treasury Board of Canada. *Theory-Based Approaches to Evaluation: Concepts and Practices*; 2012. Available at http://www.tbs-sct.gc.ca/. Accessed August 8, 2016.

Articles on Funding

1. Carline JD. Funding medical education research: opportunities and issues. *Acad Med.* 2004;79(10): 918–924.
2. Gruppen LD, Durning SJ. Needles and haystacks: finding for medical education research. *Acad Med.* 2016;91(4):480–484.
3. Nemergut EC. Resident research and graduate medical education funding. *Anesthesiology.* 2013;118(3):757–758.
4. O'Haire C, McPheeters M, Nakamoto EK, et al. Engaging stakeholders to identify and prioritize future research needs. *Methods Future Research Needs Report Number 4.* AHRQ; 2007.
5. Reed DA, Cook DA, Beckman TJ, et al. Association between funding and quality of published medical education research. *JAMA.* 2007;298(9):1002–1009.
6. Reed DA, Kern DE, Levine RB, et al. Costs and funding for published medical education research. *JAMA.* 2005;294(9):1052–1057.

AMEE Guides

1. Artino AR Jr, La Rochelle JS, Dezee KJ, et al. Developing questionnaires for educational research: AMEE Guide No. 87. *Med Teach.* 2014;36(6):463–474.
2. Bloch R, Norman G. Generalizability theory for the perplexed: a practical introduction and guide: AMEE Guide No. 68. *Med Teach.* 2012;34(11):960–992.
3. Cleland J, Scott N, Harrild K, et al. Using databases in medical education research: AMEE Guide No. 77. *Med Teach.* 2013;35(5):e1103–e1122.
4. Coverdale JH, Roberts LW, Balon R, et al. Writing for academia: getting your research into print: AMEE Guide No. 74. *Med Teach.* 2013;35(2):e926–e934.
5. Crites GE, Gaines JK, Cottrell S, et al. Medical education scholarship: an introductory guide: AMEE Guide No. 89. *Med Teach.* 2014;36(8):657–674.
6. Dolmans DH, Tigelaar D. Building bridges between theory and practice in medical education using a design-based research approach: AMEE Guide No. 60. *Med Teach.* 2012;34(1):1–10.
7. Hojat M, Erdmann JB, Gonnella JS. Personality assessments and outcomes in medical education and the practice of medicine: AMEE Guide No. 79. *Med Teach.* 2013;35(7):e1267–e1301.
8. Kuper A, Whitehead C, Hodges BD. Looking back to move forward: Using history, discourse and text in medical education research: AMEE Guide No. 73. *Med Teach.* 2013;35(1):e849–e860.
9. Laidlaw A, Aiton J, Struthers J, et al. Developing research skills in medical students: AMEE Guide No. 69. *Med Teach.* 2012;34(9):e754–e771.
10. Reeves S, Peller J, Goldman J, et al. Ethnography in qualitative educational research: AMEE Guide No. 80. *Med Teach.* 2013;35(8):e1365–e1379.
11. Ringsted C, Hodges B, Scherpbier A. 'The research compass': an introduction to research in medical education: AMEE Guide No. 56. *Med Teach.* 2011;33(9):695–709.
12. Sharma R, Gordon M, Dharamsi S, et al. Systematic reviews in medical education: a practical approach: AMEE Guide No. 94. *Med Teach.* 2015;37(2):108–124.
13. Stalmeijer RE, McNaughton N, Van Mook WN. Using focus groups in medical education research: AMEE Guide No. 91. *Med Teach.* 2014;36(11):923–939.
14. Tavakol M, Sandars J. Quantitative and qualitative methods in medical education research: AMEE Guide No. 90: Part I. *Med Teach.* 2014;36(9):746–756.
15. Tavakol M, Sandars J. Quantitative and qualitative methods in medical education research: AMEE Guide No. 90: Part II. *Med Teach.* 2014;36(10):838–848.
16. Watling CJ, Lingard L. Grounded theory in medical education research: AMEE Guide No. 70. *Med Teach.* 2012;34(10):850–861.

Index